VLSI Circuits for Biomedical Applications

For a list of related Artech House titles, please turn to the back of this book.

VLSI Circuits for Biomedical Applications

Krzysztof Iniewski

ARTECH HOUSE
BOSTON | LONDON
artechhouse.com

Library of Congress Cataloging-in-Publication Data
A catalog record for this book is available from the U.S. Library of Congress.

British Library Cataloguing in Publication Data
A catalogue record for this book is available from the British Library.

ISBN 13: 978-1-59693-317-0

Cover design by Igor Valdman

10 9 8 7 6 5 4 3 2 1

Contents

CHAPTER 3

CHAPTER 4

CHAPTER 5

Preface

Human beings historically had a short life span caused by infectious diseases, wars, and natural disasters. Considerable progress in the last century was made due to improvements in hygiene, medicine and nutrition. The longer life span, however, has led to a dramatic increase in health costs and increased efforts to deal with chronic diseases. Further progress in medicine and the confinement of exploding healthcare costs can be only expected with advances in technology, electronics in particular.

This book addresses the-state-of-the-art in integrated circuit design in the context of new technologies for biomedical applications. New and exciting opportunities in interfacing to the human body, medical implants, on-chip DNA analysis, and molecular biology are discussed. Emerging circuit design techniques, new materials, and innovative system approaches are explored. This book is a must for anyone serious about electronic design for future technologies in the healthcare sector.

Krzysztof (Kris) Iniewski
Editor
Vancouver, Canada
June 2008

CHAPTER 1

Wireless Integrated Neurochemical and Neuropotential Sensing

Mohsen Mollazadeh, Kartikeya Murari, Christian Sauer, Nitish Thakor, Milutin Stanacevic, and Gert Cauwenberghs

1.1 Introduction

Since the first use of multisite electroencephalography experiments by W. Grey Walter in the 1930s [1], instrumentation for monitoring the physiological state of the brain has undergone tremendous advances. Instrumentation, electrodes, and analysis tools are continually being developed for the basic research as well as clinical applications.

Today, among several other stellar achievements, it is possible to locate the focal origin of epilepsy with millimetric precision [2] and to control prosthetic devices with thought alone [3]. Most of the advances made both in the clinical and research fields have been based on analyzing the electrical activity of the brain. While the majority of information flow in the nervous system is electrical, neural processing and transmission also have a chemical aspect, mediated by neurotransmitters [4]. These crucial chemical messengers are an integral part of the nervous system. Deficits and imbalances in this system have serious neurological consequences such as Parkinson's disease, epilepsy, and so on.

General principles in the design of VLSI circuits for biomedical instrumentation are extensively covered elsewhere in this edited volume. This chapter describes components for a multimodal wireless monitoring system and their integration into a system capable of recording and telemetering both electrical and neurochemical activity from multiple sites.

1.2 Neurochemical Sensing

1.2.1 A Review of Neurotransmitters

Neurotransmitters are chemical messengers that conduct signals along the electrically insulating parts of nervous pathways [5] i.e. from one neuron to another, across gaps called synapses. Neurotransmitters may be either excitatory or inhibitory. That is, they may be of a type that fosters the initiation of a nerve impulse in the receiving neuron, or they may inhibit such an impulse. Within the cells, neurotransmitter molecules are packaged in vesicles and released by rapid exocytosis upon the arrival of a nerve impulse. Then they diffuse across the synaptic gap to bind neurotransmitter receptors or other ligand gated ion channels and stimulate or inhibit the firing of the postsynaptic neuron. Figure 1.1 shows a schematic of a synapse and shows how the electrical and chemical signals are related.

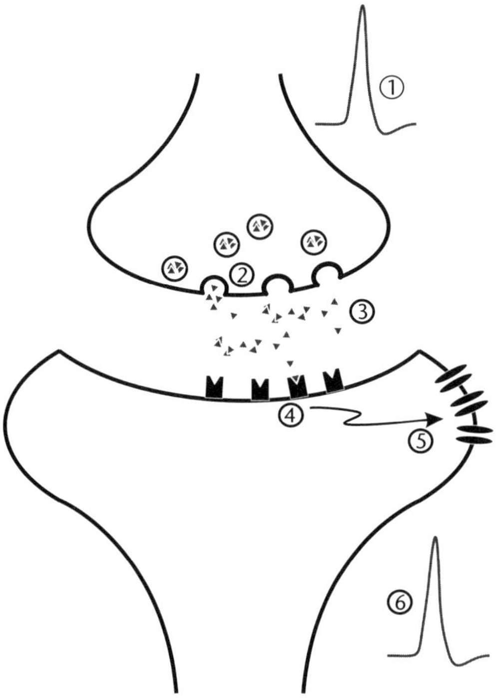

Figure 1.1 Schematic of a synapse showing the interplay between electrical and chemical signaling. Electrical signals (1), cause neurotransmitter containing vesicles to dock (2) and release the messengers (3). These bind to receptors (4) that cause downstream changes (5) in ion channels that initiate electrical signaling.

Neurotransmitters are crucial in ensuring the proper functioning of neural pathways. Imbalances or malfunctions of neurotransmitters leads to several debilitating nervous disorders like Parkinson's disease (due to lack of Dopamine [6]), bipolar depression (due to Serotonin imbalance [7]), and so on. The study of neurotransmitters is paramount in understanding the mechanism of neural pathways and diseases. Numerous methods like optical [8] (detecting light emitted by reactions), immunochemical [9] (detecting tracer compounds attached to neurotransmitters), liquid chromatography [10] (chemical separation of neurotransmitters) are used to detect and measure neurotransmitter activity. Electrochemical sensing of certain electroactive neurotransmitters (e.g. nitric oxide, dopamine) is very attractive due to high sensitivity, rapidity, and the ability to perform distributed measurements [11, 12].

1.2.2 Electrochemical Analysis and Instrumentation

Among the first applications of electrochemical analysis in biological sensing was the Clark oxygen sensor [13] patented in 1956. Electrochemical detection makes use of chemical redox reactions characterized by a transfer of electrons among the reacting species [14]. The reaction occurs at an electrode (the working electrode) surface that is held at some voltage (V_{REDOX}) with respect to a reference electrode. Usually the system requires a third electrode, a counter electrode, to maintain the voltage difference in the presence of potential drops across the solution being monitored. The transferred electrons constitute a current that is proportional to the concentration of the species being analyzed and the surface area of the electrode. Typically, in electrochemical analysis V_{REDOX} is the independent variable and the redox current is measured. There are several modes of analyses [14], two of the major kinds being cyclic voltammetry and chronoamperometry. In the former, V_{REDOX} is swept periodically over a given voltage interval while the redox current is measured. This results in an I-V signature of the species and is useful to obtain the potential difference at which the redox reaction is maximal. In chronoamperometry, or more simply, amperometry, current is measured as a function of time while the voltage difference is held constant at the optimal redox potential for maximum sensitivity obtained by cyclic voltammetry. This is the preferred mode of analysis for monitoring concentrations over time.

The instrumentation used for electrochemical analysis is called a potentiostat. There are various methods used, namely voltametry amperometry, cyclic voltametry and amperometry. As the name signifies, in the voltametric method the V_{REDOX} is held at a specified value (or waveform) while simultaneously measuring the current. The schematic of a basic potentiostat is shown in Figure 1.2. The reaction occurs between the working and the reference electrodes so the drop $V_{RE\text{-}WE}$ is the potential of interest. The output voltage of an opamp of gain A is given by:

$$e_{OUT} = A\,(e_+ - e_-) \tag{1.1}$$

Let V_{CELL} denote the drop between the counter and working electrodes and the subscripts CE, WE and RE denote the counter working, and the reference electrodes, respectively.

Since WE is grounded, single ended potentials are referred to it. Thus, $e_+ = V_{REDOX}$, $e_- = V_{RE\text{-}WE}$ and $e_{OUT} = V_{CE\text{-}WE} = V_{CELL}$. Substituting in Eqn. (1.1),

$$V_{CELL} = A\,(V_{REDOX} - V_{RE\text{-}WE}) \tag{1.2}$$

$$V_{RE\text{-}WE} = V_{REDOX} - V_{CELL} / A \tag{1.3}$$

$$V_{RE\text{-}WE} \sim V_{REDOX} \text{ as } A \to \infty \tag{1.4}$$

Thus, the potential drop between the reference and the working electrodes is forced to the preset value V_{REDOX}, which appears across the reaction media, and the redox current being forced through the counter electrode is measured.

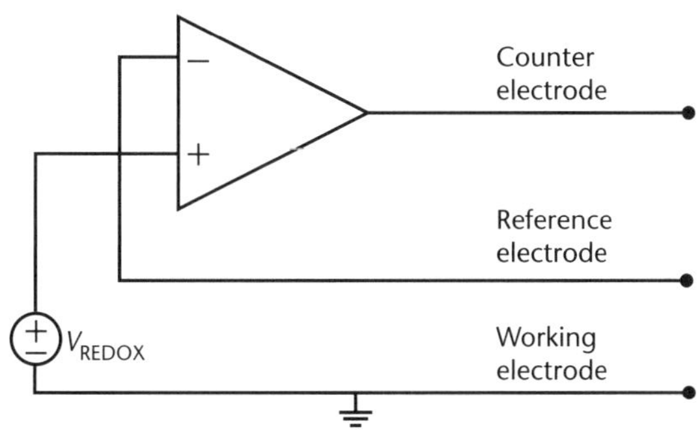

Figure 1.2 Schematic of a basic three-terminal potentiostat for neurochemical sensing by measurement of neurotransmitter-activated redox currents.

1.2.3 VLSI Multichannel Potentiostat

Typically utilized benchtop potentiostats are used for electroanalytical biosensing that offer a poor match in terms of footprint, power consumption, sensitivity, parallel scalability, etc. CMOS VLSI potentiostats having one or a few channels have been developed in the past to record from electrochemical sensors [15–19]. Custom potentiostats for biosensing applications can be reduced to a two-terminal setup, with just the working and reference electrodes. The counter electrode is not needed since the expected redox currents are very small due to very low physiological concentrations of analytes leading to negligible voltage drops across the solution.

The system diagram for one channel of a multichannel VLSI potentiostat [20] is shown in Figure 1.3.

Each channel essentially integrates the redox current for a certain conversion period and then digitizes the result. The circuit consists of a charge-mode incremental delta-sigma analog-to-digital converter [21] with time-multiplexing digital gain modulation to extend the dynamic range that is needed for physiological monitoring. Figure 1.4 shows the implementation and the timing diagram for the front end. The redox current is integrated on the capacitor C_1. C_1 can be digitally set to 100fF or 1.1pF to accommodate a wide range of redox currents while maintaining reasonable conversion times. The capacitor C_2 provides a low input impedance virtual ground node that is charged to V_{REDOX} at the beginning of a conversion period. The single bit digital to analog converter is implemented using switched current sources realized by the transistors M_1 and M_2. These transistors are always turned on to decrease the effects of charge injection noise. Transistors M_3, M_4, M_5, and M_6 are minimum size switches that direct the reference current into either the integrator or the reference voltage source. The high gain amplifier is a cascoded inverter operating in the subthreshold region. In a standard $\Delta\Sigma$ modulator, the reference current I_{ref} is either added to or subtracted from the input current I_{in} and $I_{in} \pm I_{ref}$ is integrated during the entire time. This forces the input and reference currents to be of the same magnitude. To allow for a wider range of input currents, a programmable gain of the input current is introduced by controlling the integration time of the reference current using a clock, *dsClk*, that has a programmable duty cycle. The reference current is integrated only when *dsClk* is high, while the input current is integrated through

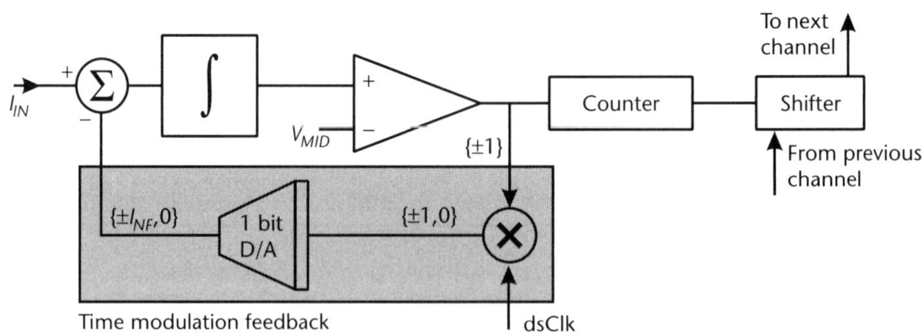

Figure 1.3 Block diagram of a single channel of the VLSI potentiostat showing the $\Delta\Sigma$ modulator with the time modulation feedback. From [18] with permission, © IEEE 2007.

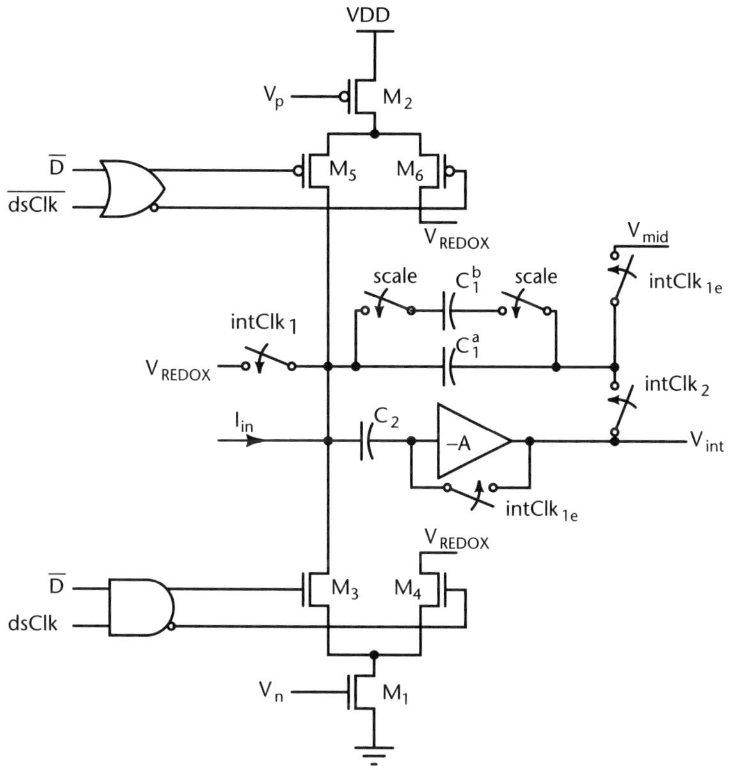

Figure 1.4 Implementation level diagram of the ΔΣ modulator. From [18] with permission, © IEEE 2007.

the whole period of the clock *dsClk*. The duty cycle of *dsClk* represents the gain of input current with respect to the reference current, enabling multiple scales with the same reference current. In Figure 1.4, this digital gain is represented by the logic gates feeding into the transistors M_3 and M_4 and M_5 and M_6. The integration period and the rate of sampling the input current are set by the clock *intClk*. The clocks $intClk_1$ and $intClk_2$ are non-overlapping clocks derived from *intClk*. $intClk_{1e}$ is a copy of $intClk_1$ with the rising edge following and the falling edge preceding those of $intClk_1$. The ratio of periods of the clocks *dsClk* and *intClk* represents the oversampling ratio (OSR) of the ΔΣ modulator. The decimator is implemented as the simple accumulate and dump circuit. The number of active (logic one) output bits of the ΔΣ modulator are counted using a 16-bit counter during one conversion period. The conversion period is programmable and is represented by the period of the programmable clock *intClk*. At the end of each conversion cycle, the counter value is written to the output parallel-in serial-out shift register and a new conversion cycle begins with the cleared counter. The registers for all the channels are daisy-chained to obtain a single output bit stream. The register is read out asynchronously at any time during the conversion cycle. Figure 1.5 (a) shows the normalized digital outputs of the chip for input currents over six orders of magnitude. An illustrative example of the operation of one channel of the chip is shown in Figure 1.5 (b). *In vitro* monitoring of the neurotransmitter dopamine was performed using commercially

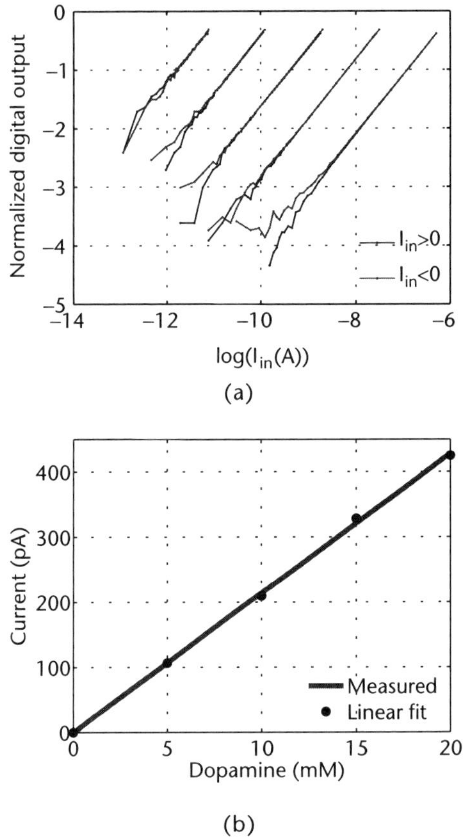

Figure 1.5 Measured results from the potentiostat chip: (a) characterization data for input currents over six orders of magnitude and (b) calibration curve obtained for monitoring micromolar dopamine concentration *in vitro*. From [18] with permission, © IEEE 2007.

available electrochemical sensors (CF30-250, WPI, FL). Different concentrations of dopamine were added to a stirred phosphate buffered saline (PBS) solution and the chip output was observed after equilibrating.

1.3 Neuropotential Sensing

While synapses transfer information locally in insulating gaps through electrochemical signaling as described in the previous section, information is transmitted over a longer range in the form of electrical action potentials traveling across the central nervous system. The electrical activity of the brain can be recorded from within the brain (spike or local field potentials), the surface of the brain (electrocorticogram or ECoG), or from the scalp (electroencephalogram or EEG). These signals encode information about the state of the brain which potentially can be extracted by signal processing methods. Thus, electrophysiology-based recording systems can be used to understand the mechanism underlying brain function as well as help paralyzed patients using a brain-computer interface [3]. Another common application area is the recording of electrocorticograms in clinical investigation of neurological disorders such as epilepsy. However, due to the large-scale instrumentation needed to implement EEG recording systems, these systems are currently mostly used inside hospitals. In all these applications, miniaturized recording systems are required so that they can be integrated into the daily lives for those who need it.

In this section, we limit the discussion to ECoG and EEG signals, and present VLSI interface circuitry for these signals. Discussion on spike signals and associated circuitry can be found in the following chapters.

1.3.1 Physiological Basis of EEG/ECoG

The brain is an extremely complex system, constantly carrying out information transfer and processing. The neural system works through the interactions between large assemblies of neurons in the central nervous system (CNS) and the peripheral neural system. At the cellular level, neurons transfer and process the information via the action potentials and neural firing (also known as spikes). When this kind of electrical activity transfers to the surface of the cortex and to the surface of the scalp, it can be recorded and processed to reveal the information contained in the signal.

EEG/ECoG is the prevailing method to record the dynamics of the brain's larger-scale electrical activity. While the origin of the activities recorded by scalp electrodes lie in the action potentials of cortical neurons, it is generally agreed that the ECoG and EEG signals are generated by excitatory postsynaptic potentials (EPSP) [22]. Yet, the origins of the generated rhythms in these electrical signals are not fully understood. The recorded electrical signals are the result of aggregation of excitatory and inhibitory postsynaptic potentials (EPSPs and IPSPs) across large volumes of neural tissue that undergo volume conduction before they reach the cortical surface for ECoG recording, and that undergo further spatial signal smearing through bone and tissue conduction before reaching the scalp for EEG recording. The effect of volume conduction is that of both spatial and temporal filtering, removing high-frequency components and masking individual spike waveforms.

The effect of this signal aggregation also reveals patterns of synchronous activity that are indicative of mental states and hence are useful in brain state monitoring. Electrical recordings from the surface of the brain demonstrate continuous oscillatory activity with different intensities and patterns. The intensities of the ECoG can be as large as 10 mV while EEG recordings are usually around 100 μV due to the attenuation through the skull and skin. The frequencies of these waves range from 0.5 to 100 Hz and their character is highly dependent on the degree of activity in the cerebral cortex. For example, brain waves change markedly between states of wakefulness and sleep. Depending on brain state and mental activity, brain waves could be irregular without discernable patterns, or distinct spatiotemporal patterns could manifest. Some of these are characteristics of specific abnormalities of the brain such as epilepsy. Others occur under normal healthy conditions and can be typically classified as belonging to one of four major wave groups, based on their frequency content: *Delta* (0.5–4 Hz), *Theta* (4–8 Hz), *Alpha* (8–12 Hz), *Beta* (12–30 Hz), and *Gamma* (>40 Hz) [23].

1.3.2 Interface Circuitry

EEG/ECoG signals have very low amplitudes in the μV voltage range that require amplification before any signal processing. The inputs to the amplifier can be connected in three different methods: between each two electrodes (bipolar), between one monopolar lead and a distant reference electrode (usually attached to one or both ear lobes), or between one electrode and the average of all. In the last method, the system reference is formed by connecting all scalp recording locations through equal high resistances to a common point [23].

The application requirements call for the following specifications on the instrumentation amplifier: low input-referred voltage noise ($< 2\ \mu V_{rms}$), low leakage current (< 1 pA), high common mode rejection ratio (CMRR > 80 dB), high input impedance (> 1 MΩ), high power supply rejection ratio (PSRR > 90 dB), and high isolation mode rejection ratio (IMRR > 120 dB). For digitized electrophysiology recording systems, control over quantization error in analog-to-digital conversion (ADC), sensitivity, and filter cutoff frequency should also be considered [24].

The amplified EEG/ECoG signals need to be filtered to remove noise and out-of-band frequency signals. EEG spectra typically span a 0–125 Hz signal bandwidth, whereas ECoG spectra extend to higher frequencies (500 Hz or larger) and require larger bandwidth filters. Routine EEG should be acquired at least at a sample rate of 250 Hz, to accommodate the 0–125 Hz signal band. Higher sampling rates are often used to account for finite roll-off of anti-alias filtering and for improved noise suppression. Further filtering may be required to remove power line artifacts (50 or 60 Hz). Accounting for the different frequency bands of interest (*Alpha*, *Beta*, *Gamma*, *Theta*) in EEG, band selection filters are typically provided by the EEG recording system. While some systems include band-selection analog filters in the recording unit, others provide digital filtering in their accompanying utility software.

In light of these considerations, we describe efficient VLSI implementation of EEG/ECoG electrophysiology recording systems for micropower implantable use. Figure 1.6 shows the functional block diagram for one channel of a multi-channel

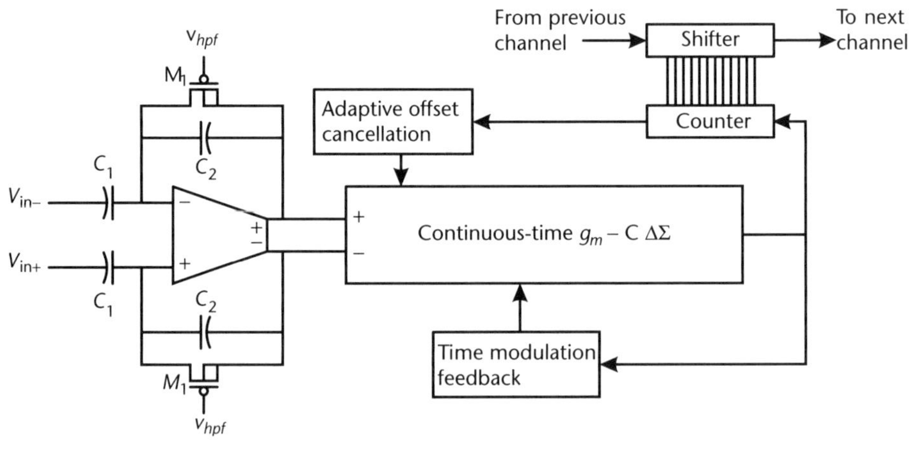

Figure 1.6 Block functional diagram for one channel of the biopotential sensing chip.

VLSI biopotential interface chip. Each channel integrates a dedicated ADC to relax the precision requirements on signal transmission over a wireless link and thus minimize the net power consumption. The channel comprises a bandpass filtering amplifier, G_m-C incremental ΔΣ analog-to-digital converter, decimating counter, and daisy-chained parallel-to-serial output register.

Amplifier

The front-end amplifier used is a fully differential version of the design presented in [25]. The amplifier midband gain is set to 40 dB by ratio of capacitors (C_1 = 20pF and C_2 = 200fF). The PMOS transistors M1 and M2 provide large resistance in the GΩ range for sub-Hz cutoff highpass filtering and AC coupling of the input [25]. Transistor sizing of the fully differential, two-stage amplifier is optimized for low input-referred noise. The gate bias V_{hpf} controls the highpass cutoff frequency, ranging from 0.2 Hz to 95 Hz. The lowpass cutoff frequency ranges from 120 Hz to 8.2 kHz, and is $g_{m1}/2\pi AC_c$ set by the transconductance of the first stage g_{m1} proportional to bias current I_{biasp}, midband gain of the amplifier A, and by the compensation capacitance C_c between first and second stage [26].

Analog-to-Digital Converter

The choice of ADC topology in the design is determined by several factors that include the nature of the signal and system level considerations in the interface. One could choose to provide a single ADC for the entire system, which requires multiplexing the output of the amplifiers at high rate. This increases the power requirements of the amplifier, which needs to drive a large load because of the high switching rate. A more energy-efficient alternative choice is to include one ADC per channel as shown in Figure 1.6. High efficiency requires the design of the ADC to be optimized for high density of integration, and for accuracy rather than speed in the conversion. Algorithmic and ΔΣ ADCs are suitable for this design, and offer a further advantage of adjustable resolution through global control of clocking waveforms. The functional diagram of a Gm-C incremental ΔΣ implementing variable-resolution ADC is shown also in Figure 1.6. The core of the ΔΣ ADC is identical to the one implemented in the potentiostat for neurochemical sensing presented in the previous section [20], offering also the benefit of a digitally selectable gain using time-modulation feedback. A transconductance element, implemented with an nMOS differential pair OTA and current mirror, converts the differential output of the EEG preamplifier to a current I_{in}, which is continuously integrated by the ΔΣ input stage. The continuous integration in the Gm-C ΔΣ avoids the need for sampling and for anti-alias filtering. A second nMOS OTA provides an offset current I_{offset} that adaptively compensates for OTA and current feedback mismatch in the ADC. The MSB from the decimator adjusts the direction of I_{offset} through an integrator implemented by a charge pump, one update per conversion cycle. Larger or more frequent updates in I_{offset} make it possible to further filter $1/f$ noise outside the signal band.

The digital output of all the channels can then be decimated and shifted out in a daisy-chain fashion for a serial readout.

To characterize the accuracy in the overall response including front-end amplification/filtering and ADC quantization, Figure 1.7 shows the power spectrum of

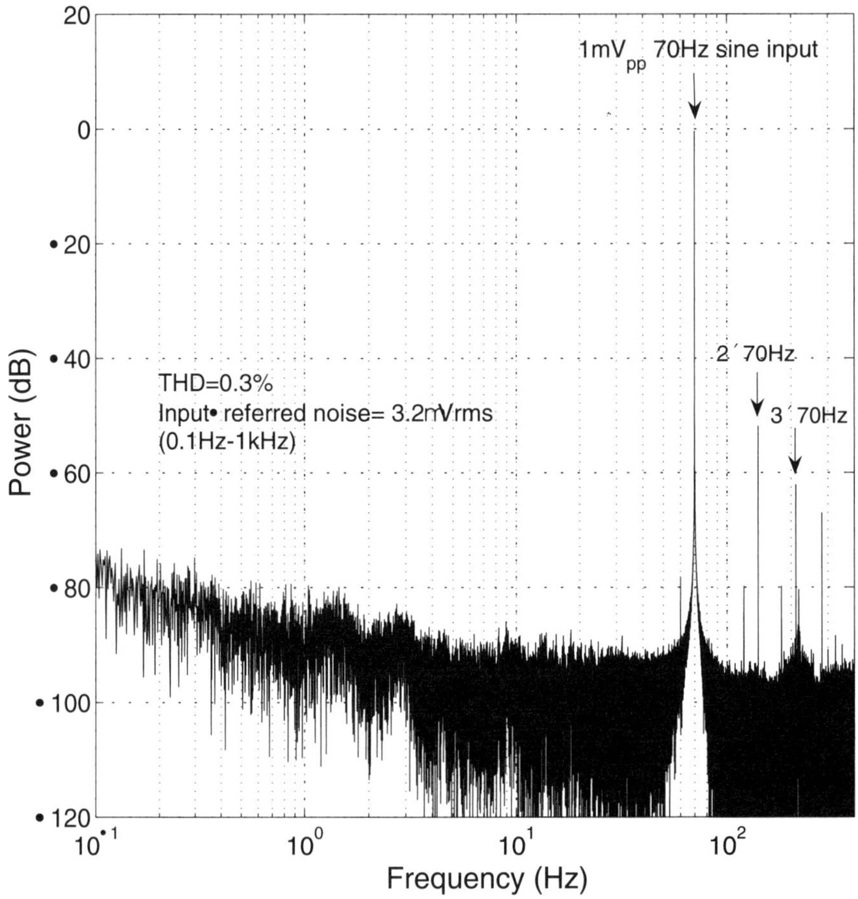

Figure 1.7 Normalized power spectrum of digital output for 1 mVpp 70 Hz sine input to the front-end amplifier. V_{hpf} = 3.3 V, I_{amp} = 12.2 μA, resolution = 10 bits, G = 4, f_s = 4 MHz (1 kS/s).

the recorded digital output with a 1mV_{pp} 70 Hz sine wave presented to the front-end amplifier input. The data indicate a THD of 0.3%, and an input-referred noise of 3.7 μVrms over the 0.1 Hz to 1 kHz range. Lower quantization noise levels can be attained by a higher gain setting for smaller signal amplitudes.

1.4 RF Telemetry and Power Harvesting in Implanted Devices

While the previous two sections describe the sensor interface circuitry for multimodal sensing, telemetry of the recorded data as well as powering the VLSI interface circuitry is a major performance-limiting factor in implanted devices. Recording from unrestrained animals requires wireless, untethered operation. Batteries are not available, since they increase the size of the device and limit implant locations. Energy harvesting makes use of the external environment as a source of energy (temperature, gradient, wind, etc.), but most of these factors are unavailable for powering an implantable system. Radio Frequency (RF) power harvesting through inductive coupling is an alternate solution to power the system. The same link can also be used to transmit data to and from the implantable system. In this section, we will review the basics of power harvesting through magnetic coupling and give circuit designs for telemetry and powering in CMOS.

1.4.1 Introduction to Inductive Coupling

The operational frequency of the telemetry system and its impact on tissue absorption in the body are important design considerations. The human body comprises different layers of tissue with variable conductivity and permeability. High-frequency energy is absorbed by the body while low-frequency energy is reflected [27]. In a frequency region between 1 and 20 MHz, maximum energy passes through the body. Therefore, the design of the telemetry system is constrained to operation frequencies in this range. As a special case of interest, assume an operation frequency of 4 MHz. The corresponding wavelength is 75 meters, precluding the use of antennas that require much larger apertures than practically possible in an implant. Power and information can however be transmitted through inductive coupling between two coils that are placed relatively close to one another. These coils can be sized significantly smaller than the wavelength since transmission of data and power is mediated through coupling in magnetic field, rather than through electromagnetic radiation and wave propagation.

In two inductively coupled coils, a current generated in the primary coil induces a current in the secondary coil, proportional to the first current. The proportion of power that is transferred is quantified by the coupling factor, k, which ranges between 0 and 1 (100%) depending on geometrical factors and material properties of the coupling medium (air, tissue, bone, hair, etc.). Typical coupling factors in transformers with optimized coupling are usually around 0.5 (50%), with parasitic coupling and absorption in surrounding media contributing to the power losses in transmission. For telemetric power and data transfer between implant and reader/host coils, the coupling is relatively weak, resulting in much lower coupling factors. In order to understand the effect of design parameters on coupling efficiency in power transfer, we need to quantify the magnetic field strength induced and carried between the two coils. The magnetic field produced by a primary circular coil of radius R_1 at distance x along the perpendicular axis is:

$$H = \frac{NIR_1^{\,2}}{2\sqrt{(R_1^{\,2} + x^2)^3}}$$

where N is the number of windings, and I is the current supplied through the coil. For a secondary coil placed parallel to the primary coil and centered along the same axis at distance x, the induced current can be derived from estimating the magnetic flux through the secondary coil, resulting in an approximate expression for the coupling factor [28]:

$$k = \frac{R_1^2 R_2^2}{\sqrt{R_1 R_2 (R_1^2 + x^2)^3}}$$

where R_2 is the radius of the secondary coil. Maximizing the power transfer efficiency amounts directly to maximizing the coupling factor k. The optimal coil radius for the primary coil, maximizing k, is thus directly given by the distance between coils:

$$R_1 = x$$

In an implantable system, the distance x between outside coil and implant is approximately 2.5 cm, which constrains the reader coil to a radius R_1 = 2.5 cm. The coupling factor is further maximized by maximizing the radius R_2 of the implant coil, subject to physical size constraints of the implant typically in the mm range. The weak inductive coupling results in relatively low coupling efficiency k, approximately 5%.

Figure 1.8 (a) shows a simplified circuit model of an inductively coupled system. The left side of this model represents the outside reader coil, while the right coil represents the implanted system. We can model the inductive link as a weakly coupled transformer as shown in Figure 1.8 (b). The induced voltage across the load R_L can be written as:

$$V_2 = \frac{V_1}{1+(j\omega L_2 + R_p)(\frac{1}{R_L} + j\omega C_1)}$$

Because of the low coupling efficiency (5%), very large values of V_1 around 100 V are required to generate sufficiently large V_2 for operating the implant circuits. A tuned LC circuit is required to generate such a large voltage from low source voltage at the generator; $V_1 = Q2V_{dd}/\pi$. Hence for a V_{dd} of at most 5 V in submicron CMOS

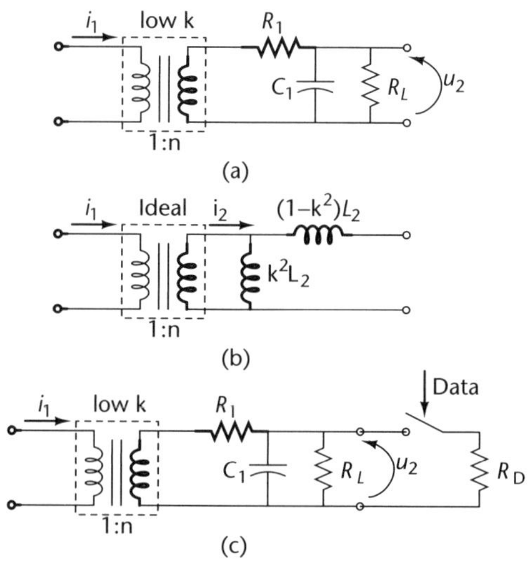

Figure 1.8 (a) Simplified model of the inductively coupled system. (b) Common model of a weakly coupled transformer. (c) System schematic with attached load modulation resistor and switch. The switch is controlled by the data sent through the system.

processes, Q should be around 100. This on the other hand limits the bandwidth of the system since $\omega_b = \omega_c/Q$, so for a center frequency of 4 MHz, the maximum bandwidth is 40 kHz. This is acceptable because of the slow sensing application targeted here. Also, note that the high voltage levels generated in the primary coil are safe for use and do not pose a danger to the subject or others handling the system because the high impedance of the high-Q telemetry system carries relatively little power.

As presented, the coupling between coils provides for inductive power transfer from the reader coil to the implant coil. Different methods for data transmission from the interface circuitry at the implant to the reader coil are available. Here, we consider ohmic load modulation, using the same inductive link to transmit the acquired data upstream as used to transmit power downstream. Other methods such as capacitive load modulation and active transmission can be used, although each has its own drawbacks.

Data transmission using ohmic load modulation in an inductively coupled system is accomplished simply by changing the load resistance of the implant. Generally, this is achieved by switching a second resistor loading the implant coil, in addition to the resistive load of the implant interface circuits, as shown in Figure 1.8 (c). The switched insertion of the resistor changes the current in the implanted coil, which in turn changes the impedance and hence the current in the reader coil. This current is sensed using transimpedance circuits at the reader, and this simple ASK data transmission scheme is further decoded.

1.4.2 Telemetry System Architecture and VLSI Design

The VLSI power harvesting and telemetry system at the minimum should include these subunits: rectifier, regulator, clock and data recovery, and data encoder. Figure 1.9 shows the block diagram of such a system. The transmitter coil can be driven by a high-efficiency class-E transmitter. A full wave rectifier followed by a low-pass circuit recovers a dc voltage. Figure 1.10 (a) shows an example of a rectifier circuit implemented in a AMI 0.5 μm CMOS process [29].

When voltage on side A of the coil is higher than that of side B, M2, and M3 are shut off while M1 and M4 are turned on. This ties the low voltage side of the coil to ground while passing the high voltage. The situation is reversed when B is higher than A. The use of pMOS transistors prevents latch-up inducing collector currents from occurring and removes the necessity of using additional components. This voltage is dependent on the load and not suitable for driving the active circuitry. A regulated supply voltage is required to ensure proper operation of the circuitry. Figure 1.10 (b) shows an example circuit diagram of a regulator. The output voltage is stabilized proportional to voltage reference through a negative feedback. The reference voltage can be generated from rectified voltage by a supply independent reference circuit made out of CMOS devices only. Note that this topology requires a minimum current to be drawn from the output for proper operation of the circuitry. Since most implantable systems are mixed-signal systems, it is preferred to have two regulators on the chip to separate analog from digital supply and minimize the switching noise in the analog part.

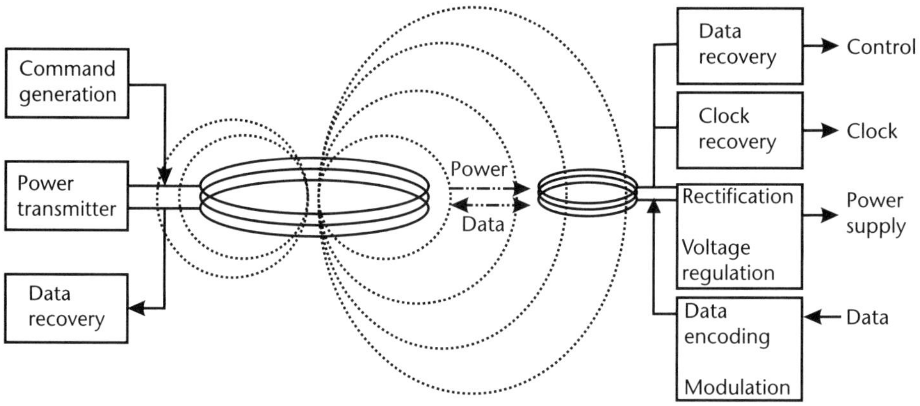

Figure 1.9 Block diagram of the RF power harvesting and telemetry system. From [29] with permission, © IEEE 2005.

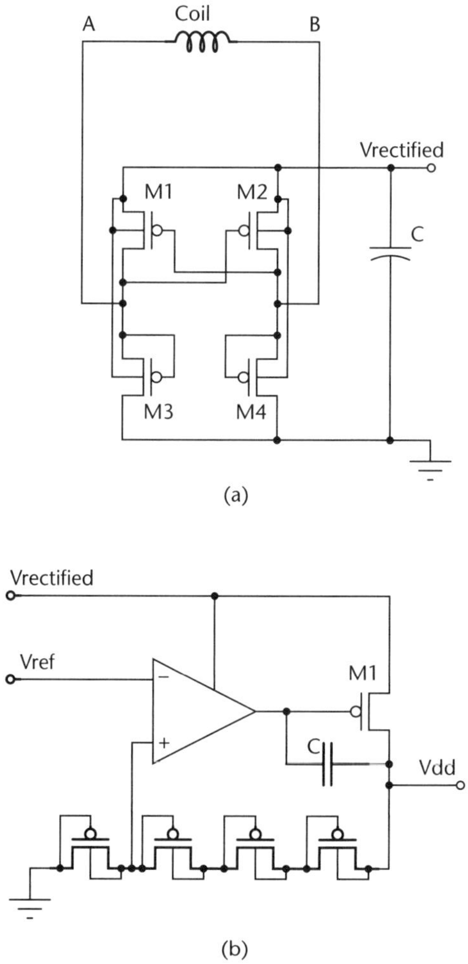

Figure 1.10 (a) Rectifier and (b) regulator circuit diagram. From [29] with permission, © IEEE 2005.

In order to test the coupling and determine the maximum power transfer, the transmitter and receiver coils were placed close together and moved apart. As shown in Figure 1.11, distances between 10 mm and 100 mm were tested. The chip was loaded such that it would produce 0.7 mA when the voltage was enough to operate the regulator. With this load the chip was able to provide the desired regulated voltage with a distance of up to 3 cm between the two coils. The RMS voltage on the coil, the rectified voltage, and the regulated voltage were recorded. At low current draw the rectified voltage follows the coil RMS voltage fairly closely. The two values diverge when more current is drawn from the regulator. When the rectified voltage drops to the regulated value, the PMOS controlling current is completely on. This ties the regulated voltage to the rectified, while affecting the coil voltage slightly less.

The next step is to recover the digital clock and commands from the induced signals. A square wave clock can be extracted from the sinusoidal signal by a chain of inverters. Slower clocks can also be obtained by dividing the main clock. Figure 1.12 shows the actual measurement of the above circuitry during operation. The largest voltage (Ch2) is the rectified voltage, followed by the regulated (Ch1) and than the reference (Ch3) voltages. The recovered 4 MHz clock (Ch4) is shown at the bottom of the trace.

Data demodulation circuitry depends on the type of modulation implemented in the base station. For an ASK scheme, an envelope detector followed by an RC filter is sufficient. Figure 1.13 shows a circuit diagram of such a circuitry. A filter circuit (C1, R1) reduces the amplitude of this signal to workable levels. The envelope recovery is performed with 2 NMOS devices (M1, M2), a transconductance amplifier (I1), and several filter circuits (C2, R2, R3) [30]. These serve to remove the carrier waveform and leave only the data signal. A high-pass filter (C3, R4) removes any

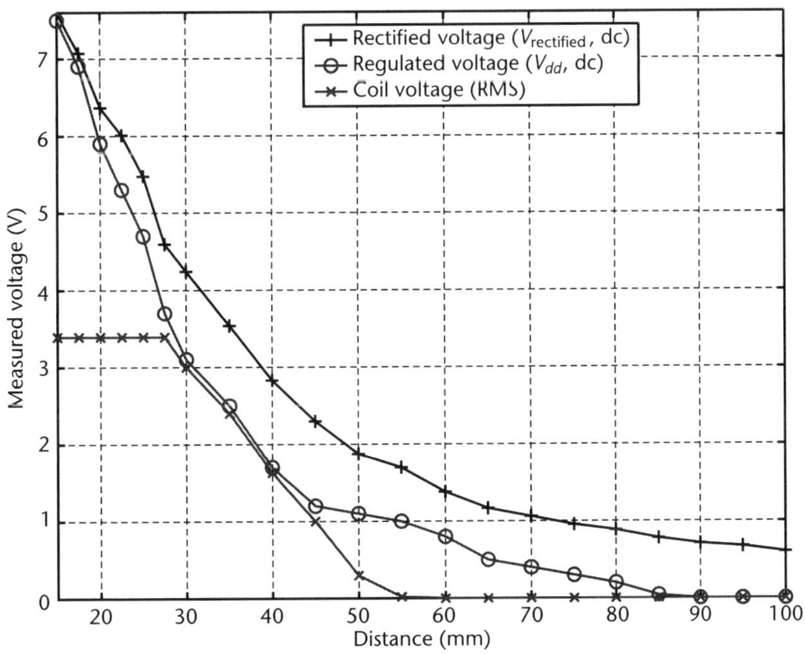

Figure 1.11 Air coupling at different distances. From [29] with permission, © IEEE 2005.

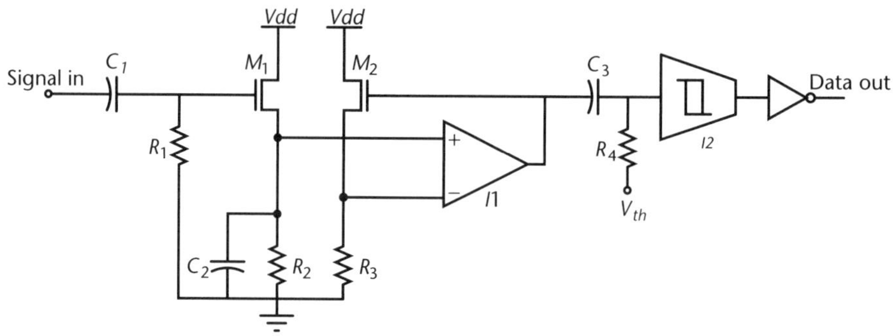

Figure 1.12 Data recovery circuitry (ASK demodulation).

DC component remaining in this signal and biases the voltage around a level for subsequent Schmitt triggering. The Schmitt trigger (I2) recovers the digital signal while suppressing noise present due to low signal amplitude or excessive noise on the envelope signal.

A finite state machine at the next level decodes this data and determines the parameters for system operation (e.g. number of channels, channel selection, and A/D resolution).

Data are accepted from the sensor in non-return to zero (NRZ) format. The data are encoded in a modified Miller encoding scheme. For every logical one in the NRZ data stream a pulse is generated. The pulse width is controlled by gating the

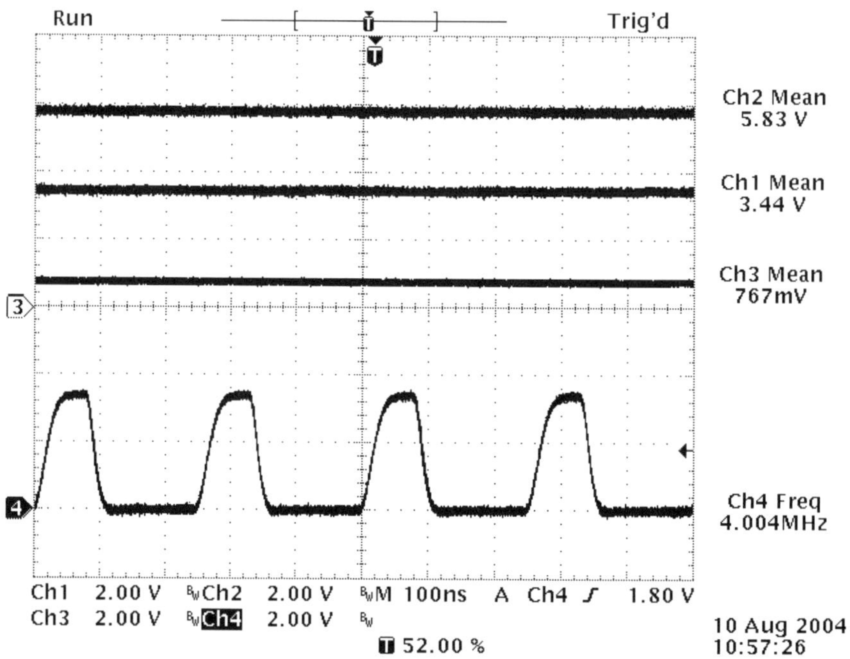

Figure 1.13 Oscilloscope trace of the microchip analog waveforms.

input clock for ease of implementation. This clock could also be supplied by clocks internally generated on chip. This encoding format transmits two signal transitions for every "one" datum, and none for a "zero" datum. The transmission of the two-level NRZ signal is accomplished by turning on an NMOS transistor that connects a resistor between the coil and ground. This modulates the impedance of the coil, a change that can be read out on the transmission coil. With the Modified Miller encoding scheme, the active time of the switched resistor load is minimized, thus reducing the power consumption. This scheme is also more tolerant to noise. It does not depend on the duration of a high pulse, but rather the occurrence of such a pulse.

1.4.3 Alternative Encoding and Transmission Schemes

Digitized data can also be transmitted via different modulation techniques for higher performance at the expense of higher complexity, where desired. As mentioned, one limitation of the simple scheme using the same coil both for power transmission as well as data telemetry, is the limited data bandwidth $\omega_b = \omega_c/Q$, which is 40 kbps in the design described. Higher rates can be achieved (where desired, e.g. for multichannel ECoG measurement) by using a dedicated reader coil in addition to the power delivery coil at the receiver end. To achieve these higher data rates further requires implementation of alternative encoding schemes to the simple ASK scheme (switching a resistor on and off across the coil), again at the expense of increased complexity and power consumption. Improvements in either data rate or error rate can also be obtained by optimizing the decoder performance at the receiver, where power consumption and complexity are less noticeable as constraining factors. Alternatives to the envelope detection scheme for ASK demodulation described above, such as synchronous detection, should be considered.

To illustrate the effect of encoding and decoding strategy on the quality of data transmission in the above system, 10 seconds of data were sent and recorded at several data rates ranging from 1 to 10 kbps. The highest theoretical data rate possible on this link is 40 kbps, as primarily determined by the quality factor of the transmitter coil (with a carrier frequency of 4 MHz). This can be lowered at the cost of increased power to operate the system over the same distance. Figure 1.14 shows data recovered by the envelope detector after modified Miller encoding and transmission at several data rates. At higher data transmission rates the signal is smaller and harder to detect. At the highest frequency (10 kbps) errors occur in both data formats (NRZ and modified Miller) with more errors in the NRZ data. This is likely due to the increased complexity of decoding such data.

A more robust scheme of ASK demodulation is coherent demodulation. This requires a phase locked copy of the carrier signal that is multiplied with the received signal and low pass filtered to remove the carrier. In order to reduce complexity and making use of the fact that in the time domain, the square of a digital bitstream is equivalent to the bitstream itself, a coherent demodulator was implemented using a four quadrant Gilbert multiplier. The received signal was squared and then filtered with a low-pass filter at 400 kHz to extract the data from the carrier. The data rate of the system could be pushed to 20 kbps without errors for both NRZ and modified Miller data using this demodulating scheme.

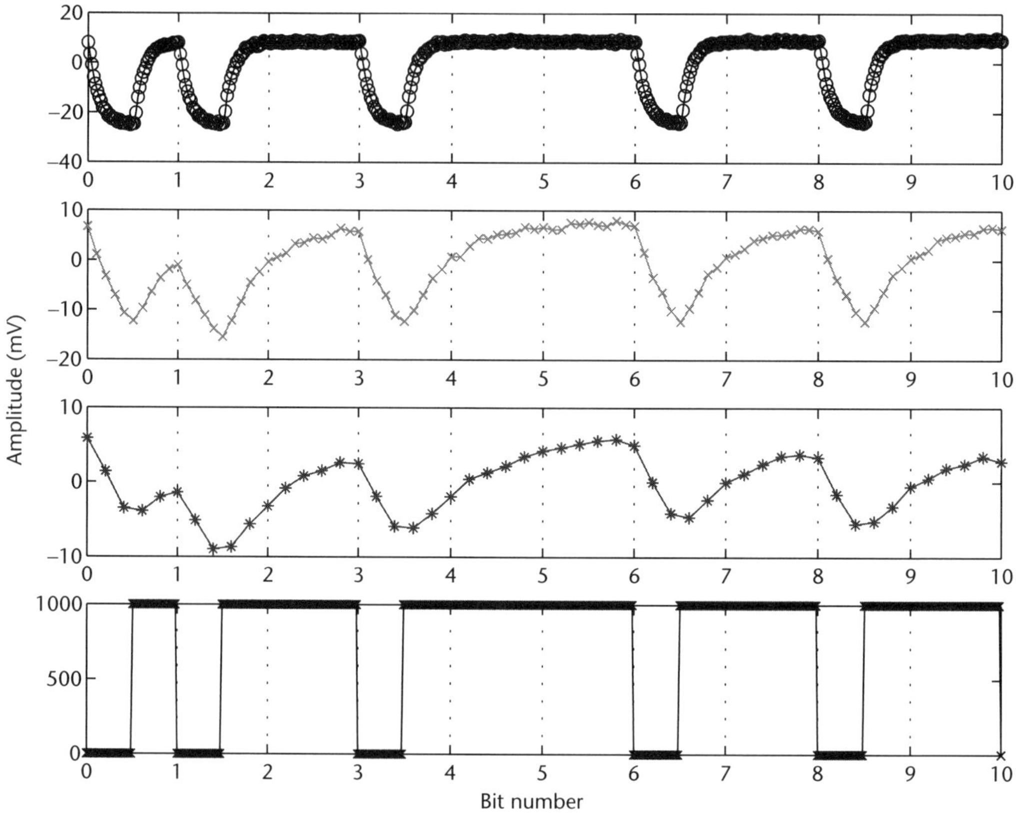

Figure 1.14 Comparison of data envelopes at frequencies tested for the Miller encoded data stream '1 101 001 010'. From the top, data at 1 kbps, data at 5 kbps, data at 10 kbps, and the ideal output Miller encoded data.

1.5 Multimodal Electrical and Chemical Sensing

Simultaneous detection and sensing of neurochemicals and electrophysiological field potentials are very useful when studying the interaction between the chemical synaptic and electrical neuronal activity, both in the healthy and the diseased brain. The capability to monitor the close interaction between electrical and chemical activity *in vivo* is crucial, as *in vitro* experimentation is deficient in studying network aspects and environmental factors in awake and behaving animals. Implantable multi-channel instrumentation with this multi-model capability could provide important information regarding neurological conditions where there is an imbalance between the chemical and electrical activity as in epilepsy [31]. The previous three sections have described the individual VLSI components that when properly combined comprise a multimodal amperometric/voltametric sensing system. This section describes the combination of the three systems and the protocol under which they co-operate. Figure 1.15 shows the schematic diagram of the system in an implantable scenario [32].

The principle is to (a) have the power harvesting chip supply power and clocks to both the potentiostat and the EEG processor; and (b) utilize the telemetry link to

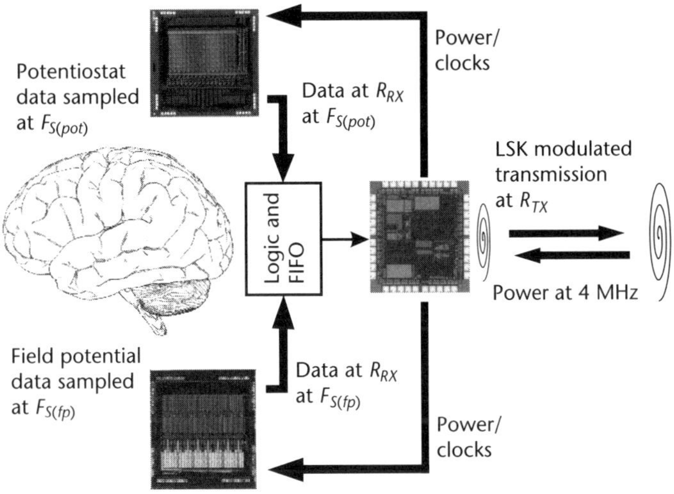

Figure 1.15 System diagram of the wireless multimodal recording system including micrographs of the constituent chips.

transmit the digitized neurochemical and electrophysiological data to a base station. This involves transmitting two simultaneous data streams over a single link, requiring additional interface circuitry. The interface circuitry serves to interleave and buffer the two data streams, equalized for a constant data rate over the telemetry link. The bandwidth assignment takes into account the sampling requirements of both signals. Neurochemical changes are generally on a much slower time scale (on the order of several hundreds of milliseconds to seconds) than EEG signals (on the order of a few tens of milliseconds), and hence are assigned proportionally lower bandwidth in data transmission. The net bandwidth in the assignment is limited by that of the telemetry module, which utilizes the same link for power and data transmission. As described above, the constraint on telemetry bandwidth is the Q-factor of the coils used for transmission. A high Q-factor benefits range of transmission, but also curtails the bandwidth of the data transmission subsystem.

Both the potentiostat and the EEG processor produce bit-serial output at variable rate and precision, as controlled by system clock, digital gain, and OSR, as described above. With a system clock of 2 MHz and a digital gain of 32, the potentiostat chip digitizes 16 channels of transduced neurotransmitter concentrations to 16 bits per sample at a sampling rate of 1Hz. The chip serially outputs the digitized data at a burst rate of R_{rx} = 64 kHz. For the EEG processor, a system clock of 4 MHz, a digital gain of 4- and 12-bit digitization over 4 channels produces EEG data sampled at 250 Hz, and output serially at the same burst rate as the neurochemical data. To combine and equalize the two data streams compatible with the constant rate bit-serial transmission by the telemetry system, the digital data from both sources is multiplexed and written in a buffer memory. Read and write operations are performed asynchronously for uninterrupted continuous data transfer.

An example recording illustrating the operation of the multimodal neurosensing system is shown in Figure 1.16. Real-time neurochemical data was obtained *in vitro* by monitoring the solution of phosphate buffered saline to which dopamine was added at timed intervals. The system shown in Figure 1.15 was set up with the power

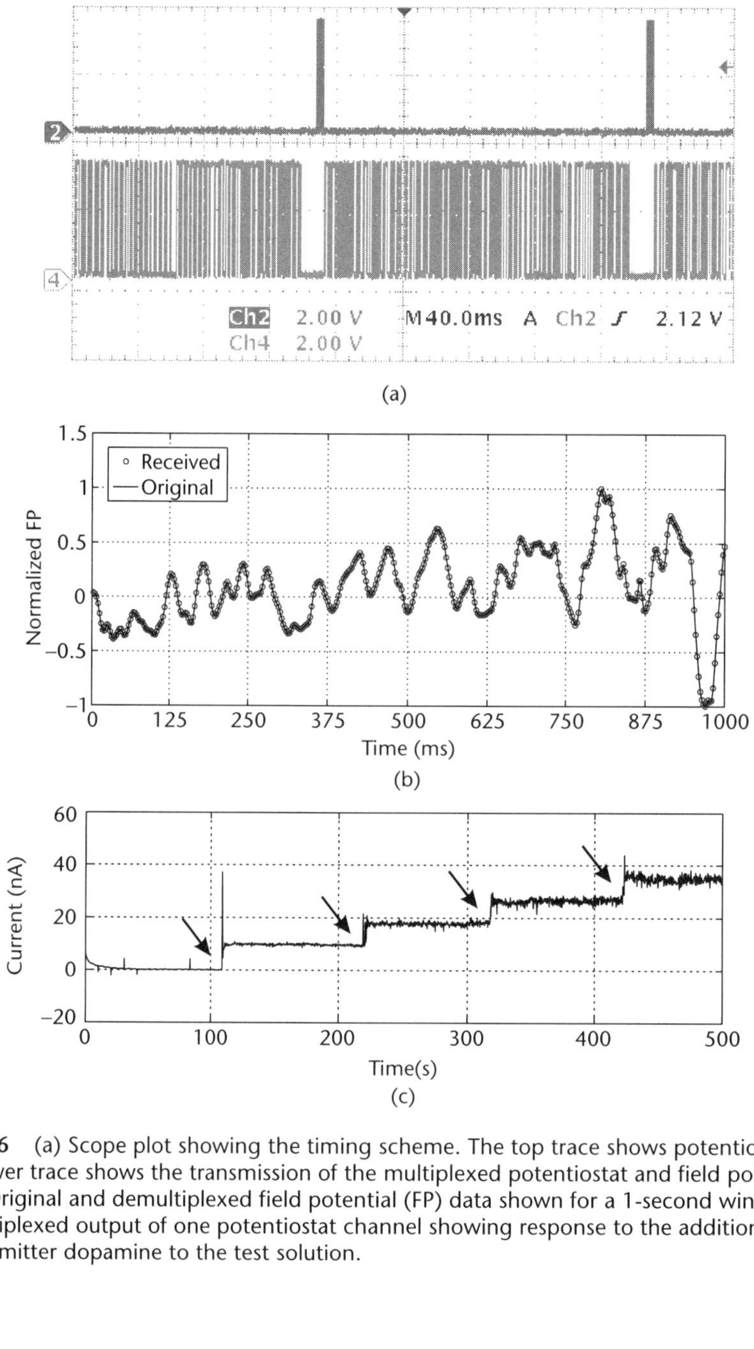

Figure 1.16 (a) Scope plot showing the timing scheme. The top trace shows potentiostat data bursts. Lower trace shows the transmission of the multiplexed potentiostat and field potential data. (b) Original and demultiplexed field potential (FP) data shown for a 1-second window. (c) Demultiplexed output of one potentiostat channel showing response to the addition of the neurotransmitter dopamine to the test solution.

harvesting chip supplying the power and system clock to the potentiostat. Discrete logic was used to implement the interface and memory. This was powered independently. The received data were demodulated using a coherent detector, read into a computer using a DAQ card and demultiplexed. Figure 1.16 (b) shows the original and received electrophysiological data. Figure 1.16 (c) shows the received data from the simultaneous *in vitro* neurochemical monitoring.

1.6 Summary

In this chapter we framed the challenges inherent in wireless monitoring of multimodal electrochemical neural activity, and presented a design methodology for an integrated solution capable of recording and telemetering both electrical and neurochemical activity from multiple sites. The following observations summarize the message of this chapter:

1. Wireless monitoring of *in vivo* neural activity using implanted passive telemetry poses stringent constraints on the available power for sensor acquisition, signal processing, and transmission of recorded neural activity. Without on-chip signal compression, signal bandwidth scales with available power. Transmitted power scales approximately inversely with the square of the distance between implant and reader, and also depends on coil geometry and coding/decoding schemes. Larger peak activity (but same average sustained activity) can be supported by including a rechargeable battery with the implant.
2. Both electrical (neuropotential) and chemical (neurotransmitter) activity are simultaneously monitored by combining voltage and current measurement with properly designed electrodes and properly controlled biasing and waveform generation. Redox currents in cyclic voltametry using a potentiostat register concentrations of cation-sensitive neurotransmitters selected by electrode coating and further identified by redox potential. Scalp and intracranial electrical recording identify EEG and ECoG neuropotentials at various spatial and temporal scales, from single-neuron spikes in extracellular electrode recording to brain waves extending across the cerebral cortex. Simultaneous monitoring of these signals at various spatial and temporal scales are important in detection of pathological neural/brain states such as epilepsy and in the study of Alzheimer's and other neurodegenerative diseases.
3. A mixed-signal VLSI circuit methodology, with analog front-end acquisition, amplification and filtering, and with digital bit-serial coding of the quantized signals, offers low noise acquisition, high fidelity transmission, and low power operation. By multiplexing and interleaving of bit-serial data streams, the available wireless transmission bandwidth can be traded between a lower number of higher bandwidth signals (such as ECoG), or a larger number of lower bandwidth signals (such as low-frequency EEG, or distributed neurochemical activity).

References

[1] P. F. Bladin, "W. Grey Walter, pioneer in the electroencephalogram, robortics, cybernetics, artificial intelligence," *Journal of Clinical Neuroscience*, vol. 13, pp. 170–177, 2006.

[2] C. Plummer, A. S. Harvey, and M. Cook, "EEG source localization in focal epilepsy: Where are we now?," *Epilepsia*, 2007.

[3] L. R. Hochberg, M. D. Serruya, G. M. Friehs, J. A. Mukand, M. Saleh, A. H. Caplan, A. Branner, D. Chen, R. D. Penn, and J. P. Donoghue, "Neuronal ensemble control of prosthetic devices by a human with tetraplegia," *Nature*, vol. 442, pp. 164–171, 2006.

[4] S. H. Dale, "Nobel Lecture "Some Recent Extensions of the Chemical Transmission of the Effects of Nerve Impulses"," 1936.

[5] E. R. Kandel, J. H. Schwartz, and T. M. Jessell, *Principles of Neural Science*: McGraw-Hill Medical, 2000.

[6] T. Wichmann and M. R. Delong, "Pathophysiology of parkinsonian motor abnormalities," *Advances in Neurology*, vol. 60, p. 53, 1993.

[7] M. E. Thase and G. S. Sachs, "Bipolar Depression: pharmacotherapy and related therapeutic strategies," *Biological Psychiatry*, vol. 48, p. 558, 2000.

[8] R. S. Braman and S. A. Hendrix, "Nanogram nitrite and nitrate determination in environmental and biological materials by vanadium(III) reduction with chemiluminescence detection," *Analytical Chemistry*, vol. 61, pp. 2715–2718, 1989.

[9] K. Nakai and R. P. Mason, "Immunochemical detection of nitric oxide and nitrogen dioxide trapping of the tyrosyl radical and the resulting nitrotyrosine in sperm whale myoglobin," *Free Radic Biol Med*, vol. 39, pp. 1050–8, Oct. 15, 2005.

[10] I. Baranowska and M. Zydron, "Liquid chromatography in the analysis of neurotransmitters and alkaloids," *Journal of Chromatographic Science*, vol. 40, pp. 224–228, 2002.

[11] R. B. Kawade and K. S. V. Santhanam, "An in vitro electrochemical sensing of dopamine in the presence of ascorbic acid," *Biochemistry and Bioenergetics*, vol. 38, p. 405, 1995.

[12] T. Malinski, Z. Taha, S. Grunfeld, and A. Burewicz, "Measurement of nitric oxide in biological materials using a porphyrinic microsensor," *Analytica Chimica Acta*, vol. 279, p. 135, 1994.

[13] L. Clark, R. Wolf, D. Granger, and Z. Taylor, "Continuous recording of blood oxygen tensions by polarography," *Journal of Applied Physiology*, vol. 6, p. 189, 1953.

[14] A. J. Bard and L. R. Faulkner, *Electrochemical Methods*: John Wiley & Sons, 1980.

[15] A. Gore, S. Chakrabartty, S. Pal, and E. C. Alocilja, "A multichannel femtoampere-sensitivity potentiostat array for biosensing applications," *IEEE Trans. Circuits and Systems I: Fundamental theory and applications*, vol. 53, pp. 2357–2363, 2006.

[16] R. G. Kakerow, H. Kappert, E. Spiegel, and Y. Manoli, "Low power single-chip CMOS potentiostat," in *Solid-State Sensors and Actuators, Eurosensors IX*, 1995.

[17] M. Roham and P. Mohseni, "Wireless amperometric neurochemical monitroing using an integrated FSK telemetry circuit," in *3rd International Conference on Neural Engineering*, Kohala Coast, Hawaii, 2007, pp. 159–162.

[18] M. Stanacevic, K. Murari, A. Rege, G. Cauwenberghs, and N. V. Thakor, "VLSI potentiostat array with oversampling gain modulation for wide-range neurotransmitter sensing," *IEEE Trans. Biomedical Circuits and Systems*, vol. 1, pp. 63–72, March 2007.

[19] R. B. F. Turner, D. J. Harrison, and H. P. Baltes, "A CMOS potentiostat for amperometric chemical sensors," *IEEE Journal of Solid-State Circuits*, vol. SC-22, p. 473, 1987.

[20] K. Murari, "Electrochemical detection of neurotransmitters with a VLSI interface," in *Biomedical Engineering*, Baltimore: Johns Hopkins University, 2004.

[21] J. Candy and G. Temes, *Oversampling delta-sigma data converters*: IEEE Press, 1991.

[22] K. E. Misulis, *Essentials of Clinical Neurophysiology*. Boston: Butterworth-Heinemann, 1997.

[23] J. G. Webster, *Medical Instrumentation, application and design*, third ed.: John Wiley & Sons, 1998.

[24] S. K. Yoo, N. H. Kim, S. H. Kim, and J. L. Kim, "The developement of high precision EEG amplifier for computerized EEG analysis," in *IEEE Annual Conf. Eng, Medicine Biology Society*, Montreal, Quebec, 1995.

[25] R. Harrison and C. Charles, "A low-power low-noise CMOS amplifier for neural recording applications," *IEEE Journal of Solid-State Circuits*, vol. 38, pp. 958–965, 2003.

[26] D. A. Johns, *Analog integrated circuit design*: John Wiley & Sons, 1997.

[27] P. Vaillancourt, A. Djemouai, J. Harvey, and M. Sawan, "EM radiation behavior upon biological tissues in a radio-frequency power transfer link for a cortical implant," in *IEEE Eng. in Medicine & Biology*, 1997, pp. 2499–2503.

[28] K. Finkenzeller, *RFID Handbook*. London, U.K.: Wiley, 2003.

[29] C. Sauer, M. Stanacevic, G. Cauwenberghs, and N. V. Thakor, "Power harvesting and telemetry in CMOS for implanted devices," *IEEE Trans. Circuits and Systems I: Fundamental theory and applications*, vol. 52, pp. 2605–2613, 2005.

[30] D. Su and W. McFarland, "An IC for linearizing RF power amplifiers using envelope elimination and restoration," *IEEE Journal of Solid-State Circuits*, vol. 33, pp. 2252–2258, 1998.

[31] I. Fried, C. L. Wilson, N. T. Maidment, J. J. Engel, E. Behnke, T. A. Fields, K. A. MacDonald, J. W. Morrow, and L. Ackerson, "Cerebral microdialysis combined with single-neuron and electroencephalographic recording in neurosurgical patients. Technical note," *Journal of Neurosurgery*, vol. 91, pp. 697–705, 1999.

[32] M. Mollazadeh, K. Murari, C. Sauer, M. Stanacevic, N. V. Thakor, and G. Cauwenberghs, "Wireless integrated voltametric and amperometric biosensing," in *Life Science Systems and Applications Workshop*, Bethesda, MD, 2006.

CHAPTER 2

Visual Cortical Neuroprosthesis: A System Approach

Moisés Piedade, José Gerald, Leonel Sousa, and Gonçalo Tavares

2.1 Introduction

In the last few years there has been a huge effort to develop implantable integrated stimulators for biomedical applications. Most of these stimulators are in the area of muscular stimulation (for instance, for heart or limb diseases) [1–5] and in the area of cortical or nerve stimulations (e.g., for blind/partially blind people or hearing diseases) [6–12]. In all these stimulators, information has to be coded in a format somewhat similar to the way stimulation is performed prior to the development of each of the particular diseases. Moreover, with the exception of a few applications (e.g., pacemakers), long-time performance of the implanted stimulator implies the power to be provided by the outside unit. It avoids future operations to replace old batteries, reduces the risk of infections and therefore improves the patient health level. This poses the need for wireless remote delivery of power and data [10–12].

Microelectronic prostheses that interact with the remaining healthy retina have been developed to restore some vision to those who suffer from eye diseases, such as *Retinitis Pigmentosa*. This type of prosthesis can use sub-retinal devices [13] (to replace the photoreceptors) or more complex epiretinal devices [14] (for capturing and processing images that are transmitted to the ganglion cells through an electrode array) but requires that output neurons of the eye and the optical nerves are in a healthy state. When this is not the case, these microelectronic prostheses are not useful and the stimulation has to be performed in the primary visual cortex, directly to the neurons in higher visual regions of the brain. This is a challenge, because visual information has to be encoded in a format somewhat similar to the way stimulation was done prior to the development of total blindness. It is expected that neurons will adapt to the stimulus in a way that a blind individual will be able to extract from it information on the physical world [15].

Brindley [16] and Dobelle [17] showed that simultaneous stimulation of multiple electrodes allowed blind volunteers to recognize simple patterns. This research, however, also showed that a cortical prosthesis based on a relatively large number of superficial implanted electrodes requires high currents to produce phosphenes (more than 1 mA), which leads to problems such as epileptic seizures. To avoid this, deep intracortical neuro-stimulation should be used, exciting the neurons at a depth between 1 mm and 2 mm, which corresponds to the cortical layers 4 (namely, C_α and C_β), where signals from the Lateral Geniculate Nucleus (LGN) arrive.

This chapter presents a cortical visual neuroprosthesis for profoundly blind people which has been developed within the scope of the CORTIVIS project and supported by the European Commission [18] and by the Portuguese Foundation for Science and Technology (FCT) [19].

Figure 2.1 illustrates the basic components of our Cortical Visual Neuroprosthesis approach. The whole system uses a bioinspired visual processing front-end, the *Neuromorphic Encoder*, which generates the electrical signals that are transferred to inside the skull through a RF link, for stimulating an array of penetrating electrodes implanted into the primary visual cortex. Power to operate the stimulating circuitry is also provided from the outside through the RF link. This visual neuroprosthesis is expected to recreate a limited, but useful visual sense in blind individuals, by applying the electrical signals up to 1024 microelectrodes. In what concerns the neuromorphic encoder, the simplest models assume that the neural coding can be reduced to predicting the firing rate as a function of the sensory stimulus. This assumption may be justified in certain brain areas, e.g. deep in the cortex [20]. On the other hand, neurons in the early visual system, for example from the retina to the LGN, can deliver reproducible spike trains, whose trial-to-trial variability is clearly lower than the one predicted from the simple firing rate approach [21]. To predict individual spikes, spike patterns with higher timing accuracy and also to account for the stochastic variability of these responses other approaches have to be considered. A first experimental work comparing the performance of these models has been recently published [22].

The wireless radio frequency (RF) link must provide both power and bidirectional data transmission between the outside and the implant. While the visual neuroprosthesis requires a few tenths of milliwatts of power, the actual power provided from the outside must be somewhat higher, in order to account for the coupling

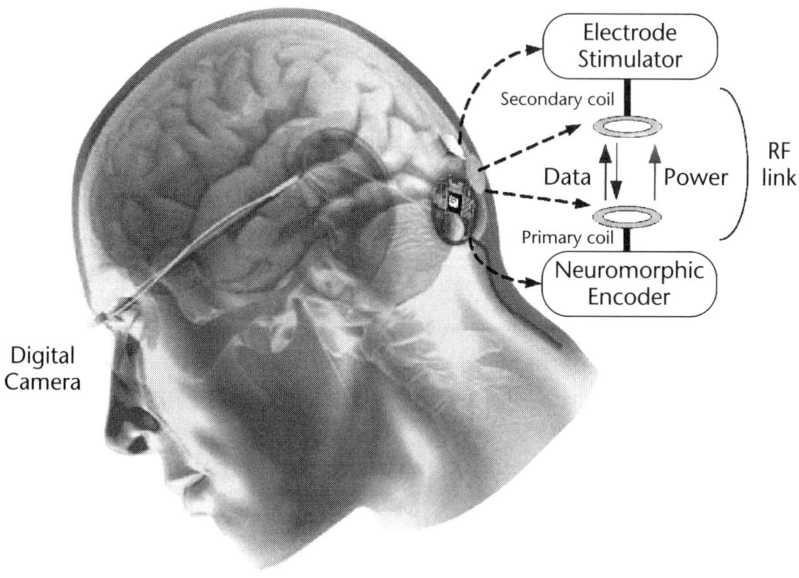

Figure 2.1 Cortical visual neuroprosthesis concept. From [37] with permission, © IEEE 2005.

losses. The most common solutions proposed in literature for the RF link are Amplitude Shift Keying (FSK) modulation [23–26], FSK [23, 27] and Binary Phase Shift Keying (BPSK) modulation [23, 28]. The ASK signal is usually demodulated in a noncoherent fashion, using a very simple receiver. However, the performance of the ASK receiver is highly dependent on the amplitude of the received signal, which is unknown and depends on the relative position between the implant and the outside unit. Therefore, an ASK solution requires high-efficient gain-monitoring and level-controlling devices. This is not the case with either FSK or BPSK, which are constant amplitude modulations. Within reasonable limits, the FSK and BPSK receivers are insensitive to the amplitude of the received signal, making these circuits more robust with respect to the high variability of the RF channel. Demodulation of FSK and BPSK is usually done coherently, thus requiring more complex and power-consuming receivers.

After careful analysis of the different modulation characteristics, FSK was chosen as the modulation to use in the forward link. For monitoring purposes a reverse data link has also been implemented. It uses BPSK, which is implemented with a very simple transmitter. BPSK was not selected for the forward link because the receiver (which is based on a Costas Loop demodulator) is more complex than the FSK receiver.

This chapter is organized as follows. In Section 2.2 the main components of the system are specified and an architecture is proposed to fulfill those specifications. Section 2.3 presents the prosthesis external body (primary) unit, which includes the neuromorphic encoder and the wireless communication link. Section 2.4 presents some circuits of the body implantable (secondary) unit. Experimental results of the system prototype are reported in Section 2.5. Section 2.6 concludes the chapter and summarizes the main results achieved.

2.2 System Architecture

The system architecture of the proposed visual neuroprosthesis is represented in Figure 2.2. It is physically divided in two units: a primary unit located outside the body and a secondary unit consisting of an implant located inside the body. The units are connected by means of a low-coupling two-coil transformer, which establishes a magnetic RF link between the two devices. The purpose of this RF link is twofold: (1) to remotely power the secondary unit, a mandatory requirement to avoid the use of batteries in the implant and (2) to allow bidirectional data communication between the units. The primary unit interfaces with a miniature digital video camera

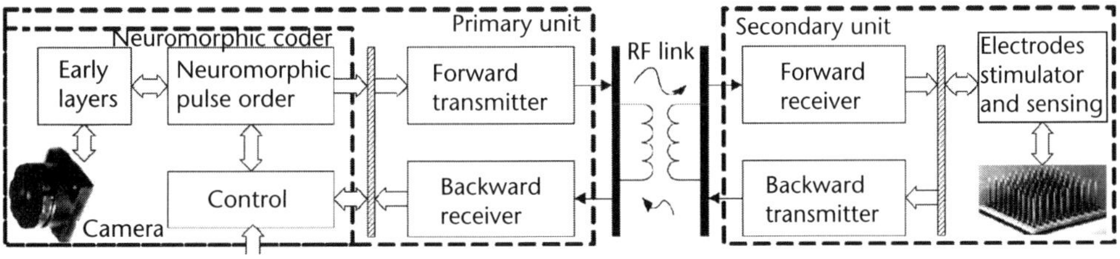

Figure 2.2 Prosthesis system architecture. From [37] with permission, © IEEE 2005.

and with a personal computer (PC) used for system configuration, patient visual training, and prosthesis performance analysis purposes.

The *Neuromorphic Encoder* translates the visual signal captured in the miniature digital camera into a sequence of electrical pulses, a spike train, capable of being recognized by the brain. It is composed of two main modules connected in series. The *Early Layers* are responsible for processing the visual signal and for its conversion into a spike rate. This rate is then taken as input by the *Neuromorphic Pulse Coding* module and is translated into the actual spike events by using a simplified version of the integrate-and-fire spiking neuron [29]. The access to the RF link is then arbitrated by the latest module using a First-In First-Out (FIFO) buffer to store the events until the link is able to send more spike events. In the visual neuroprosthesis presented in this chapter, the *Neuromorphic Encoder* is required to process visual images at a rate of 30 frames per second (fps), generating spikes at a rate up to 100 Hz and stimulating a number of microelectrodes equivalent to an array with up to 32 × 32.

The *Forward Transmitter* receives the multiplexed spike data from the *Neuromorphic Pulse Coding* in a synchronous serial bit stream format at a rate of f_b = 1 Mbps. This data is modulated using FSK modulation with a center frequency of f_c = 10 MHz and a frequency deviation Δf = ±323 kHz. On the secondary unit, power is extracted from the received signal by a power supply generator circuit (considered to be part of the *Forward Receiver* in Figure 2.2) which will be described later in Section 2.4. Because the integrity of brain tissue does not allow the use of high-power circuitry, the secondary unit is required to operate with only tenth's of milliwatts of remotely delivered power. The spike data is recovered by the *Forward Receiver*, which consists of a FSK demodulator, bit synchronizer, and frame disassembly circuit. The recovered data and clock are then forwarded to the microelectrodes stimulator circuit.

To accomplish implant monitoring (e.g. electrode impedance measurement and calibration) a reverse data link has been developed. In the secondary unit, maintenance data is modulated and transmitted using BPSK at a data rate of f_b = 156.25 kbps using low amplitude (≈1 V) and a carrier frequency f_c = 5 MHz. The main objective of the *Electrode Stimulators and Sensing* module is to stimulate the primary visual cortex and to measure the connectivity between the electrodes and cortex. Extensive experiments have shown that in order to safely induce phosphenes a current of 20μA is required. Electrode sensing is achieved by injecting a fixed current value to a microelectrode and then measuring the induced voltage value. This allows for measuring the connectivity between the microelectrode and the visual cortex cells.

The *Electrode Stimulators and Sensing* module is composed of a set of Digital to Analog Converters (DACs) [30], which are used to stimulate up to 32 × 32 microelectrodes in the visual cortex with the spike events received from the *Neuromorphic Encoder*. Each DAC has a current-steering type architecture, using scaled currents added at an output node, in order to ensure the desired linear DAC operation. The main difference with respect to the common current-steering DAC is that it allows for the removal of the charge from the brain: it can inject current (positive sign) or remove current (negative sign) from the electrode. The DAC reference current is around 29μA and the overall power consumption for stimulating and sensing the 1024 electrodes is expected to be under 50 mW. The amplitude and duration of the stimulus is pre-recorded in dedicated registers on the *Electrodes Stimulator and Sensing* module, which can be accessed by means of the RF link for both reading and writing.

The overall system is presently under development in VLSI technology. The *Electrode Stimulator and Sensing* block is to be implemented in a modular way in AMS CMOS 0.35μm technology: each module (except for the power supply generator) drives a 100-microelectrode array, which will be attached directly to the VLSI chip (flip chip technology) [30]. The Forward and backward emitters and receivers are also being developed using AMS CMOS 0.35μm technology. Moreover, in order to evaluate the circuit requirements when implementing the in-deep sub-micron technology, the *Neuromorphic Encoder* is now being synthesized using the UMC 0.13μm CMOS technology process [31]. The UMC L130E SG-HS 1P8M process is a single poly, 8 metal layer with an operating voltage of 1.2 V.

However, to rapidly prove the concepts involved in the RF link, a scaled-frequency prototype operating 10 times slower was built using conventional integrated circuits and discrete components: the forward data rate is 100 kbps with a carrier frequency of 1 MHz; the backward data rate is 15.625 kbps with a carrier frequency of 500 kHz. Also a neuromorphic encoder was developed using FPGA technology. The visual neuroprothesis system was planned to support the driving of 1024 electrodes. However, the stimulator chip that is being developed will be flipped directly over the back of one microelectrodes array (100 microelectrodes).

2.3 Prosthesis Exterior Body Unit and Wireless Link

2.3.1 Neuromorphic Encoder

The block diagram of the *Neuromorphic Encoder* in Figure 2.3 includes the spatio-temporal receptive fields of the retina ganglion cells. The neuromorphic encoder is organized in three main blocks: (1) *Early Layers* that perform both spatial and temporal processing of the visual signal, (2) *Neuromorphic Pulse Coder*, responsible for converting the pre-processed visual information to a sequence of pulses that can be interpreted by the brain, and (3) *Spike Multiplexing* that applies Address Event Representation (AER) [32] to convey information about the pulses through a serial link, without timestamps, to the microelectrode stimulator. The *Neuromorphic Encoder* translates a visual stimulus $s(r,t)$ described by the intensity of each of the three basic (R)ed, (G)reen and (B)lue color components, as a function of space $r = [x\ y]^T$ and time t, into a sequence of pulses. This encoder was designed to allow a blind individual to recognize patterns up to 32 × 32 points, corresponding to 1024 microelectrodes.

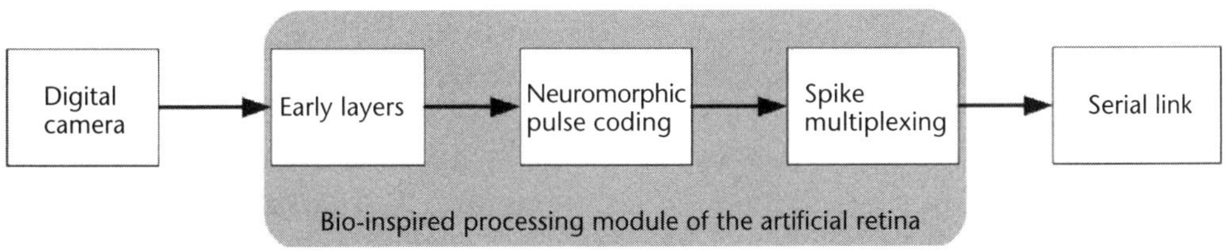

Figure 2.3 Neuromorphic encoder.

2.3.1.1 Early Layers

The *Early Layers* block represented in Figure 2.4 is responsible for spatio-temporal filtering. This block is an extension to the chromatic domain, by considering independent filters for each basic color component. The first filtering element of the *Early Layers* is an edge detector implemented by a two-dimensional Difference-of-Gaussians (DOG) per color channel (see Figure 2.4). As it is well known, DOG functions can be used for edge detection when the gains of the two Gaussians have opposite signs and different standard deviations.

The output of the edge detection modules, corresponding to the different color components, are integrated by applying the desired relative weights (* represents the convolution operator):

$$m(r,t) = \sum_{i=R,G,B} \alpha_i \left(s_i(r,t) * \mathrm{DOG}_i \right) \tag{2.1}$$

The $m(r,t)$ signal is then convolved with the impulse response of a first order high-pass filter h_{HP} with the pole at $-\alpha$ rad/s to perform motion detection. The resulting activation function $u(r,t) = m(r,t) * h_{HP}(r,t)$ is then modulated by the Contrast Gain Controller (CGC) that models the strong modulation effect exerted by stimulus contrast. The CGC non-linear approach is also used in order to model the motion anticipation effect [33]: the CGC output $w(r,t)$ is convolved with the impulse response of a lowpass temporal filter h_{LP} with a single pole at $-\gamma$ rad/s; the resulting signal $v(r,t) = y(r,t) * h_{LP}(r,t)$ is then processed by the non-linear function:

$$g\left(v(r,t)\right) = \frac{1}{1 + \left[v(r,t) \cdot H\left(v(r,t)\right) \right]^4} \tag{2.2}$$

before being applied to modulate the amplitude of the CGC input signal ($H(\cdot)$ represents the Heaviside step function). Finally, the last processing step of the Early Layers block is a rectifier operation represented in Figure 2.4. It yields the firing rate $f(r,t)$ of the ganglion cells response to the input stimuli:

$$f(r,t) = \Psi \cdot H(y(r,t) + \theta) \cdot [y(r,t) + \theta] \tag{2.3}$$

where Ψ and θ define the scale and baseline values of the firing rate.

The bilinear approximation was used in order to implement the temporal filters, resulting in first-order Infinite Impulse Response (IIR) digital filters. Also, to reduce the amount of memory needed, the temporal filters were implemented in a transposed form where the output is calculated by adding the input $x[n]$ to a stored value $l[n]$ that is computed in the previous cycle.

The diagram of the visual encoder computational architecture is depicted in Figure 2.5 (the notation $x[q,n]$ stands for the discrete space/time equivalent of the signal $x(r,t)$).

Folding techniques were applied to the architecture directly derived from the Signal Flow Graph (SFG), in order to comply with restrictions, such as low power consumption and area circuit. The complete *Early Layers* circuit was folded 1024 times and the firing rate for each microelectrode is computed in series. Moreover,

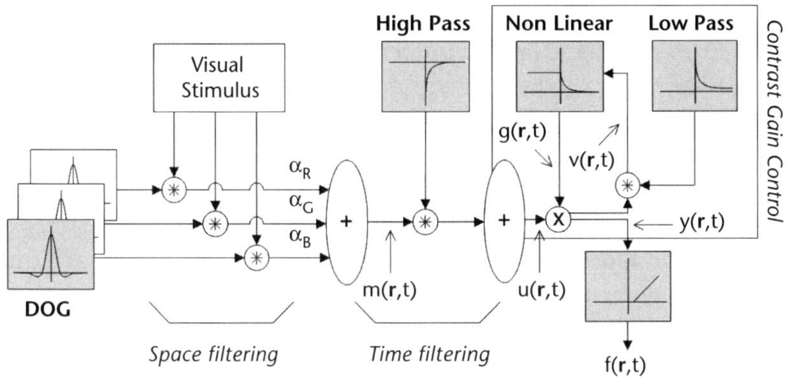

Figure 2.4 Early layers block.

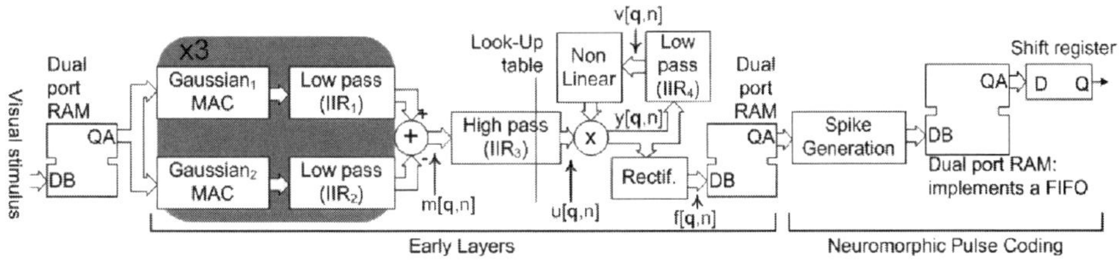

Figure 2.5 Diagram of the visual encoder computational architecture. From [37] with permission, © IEEE 2005.

assuming a Gaussian kernel of 7×7, edge detection requires a total of 98 multiplications and 98 additions. The folding technique has been applied to the Gaussian filters by a factor equal to the kernel size. Therefore, as shown in Figure 2.5, only one multiply-and-accumulate (MAC) unit is needed to compute each Gaussian filter. The non-linear processing modules, namely the non-linear function applied in the CGC and the rectifier, were implemented by means of a look-up table and a comparator, respectively.

2.3.1.2 Neuromorphic Pulse Coding

The *Neuromorphic Pulse Coding* (NPC) block performs two operations: (1) converts the continuous time-varying representation of the signal produced in the *Early Layers* of the retina into a neural pulse representation, and (2) arbitrates the access of the generated spikes to the serial bus at the input of the *Forward Emitter*. We have considered a representation in which the signal provides information only when a new pulse begins. This block then stores the information about spike events and sends them to the implant at the maximum rate allowed by the channel. The model adopted for the Spike Generation is a simplified version of an integrate-and-fire spiking neuron [29]: the neuron accumulates input values from the respective receptive field (output firing rate determined by the *Early Layers*) until it reaches a threshold ϕ; then it fires a pulse and discharges the accumulated value; a leakage term is included to force the accumulated value to diminish for low or null input values.

The implementation of the pulse generation circuit operates in a two-stage pipeline: in the first stage the input firing rate is added to the accumulated value; in the second stage, the leakage value is subtracted and, if the result is higher than a threshold ϕ, a pulse is fired and the accumulator returns to zero. This block is connected to the *Early Layers* by means of a dual-port memory bank, as represented in Figure 2.5. This allows for the *Early Layers* block to write data onto one port while the *Neuromorphic Pulse Coding* block reads data from the other port. The *Spike Multiplexing* block uses a first-in first-out (FIFO) buffer to arbitrate the access of the spikes generated in the *Spike Generating* block to the RF link (see Figure 2.5). When a spike is generated, it is stored in the buffer until the channel becomes available. The buffer allows the system to respond well to short periods in which the spike rate is high.

2.3.1.3 Model Evaluation

To evaluate the performance of this model, an experimental analysis was made by using real experimental data from salamander retinal responses [22]. This work has compared the performance of the presented model to the one of a recently published stochastic model, which attempts to predict the temporal occurrence of spikes and spike patterns [20]. Model performance was assessed based on the mean squared error (MSE) of the firing rate. The MSE for the firing rate of the presented model is about 1.11, while for the stochastic model is 1.13 [22]. These results show that by using a deterministic model, it is possible to approximate the real neural retina response with an accuracy similar to that of the stochastic model. However, deterministic models are less demanding in terms of computational capacity, thus making them a more suitable approach for developing a visual neuroprosthesis.

2.3.2 External Body Unit (Primary RF Unit)

The RF link block diagram is shown in Figure 2.6. The RF link circuitry can be divided into three parts: the primary RF unit (located outside the body), the secondary RF unit (located inside the body, but not necessarily inside the head), and the transformer, which establishes inductive coupling between the two previously mentioned units (one coil is external and another is internal). A bidirectional RF link is established: the primary (forward) link and the secondary (backward) link. In the

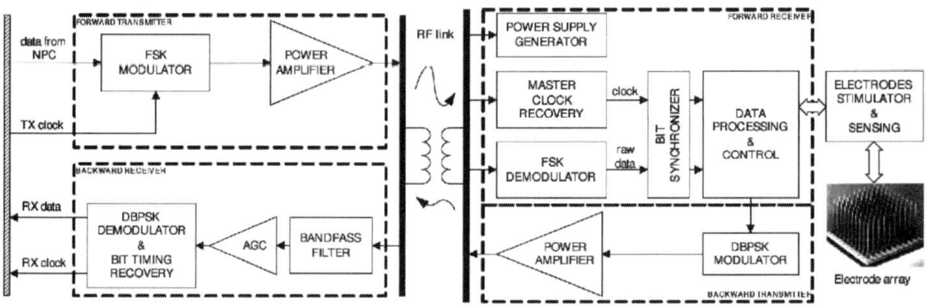

Figure 2.6 RF link circuitry diagram. From [37] with permission, © IEEE 2005.

main link, the data bit rate is up to 1 Mbps, and a power/data signal is transmitted using FSK modulation with a 10 MHz frequency carrier. In the secondary link, the data bit rate is up to 156.25 kbps (which is enough for maintenance and initial configuration purposes) and data is transmitted using BPSK modulation with a 5 MHz frequency carrier. Initially, in order to implement a very compact low-power wireless communication link, some integrated circuits were designed using AMS CMOS 0.8 μm technology. However, new circuits currently in development use AMS CMOS 0.35 μm technology [30].

The transmitter is shown in Figure 2.7(a) and includes a FSK modulator (implemented by means of a counter, driven by an oscillator f_{CLK}) and a signal amplifier. The data is modulated with frequencies $\frac{f_{CLK}}{16}$ (data bit '0') and $\frac{f_{CLK}}{15}$ (data bit '1'). This signal feeds a class E switching-mode tuned power amplifier, as shown in Figure 2.7(a), whose configuration was chosen to optimize the efficiency at the transmitter [34].

The primary RF unit receiver is a Costas-Loop [23] BPSK coherent demodulator. This receiver is placed after a 6th order bandpass filter and a RF Automatic Gain Control (AGC) circuit.

2.3.3 RF Transformer

The coupling transformer is of major importance in the RF link since it has a strong influence on the overall performance of the internal unit. Its design must allow proper system operation regardless of the intercoil distance (within reasonable limits, say 1 to 2 cm). It must be noticed that the real transformer, at the desired operation frequencies, exhibits a distributed parameter behavior (as represented in the model in

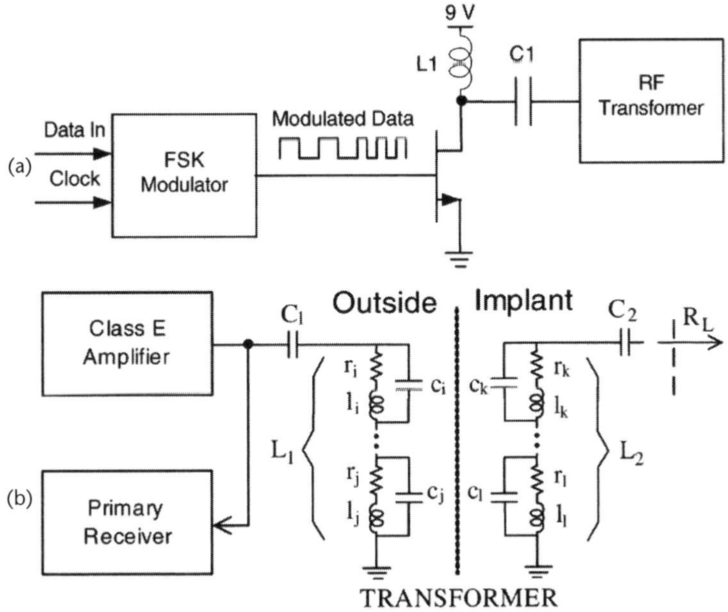

Figure 2.7 RF unit: (a) transmitter; (b) coupling transformer model. From [37] with permission, © IEEE 2005.

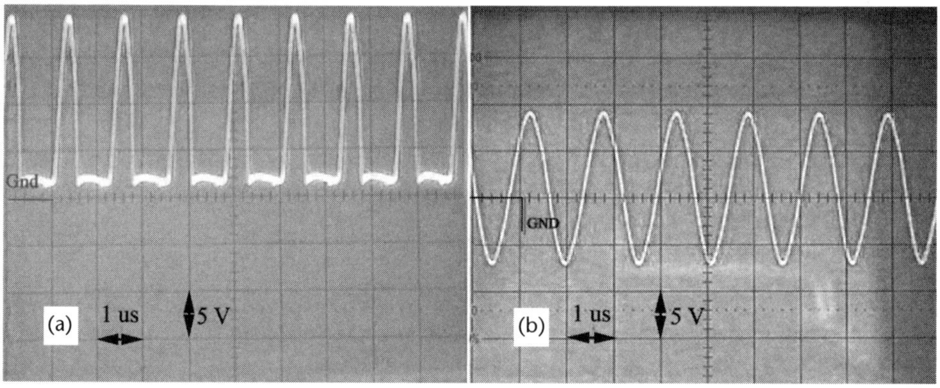

Figure 2.8 Transmitted signal for an intercoil distance of 1 cm: (a) before the transformer; (b) after the transformer.

Figure 2.7(b)). Due to the coil separation, there is a high magnetic flux dispersion (not connected with the secondary coil), which makes the coupling weak and a significant amount of energy is lost. To maximize the efficiency, it is important to perform an appropriate design of the coils. In order to compensate the equivalent inductances relative to the primary and secondary magnetic flux dispersions, capacitors C_1 and C_2 are connected in series with the respective coil, resonating at the 10 MHz carrier frequency. As a consequence, the RF transformer behaves like a double-tuned bandpass filter. Both circular coils have a cylindrical powerful neodymium magnet inside, used for coil self-attracting and fixing purposes [35, 36].

Experiments confirmed the importance of taking into account the distributed capacitance and the skin effect in the transformer. In fact, the absence of an iron core makes it impossible to have a strong magnetic coupling: the measured coupling factor was 0.3 for an intercoil distance of 1 cm using carefully designed planar coils of Litz wire with about 3 cm of diameter. Figure 2.8 illustrates the transmission of an unmodulated carrier before and after the transformer for a 16 times lower frequency-scaled prototype. As one can see, some attenuation is introduced by the transformer, as the result of the very weak magnetic coupling. Nevertheless, the signal delivered to the receiver still allows satisfactory power and data recovery.

2.4 Body Implantable Unit

The body implantable unit is shown in Figure 2.6 and includes the secondary RF unit. The power recovery circuit is comprised of a half-wave rectifier, protection circuits, and a series regulator. It recovers the required power from the received signal, with a power efficiency of about 30% for an intercoil distance of 1 cm.

The binary *FSK Demodulator* is based on a Phase Locked Loop (PLL) circuit and a comparator and provides a stream of Non-Return-to-Zero (NRZ) data. This bit stream is fed to the *Bit Synchronizer*, which provides a synchronized clock and retimed data to the *Data Processing and Control* unit. The *Data Processing* and *Control* unit performs bit and frame synchronization and frame disassembly. Finally, the formatted data is forwarded to the *Electrode Stimulator and Sensing* block.

The master clock recovery task is accomplished in the *Master Clock Recovery* block (see Figure 2.6), which is implemented by means of a narrow-band PLL designed to produce a 10 MHz reference clock from the received signal.

2.4.1 Bit Synchronizer

The signal received from the primary system is used to extract the system master clock, with frequency $f_{CLK} = \frac{1}{T_{CLK}} = N \times R_b$ where $R_b = \frac{1}{T_b} = 1$ Mbit/s is the raw bit-rate and $N = 10$ (corresponding to a RF carrier frequency of 10 MHz). Since the master clock is derived from the transmitted signal, it follows that the data stream is frequency synchronized (i.e., frequency-locked) with the master clock; a data clock could therefore be obtained by suitable division (by a factor N) of f_{CLK}. This is because there is no frequency offset between transmitter and receiver in this system. However, the (lead or lag) *phase difference* between the positive-going clock transitions and the optimum time epoch for sampling the data, which is the middle time of the data bit, is unknown and varies significantly. In fact, even small disturbances in the relative position of both coils lead to important phase offsets which have to be properly estimated and compensated by the bit synchronizer. The task performed by the bit synchronizer is thus of fundamental importance to establish a proper time reference in the receiver. The positive-going transitions in this reference clock should accurately signal the optimum instants to sample and detect the received data bits. The bit synchronizer and its interaction with the receiver is shown in Figure 2.9(a).

The bit synchronizer has a feed-forward structure that avoids the annoying loop behavior known as hang-up [36,37]. This phenomenon is typical in feedback synchronizer operation and manifests itself has an unacceptably long synchronizer acquisition period, compromising receiver operation. Suppose that we have a binary counter being driven with the master clock frequency f_{CLK}; then, it will advance N states within each bit period. If, at time t_0, the counter is in state i then, at time $t_0 + \frac{T_b}{2}$, it will have advanced $\frac{T_b}{2 \times T_{CLK}} = \frac{f_{CLK}}{2 \cdot R_b} = \frac{N}{2}$ and be in state $i + \frac{N}{2}$ (on average); this is the time epoch at which the recovered clock should have a positive transition, marking the middle of the data bit. This reasoning justifies the bit synchronizer block diagram represented in Figure 2.9(b): the positive-going transition on the raw, unsynchronized data signal latches the counter state i, at reference time t_0, and marks the start of a bit. When the counter reaches the state $S = i + \frac{N}{2}$, then $\left(S + \frac{N}{2}\right) \bmod N = (i + N) \bmod N = i$ and the comparator will signal this event to the final processing block, which in turn samples the raw data and produces a clock pulse synchronized with the master clock. Note that after a positive-going transition of the raw data, the synchronizer operates in a free-running fashion. The phase offset, which eventually accumulates after this event is corrected when the next positive-going transition occurs. Thus the raw data should not have long sequences of equal bits. This is guaranteed by the use of self-synchronizing scrambler and descrambler circuits. The developed bit synchronizer has the following desirable properties, namely (1) due to

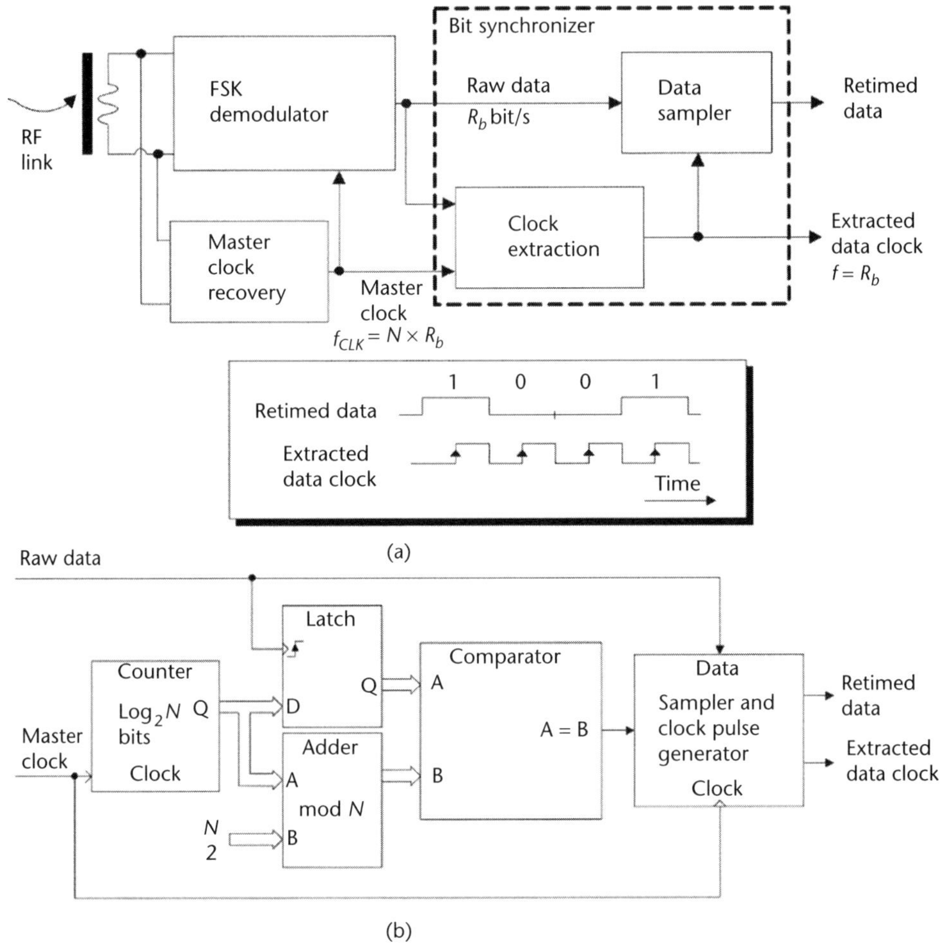

Figure 2.9 Bit synchronizer: (a) data clock recovery and clock extraction; (b) block diagram of the developed feed-forward bit synchronizer. From [37] with permission, © IEEE 2005.

the absence of frequency offset between transmitter and receiver the recovered clock is *jitter-free* (no dynamic phase error), (2) avoids the hang-up phenomenon, and (3) is easily implemented with very simple digital logic.

2.4.2 Reverse Link

A reverse link is used for monitoring tasks, electrode calibration, and voltage measurement. It is established from the secondary to the primary system at a lower data rate of 156.25 kbps, using BPSK modulation. This modulation was chosen because the transmitter is very simple and requires very low power. The operation of this reverse link is in half-duplex mode, i.e., while data is being sent on this link to the external body unit, no useful data is transmitted in the forward link (to the implantable body unit). However, to keep the implantable body unit conveniently powered, the exterior unit continually transmits an unmodulated carrier (at 10 MHz). As mentioned before, in the external unit, the BPSK data is recovered by means of a

Costas-Loop demodulator, which performs satisfactorily with intercoil distances up to 2 cm.

2.4.3 Communication Protocol

A data protocol, developed specifically for this system, is used in both forward and backward communication links. Three operation modes are specified for the forward transmission. In the *normal mode*, the RF link is used to transmit spike information to the *Electrodes Stimulator and Sensing* block, and each data field contains the address of the electrode to be stimulated. In the other operation modes one can read from or write to the internal registers, for controlling the amplitude and duration of the electrical pulses. In the write operation mode two pairs of data are sent: the address of the register being configured and the new value to be written. The read operation is needed to measure the impedance of the microelectrodes (through the developed voltage and known drive current), in order to evaluate the microelectrode-cortex interface.

The protocol was implemented using four blocks, a transmitter and a receiver, for both exterior and implantable body units. The transmitters, or data packagers, are built around a 13-bit shift register with parallel load and serial output. The output is scrambled and sent to the RF link. On the other side, data unpackagers for the receivers were also designed.

2.5 System Prototype

A prosthesis demonstrator was built around a motorized human model head named Elonica; see Figure 2.10.

Figure 2.10(a)–(d) shows photographs of the VGA monitor on an experimental test of the *Neuromorphic Pulse Coding* block and *Serialization and Data Packing* module. Elonica is controlled by a PC through a VGA touch screen monitor driven by a Web multimedia application. The idea is to remotely control Elonica in order to look for different target objects to illustrate the visual effects of each artificial retina processing phase. The artificial retina and prosthesis low-power circuitry is power fed by a solar cell "graduation hat" illuminated by an artificial sun that recharges two lithium ion batteries placed under the hat top.

A CMOS XVGA (1280 × 1024 pixel) digital color microcamera placed behind Elonica glasses is connected to the retina processor by a flat cable digital bus placed within a tissue strap.

The designed artificial retina processing board is based on a XILINX SPARTAN XC3S400 FPGA [38]. The retina processor (depicted in Figure 2.11(a)) controls the microcamera, through the *Register Configuration* module, decimates the input image and generates four images (32 × 32 pixel): (i) low pass filtered and decimated original color image (Figure 2.10(a)) in *Image Capture and Resize* module, (ii) retina processed black and white spatial image (Figure 2.10(b)), (iii) retina time filtered image (Figure 2.10(c)) used to generate retina spikes using a neuromorphic integrate-and-fire spiking neuron model in *Neuromorphic Encoder*, and (iv) recovered black and white image (Figure 2.10(d)) obtained by onboard decoding of the generated

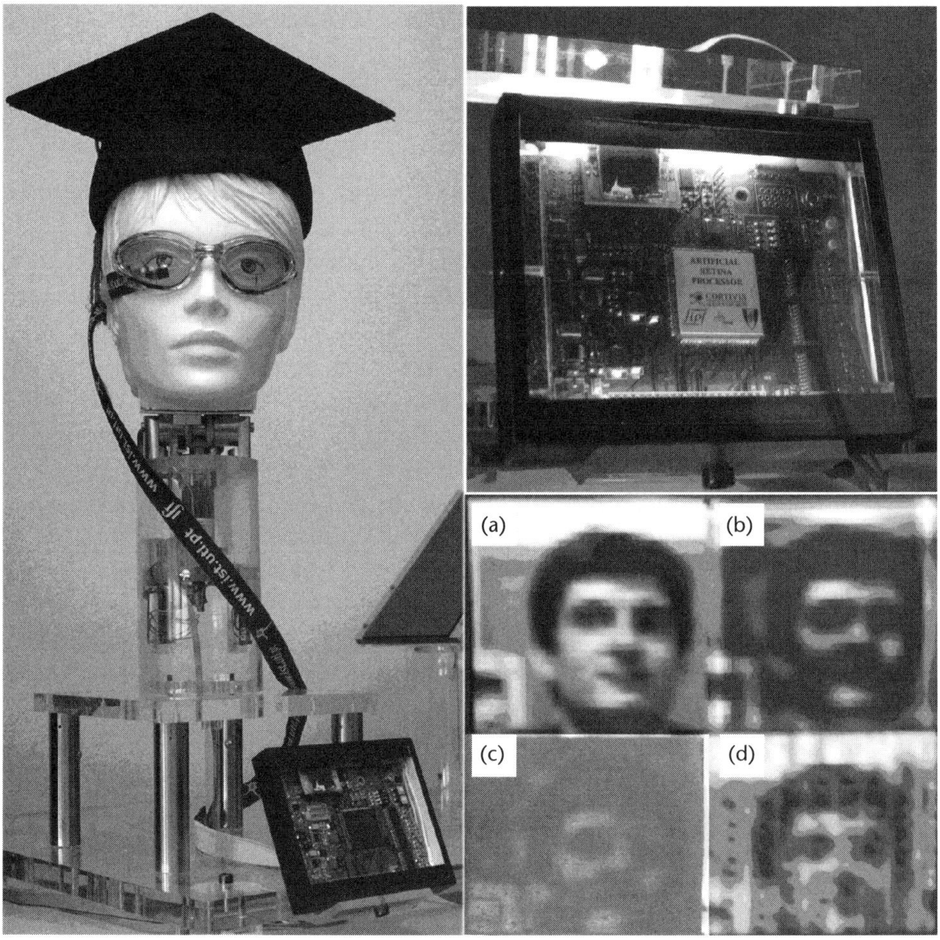

Figure 2.10 Elonica (left), retina processor (upper right) and VGA monitor output (lower right): (a) decimated original image; (b) spatial filtered image; (c) time filtered image; (d) recovered image from spike coded image.

spikes. These four images are composed by the *Image Display* module in a full-frame VGA compatible image that is fed to a standard VGA LCD monitor. The retina processor also includes the *Serialization and Data Packing* module that corresponds to the forward transmitter data packager, as described in Section 2.4.3.

The artificial retina blocks were described in VHDL and, by using the XILINX WEBPACK 6.2 tool, synthesized and mapped to the chosen XC3S400 FPGA. The resource occupancy of the FPGA for the implemented modules is shown in Figure 2.11(b). As can be seen, the complete system was able to be mapped in the chosen FPGA using only 26% of the total resources, operating at a maximum frequency of 85 MHz and consumes ≈500 mW at 5 V. This largely exceeds the required ≈1.5 MHz for the implementation of the *Early Layers* block (processing of an image of size 32 × 32 at a rate of 30 fps executing 49 operations per cycle due to hardware folding) and ≈1 MHz for the *Neuromorphic Pulse Coding* block (generation of spikes at a maximum rate of 100 Hz to an equivalent microelectrode array of size 32 × 32).

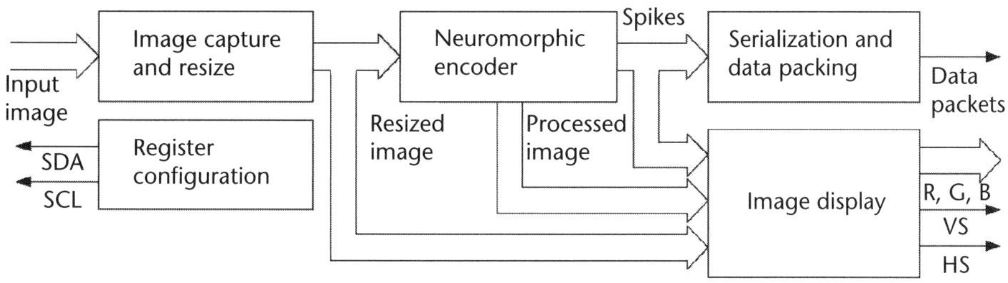

(a)

Modules	Slice Occupation		RAM blocks	Mult.
Total available resources	3584	100%	16	16
Image Capture and Resize	108	3%	0	2
Register Configuration	142	4%	0	0
Classic Model	420	12%	5	3
Serialization and Data Packing	60	2%	2	0
Image Display	218	6%	8	9
Complete System	948	26%	15	12

(b)

Figure 2.11 Retina processor: (a) block diagram; (b) table of FPGA resources used. From [37] with permission, © IEEE 2005.

In order to study the important magnetic coupling issues through the cranium wall, an RF link board level prototype was implemented [37]. This prototype is a ten times down frequency scaled version of the system, operating with a forward data rate 100 kpbs and carrier frequency 1 MHz and with backward data rate 15.625 kbps with carrier frequency 500 kHz. The maximum power output capability, see Figure 2.12, occurs for intercoil distances below 1 cm (this is the target distance for which the RF transformer design was optimized). For a primary RF unit power consumption of 180 mW (from a 9 V power supply) it was possible to obtain 50 mW of power at the secondary receiver output, which leads to an efficiency of about 28% for intercoil distances up to 1 cm. Note that, to avoid cortex heating effects, the maximum power consumption of VLSI circuits in the secondary system is limited to 100 mW.

Figure 2.13(a) illustrates the variation of the frequency response of the transformer with respect to the distance between the primary and secondary coils. The transformer pass band is centered at 1 MHz, as desired and has always enough bandwidth BW (greater than 200 kHz) for the transmitted data. Besides the significant attenuation introduced by the transformer resulting from its very weak magnetic coupling [37], the signal delivered to the receiver still allows satisfactory power and data recovery. The overall transmitted and received data are illustrated in Figure 2.13(b) (the bit rate is 100 kpbs and the intercoil distance is 1 cm). As one can see from this figure, scrambled data is properly recovered at the receiver after crossing all the RF link: primary modulator, RF transformer, and FSK secondary demodulator. In this experiment, 50 mW of a 3.3 V DC power supply are being extracted by the secondary power recovering circuitry, simultaneously with the secondary data demodulation. The oscilloscope traces correspond to the data from the NPC (top) and the recovered data in the secondary unit (bottom), respectively.

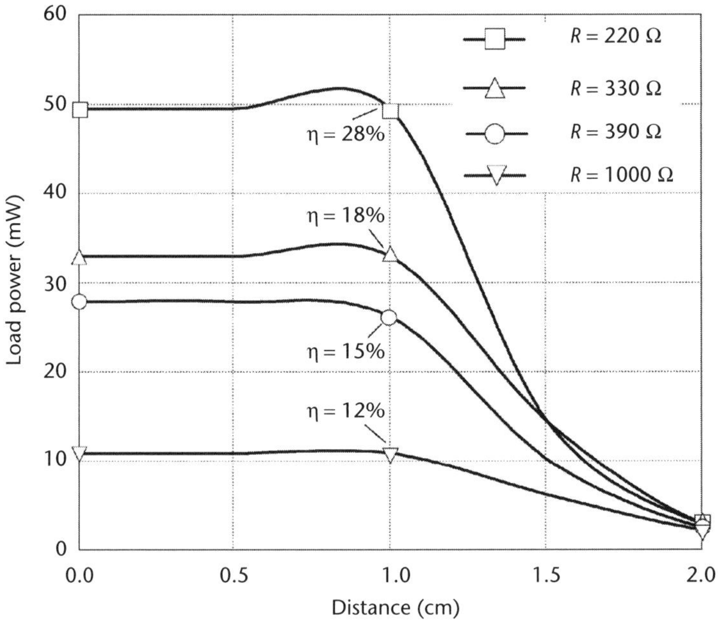

Figure 2.12 Power and efficiency variation with the coil distance and load resistor. From [37] with permission, © IEEE 2005.

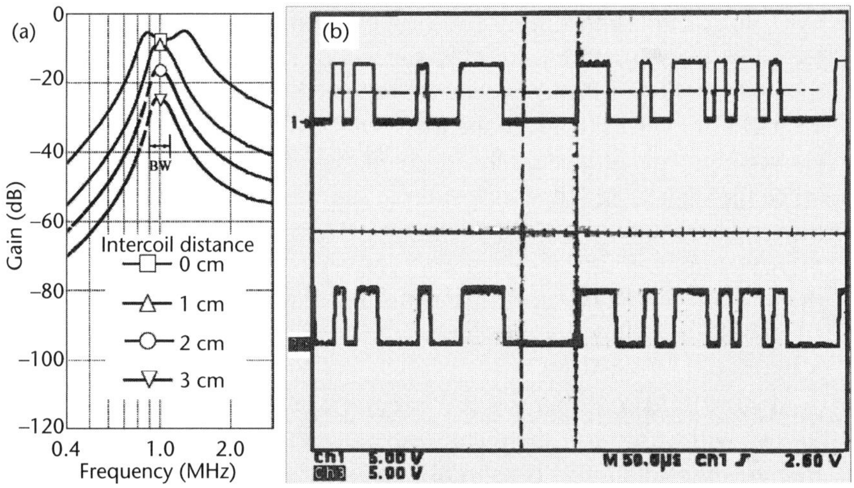

Figure 2.13 RF link : (a) frequency response; (b) FSK demodulator operation: transmitted NRZ data (top) and recovered data (bottom). From [37] with permission, © IEEE 2005.

2.6 Conclusions

This chapter proposes an architecture for a visual neuroprosthesis and demonstrates its feasibility using nowadays technology. The primary goal of this system is to restore a limited but useful visual sense to profoundly blind people. This neuroprosthesis is based on a *Neuromorphic Encoder* and a non-invasive system for intracortical stimuli of the visual cortex. The developed *Neuromorphic Encoder* receives the visual stimulus from a miniature digital video camera, performs the spatial and temporal processing corresponding to the early layers of the retina and implements a simplified version of an integrate-and-fire spiking neuron to model the spike generation.

To achieve a non-invasive system for intracortical stimulation, a bidirectional RF link was designed. The system uses FSK modulation in the forward link and BPSK modulation in the backward link. These modulation formats were chosen since, due to their constant-amplitude characteristic, they can offer significant robustness against the severe amplitude variations which are expected in this system. Because of its high efficiency, a class E tuned power amplifier was chosen to transmit at 1 Mbps over a 10 MHz carrier.

The Neuromorphic Encoder, which generates the spikes delivered to the RF link, was implemented in a video processing board based on a XILINX Spartan XC3S400 FPGA. The encoder occupies about 26% of the FPGA resources, exhibiting a power consumption of about 500 mW for a clock frequency of 50 MHz.

A frequency scaled prototype was also built in order to test the performance of the data and power communication system. The transmitted signal also carries the power for the secondary unit (≈50 mW) with an average efficiency of 28% for 1 cm intercoil distance. The system operates very well with power, data, and clock recovery for distances up to 2 cm.

Based on the developed prototype, a complete system is now being designed in ASIC technology. The *Neuromorphic Encoder* is being synthesized using the UMC 0.13 μm CMOS technology process. For the *Wireless Communication Link* and the *Electrode Stimulators and Sensing* modules, a 0.35 μm AMS CMOS technology is required to allow for the high voltage levels being used. The work presented here contains several significant innovations, namely: (1) it is the first known complete architecture designed and implemented of the intracortical visual neuroprosthesis; (2) a new full-directional RF link carrying data and power was proposed with significant contributions, namely: a new feed-forward bit synchronizer and a new communication protocol appropriated for cortical prosthesis; and (3) a new video neuromorphic encoder system. It is expected that these innovations contribute to help the development of future practical and compact visual prosthesis.

Acknowledgments

This work was partially supported by the Portuguese Foundation for Science and Technology (FCT) through the FEDER program.

References

[1] M. R. Shah, R. P. Phillips, and R. A. Normann, "A transcutaneous power and data link for neuroprosthetic applications," *Paper presented at the annual meeting of the IEEE-EMBS*, pp. 1357–1358, 1993.

[2] T. Cameron, G. Loeb, R. Peck, J. Schulman, P. Strojnik, and P. Troyk, "Micromodular implants to provide electrical stimulations of paralyzed muscles and limbs," *IEEE Transactions on Biomedic Engineering*, vol. 44, no. 9, pp. 781–790, 1997.

[3] B. Smith, Z. Tang, M. Johnson, S. Pourmehdi, M. Gazdik, J. Buckett, and P. Peckham, "An externally powered, multichannel, implantable stimulator-telemeter for control of paralyzed muscle," *IEEE Transactions on Biomedic Engineering*, vol. 45, no. 4, pp. 463–475, 1998.

[4] Q. Bai and K.D.Wise, "Single-unit neural recording with active microelectrode arrays," *IEEE Transactions on Biomedic Engineering*, vol. 48, pp. 911–920, August 2001.

[5] R. A. Andersen and C. A. Buneo, "Intention maps in posterior parietal cortex," *Annual Revision of Neuroscience*, vol. 25, pp. 189–220, 2002.

[6] W. H. Dobelle, "Artificial vision for the blind by connecting a television camera to the brain," *American Society for Artificial Internal Organs (ASAIO) Journal*, no. 46, pp. 3–9, 2000.

[7] W. Liu, E. McGucken, K. Vitchiechom, and M. Clements, "Dual unit visual intraocular prosthesis," *Proc. of the 19th International Conference on IEEE-EMBS*, pp. 2303–2306, 1997.

[8] T. Stieglitz, H. Beutel, R. Keller, C. Blau, and J.-U. Meyer, "Development of flexible stimulation devices for a retina implant system," *Proc. of the 19th International Conference on IEEE-EMBS*, pp. 2307–2310, 1997.

[9] W. Dobelle, J. L. Antunes, D. Coiteiro, and J. Girvin, "The first artificial vision system in commercial distribution," http://www.dobelle.com/news.html.

[10] G. A. Kendir, W. Liu, R. Bashirullah, G. Wang, M. Humayun, and J. Weiland, "An efficient inductive power link design for retinal prosthesis," *Proc. of the IEEE International Symposium on Circuits and Systems IEEE ISCAS'04*, pp. 41–44, 2004.

[11] M. Mojarradi, D. Binkley, B. Blalock, R. Andersen, N. Ulshoefer, T. Johnson, and L. D. Castillo, "A miniaturized neuroprosthesis suitable for implantation into the brain," *IEEE Transactions on Neural Systems and Rehabilitation Engineering*, vol. 11, no. 1, pp. 38–42, March 2003.

[12] Cochlear hearing implants, http://www.cochlear.com/.

[13] E. Zrenner, A. Stett, S. Weiss, R. Aramant, E. Guenther, K. Kohler, K. Miliczek, M. Seiler, and H. Haemmerle, "Can subretinal microphotodiodes successfully replace degenerated photoreceptors?" *Vision Research*, vol. 39, no. 15, pp. 2555–2567, 1999.

[14] R. Eckmiller, "Learning retina implants with epiretinal contacts," *Ophthalmic Research*, vol. 29, no. 5, pp. 281–289, 1997.

[15] J. Eggermont, "Is there a neural code?" *Neuroscience & Biobehavioral Reviews*, vol. 22, no. 2, pp. 355–370, 1998.

[16] G. Brindley, "Effects of electrical stimulation of the visual cortex," *Human Neurobiology*, vol. 1, no. 4, pp. 281–283, 1982.

[17] W. Dobelle and M. Mladejovsky, "Phosphenes produced by electrical stimulation of human occipital cortex, and their application to the development of a prosthesis for the blind," *The Journal of Physiology*, vol. 243, no. 2, pp. 553–576, 1974.

[18] European Project "Cortical visual neuroprosthesis for the blind (CORTIVIS)," RTD programme "Quality of life and management of living resources," QLK6-CT-2001-00279. http://cortivis.umh.es.

[19] National Project "Intracortical neuronal stimulator (ICONS)," FCT Project PTDC/EEA-ELC/68972/2006 and National Project "Retina Neural Code: Accurate Modeling Towards and Artificial Visual System (RNC)," FCT Project POSI/EEA-CPS/61779/2004. http://sips.inesc-id.pt/projects.php.

[20] J. Keat, P. Reinagel, R. C. Reid, and M. Meister, "Predicting every spike: a model for the responses of visual neurons," *Neuron*, vol. 30, pp. 803–817, June 2001.

[21] M. Merry and M. Meister, "Refractoriness and neural precision," *The Journal of Neuroscience*, vol. 18, no. 6, pp. 2200–2211, March 1998.

[22] J. Martins and L. Sousa, "Performance comparison of computational retina models," *Proc. of the 5th IASTED International Conference on Visualization, Imaging and Image Processing*, Benidorm, Spain, September 2005.

[23] J. G. Proakis, *Digital Communications*, McGraw-Hill, 1983.

[24] W. Liu, K. Vichienchom, M. Clements, S. DeMarco, C. Hughes, E. McGucken, M. Humayun, E. D. Juan, J. Weiland, and R. Greenberg, "A neuro-stimulus chip with telemetry unit for retinal prosthetic device," *IEEE Journal of Solid-State Circuits*, vol. 35, pp. 1487–1497, October 2000.

[25] A. Abrial, J. Bouvier, M. Renaudin, P. Senn, and P. Vivet, "A new contactless smart card IC using an on-chip antenna and an asynchronous microcontroller," *IEEE Journal of Solid-State Circuits*, vol. 36, pp. 1101–1107, July 2001.

[26] Q. Huang and M. Oberle, "A 0.5-mW passive telemetry IC for biomedical applications," *IEEE Journal of Solid-State Circuits*, vol. 33, no. 7, pp. 937–946, July 1998.

[27] K. N. M. Ghovanloo, "A wideband frequency-shift keying wireless link for inductively powered biomedical implants," *IEEE Transactions on Circuits and Systems—I: Regular Papers*, vol. 52, no. 12, pp. 2374–2383, December 2004.

[28] M. Sawan, Y. Hu, and J. Coulombe, "Wireless smart implants dedicated to multichannel monitoring and microstimulation," *IEEE Circuits and Systems Magazine*, vol. 5, no. 1, pp. 21–39, first quarter 2005.

[29] W. Gerstner and W. Kistler, *Spiking Neuron Models*. Cambridge University Press, 2002.

[30] M. Santos, J. Fernandes, and M. Piedade, "A microelectrode stimulation system for a cortical neuroprosthesis," *Proc. of Conference Design of Circuits and Integrated Systems (DCIS'06)*, November 2006.

[31] P. Malisse, *UMC L130E FSG-HS 1P8M logic process with VST libraries*, Europractice IC Service, December 2003.

[32] L. J. and W. J., "A multi-sender asynchronous extension to the address event protocol," in *Proc. of 16th Conference on Advanced Research in VLSI*, pp. 158–169, 1995.

[33] S. D. Wilke, A. Thiel, C. W. Eurich, M. Greschner, M. Bongard, J. Ammermüller, and H. Schwegler, "Population coding of motion patterns in the early visual system," *Journal of Comparative Physiology A*, vol. 187, no. 7, pp. 549–558, March 2001.

[34] N. O. Sokal and A. D. Sokal, "Class E—A new class of high-efficiency tuned single-ended switching power amplifiers," *IEEE Journal of Solid-State Circuits*, vol. 10, pp. 168–176, June 1975.

[35] J. Gerald, G. Tavares, M. Piedade, E. Varela, and R. Ribeiro, "RF-link for cortical neuroprosthesis," *Proc. of IEEE International Symposium on Circuits and Systems, IEEE ISCAS'05*, Kobe, Japan, May 2005.

[36] J. Gerald, G. Tavares, M. Piedade, and E. Varela, "Wireless transmission of power and data to implants," *Proc. of the 5th Conference on Telecommunications, CONFTELE'05*, Tomar, Portugal, April 2005.

[37] M. Piedade, J. Gerald, L. Sousa, G. Tavares, and P. Tomás, "Visual neuroprosthesis: a non-invasive system for stimulating the cortex," *IEEE Transactions on Circuits and Systems I—Regular papers, IEEE*, vol. 6, no. 12, pp. 2648–2662, December 2005.

[38] Xilinx, "Spartan-3 FPGA family: complete data sheet," http://direct.xilinx.com/bvdocs/publications/ds099.pdf.

CHAPTER 3

CMOS Circuits for Biomedical Implantable Devices

Mohamad Sawan and Benoit Gosselin

3.1. Introduction

With the rapid development of biomedical circuits and systems during the last few years, high-performance implantable medical devices (sensors and neuromuscular stimulators) play a more and more important role in modern medicine. Implanted sensors and actuators are most often in contact with sensitive organs such as the heart, arteries, nerves, or the brain, and therefore must rigorously address requirements and design parameters for safety. At present, manifold engineering efforts are deployed to increase the reliability of these devices for everyday utilization by patients.

The purpose of transcutaneous energy transfer is to provide a safe and effective method for the remote delivery of energy to implanted biomedical devices. In general, such wireless power supplies are based on a modulated carrier that is rectified to transcutaneously power the implant. This technology allows patient mobility, improves quality of life, and reduces risk of infection compared to percutaneous wires. Electromagnetic radio-frequency (RF) inductively coupled link is a commonly used technique to deliver power to implanted prosthetics. Adequate power transfer leaves skin intact; however, high power consumption increases a tissue's temperature because of heat dissipation and implies higher electromagnetic field density through tissues when powering the devices. These drawbacks can arm biological tissues, thus the external part of such a link must transmit power to the implanted part at field levels below government safety standards (10 mW/cm^2) [1]. At present, inductively coupled link technique is certainly the most desirable method for patients, because of its safety, and high power transfer efficiency. However, it still lacks some characteristics such as wide bandwidth, and better tolerance to displacement.

Meanwhile, such a link is also employed as a media to transmit data between the external controller and the implanted unit. This chapter will describe a typical biotelemetry link, which consists of two coils, one implanted in the human body and another one being put close but outside the body. The link is intended to power up the receiver, and bidirectionally transmit data at various speeds, within various modulation/demodulation schemes. Among other building blocks, binary and quadrature phase-shift-keying (BPSK) demodulators based on a hard-limited Costas loop topology will be presented. Regarding the power transfer, circuit topologies will be considered and discussed to achieve high-power efficiency. In most cases, the primary circuit of the link is a tuned-in series to provide a low-impedance load to the driving transmitter, whereas the secondary is almost invariably a parallel LC circuit that drives a nonlinear rectifier load.

Modern implanted circuits and systems must make appropriate use of the supplied energy and available bandwidth by means of dedicated techniques. A case study related to inductively powered brain interfacing circuits will be discussed. Integrated devices that present increasing densities are necessary for tackling the central nervous system and gather invaluable information about neurodynamics. In such devices, design trade-offs must be made for a safe usage and continuous operation. The proposed case study will illustrate these trade-offs and address them with power-aware circuit techniques.

On the other hand, neural recording sensors generate huge data rates, and present telemetry links are merely able to transmit 10 % of the recorded raw data for 100 channels. Therefore, a mechanism for data reduction must be provided within such applications to overcome bandwidth limitations. Techniques using integrated signal processing circuits for real-time data compression can increase the link capacity by several orders of magnitude. Such methods work side by side with an efficient telemetry system. Details and comparison regarding low-power CMOS circuits intended for such a purpose will be given. In addition, challenges in terms of power consumption and silicon area will be addressed.

This chapter is organized as follows: We first introduce the characteristics of the required inductive link. Then, Section 3.2 describes the background theory and design principles that allow high-energy transfer to an implant. Section 3.3 presents efficient communication systems for high data rate over such a link. Section 3.4 proposes a case study illustrating the design of implanted circuits and systems to be powered by the presented inductive link. Section 3.4.1 describes the implementation of low-power, low-noise bioamplifiers dedicated to massive integration in biomedical devices. Section 3.4.2 introduces low-power analog circuits and digital building blocks to perform real-time data compression in implants. Finally, a summary of the chapter and conclusions are given in Section 3.5.

3.2 Inductive Link to Deliver Power to Implants

Figure 3.1 depicts a block diagram of a typical system dedicated to power implanted electronic devices using an inductive link. A power amplifier drives an external coil in the RF transmitter (the primary). The implanted coil (the secondary) receives the necessary energy through inductive coupling. A voltage rectifier and a voltage regulator follow for delivering an adequate dc supply voltage to the implanted circuits. The ac voltage induced at the secondary should be high in order to allow the voltage rectifier and voltage regulator blocks to extract the expected dc voltage as well as the energy to power on the whole implant. The most important characteristics to be considered when designing inductively coupled link to transfer energy are the ratio of the output voltage to the input voltage, the power efficiency, the bandwidth, the external power amplifier characteristics, and the load of the implant.

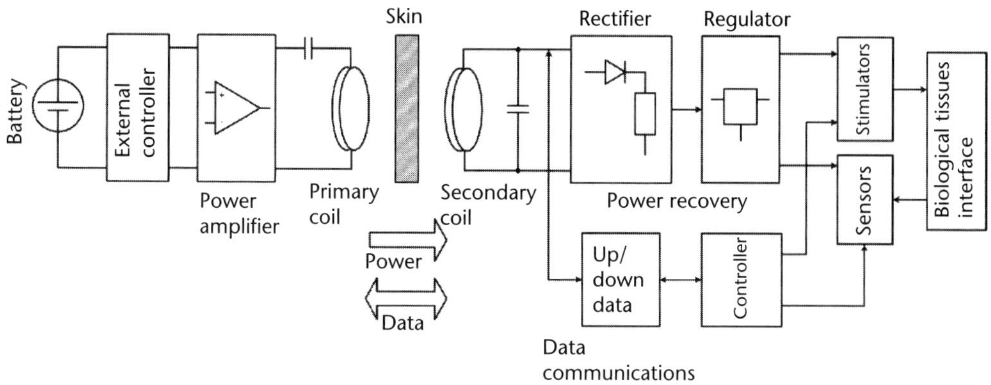

Figure 3.1 Inductive link to transmit power/data to an implant.

3.2.1 Inductive Link Fundamentals

A typical inductive link is composed of two resonant circuits, a primary circuit (R_p, C_p, L_p) and a secondary one (R_s, C_s, L_s). A model of the loaded inductively coupled link is shown in Figure 3.2. The resistor R_p includes the series resistance of the primary inductor and the source resistor, which depends on the power amplifier output. R_L is the ac series resistor equivalent to the load resistance of the implanted circuits, noted R_{ac}. R_{ac} dissipates an ac power equivalent to the dc power dissipated in a parallel resistor R_{dc}, thus $R_{ac} = R_{dc}/2$. R_{ac} is replaced by its series equivalent for convenience, thus at resonance frequency, $R_L = (\omega L_s)^2/R_{ac}$. The transfer function of the link is obtained from the following network equations:

$$V_{in} = \left[R_p + j\left(\omega L_p - \frac{1}{\omega C_p} \right) \right] I_p + j\omega M I_s \tag{3.1a}$$

$$0 = j\omega M I_p + \left[R_s + R_L + j\left(\omega L_s - \frac{1}{\omega C_s} \right) \right] I_s \tag{3.1b}$$

where the mutual inductance between L_p and L_s is defined as

$$M = k\sqrt{L_p L_s} \tag{3.2}$$

and k is the coupling coefficient. The primary and secondary circuits are assumed to be tuned to the same resonant frequency ω_o, so that

$$\omega_o = \frac{1}{\sqrt{L_p C_p}} = \frac{1}{\sqrt{L_s C_s}} \tag{3.3}$$

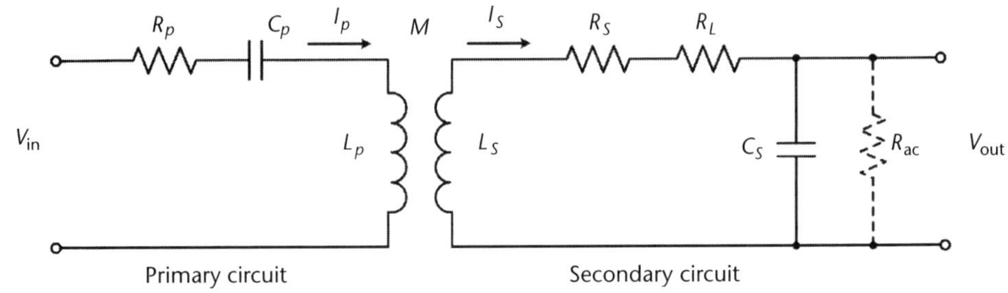

Figure 3.2 Model of the simplified loaded inductive link.

The transfer function of the link is obtained from (3.1a) and (3.1b)

$$\frac{V_{out}}{V_{in}} = -\frac{\omega^2}{\omega_o^2}\frac{k\sqrt{L_s / L_p}}{\left[k^2 + \frac{1}{Q_pQ_s} - \left(1 - \frac{\omega^2}{\omega_o^2}\right) + j\left(1 - \frac{\omega^2}{\omega_o^2}\right)\left(\frac{1}{Q_p} + \frac{1}{Q_s}\right)\right]} \tag{3.4}$$

where $Q_p = \omega L_p/R_p$, and $Q_s = \omega L_s/(R_s+R_L)$ are the quality factors of L_p and L_s respectively, and ω is the operating frequency. The maximum ratio V_{in}/V_{out} is reached when k is equal to the critical coupling coefficient k_c, which is given by

$$k_c = \frac{1}{\sqrt{Q_pQ_s}} \tag{3.5}$$

3.2.2 The Power Efficiency

The power efficiency of the link can be determined considering the fact that the reflected impedance from the secondary (receiving coil) to the primary coil adds in series with the primary circuit. At resonance, and at critical coupling coefficient, the reflected impedance is purely resistive, and the corresponding dissipated power in the primary circuit is obtained from

$$P_{in} = \frac{V_{in}^2}{R_p + (\omega M)^2 / (R_s + R_L)} \tag{3.6}$$

Also, for these same conditions ($\omega = \omega_o$ and $k = k_c$), the secondary current is maximal, and the maximal voltage ratio V_{out}/V_{in} can be obtained from

$$\left(\frac{V_{out}}{V_{in}}\right)_{\max} = \frac{1}{2k_c}\sqrt{\frac{L_s}{L_p}} = \frac{1}{2}\sqrt{Q_pQ_s}\sqrt{\frac{L_s}{L_p}} \tag{3.7}$$

Then, using the fact that the power transferred to the secondary is equivalent to the same amount of power delivered to the reflected impedance, the power efficiency η_{link} of the inductive link is expressed as [1]

$$\eta_{link} = \frac{(\omega M)^2 / (R_s + R_L)}{R_p + (\omega M)^2 / (R_s + R_L)} \cdot \frac{R_L}{R_s + R_L} \tag{3.8}$$

Then, we can show that the link behaves as a narrow-band bandpass filter due to relatively high Q factors in the resonant circuitries often using off-chip coils. The bandwidth of the tuned inductively coupled link can be derived from (3.4). At critical coupling factor, and assuming identical quality factors for coils ($Q_p = Q_s = Q$), the bandwidth of the link can be estimated with [2]

$$\Delta f = \frac{\omega_o}{2\pi \cdot Q}\sqrt{2} \tag{3.9}$$

Besides, the coupling coefficient k depends on the mutual inductance M, and inductors L_p and L_s. Low k (< 0.1) are typically achieved because the primary and secondary coils are usually small, and because they are separated by a skin layer of a few centimeters. Since L_p and L_s are small in general, they can be obtained with coils of only a few metal loops. Therefore, they can be approximated by two aligned one-turn circular loops of specific radi, separated with distance d. An expression for the mutual inductance as a function of d is easily obtained using Neuman formula [3]. Thus, changing the distance between the coils has a direct impact on the mutual inductance, the coupling factor, and the transmitted power. Lateral and angular displacements also affect the inductively coupled link. A discussion and approximation formulas for the mutual inductance in the presence of lateral or angular misalignments can be found in [4, 5].

A class E power amplifier is recommended for high-power transfer efficiency to the primary. Such amplifier theoretical efficiency reaches 100%. A class E amplifier uses a shunt inductor, a capacitor, and only one power transistor, followed by the series resonant circuit of the link primary [6, 7]. The power transistor acts as a low-loss switch whose switching frequency is tuned close to the resonant frequency of the link primary circuit. This results in a sinusoidal output waveform.

For instance, a typical application would use a f_{carrier} = 13.56 MHz carrier frequency in the regulated industrial, scientific, and medical (ISM) applications frequency band. The primary and the secondary circuits of such a link are tuned to $\omega_o = 2\pi f_{\text{carrier}}$. The link parameters arc R_p = 3 Ω, R_s = 10 Ω, k = 0.07, Q_p = 100, and Q_s = 20. Also, the implantable part typically drains 5.0 mA from a 1.8 V power supply, which results in a load resistor R_{dc} of 360 Ω. Assuming that a class E power amplifier with 100% efficiency, and a voltage supply of 5 V are used at the primary, we can evaluate, P_{in}, $V_{\text{out}}/V_{\text{in}}$ (max), η_{link}, and $\Delta\omega$. First, the coupling factor k, and inductors L_s, and L_p are evaluated:

$$L_p = \frac{100 \cdot 3\Omega}{2\pi \cdot 13.56MHz} = 3.52\mu H \text{ and } L_s = \frac{20 \cdot 10\Omega}{2\pi \cdot 13.56MHz} = 2.35\mu H$$

Then, the critical coupling factor and the mutual inductance are

$$k_c = \frac{1}{\sqrt{100 \cdot 20\Omega}} = 0.0224 \text{ and } M = 0.07\sqrt{3.52\mu H \cdot 2.35\mu H} = 0.20\mu H$$

From (3.7), the maximum ratio V_{out}/V_{in} is

$$\left(\frac{V_{out}}{V_{in}}\right)_{\max} = \frac{1}{2 \cdot 0.0224}\sqrt{\frac{3.52\mu H}{2.35\mu H}} = 18.3$$

So, using (3.6) the power available at the primary is

$$P_{in} = \frac{(5V)^2}{3\Omega + (13.56MHz \cdot 0.20\mu H)^2 / (10\Omega + 222\Omega)} = 5.86\ W$$

The value of the equivalent ac load series resistor is $R_L = (2\pi \cdot 13.56\ MHz \cdot 3.52\ \mu H)^2/180\ \Omega = 222\ \Omega$, and we can then obtain the efficiency of the link from (3.8):

$$\eta_{link} = \frac{(13.56MHz \cdot 0.20\mu H)^2 / (10\Omega + 222\Omega)}{3\Omega + (13.56MHz \cdot 0.20\mu H)^2 / (10\Omega + 222\Omega)} \cdot \frac{222\Omega}{10\Omega + 222\Omega} = 0.28$$

and the bandwidth using (3.9):

$$\Delta f = \frac{13.56MHZ}{1/k_c^2}\sqrt{2} = 60.4\ kHz$$

Figure 3.3 shows the efficiency of such a link according to the current drained by the implanted part. The implanted circuits are assumed to be powered by a 1.8 V voltage supply.

3.2.3 Power Recovery and Voltage Regulation

Then, the carrier recovered at the secondary is rectified and regulated in order to power up the implant with a stable dc voltage. These steps affect the overall power efficiency of the inductive link. For instance, the voltage regulator power efficiency is calculated as

$$\eta_{reg} = \frac{I_L V_{in\_reg}}{(I_q + I_L)} \approx \frac{V_{in\_reg}}{V_{out\_reg}} \tag{3.10}$$

where, I_q is the quiescent current drained by the regulator, and I_L is the load current. Since I_q is usually much less than I_L, the efficiency η_{reg} mostly relies on the dropout

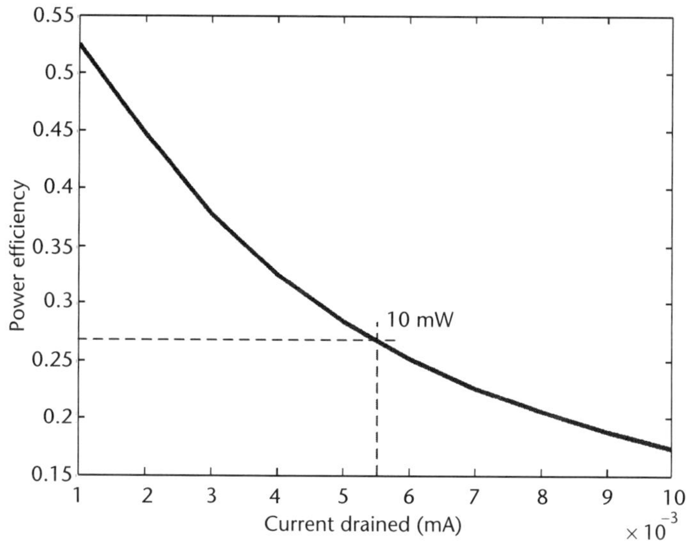

Figure 3.3 Efficiency of the link according to the current drained by the implanted circuits. A 1.8 V voltage supply is assumed in the implanted part.

voltage (V_{in_reg}–V_{out_reg}). This entails needs for low dropout voltage in the regulator. A low dropout (LDO) linear regulator is depicted in Figure 3.4 [8]. It generates two supply voltage levels. A high-level voltage (V_H) is provided for higher-voltage applications, such as stimulators, and a lower one (V_L) supplies other circuitry, such as low-power sensors. Such a regulator employs a pass transistor (NM_1) to isolate the input and output voltages, and an error amplifier with resistive feedback to correct the difference between the input and output voltages. Regulators using n-type pass devices are often preferred because they show fewer stability problems, better regulation, and lower Ohmic output impedance than their p-type counterparts. However, conventional n-type regulators suffer from higher dropout voltage because a higher gate-to-source voltage is required in the pass device. This problem can be alleviated by using a native transistor (NM_1 in Figure 3.4), for which the threshold voltage (V_{th}) adjustment step is omitted in the fabrication process. These transistors, available in most modern processes, have a much lower V_{th} than regular devices. By contrast, a regular transistor can be used at the second stage of the dual output regulator since the high-regulated voltage V_H provides sufficient voltage swing at the output of the feedback amplifier.

Besides, better power efficiency, larger bandwidth, and tolerance to coils displacement are among the remaining design challenges for the implementation of better inductively coupled links. At present, it is possible, with the presented circuits, to build a wireless power supply delivering one mA to the implant with an efficiency above 50%, which is sufficient for several biomedical applications.

3.3 High Data Rate Transmission Through Inductive Links

In addition to transmitting the needed energy to power up the implantable part, the inductive link is used to bidirectionally transmit the data at different rates and in

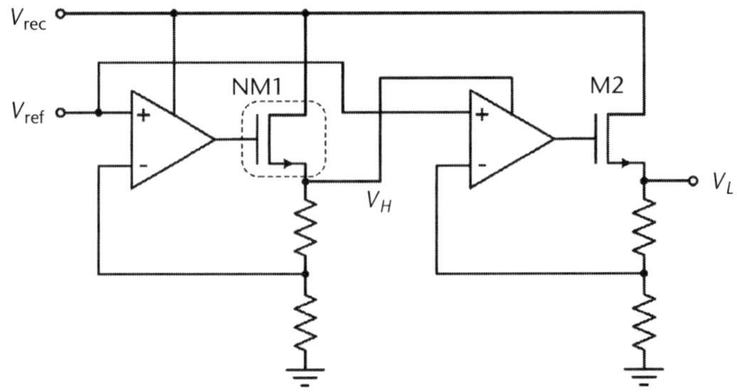

Figure 3.4 Dual output LDO regulator using a native transistor NM_1 with a reduced V_{th}. The first stage is supplied by the rectified voltage (V_{rec}), whereas the second stage is supplied by V_H, the regulated output voltage taken from the first stage.

various modulation formats. In order to improve the data transmission rate, we proposed recently two types of bidirectional data communication systems. The first one, the digital demodulator [2], is used to recuperate ASK modulated data instead of the conventional Manchester decoder. The second technique, the binary phase shift keying (BPSK) demodulator, is employed to retrieve the modulated data [9]. These two techniques are employed to downlink the data to the implant. Also, load shift keying (LSK) modulation is used as uplink data transmission. The later technique is based on the property of inductive coupling in which the impedance of the primary coil reflects the effective secondary load [10]. Such a scheme does not need a carrier signal, and its circuitry does not include a power amplifier. The design details regarding these two transmission methods can be found in our previous work [2].

Table 3.1 summarizes the main modulation methods used in wireless implantable systems. In the next sections, a reminder of the BPSK characteristics is given, and we then focus on the QPSK structure.

Table 3.1 Modulation Methods and Characteristics of the Reported Inductive Link Circuits.

	Data Transmission				
References	*Downlink (rate)*	*Uplink (rate)*	*Carrier (Hz)*	*Power Consumption*	*Technology*
[9]	BPSK (1.6 Mbps)	LSK (200 kbps)	13.56 M	600 μW	0.18 μm CMOS
[49]	Packet detect RF energy	Burst of	2.5 M	— CMOS	2 μm
[50]	PWM-ASK (250 kbps)	ASK	1~10 M	5 mW	1.2 μm CMOS
[51]	ASK (125 kbps)	PWM-ASK	4 M	10–90 mW BiCMOS	3 μm
[52]	ASK (120 k) (117–234 k)	BPSK	10 M	4.5 mA BiCMOS	2.5 μm
[53]	OOK (100 kbps)	No	5 M	0.5 mA, 10 V	2 μm CMOS
[54]	OOK (200 kbps)	LSK	6.78 M	< 120 mW CMOS	1.2 μm

Source: [2].

3.3.1 The BPSK Demodulator

A mixed-signal (analog/digital) modulation/demodulation module is used for extracting clock and data signals from a PSK modulated 13.56-MHz carrier. BPSK is a modulation process whereby the input signal shifts the phase of the output waveform between 0° and 180°, which is equivalent to multiplying the carrier with a bit stream of '1' and '–1' representing high and low states, respectively. This demodulation technique is based on the Costas loop due to its especially practical feasibility. It consists of two parallel phase-locked-loops (PLL), whose phase error outputs are multiplied to control the frequency of the oscillator.

The main drawback of the conventional Costas loop demodulator is its complexity. Normally, a four-quadrant analogue multiplier is adopted to realize the I/Q arm phase detector and the multiplier in the center branch. Recently, digital techniques are employed to implement such demodulator, including multiplication, filter, phase shifting, and digital controlled oscillator. However, the all digital Costas loop demodulator suffers from a high power consumption, which is intolerable for implantable applications.

The block diagram of a BPSK demodulator is shown in Figure 3.5. First, a comparator converts the received carrier in a square waveform. This allows the use of simple digital phase detectors in the two arms of the circuit, because a sinusoidal input signal is considered in place of the square wave, since the low-pass loop filters reject the high-order harmonics. In addition, another comparator is added into the lower branch, which forms a hard-limited Costas loop. A fully differential architecture is adopted in all branches to improve the circuit's reliability, power supply rejection ratio (PSRR), and noise immunity. The BPSK demodulator has been fabricated in a TSMC 0.18-μm CMOS technology.

3.3.2 The QPSK Demodulator

In Table 3.2, the characteristics of three main PSK modulation methods are compared. From BPSK to QPSK, a doubled transmitted data rate is achieved within a given bandwidth, at the expense of noise or distortion immunity. BPSK and QPSK have a 3-dB bit error rate (BER) advantage over BFSK. In BFSK, the carrier frequency is changed between two discrete values. Although easier to implement, BFSK has a

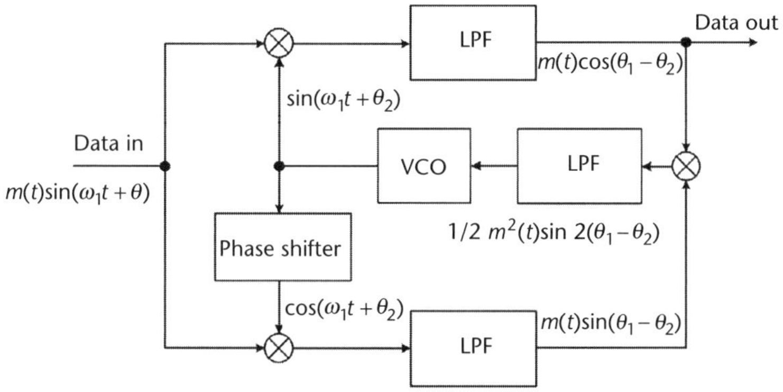

Figure 3.5 Block diagram of the Costas loop-based BPSK demodulator.

Table 3.2 Comparison of Common Modulation Schemes

Mod. Scheme	*Bit Error Rate*	*Advantages*	*Disadvantages*
BPSK	3 dB better than BFSK	Increased noise immunity	1 bit/symbol
QPSK	Same as BPSK	2 bits/symbol Better bandwidth efficiency	Increased susceptibility to phase noise
BFSK	3 dB worse than BPSK or QPSK	Easy to implement	Poor bandwidth efficiency High power demand

poor bandwidth efficiency, which in turn limits the data rate for a given bandwidth. So, BFSK is widely used in low data rate applications.

On the other hand, PSK is the most widely used digital modulation scheme. More particularly, the QPSK scheme improves our previous results with BPSK [9], because of its bandwidth efficiency and higher data rate [11]. In both modulation methods, a carrier frequency of 13.56 MHz, which is legally designated for ISM applications, is used [12]. The QPSK is based on two carriers, one in-phase and another in 90° quadrature phase. Their polarities are switched respectively by two binary signals (two-bit data streams). Hence, QPSK has four possible transmitted phases, and it doubles the data rate of BPSK, but without requiring additional bandwidth.

In order to apply QPSK modulation, a series sequence should be partitioned into two independent data streams: the even bits data stream modulates the in-phase carrier, while the odd bits modulate the quadrature carrier. In standard QPSK, the even and odd bit streams are both transmitted at the rate of $1/2T$ bit/s, where T is the symbol period of the source signal, and are synchronously aligned, such that their transitions coincide. Since the modulated carrier temporarily fades away whenever a data signal changes polarity, the demodulator temporarily loses the signal that it tries to lock onto. The aligned data transitions make this effect worse. In offset QPSK (OQPSK), the odd data stream is offset by T. The two data streams no longer change their states simultaneously, but are staggered in time. This timing change makes the effect less severe and does not have any impact on channel capacity or bandwidth. In our design, the input signal of the proposed demodulator is a OQPSK modulated signal.

The proposed QPSK demodulator also uses the Costas loop method. The modified hard-limited Costas loop is shown in Figure 3.6 [11]. The two low-pass filters in the I and Q branches of the QPSK demodulator are followed by limiters, which directly change the filter output voltages to the highest level or lowest level when there is a phase error, and thus speed up the tracking process of the loops.

Providing that two independent binary messages $x(t)$ and $y(t)$ modulate the two orthogonal components of the carrier, where $x(t)$ and $y(t)$ take values of +1 or −1, for representing a one or a zero respectively, then the transmitted signal can be represented as

$$V_s(t) = x(t)\cos(\omega_1 t + \theta_1) - y(t)\sin(\omega_1 t + \theta_1) \tag{3.11}$$

When the loop has locked, the voltage controlled oscillator (VCO) generates a signal of the form

$$u_{\text{vco}}(t) = \sin(\omega_1 t + \theta_2) \tag{3.12}$$

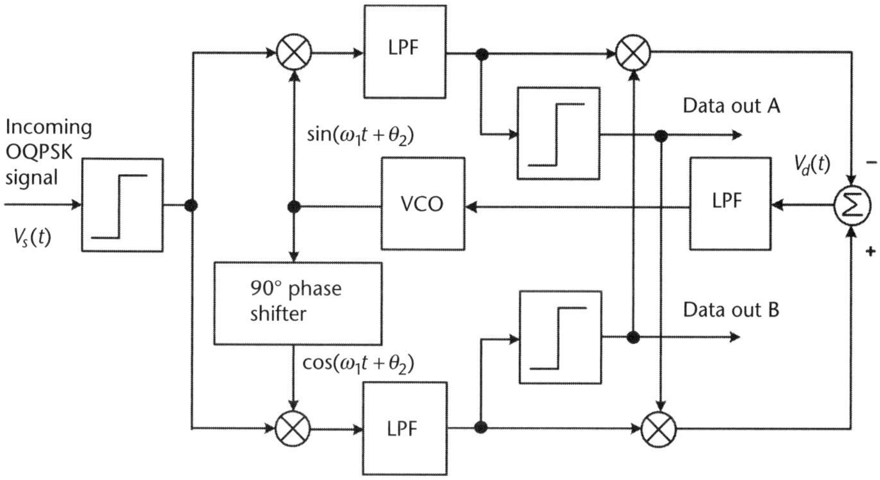

Figure 3.6 Block diagram of the Costas loop based QPSK demodulator.

After applying usual multiplications and trigonometric identities, the low-frequency output of the adder is

$$
\begin{aligned}
V_d(t) = & \left[x(t)\sin(\theta_e) + y(t)\cos(\theta_e)\right] \cdot \mathrm{sgn}\left[x(t)\cos(\theta_e) - y(t)\sin(\theta_e)\right] \\
& -\left[x(t)\cos(\theta_e) - y(t)\sin(\theta_e)\right] \cdot \mathrm{sgn}\left[x(t)\sin(\theta_e) + y(t)\cos(\theta_e)\right]
\end{aligned}
\tag{3.13}
$$

where $\theta_e = \theta_1 - \theta_2$ is the phase error, and $sgn(\cdot)$ is the hard limiting operation. For rectangular data signals, the average dc outputs can be calculated as if

$$
V_d(t) = \begin{cases}
\sin\theta_e, \; if \; -45° < \theta_e < 45° \\
-\cos\theta_e, \; if \; 45° < \theta_e < 135° \\
-\sin\theta_e, \; if \; 135° < \theta_e < 225° \\
\cos\theta_e, \; if \; 225° < \theta_e < 315°
\end{cases}
\tag{3.14}
$$

When $\theta_e = 0$, we have $V_d(t) = sin(\theta_e)$, which can be approached by θ_e. The Costas loop then operates like a conventional PLL, and locks at $\theta_e = 0°$. Similarly, the loop can also lock at $\theta_e = 90°$, 180°, and 270°. Hence, there is an inherent fourfold phase ambiguity that must be resolved by other means.

The phase ambiguity stems from an inability of the PSK demodulator's carrier recovery circuitry to select the correct reference phase from the four possible stable lock points. With this phase ambiguity, the loop can lock to any of four possible phase points, only one of which has the correct phase relationship with the carrier. The QPSK fourfold phase ambiguity can be resolved by using differential coding techniques, at the cost of a reduced power efficiency.

3.3.3 Validation of the Demodulator Architecture

A MATLAB® simulation of the OQPSK topology illustrates that the modified hard-limited Costas loop can effectively perform both carrier reconstruction and synchronous data detection. In this simulation, the total data transmission rate of the two data streams can be up to 8 Mbps with the carrier frequency of 13.56 MHz.

The design of the demodulator is realized by pure analog circuits to achieve high speed and low-power consumption. In fact, an input comparator is adopted to convert the input OQPSK modulated signal into square waveform, allowing a XOR phase detector to be used in each branch. Figure 3.6 shows the block diagram of the proposed QPSK demodulator. In order to achieve better noise immunity and higher PSRR, the actual structure is fully differential. Most of the building blocks are similar to those of the BPSK demodulator, except for the subtracter, which is easily realized using opamp and resistor network.

This demodulator has been implemented in a TSMC 0.18-μm CMOS process and simulated using *spectre*. A data rate of up to 4 Mbps is achieved with a 13.56 MHz carrier at a total power dissipation of 0.75 mW. In Table 3.3, the performance of this QPSK demodulator is compared with other demodulators.

3.4 Energy and Bandwidth Issues in Multi-Channel Biopotential Recording: Case Study

A seen in this chapter, the presented telemetry link can supply a broad variety of biomedical devices in sensor and actuator applications. This includes data acquisition circuits, amplifiers, filters, data converters, digital signal processors, controllers, and transceivers. Moreover, the link must accommodate various applications with a sufficient bandwidth to permit bidirectional digital communications. However, the power generated by such a link is restricted because of safety constraints and finite coupling coefficients. In addition, the link exhibits a narrow bandwidth, which limits data communication rates. Thus, the design of complex implantable systems using such a medium requires special attention.

For example, neuroscience research and neuroprosthetics necessitate devices of high complexity. High-channel count sensors are needed to simultaneously record biopotential events from several neurons. Developments in this area have been stim-

Table 3.3 Comparison of Results for the Presented BPSK Modulator and Other Topologies

	FDSFSK [55]	*RDFSK [56]*	*DFSK [57]*	*BPSK [9]*	*QPSK [49]*
CMOS Process (μm)	3	1.5	1.5	0.18	0.18
Carrier (MHz)	2 ~ 20	2 ~ 20	5/10, 50.5 based clock	13.56	13.56
Max. data rate (Mbps)	2.5 (S*) 1 (M**)	4 (S) 1.5 (M)	4 (S) 2.5 (M)	1.12 (S)	8 (MATLAB) 4 (S)
Power dissipation (mW)	0.55 at 100 kbps	0.45 at 200 kbps	0.38	0.414 at 1.12 Mbps	0.75 at 4 Mbps

*S = Simulated, **M = Measured

ulated by astonishing emerging clinical applications including mind-driven rehabilitation systems and implants for treating diseases such as epilepsy [13, 14]. Efforts toward the development of fully implantable systems have led so far to the implementation of devices featuring up to a hundred recording channels [15, 16]. But, systems including larger channel-count are required to address future needs. In this case, dedicated power-aware design techniques, and advanced on-chip data processing are mandatory to overcome limitations in the wireless link.

This case study addresses power and bandwidth issues in wireless neural sensors using an inductive link. In the first part of the study, we put emphasis on low-power circuits design techniques for implementing dense devices. In the second part of the study, we describe analog and digital building blocks to realize real-time on-chip data compression for increasing the link capacity.

3.4.1 Micropower Low-Noise Bioamplifier

Bioamplifiers are fundamental building blocks in biomedical sensing devices [16–24]. They are needed to retrieve the weak bioelectrical signals from the background activity. Amplifiers intended for use in implantable devices must dissipate low power for safe permanent usage, and present small size for realizing compact devices. In addition, bioamplifiers must present a bandpass characteristic to remove low-frequency components such as the dc offset across differential sensing electrodes. Electrode potential mismatches are responsible for input offsets that can reach hundreds of millivolts. This can saturate the output of the amplifier if nothing is done. Therefore, a low-frequency suppression scheme must be adopted. However, additional circuits needed to achieve this requirement can increase the power consumption and the area of the bioamplifier, and reduce the manageable number of recording channels.

A suitable low-frequency suppression scheme must be a candidate for full on-chip integration in area- and power-constrained sensors. In addition, the adopted scheme must not degrade the input-referred noise, nor lower the input impedance of the amplifier, or attenuate the input signal.

Active schemes based on closed-loop control of dc levels have been proposed to address these limitations [25, 26]. Such schemes provide enhanced suppression of the low-frequency content, whereas they allow for high input impedance.

Figure 3.7 presents the schematic of a compact bioamplifier design using an active low-frequency suppression scheme [27]. Such a bioamplifier features a bandpass characteristic, whereas it avoids passive ac couplings input networks. The depicted topology consists of a low-noise amplifier ($A1$) featuring an inverting Miller integrator within its feedback path. The active Miller integrator uses a second amplifier ($A2$), a capacitor (C_I), and a high-value resistor (R_{eq}). Its time constant (τ) sets the –3 dB high-pass cutoff frequency (f_{hp}) of the bioamplifier ($\tau = R_{eq}C_I$). The midband gain of the bioamplifier equals the low-frequency open-loop gain of $A1$, noted A_{v1}, and the –3 dB low-pass cutoff frequency (f_{lp}) is defined by $A1$ dominant pole. The transfer function of the ideal bioamplifier is

$$\frac{v_{out}(s)}{v_{in}(s)} = \frac{-s\tau A_{v1}}{s\tau + A_{v1}} \tag{3.15}$$

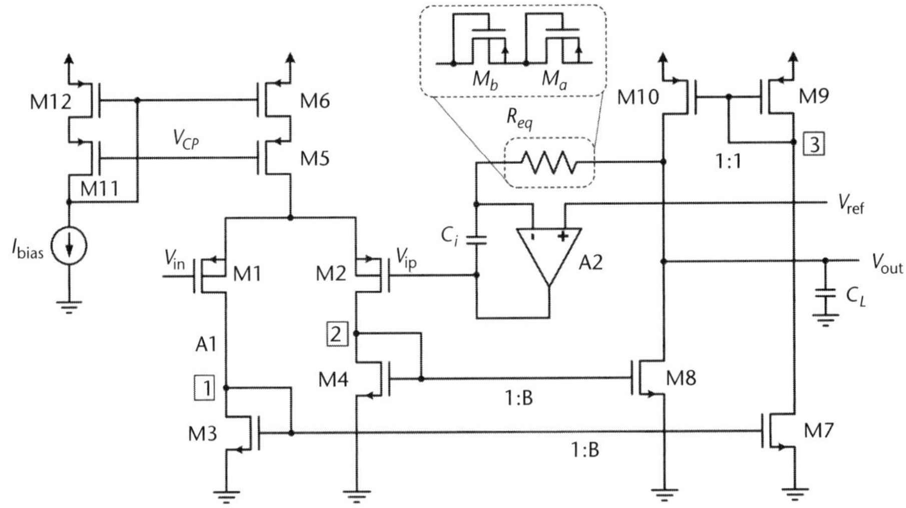

Figure 3.7 Bioamplifier schematic. The low-noise current mirror operational transconductance amplifier *A*1 features a Miller integrator-based low-frequency suppression circuit within its feedback path.

This transfer function yields –3 dB high-pass cutoff frequency given by

$$f_{hp} = \frac{1}{2\pi} \frac{A_{v1}}{R_{eq} C_I} \tag{3.16}$$

This high-pass cutoff frequency rejects the unwanted low-frequency content, but passes the useful neural signal with bandwidth that starts at a few tens of hertz. The frequency and phase responses of the bioamplifier are depicted in Figure 3.8.

The low-frequency gain of the current mirror operational transconductance amplifier (OTA) *A*1 is defined as

$$A_{v1} = B\frac{g_{m1}}{g_o} = \frac{Bg_{m1}}{(g_{ds8} + g_{ds10})} \tag{3.17}$$

where the output conductance g_o results from the summation of transistors $M_{8,10}$ output conductances. The gain-bandwidth product (noted *GBW)* of the current mirror OTA is determined by the dominant pole of the OTA. This pole is realized at the output node which exhibits the highest conductance (g_o) and the biggest capacitive load C_L. Its value is given by

$$f_d = \frac{g_o}{2\pi(C_{no} + C_L)} \tag{3.18}$$

in which C_{no} includes all capacitances connected to the output node, and parameter *B* equals the ratio of drain currents $(I_{D1,2} = I_{D3,4}) / (I_{D7,8} = I_{D9,10})$ in the current mirrors OTA (Figure 3.7). The *GBW* is expressed as

$$GBW = A_{v1}f_d = \frac{Bg_{m1}}{2\pi(C_{no} + C_L)} \tag{3.19}$$

A unitary ratio B is considered for the rest of this example. Other non-dominant poles occur at nodes 1, 2, and 3. Poles at nodes 1 and 2 are the same, therefore, they form together a single nondominant pole f_{nd2}, which is

$$f_{nd2} = \frac{g_{m4}}{2\pi C_{n2}} \tag{3.20}$$

Another nondomimnant pole occurs at node 3 but acts only on half of the output signal (only the path formed by transistors $M_{1,3,7,9}$ is subject to this pole). As demonstrated in [28], when a pole acts only on half of the signal, a zero must be added at twice the pole frequency. Thus, the following pole-zero doublet is formed:

$$f_{nd3} = \frac{g_{m9}}{2\pi C_{n3}} \tag{3.21}$$

$$f_{z3} = 2f_{nd3} \tag{3.22}$$

Then, considering the bioamplifier low-frequency suppression circuit, we see in Figure 3.7 that the Miller integrator samples the main amplifier ($A1$) output voltage at node v_{out}, integrates it, and applies a correction voltage at terminal v_{ip}. As a result, node v_{ip} tracks the dc level seen by $A1$ at v_{in}, which effectively cancels any dc offset, drift, and other low-frequency input voltages. A high-value equivalent resistor R_{eq} is needed for the integrator (Figure 3.7). A MOS-bipolar device composed

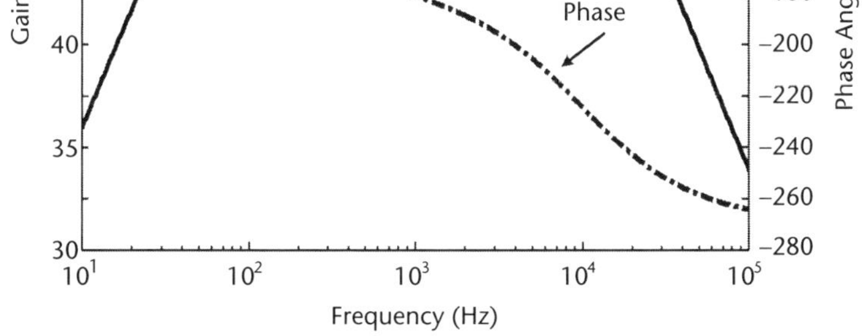

Figure 3.8 Phase and frequency responses of the bioamplifier. The bioamplifier presents a bandpass characteristic for amplifying the neural signal and rejecting the unwanted content.

of two stacked diode-connected PMOS transistors, whose bulk terminals are tied to their sources, can be used to implement R_{eq}. Equivalent resistors greater than 10^{13} Ω are achieved for small input signals with this configuration [27]. Therefore, a very long time constant that requires only a small-integrated capacitor size can be implemented. Typically, an integrated metal-to-metal (MiM) capacitor of 1 pF can be used.

Despite the fact that the feedback loop is connected from $A1$ output to its positive input terminal (v_{ip}), it is worth it to see that the bioamplifer uses negative feedback since the inverting integrator attaches a negative sign to its output voltage. $A2$ senses the reference voltage at node v_{ref} and replicates it at v_{ip} for providing common mode voltage rejection in the bioamplifier.

Next, the bioamplifier design must address the noise versus power consumption trade-offs. For that purpose, amplifiers $A1$ and $A2$ can be optimized through a transconductance efficiency-based design methodology for the best performances. The adopted design strategy allows for optimal sizing of transistors, and for operation over the entire continuum of channel inversion levels, with respect to a pre-selected drain current, and an inversion coefficient (IC). The later results from the normalized drain current I_D divided by the specific current I_S, and is proportional to the level of channel inversion of a MOS transistor [29],

$$IC = \frac{I_D}{2n\mu C_{ox}(W / L)U_T} \tag{3.23}$$

where n is the slope factor, μ is the carrier mobility, C_{ox} is the gate-oxide capacitance per unit area, W and L are the channel width and length, and U_T is the thermal voltage (kT/q). The MOS transconductance efficiency (g_m/I_D) is maximum for transistors operating in weak inversion (IC < 0.1), and reaches its minimum for transistors in strong inversion (IC > 10). Specifically, operation at very low IC results in optimally high transconductance for a given current, but requires large W/L ratios. Conversely, operating at high IC yields low transconductance, but offers larger bandwidth. The transconductance ratio valid for all levels of inversion is defined as

$$g_m/I_D \cong \frac{1}{nU_T}\varphi(IC) \tag{3.24}$$

where

$$\varphi(IC) = \frac{1}{0.5 + \sqrt{0.25 + IC}} \tag{3.25}$$

is taken from the EKV model [30], and yields values between 0 and 1. The design method first consists in choosing transistor drain currents according to power and noise specifications. Then, the amplifier parameters such as input-referred noise, low-frequency gain, output resistance, and bandwidth are optimized through careful selection of device size according to the required channel inversion level.

The input-referred thermal noise power achieved by the current mirror OTA $A1$ is

$$v^2_{ni,thermal(A1)} = 2v^2_{n1} + 4v^2_{n3}(g_{m3} / g_{m1})^2 + 2v^2_{n9}(g_{m9} / g_{m1})^2 \tag{3.26}$$

where v^2_{ni} equals $4kTn\Gamma_i/g_{mi}\Delta f$, and the thermal noise factors Γ_i take values 1/2, or 2/3, whether the device operates in weak or in strong inversion. Then, assuming n constant for all regimes of operation, and replacing v^2_{ni} and (3.24) in (3.26) gives

$$v^2_{ni,thermal(A1)} = \left[8kT\frac{n^2U_T}{I_{D1}}\frac{1}{\varphi(IC_1)} \cdot \left(\Gamma_1 + 2\frac{\varphi(IC_3)}{\varphi(IC_1)}\Gamma_3 + \frac{\varphi(IC_9)}{\varphi(IC_1)}\Gamma_9 \right) \right] \Delta f_{(A1)} \tag{3.27}$$

Equation (3.27) shows that, for minimizing the noise, high IC are required in the differential pair, whose transistors are related to $\varphi(IC_1)$, whereas low IC are needed for the current mirrors, whose transistors are related to $\varphi(IC_{3,9})$. Operating $M_{1,2}$ in weak inversion pushes $\varphi(IC_1)$ toward 1, whereas operating the remaining transistors in strong inversion pushes $\varphi(IC_3)$ and $\varphi(IC_9)$ downward toward 0, for fulfilling the requirements. IC are adjusted by picking large $(W/L)_{1,2}$ and low $(W/L)_{3,4,7,8,9,10}$ ratios, with respect to a fixed drain current.

Similar design considerations apply for the two-stage OTA $A2$, but in this case, the noise power only depends on two IC (related to transistors in the differential pair, and in the active load respectively [31]. Under these design considerations, both OTAs ($A1$ and $A2$) input thermal noises simplify to

$$v^2_{ni,thermal(OTA)} = 4kT\frac{n^2U_T}{I_{D1}}\frac{1}{\varphi(IC_1)}\Delta f \tag{3.28}$$

Equation (3.28) is used as a design insight to set the transistor's drain current according to satisfactory noise performance. For example, bias currents (I_{bias}) of 1 μA and 2 μA can be used in the cascode current sources for biasing $A1$ and $A2$, respectively (Figure 3.7). This yields an input noise voltage of around 3 μVrms for $A1$ at body temperature, according to (3.28). A slightly higher bias current can be used in $A2$, for ensuring stability of the Miller integrator working in closed-loop.

Besides, large area transistors with small inversion coefficients must be used in the differential input pairs of both OTAs for minimizing the $1/f$ noise in the bioamplifier. In general, PMOS transistors exhibit less $1/f$ noise than NMOS devices as long as their gate voltage overdrive ($V_{eff} = V_{GS} - V_{TH}$) stays low. Even though this effect appears to be more substantial in larger geometry processes [32], the $1/f$ noise level at low V_{eff} is approximately half an order of magnitude less in PMOS devices than in NMOS in a 0.18-μm bulk CMOS technology [33]. Corner frequencies of a few hundred hertz can be achieved for both OTAs using large input transistors ($L_{1,2}$ = 800 μm, $W_{1,2}$ = 4 μm, for instance). Having such low corner frequencies reduces the impact of the $1/f$ noise and makes the overall input noise to mainly depend on the transistor's thermal noise.

This bioamplifier design has been fabricated in a TSMC 0.18-μm one-metal one-poly CMOS process for performing *in vivo* neural recordings. It was designed for a gain of 400 and a bandwidth of 9.2 kHz, with bias currents of 1 μA for $A1$, and 2 μA for $A2$. The fabricated bioamplifier fits in a 0.260 mm Δ 0.190 mm chip area, and dissipates less than 9 μW. The midband gain is 50.25 dB and cutoff frequencies f_{hp} and f_{lp} are located at 102 Hz and 9.1 kHz, respectively, which yields a bandwidth of 9 kHz. Figure 3.8 presents neural waveforms obtained with the presented bioamplifier in an *in vivo* experiment. To summarize, we illustrate the benefit of the presented design by referring back to the practical example given in Section 3.2. The link described in this example achieves an efficiency of 30%, and provides a power of 5.86 W at the primary. Assuming ideal rectifier and regulator circuits in the implantable part, we see that such a link could supply up to 1000 instances of the presented bioamplifier design. Moreover, all amplifiers can be integrated within a 0.5 cm^2 silicon die. A sensor presenting such density would be highly profitable for *in vivo* experimentations in various branches of neuroscience. However, other required implanted circuitry, and tools for signal processing and data analysis are still missing for managing such device.

3.4.2 Real-Time Data Reduction and Compression

Bandwidth limitation is among the most troublesome bottlenecks in wireless biomedical devices. A typical neural recording application requires 100 channels, a minimum sampling frequency of 20 kHz per channel, and a sample representation of 8 bits. An implanted sensor that continuously records the raw neural signals from 100 channels would generate an overwhelming data rate of 16 Mbits/s. Present low-power implantable biotelemetry links are merely able to transmit a small subset of this total amount of channels, whereas sensors that incorporate more and more channels are needed for expansion. Consequently, such interface requires an on-chip mechanism for bandwidth reduction; otherwise, the data rate would be prohibitive and prevent wireless recording from several channels.

In that respect, embedded signal processing circuitries are used for performing *in vivo* data reduction in implants [16, 34–39]. Data reduction is intended to decrease the volume of data that must be handled by low-power telemetry. Such a procedure extracts relevant content from the raw signal by means of real-time waveform detection and rejects the remaining parts of the signal to achieve smaller data rates.

Such a scheme is highly profitable in multi-channel neural recording devices because of a neural signal's nature in general. The principal mechanism of information transmission in extracellular neural recording waveforms is a change in AP generation rate by individual neurons. APs are short waveforms of a few ms of duration whose rate of occurrence ranges between 10 to few hundreds per second. Therefore, automatic biopotentials detection makes it possible to detect AP waveforms and to transmit only the necessary information, instead of the entire raw neural signal. For example, an implanted sensor could detect APs and send only their times of occurrence. Figure 3.9 illustrates this scheme.

Note that, in addition to reducing the volume of data, a suitable detection scheme must preserve the information content in the useful neural signal and conserve its

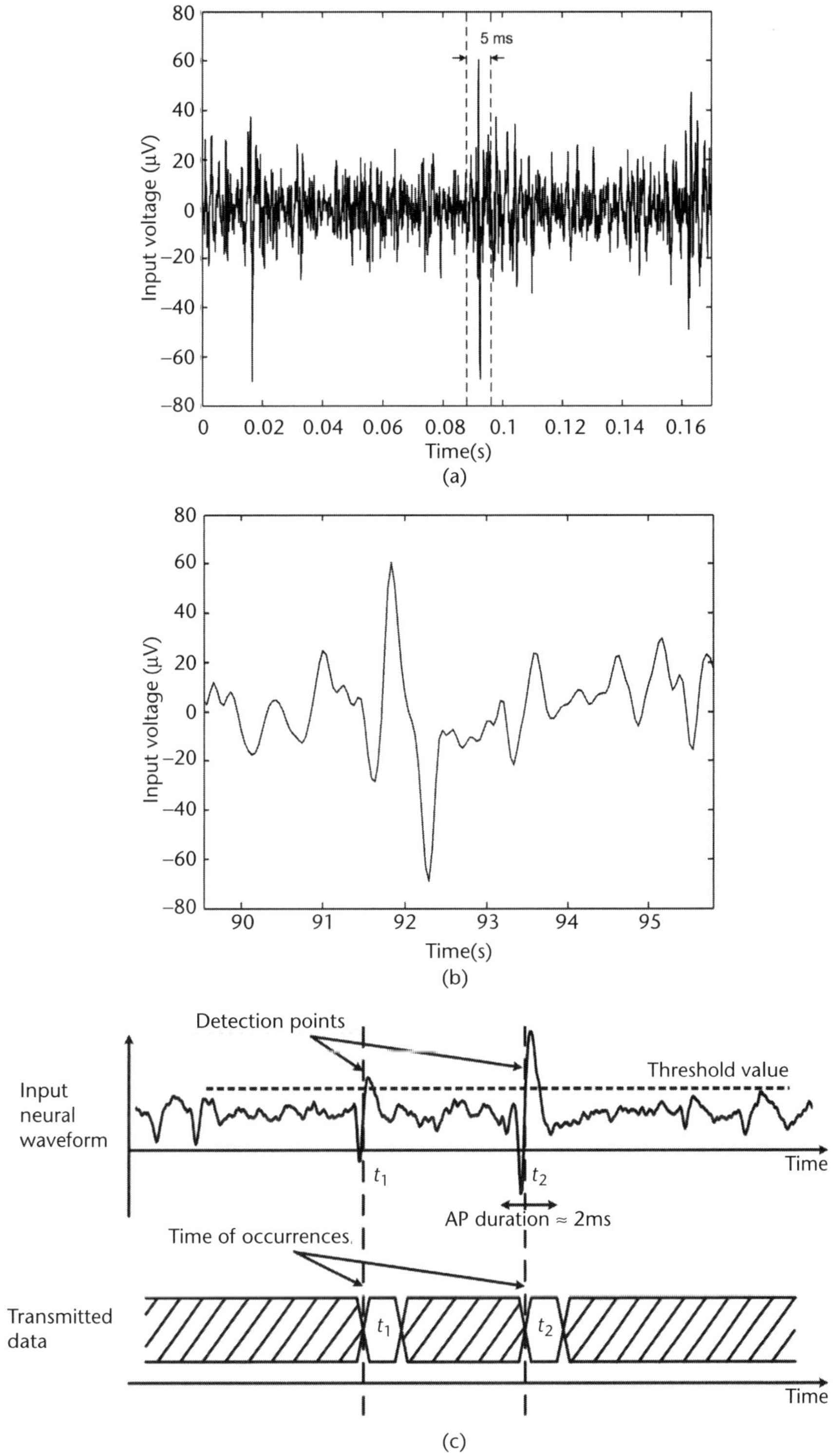

Figure 3.9 A possible data reduction scheme with automatic biopotentials detection. The time of occurrence of APs are sent to a remote host upon detection. (a) Raw neural signal. (b) Zoom of a part of the raw signal. (c) Detected Action Potentials.

integrity. Moreover, it must imply a minimum circuits and power overhead for its implementation.

Several types of hardware biopotential detectors can be used for performing *in vivo* detection. The most direct detector scheme uses simple thresholding. Within such a scheme, detection occurs when the biopotential's amplitude crosses a specified threshold. This detector can easily be implemented with digital blocks or analog circuits requiring minimal overhead. In fact, an optimized analog implementation can, in general, achieve lower power densities and smaller chip area. Likewise, thresholding is relatively straightforward for an analog implementation, as the detector can be built from a low-power voltage comparator.

Several types of comparator topologies are available. Although some applications can use a simple open-loop op-amp as a voltage comparator, this approach is usually not accurate and fast enough. For a superior sensitivity, important design characteristics need to be targeted: high precision, low offset, low input-referred noise, high slew rate, high speed, and low propagation delay are required. High performance multi-stages comparators are more suited for a fast operation and high precision. Figure 3.10 shows the schematic of a multi-stages latched comparator used in this example. This design includes a preamplifier and a latch made from the cross-gate connected transistors M_{L1}, M_{L2}. The latch acts as a decision element and presents positive feedback to increase the comparator gain and avoid metastability. The preamplifier is used to achieve a high resolution and to minimize kickback noise related to the latch operation. This design can resolve mV-level signals with tail currents on the order of a few tens of nA, thus achieving very low-power consumption. Note that the weak-amplitude neural signals must be amplified before being resolved by the voltage comparator. A suitable low-noise amplifier, such as the one described in Section 3.4.1 of this chapter, should be used for that purpose.

However, accurate detection with thresholding is only possible for a relatively high signal-to-noise ratio (SNR). The error rate increases with the noise as more false positives and false negatives occur. Using a preprocessor module can improve detection of biopotentials in noise. For a detector based on such a scheme, first use a preprocessor to accentuate biopotentials shapes and attenuate noise. Then, the preprocessor output is passed through a threshold function for determining the biopotentials' locations. Figure 3.11 depicts a block diagram of this detection strategy.

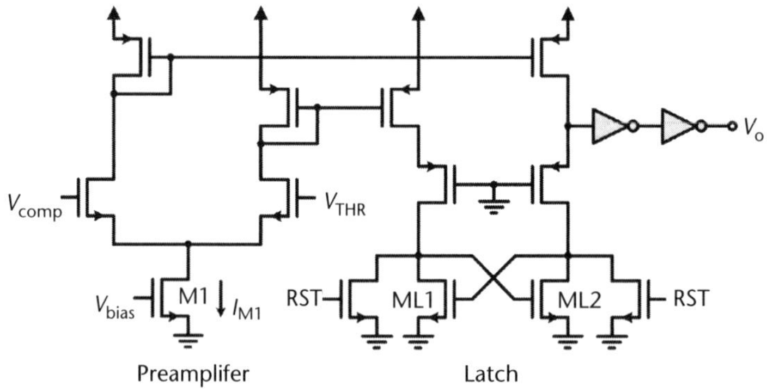

Figure 3.10 Schematic of a high-precision latched comparator for the decision block.

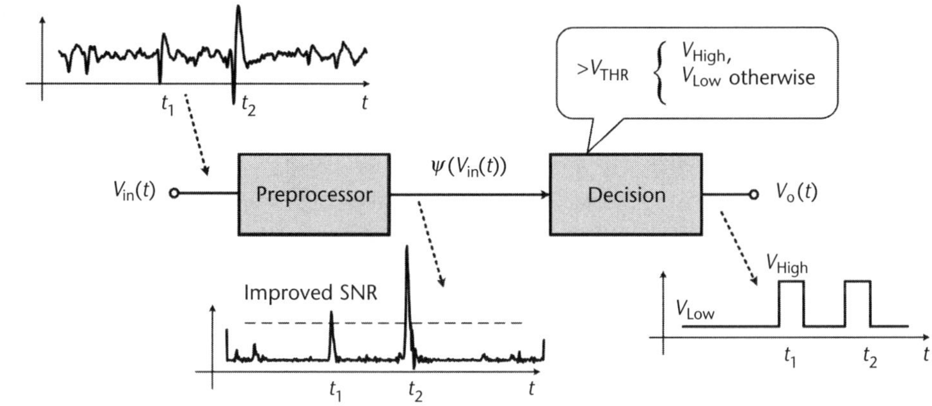

Figure 3.11 Block diagram of a detector using a preprocessor and a decision block. The times of occurrence of biopotentials are captured on threshold crossing. Typical input signals and output waveforms are shown for each block.

Low-complexity preprocessing methods are preferred for integration in implants over computationally demanding ones. Accordingly, very reliable but intensive techniques such as template matching, matched filtering, or artificial neural networks-based methods would be hardly portable in implantable devices. Moreover, those techniques require *a priori* knowledge of the targeted waveforms, which is not convenient in real-time, in a varying environment.

Low-power analog computation can contribute to implementing preprocessors. Analog building blocks such as filters, multipliers, differentiators, integrators, and translinear circuits can be used to realize various types of functions [40, 41]. Obviously, algorithms intended for an analog implementation must be computationally simple and suitable for continuous-time operation.

For instance, mathematical operators–based detectors can yield low-overhead implementations and reach the expected performances. Energy-based detectors are often used for real-time detection in neural recording. For such a task, the power of a signal is estimated by calculating its root mean square value over a sliding window. The variance and mean of the processed signal are often used to adaptively adjust the detection threshold in real-time [42].

The Teager energy operator (TEO) is an energy-based detector that can precisely estimate the energy of a signal. This operator calculates the square of the instantaneous product of a signal amplitude and frequency [43, 44]. The TEO is considered superior to other energy estimators, because it is simultaneously sensitive to frequency and amplitude. This detector is used as a kind of time-frequency analyzer. Moreover, the TEO is robust at low SNR, and exhibits excellent sensitivity to transients, which makes it very well suited for the detection of AP waveforms. Besides, its low complexity makes the TEO naturally suitable for an analog implementation. For a continuous-time signal $x(t)$, the TEO operator is defined as

$$\psi(x(t)) = \left(\frac{dx(t)}{dt}\right)^2 - x(t)\left(\frac{d^2x(t)}{dt^2}\right) \tag{3.29}$$

Figure 3.12 shows a schematic of an analog implementation of a TEO-based preprocessor circuit. Three analog blocks are required: a differentiator, a four-quadrant multiplier, and a summer. Figure 3.12b presents the three building blocks that constitute the TEO preprocessor. The differentiator employs two OTA and a small capacitor [40]. The capacitor can be sized to 1 pF, if sufficiently small transconductances are used (Figure 3.12b). The differentiator transfer function is

$$\frac{V_{in}}{V_o} = \frac{sC}{sC + g_{m1}} \cdot \frac{g_{m2}}{g_{m3}} \tag{3.30}$$

The multiplier uses a crossed-coupled quad structure in which a differential multiplication is obtained by driving the gate and bulk of four PMOS devices (Figure 3.12c). When the differential inputs v_1 and v_2 are within the circuit linear range ($\leq$ 200 mV), the four-quadrant multiplier operation is described by

$$i_o = \frac{\kappa(1-\kappa)I_{bias}}{4U_T^2} v_1 v_2 \tag{3.31}$$

where κ is the inverse of the slope factor ($\kappa = 1/n$). Source degeneration transistors $M_{6,7,8,9}$ are used to extend the multiplier linear range. OTA and capacitors (OTA-C) circuits whose transistors are biased in the weak inversion regime are used in each block to achieve ultra-low power consumption. Bandwidth, transconductance gain, linearity, and power consumption are optimized using the transconductance efficiency-based design methodology introduced in Section 3.4.1. In addition, source degeneration, bulk injection, and bump linearization techniques can be combined to extend the linear operating range of subthreshold OTAs [45]. This analog TEO preprocessor was implemented in a CMOS 0.18 μm process and simulated under *spectre*. The simulated circuit dissipates as low as 170 nW and presents a dynamic range of 200 mV.

Similar to the TEO, several other types of low-power analog preprocessors can be implemented. For example, bandpass filters that highlight activity levels in specific frequency bands can be used to detect biopotentials whose energy is contained in specific frequency ranges. Another method consists in using low-power low-pass filters to implement a moving average and adjust a threshold value [46].

After preprocessing, the resulting waveform is passed through a threshold function to determine biopotentials locations. The threshold value must be set above the background activity level and optimized to minimize detection errors (minimize false positives and false negatives). Normally, the threshold value is taken as a scaled version of the preprocessor average output [43]. Therefore, automatic adjustment of the threshold value can easily be realized using basic analog circuit blocks, such as a low-pass filter.

With the presented schemes, the times of occurrence of biopotentials can be resolved upon threshold crossing and sent to a remote host for further processing or storage. This strategy allows for a high data reduction factor, but implies a major drawback: most of the detected biopotentials characteristics are irreversibly lost.

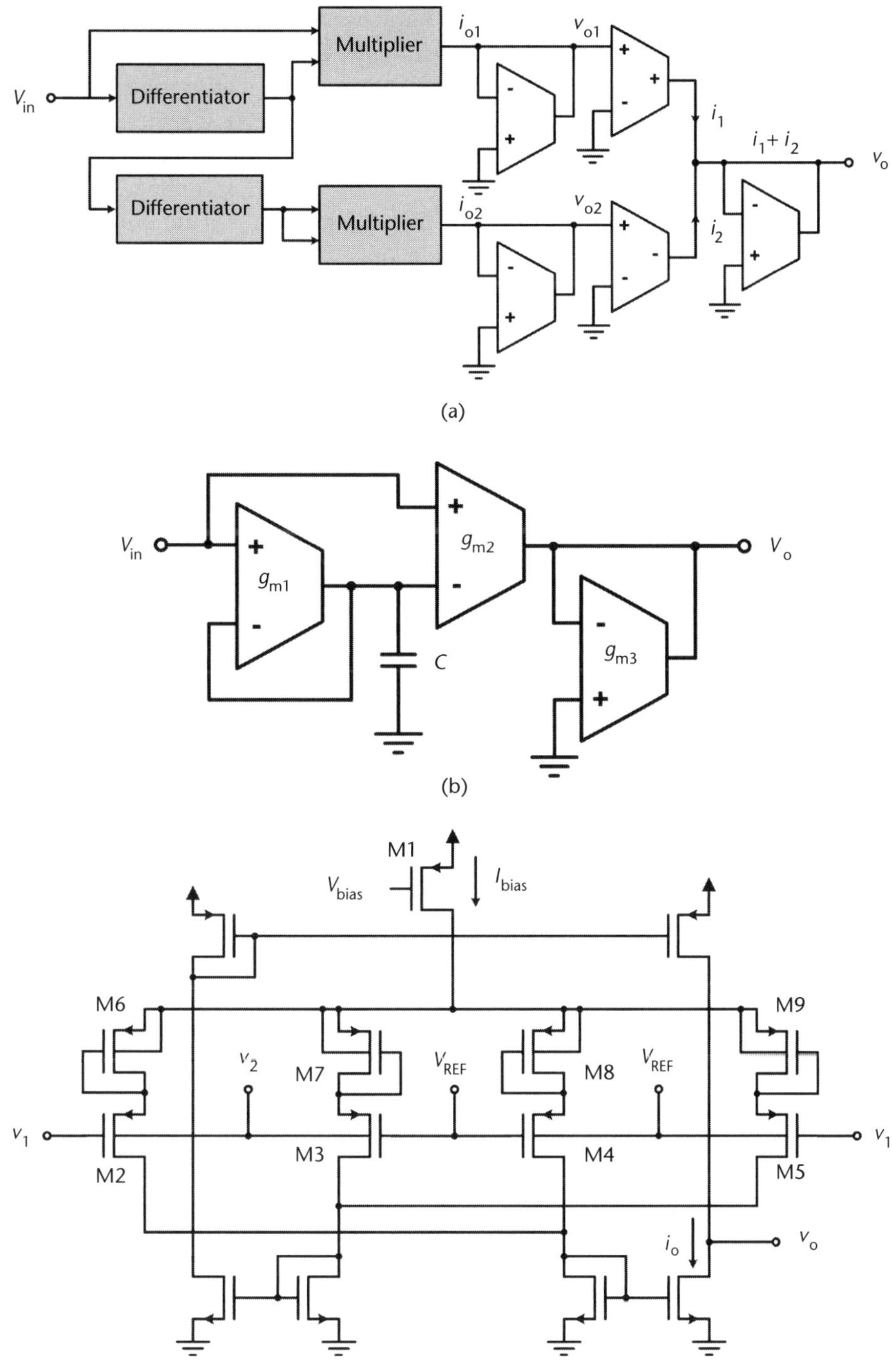

Figure 3.12 The analog TEO–based preprocessor. (a) Top-level schematic. (b) Differentiator circuit. (c) Four-quadrant analog multiplier.

Commonly, detected biopotentials characteristics must be preserved for further processing. In fact, one microelectrode records APs from several neurons at a time. Therefore, detection is a necessary first step for the classification of multi-unit waveforms into single-units. The ability to distinguish between AP waveforms on a single channel is critical for assigning units to distinct neurons. Further, well-separated neurons allow for improved performances in neuroprosthetics applications [39].

Techniques that extract specific biopotential features are used [16, 35, 36]. Parameters such as peak-to-peak amplitude, duration, peak-to-zero-crossing time, or peak length can be used [47, 48]. Such a scheme can achieve a high reduction factor, but may lack reliability, because an acceptable classification error may be difficult to reach within the discrimination task using only a small set of parameters. Besides, neuroscience investigations that aim to understand the cooperative behavior of neurons require well-separated units. Contaminated single-unit recordings are of no interest in such cases [42]. Normally, using more features lowers the classification error rate by enabling fine processing methods such as automatic feature extraction with a principal component technique. In general, the more features that are available, the better the AP shapes can be distinguished.

Thus, a scheme that consists in transmitting the biopotential waveshape in its entirety preserves the information content and allows for superior accuracy in the discrimination task. For that purpose, digital thresholding can be combined with synchronized data buffering to detect and to keep the integral biopotential waveforms. A digital threshold can be implemented in a very straightforward way in a hardware description language. Figure 3.13 illustrates a possible implementation of such a strategy. First, incoming samples are buffered in first-in-first-out (FIFO) buffers of appropriate length. Then, a detector compares each sample value with a programmable threshold. Upon threshold crossing, the content of the corresponding FIFO is copied and accumulated in an output memory buffer for data fusion.

The output memory buffers must accommodate as many samples as necessary for representing an entire AP waveform. A suitable memory size should make it pos-

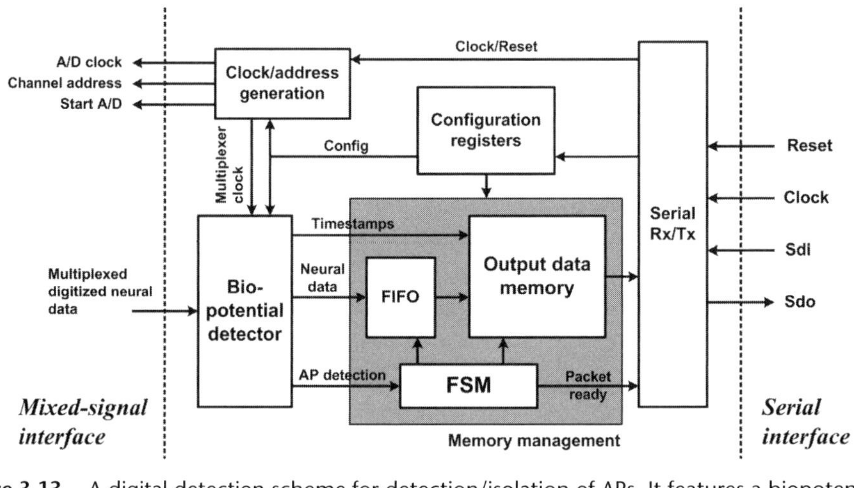

Figure 3.13 A digital detection scheme for detection/isolation of APs. It features a biopotentials detector, buffering memory, and a digital interface for serial communications.

sible to store AP waveforms typically lasting 2 ms, and sampled at 30 kHz. The size of the required output memory buffer in kilobytes is at least

$$MBuf_{size} = f_e \cdot AP_{Len} \cdot NbCh \tag{3.32}$$

where f_e is the sampling frequency, AP_{Len} is the duration of a biopotential in seconds, and $NbCh$ is the number of channels included in the device. Then, a 100-channel system with f_e = 30 kHz requires an output memory size of 5.86 kB. After data buffering, samples are assembled in packets and transmitted to a remote host over the inductive link. Figure 3.14 illustrates the memory usage in this scheme.

Such a bandwidth reduction scheme promotes better post-processing results, but yields higher data rates than other detectors that only focus on specific parameters. With typical neurons firing rates between 10 to 100 AP/s, a variable data reduction factor between 5 and 50 is expected for this scheme. This corresponds to a bandwidth reduction of up to 98% compared with integral transfer of data, whereas AP waveshapes are preserved completely. This corresponds to approximately 5 to 50 kbits/s per channel (or a maximum of 0.046 Mbits/channel), depending on the neuron firing rates and the global activity level. This reduction factor makes it possible to transmit several hundreds of recording channels over an inductive telemetry link compared to only a few without data reduction. For example, a hundred-channel system that records from an ensemble whose neurons all fire at the very high rate of 100 AP/s would generate a maximum of 4.6 Mbits/s. This worst-case data rate is clearly in the range of operation of present inductively coupled link techniques.

On the other hand, more computationally demanding preprocessors can be used for improving the detection rate and for performing enhanced data compression. For example, wavelet transform is a very effective approach to perform biopotential detection and compression [46, 58]. The discrete wavelet transform (DWT) produces approximate and detail transform coefficients that give a sparse representation of an original signal. Coefficients whose values are below a specific threshold can be ignored (set to zero) to reduce the number of bits to send toward the remote host. The resulting non-zero DWT coefficients represents the original signal with a reduced volume of data. The DWT can be implemented in an embedded dig-

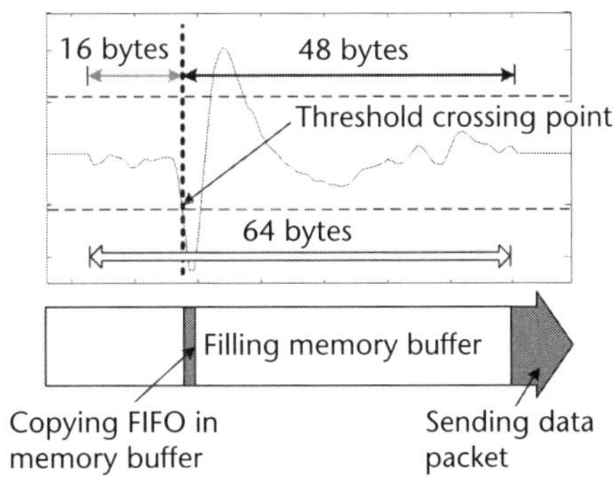

Figure 3.14 Detection/isolation of digitized AP. The first 16 samples are buffered in a FIFO and copied in the output memory upon detection. Then, the remaining 48 samples are added in memory for forming a data packet. From [58] with permission, © IEEE 2007.

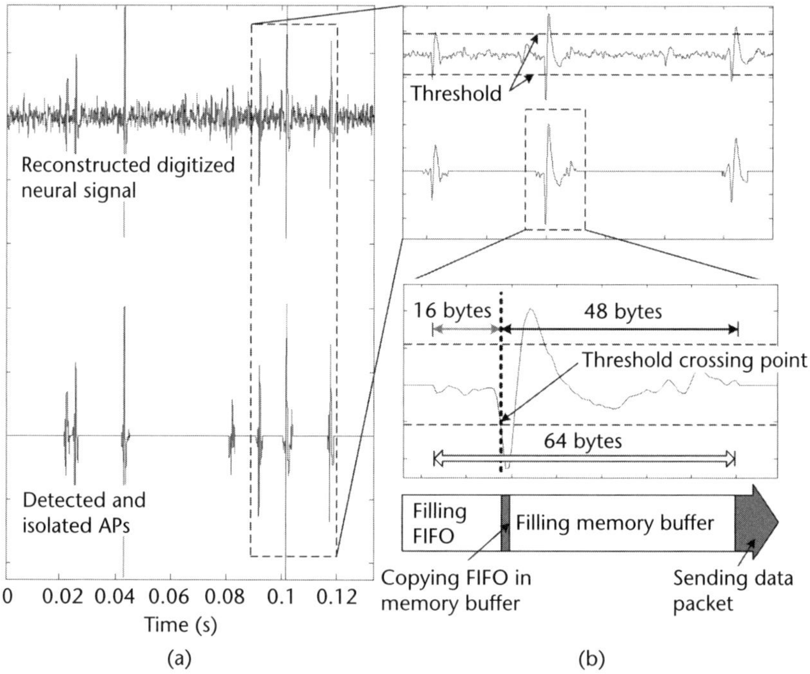

Figure 3.15 Extracellular recording from the hippocampus of a rat. (a) Sample waveform recorded with the presented bioamplifier. (b) A closer view on a recorded action potential. (Waveforms are referred to the amplifier input). From [58] with permission, © IEEE 2007.

ital processing system for operation in implantable devices. However, such intensive preprocessors are inevitably more difficult to design under restricted size and power budget.

3.5 Summary

In this chapter, we described a typical inductively coupled biotelemetry link used to wirelessly power various implanted biomedical devices, and to provide them with a medium for high-data rate bidirectional communications. Although tremendous progress has been made in this important area, there are still critical needs for increased performances. Wireless operation of implants is a necessity because it avoids batteries and percutaneous connections, which in turn reduces risks of infection and gives more flexibility to patients. There is an urgent need to build better wireless systems for the long-term powering of fully implanted devices, because the complexity of biomedical implants required in several emerging experimental and clinical areas is growing. As demonstrated in the case study, recent advances in neuroscience have brought the necessity to build dense implantable devices to record from several neurons in the cortex. However, these new neuro-interfacing circuits exacerbate needs for more power, density, and bandwidth. The power and size bottlenecks are efficiently addressed by a power-aware circuit design approach. Such strategy saves energy to supply devices of high density. The design of a custom bioamplifier topology suitable for massive integration has been presented. A transconductance-efficiency based design strategy has been applied to achieve low-noise and low-power performances. For the bandwidth issue, real-time signal processing is employed to increase the link capacity. Automatic detection of biopotentials considerably reduces the volume of data that must be handled by the transceiver. Digital building blocks and analog circuits are used to implement such detectors with minimal overhead.

Acknowledgments

The materials in this chapter are research projects supported by a Canada Research Chair on smart medical devices. Also acknowledgments are due to NSERC Canada for financial support, CMC Microsystems for the design tools and chips fabrication facilities, and the graduate students of Polystim Neurotechnologies Laboratory, more particularly Y. Hu and S. Deng for their contributions in the presented projects.

References

[1] A. Djemouai and M. Sawan, "Prosthetic power supplies," *Wiley Encyclopedia of Electrical and Electronics Engineering*, vol. 17, pp. 413–421, 1999.

[2] M. Sawan, H. Yamu, and J. Coulombe, "Wireless smart implants dedicated to multichannel monitoring and microstimulation," *IEEE Circuits and Systems Magazine*, vol. 5, pp. 21–39, 2005.

[3] C. M. Zierhofer and E. S. Hochmair, "Geometric approach for coupling enhancement of magnetically coupled coils," *IEEE Transactions on Biomedical Engineering*, vol. 43, pp. 708–714, 1996.

[4] E. S. Hochmair, "System Optimization for Improved Accuracy in Transcutaneous Signal and Power Transmission," *IEEE Transactions on Biomedical Engineering*, vol. BME-31, pp. 177–186, 1984.

[5] M. Soma, D. C. Galbraith, and R. L. White, "Radio-Frequency Coils in Implantable Devices: Misalignment Analysis and Design Procedure," *IEEE Transactions on Biomedical Engineering*, vol. BME-34, pp. 276–282, 1987.

[6] P. R. Troyk and M. A. K. Schwan, "Closed-loop class E transcutaneous power and data link for MicroImplants," *IEEE Transactions on Biomedical Engineering*, vol. 39, pp. 589–599, 1992.

[7] S. H. J. Tu, "Class E RF tuned power amplifiers in CMOS technologies: theory and circuit design considerations," *IEEE Communications Magazine*, vol. 42, pp. 6–11, 2004.

[8] Y. Hu, "Wireless interface dedicated to improve power transfer efficiency and bi-directional data communication of implantable electronic devices," in *Electrical Engineering*. vol. Ph.D. Montreal: École Polytechnique de Montréal, 2006, p. 180.

[9] Y. Hu and M. Sawan, "A fully integrated low-power BPSK demodulator for implantable medical devices," *IEEE Transactions on Circuits and Systems I: Regular Papers*, vol. 52, pp. 2552–2562, 2005.

[10] Z. Tang, B. Smith, J. H. Schild, and P. H. Peckham, "Data transmission from an implantable biotelemeter by load-shift keying using circuit configuration modulator," *IEEE Transactions on Biomedical Engineering*, vol. 42, pp. 524–528, 1995.

[11] S. Deng, Y. Hu, and M. Sawan, "A high data rate QPSK demodulator for inductively powered electronics implants," in *The 2006 IEEE International Symposium on Circuits and Systems (ISCAS)*, 2006, pp. 4–7.

[12] "Canadian Table of Frequency Allocations 9 kHz to 275 GHz," by Industry Canada, http://strategis.gc.ca/spectrum.

[13] L. R. Hochberg, M. D. Serruya, G. M. Friehs, J. A. Mukand, M. Saleh, A. H. Caplan, A. Branner, D. Chen, R. D. Penn, and J. P. Donoghue, "Neuronal ensemble control of prosthetic devices by a human with tetraplegia," *Nature*, vol. 442, pp. 164–171, 2006.

[14] M. A. Lebedev and M. A. Nicolelis, "Brain-machine interfaces: past, present and future," *Trends Neurosci*, vol. 29, pp. 536–146, 2006.

[15] R. R. Harrison, P. T. Watkins, R. J. Kier, R. O. Lovejoy, D. J. Black, B. Greger, and F. Solzbacher, "A Low-Power Integrated Circuit for a Wireless 100-Electrode Neural Recording System," *IEEE Journal of Solid-State Circuits*, vol. 42, pp. 123–133, 2007.

[16] R. H. Olsson, III and K. D. Wise, "A three-dimensional neural recording microsystem with implantable data compression circuitry," *IEEE Journal of Solid-State Circuits*, vol. 40, pp. 2796–2804, 2005.

[17] A. P. Chandran, K. Najafi, and K. D. Wise, "A new dc baseline stabilization scheme for neural recording microprobes," in *Proceedings of the First Joint BMES/EMBS Conference*, 1999, p. 386.

[18] Q. Bai and K. D. Wise, "Single-unit neural recording with active microelectrode arrays," *IEEE Transactions on Biomedical Engineering*, vol. 48, pp. 911–920, 2001.

[19] R. R. Harrison and C. Charles, "A low-power low-noise CMOS amplifier for neural recording applications," *IEEE Journal of Solid-State Circuits*, vol. 38, pp. 958–965, 2003.

[20] M. Mojarradi, D. Binkley, B. Blalock, R. Andersen, N. Ulshoefer, T. Johnson, and L. Del Castillo, "A miniaturized neuroprosthesis suitable for implantation into the brain," *IEEE Transactions on Neural Systems and Rehabilitation Engineering*, vol. 11, pp. 38–42, 2003.

[21] C. Du, J. G. Harris, and J. C. Principe, "A bio-amplifier with pulse output," in *The 26th Annual International Conference of the Engineering in Medicine and Biology Society (EMBS)*, 2004, pp. 4071–4074.

[22] P. Mohseni and K. Najafi, "A fully integrated neural recording amplifier with DC input stabilization," *IEEE Transactions on Biomedical Engineering*, vol. 51, pp. 832–837, 2004.

[23] S. Yoon-Kyu, W. R. Patterson, C. W. Bull, J. Beals, H. Naejye, A. P. Deangelis, C. Lay, J. L. McKay, A. V. Nurmikko, M. R. Fellows, J. D. Simeral, J. P. Donoghue, and B. W. Connors, "Development of a chipscale integrated microelectrode/microelectronic device for brain implantable neuroengineering applications," *IEEE Transactions on Neural Systems and Rehabilitation Engineering*, vol. 13, pp. 220–226, 2005.

[24] Y. Perelman and R. Ginosar, "An Integrated System for Multichannel Neuronal Recording With Spike/LFP Separation, Integrated A/D Conversion and Threshold Detection," *IEEE Transactions on Biomedical Engineering*, vol. 54, pp. 130–137, 2007.

[25] E. M. Spinelli, N. Martinez, M. A. Mayosky, and R. Pallas-Areny, "A novel fully differential biopotential amplifier with DC suppression," *IEEE Transactions on Biomedical Engineering*, vol. 51, pp. 1444–1448, 2004.

[26] T. Degen and H. Jackel, "A pseudodifferential amplifier for bioelectric events with DC-offset compensation using two-wired amplifying electrodes," *IEEE Transactions on Biomedical Engineering*, vol. 53, pp. 300–310, 2006.

[27] B. Gosselin, A. E. Ayoub, and M. Sawan, "A Low-Power Bioamplifier With a New Active DC Rejection Scheme," in *The 2006 IEEE International Symposium on Circuits and Systems (ISCAS)*, 2006, pp. 2185–2188.

[28] K. R. Laker and W. M. C. Sansen, *Design of Analog Integrated Circuits and Systems*: McGraw-Hill Companies, 1994.

[29] E. A. Vittoz, "Micropower Techniques" in *Design of analog-digital VLSI circuits for telecommunications and signal processing*, José E. Franca and Y. Tsividis, Eds. Upper Saddle River, NJ, USA: Prentice-Hall, Inc., 1994, pp. 53–96.

[30] C. Enz, F. Krummenacher, and E. A. Vittoz, "An analytical MOS transistor model valid in all regions of operation and dedicated to low-voltage and low-current applications," *Analog Integrated Circuits and Signal Processing*, vol. 8, pp. 83–114, 1995.

[31] D. Johns and K. Martin, *Analog Integrated Circuit Design*: Wiley, 1996.

[32] D. M. Binkley, B. J. Blalock, and J. M. Rochelle, "Optimizing Drain Current, Inversion Level, and Channel Length in Analog CMOS Design," *Analog Integrated Circuits and Signal Processing*, vol. 47, pp. 137–163, 2006.

[33] A. J. Scholten, L. F. Tiemeijer, R. van Langevelde, R. J. Havens, A. T. A. Zegers-van Duijnhoven, and V. C. Venezia, "Noise modeling for RF CMOS circuit simulation," *IEEE Transactions on Electron Devices*, vol. 50, pp. 618–632, 2003.

[34] R. Chandra and L. M. Optican, "Detection, classification, and superposition resolution of action potentials in multiunit single-channel recordings by an on-line real-time neural network," *IEEE Transactions on Biomedical Engineering*, vol. 44, pp. 403–412, 1997.

[35] K. S. Guillory and R. A. Normann, "A 100-channel system for real time detection and storage of extracellular spike waveforms," *Journal of Neuroscience Methods*, vol. 91, pp. 21–29, 1999.

[36] R. R. Harrison, "A low-power integrated circuit for adaptive detection of action potentials in noisy signals," in *The 25th Annual International Conference of the IEEE Engineering in Medicine and Biology Society (EMBS)*, 2003, pp. 3325–3328.

[37] K. Kyung Hwan and K. Sung June, "A wavelet-based method for action potential detection from extracellular neural signal recording with low signal-to-noise ratio," vol. 50, pp. 999–1011, 2003.

[38] I. Obeid and P. D. Wolf, "Evaluation of spike-detection algorithms for a brain-machine interface application," *IEEE Transactions on Biomedical Engineering*, vol. 51, pp. 905–911, 2004.

[39] Z. S. Zumsteg, C. Kemere, S. O'Driscoll, G. Santhanam, R. E. Ahmed, K. V. Shenoy, and T. H. Meng, "Power feasibility of implantable digital spike sorting circuits for neural prosthetic systems," *IEEE Transactions on Neural Systems and Rehabilitation Engineering*, vol. 13, pp. 272–279, 2005.

[40] C. Mead, *Analog VLSI and Neural Systems*: Addison Wesley Publishing Company, 1989.

[41] R. Fried and C. Enz, "A family of very low-power analog building blocks based on CMOS translinear loops," in *The 2nd IEEE-CAS Workshop on Analog and Mixed IC Design*, 1997, pp. 73–78.

[42] K. D. Harris, D. A. Henze, J. Csicsvari, H. Hirase, and G. Buzsaki, "Accuracy of tetrode spike separation as determined by simultaneous intracellular and extracellular measurements," *Journal of Neurophysiology*, vol. 84, pp. 401–414, July 2000.

[43] S. Mukhopadhyay and G. C. Ray, "A new interpretation of nonlinear energy operator and its efficacy in spike detection," *IEEE Transactions on Biomedical Engineering*, vol. 45, pp. 180–187, 1998.

[44] C. Joon Hwan, J. Hae Kyung, and K. Taejeong, "A new action potential detector using the MTEO and its effects on spike sorting systems at low signal-to-noise ratios," *IEEE Transactions on Biomedical Engineering*, vol. 53, pp. 738–746, 2006.

[45] R. Sarpeshkar, R. F. Lyon, and C. Mead, "A Low-Power Wide-Linear-Range Transconductance Amplifier," *Analog Integrated Circuits and Signal Processing*, vol. 13, pp. 123–151, 1997.

[46] C. L. Rogers and J. G. Harris, "A low-power analog spike detector for extracellular neural recordings," in *The 2004 11th IEEE International Conference on Electronics, Circuits and Systems*, 2004, pp. 290–293.

[47] B. C. Wheeler and W. J. Heetderks, "A Comparison of Techniques for Classification of Multiple Neural Signals," *IEEE Transactions on Biomedical Engineering*, vol. BME-29, pp. 752–759, 1982.

[48] M. S. Lewicki, "A review of methods for spike sorting: the detection and classification of neural action potentials," *Network: Computation in Neural Systems*, vol. 9, pp. 53–78, 1998.

[49] G. J. Suaning and N. H. Lovell, "CMOS neurostimulation ASIC with 100 channels, scaleable output, and bidirectional radio-frequency telemetry," *IEEE Transactions on Biomedical Engineering*, vol. 48, pp. 248–260, 2001.

[50] W. Liu, K. Vichienchom, M. Clements, S. C. DeMarco, C. Hughes, E. McGucken, M. S. Humayun, E. De Juan, J. D. Weiland, and R. Greenberg, "A neuro-stimulus chip with telemetry unit for retinal prosthetic device," *IEEE Journal of Solid-State Circuits*, vol. 35, pp. 1487–1497, 2000.

[51] H. Qiuting and M. Oberle, "A 0.5-mW passive telemetry IC for biomedical applications," *IEEE Journal of Solid-State Circuits*, vol. 33, pp. 937–946, 1998.

[52] J. Parramon, P. Doguet, D. Marin, M. Verleyssen, R. Munoz, L. Leija, and E. Valderrama, "ASIC-based batteryless implantable telemetry microsystem for recording purposes," in *The 19th Annual International Conference of the IEEE Engineering in Medicine and Biology Society*, 1997, vol. 5, pp. 2225–2228.

[53] G. Gudnason, E. Bruun, and M. Haugland, "A Chip for an Implantable Neural Stimulator," *Analog Integrated Circuits and Signal Processing*, vol. 22, pp. 81–89, 2000.

[54] B. Smith, T. Zhengnian, M. W. Johnson, S. Pourmehdi, M. M. Gazdik, J. R. Buckett, and P. H. Peckham, "An externally powered, multichannel, implantable stimulator-telemeter for control of paralyzed muscle," *IEEE Transactions on Biomedical Engineering*, vol. 45, pp. 463-475, 1998.

[55] M. Ghovanloo and K. Najafi, "A high data transfer rate frequency shift keying demodulator chip for the wireless biomedical implants," in *The 45th Midwest Symposium on Circuits and Systems (MWSCAS)*, 2002, vol. 3, pp. 433–436.

[56] M. Ghovanloo and K. Najafi, "A high-rate frequency shift keying demodulator chip for wireless biomedical implants," in *The 2003 International Symposium on Circuits and Systems (ISCAS)*, 2003, vol. 5, pp. 45–48.

[57] M. Ghovanloo and K. Najafi, "A wideband frequency-shift keying wireless link for inductively powered biomedical implants," *IEEE Transactions on Circuits and Systems I: Regular Papers*, vol. 51, pp. 2374–2383, 2004.

[58] B. Gosselin, A. E. Ayoub, and M. Sawan, "A Mixed-Signal Multi-Clip Neural Recording Interface with Bandwidth Reduction," *International Workshop on Biomedical Circuits and Systems (BIOCAS)*, Montreal, 2007.

CHAPTER 4

Toward Self-Powered Sensors and Circuits for Biomechanical Implants

Shantau Chakrabartty, Nizar Lajnef, Niell G. Elvin, and Alex Elvin

4.1 Introduction

This chapter describes VLSI circuits and sensors that can be used for long-term fatigue monitoring in biomechanical implants.* Biomechanics refers to the study of the mechanical behavior of living structures, which includes bone, muscles, ligaments, or soft tissue. Examples of biomechanical studies range from understanding the impact of loading on bone density to investigating effects of elevated blood pressure on cardiac muscles. Over the last few decades, this area has been in the forefront of biomedical research due to the success of arthroplasty, which refers to a surgical procedure for replacing dysfunctional joints and bones by prosthetic implants.

In Figure 4.1 candidate regions on a human skeletal system are shown in which arthroplasty has been successfully applied. In 2003, approximately 600,000 hip and knee replacement surgeries were performed in the United States, and it is expected that the demand will grow by 174% for hip replacements and by 673% for knee replacements between 2005 and 2030 [1, 2]. Even though most of these prosthetic implants are expected to last for at least 20 years, many of them suffer premature failures [3–7]. A study by McGee [8] reported wear and loosening of artificial joints as the major cause for replacement of 10–20% of implants within 15–20 years. Another study has shown that excessive wear of artificial knees led to joint swelling (synovitis), bone loss (osteolysis), and ultimately to fatigue due to misalignment or instability of the joint [9]. In such complications, a revision surgery is typically required that has proved to be more traumatic and less successful than the initial surgery [6]. Monitoring these mechanical implants for excessive wear and fatigue is therefore essential for preventing premature failures and for significantly reducing patient discomfort and risk. Unfortunately, current patient follow-ups (i.e., regular check-up routines every 5 years) cannot be uniformly applied to all patients due to the differences in their lifestyles and level of physical activity. An ideal solution is the use of sensors and integrated circuits that can be embedded in the implant. Such sensors can monitor wear and onset of fatigue before the occurrence of any catastrophic mechanical failure.

*An abridged portion of this chapter is currently under review for *IEEE Trans. on Biomedical Circuits and Systems*.

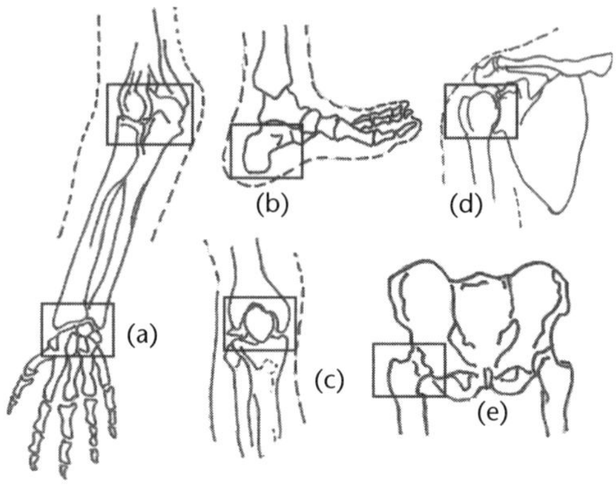

Figure 4.1 Potential candidate regions in-vivo for monitoring fatigue and wear: (a) carpals, (b) tarsals, (c) patella/knee joint, (d) scapula, and (e) acetabular (hip-socket) joint.

4.2 Stress, Strain, and Fatigue Prediction

This section will review some of the basic concepts that will be useful for understanding mechanical loading and fatigue in implants. Stress and strain are two important quantities that characterize the mechanical response of any structure when an external force is applied. Stress is a material's ability to resist any external force whereas strain quantifies the geometrical deformation of a material in response to the external force. Stress can be expressed as the ratio of the external force (F) applied per unit area (A) as

$$\sigma = \frac{F}{A} \tag{4.1}$$

Strain is expressed as a normalized change in shape or size along a direction of measurement:

$$\varepsilon = \frac{\Delta L}{L} \tag{4.2}$$

where $\Delta L, L$ denotes a change in length and original length of the material along the measurement direction. When the change in length is positive, the strain is considered to be a tensile strain, whereas for a negative change in length the strain is considered to be compressive. Due to its dimensionless nature, strain can be expressed either in percentage units or in micro-strain ($\mu\varepsilon$) units as given by $\mu\varepsilon = \mu \times 10^6$. Another important parameter useful for understanding the mechanical property of a material is the Young's modulus (Y) that links stress and strain according to

$$Y = \frac{\sigma}{\varepsilon} \tag{4.3}$$

In practice, the linear relationship between stress and strain in equation (4.3) is valid only for stresses less than yield-stress, a quantity that determines the upper limit beyond which the material looses its elastic properties. Also, the fundamental equations (4.1–4.3) represent measurements only along a single direction. These concepts have, however, been extended to higher dimensions through the use of matrix algebra and tensor calculus. A detailed treatment of multi-dimensional stress and strain, can be found in standard structural engineering texts. With this basic understanding of stress and strain, we can now define fatigue in a material.

The definition of fatigue as adapted from [10] states: "*the progressive, localized, and permanent structural damage that occurs when a material is subjected to cyclic or fluctuating strains at nominal stresses that have maximum values less than (often much less than) the static yield strength of the material. The resulting stress may be below the ultimate tensile stress, or even the yield stress of the material, yet still cause catastrophic failure.*"

In general, the fatigue life of a mechanical component under cyclic load (periodic load) is dependent on the level of the stress in that component and the number of fatigue cycles applied to the specimen [11, 12]. This relationship is typically expressed using an S-N curve, which is used for determining the life of a structural component for constant amplitude low stress levels (within the elastic limit of the material). An example of an S-N curve as shown in Figure 4.2, summarizes the approximate number of cycles required to cause ultimate failure of a component as a function of the magnitude of the applied cycling load (in terms of unit strain). Higher strain levels require fewer cycles to cause damage, whereas low strain levels that are typical in most orthopedic implants require many more cycles to cause damage. An important consequence of the S-N curve is that stress cycles less than the so-called fatigue limit stress should not cause the material to fail (often taken as a stress level that can withstand 10^7 cycles). In the context of fatigue monitoring, it is therefore unimportant to measure loading strains less than the fatigue limit of the material since they do not contribute to overall damage of the material. For many steels, the fatigue strain limit is greater than 1500 $\mu\varepsilon$. However, the S-N curve cannot be directly used to

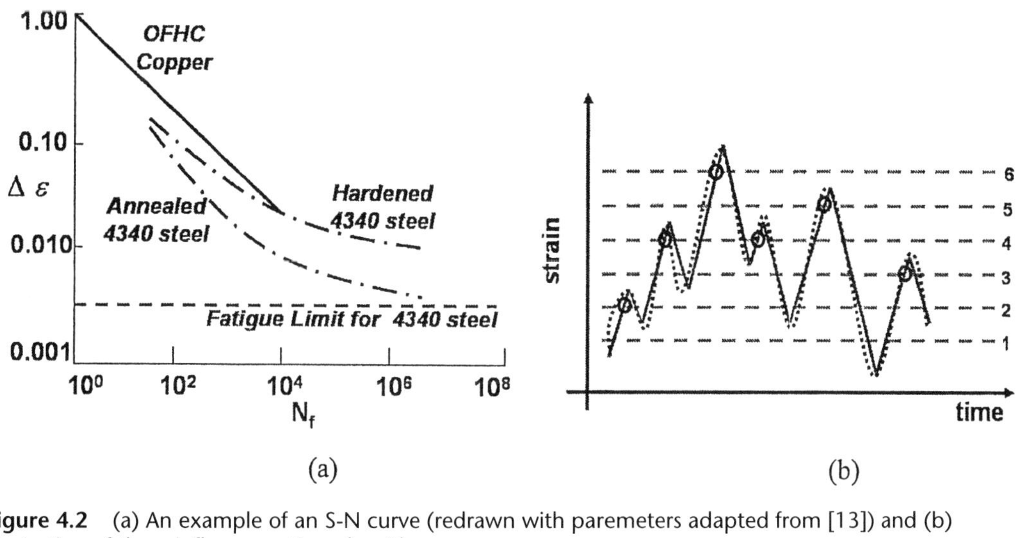

Figure 4.2 (a) An example of an S-N curve (redrawn with paremeters adapted from [13]) and (b) illustration of the rainflow counting algorithm.

determine the fatigue in an implant, as in real-world conditions the magnitude of the applied cyclic loads varies depending on the environmental conditions. For example, walking, running, or climbing can produce significantly different loading conditions in a knee or hip implant. Several algorithms have been proposed in literature for fatigue life-time predictions under non-periodic loading conditions. The most common and widely used algorithm is the Palmgren-Miner's Rule [20] often simply called the Miner's rule. In its basic form, the Miner's rule assumes that each strain cycle with magnitude i consumes $1/N_i$ of the total fatigue life, where N_i is the number of fatigue cycles taken to fail the material at a strain level of i. Algebraically this can be stated as

$$\sum \frac{n_i}{N_i} = 1 \tag{4.4}$$

The Miner's rule algorithm is by no means perfect and was not developed for all possible loading conditions. However, it is still routinely used in practice to estimate the fatigue life for structural components.

A pre-processing step is required before Miner's rule can be applied to calculate statistics of the arbitrary loading cycles. One of the popular pre-processing techniques is the rainflow-counting method that reduces a spectrum of varying stress-strain measurements into a set of simple stress-strain reversals [14, 15, 16]. This is illustrated in Figure 4.2(b), where the measured strain (denoted by the dotted curve) is simplified by a strain reversal curve shown by the solid line. The algorithm then counts the total occurrence of events when the magnitude of strain exceeds a predefined threshold. The thresholds are typically quantized strain levels as shown in Figure 4.2(b), which also shows the events (denoted by circles). The total count of events denoted by $n_i : i = 1,\ldots,6$ is then normalized by N_i (from the S-N curve) according to the Miner's rule.

4.3 In Vivo Strain Measurement and Motivation for Self-Powered Sensing

To date, the most popular approach for measuring strain, whether compressive or tensile, is using a strain gauge. Strain gauges are typically made of a piezoresistive material (Constantan, NichromeV, tungsten, Karma-type alloy wires, or even semiconductor materials) [17] which when subjected to mechanical strain leads to a change in electrical resistance. Since its first application in the 1930s, strain gauges have not only shrunk in size but have become more sensitive (quantified by gauge factor, which is the normalized change in resistance for an applied strain) [18, 19]. Metallic strain gauges can demonstrate a gauge factor up to 10 but the next generation of gauges fabricated using nanocomposites promise gauge factors beyond 30 [20–23]. Several studies have incorporated strain sensors in orthopedic implants for continuous monitoring under laboratory conditions. In [52] temporary implants containing four load cells were used to measure knee joint forces and in another study [53] a similar setup was used to measure tibial forces. In vivo strain gauges have also been in distal femoral replacements and in hip implants [51–57]. Most of these experiments have been used for logging data only for short duration and have either used remote power delivery or have used external leads through the skin to provide power. However, both power delivery mechanisms limit the mobility of the patient and are therefore unrealistic for autonomous monitoring.

One of the attractive solutions towards achieving long-term monitoring is "self-powered sensing," where electrical energy can be directly harvested from the signal being sensed. Energy harvesting has received a lot of attention in recent years [24, 25, 26, 27, 28, 29] primarily driven by the need to power networks of broadly distributed autonomous sensors. Even though a number of potential self-powering energy sources can be employed (e.g., solar, thermal, and vibrational), only a few are capable of providing the ~100 μW of continuous power typically required to operate a single sensor ([30], PicoRadio Project UC Berkeley).

Piezoelectric transducers not only provide a mechanism for sensing strain in a structure but also can be used for self-powering of the sensors through energy harvesting [35]. Piezoelectric-based "self-powered sensing" for medical implants have several advantages over traditional battery-powered techniques that suffer from limited life, large form factor, and complications due to biocompatibility. Polyvinylidene diflouride (PVDF) is a piezoelectric plastic that is currently used for suture materials and has proven to be biocompatible [36]. However, a major disadvantage of PVDF is its very low mechano-electrical energy conversion. Given the typical strain levels experienced by biomechanical structures (Table 4.1), and using the generator model, the extractable power was estimated to be less than 1 μW for a PVDF sheet of dimensions "31mm × 16mm × 0.028mm" loaded at a 1 Hz frequency. We have also shown experimentally that the power generated from a PVDF sensor for a hip-implant monitoring is indeed 1 μW [37]. This is well below the current wireless-sensor nodes power consumption of approximately 50 mW that is required for commercially available, ultra-low power wireless sensor nodes (Telos-Mote). Several research groups [30, 38] are currently working on decreasing the power requirement for wireless motes, but even these low-power wireless sensor network nodes would require a minimum energy level of 100 μW. Arms et al. [39] have shown feasibility of a self-powered wireless strain sensor requiring power levels of 1 mW (they claim this is a 20 times improvement over all previous designs). Even these low-power designs still require 100 times more power than would be available in a typical biomedical implant. Table 4.2 summarizes the state-of-art energy efficient computation and storage techniques reported in the literature, illustrating that most technologies fall short of the energy efficiency constraints imposed by self-powered fatigue sensing.

Table 4.1 Typical Strain Levels in In Vivo Biological Tissue

Structures	*Typical Strain Levels*
Nerves	0.1%–20% [31]
Bones	0.04%–0.16% [32]
Ligaments	0.1%–4% [33]
Muscles	0.1%–5% [34]

Table 4.2 Approximate Energy Consumption in a Wireless Sensor Node

Operation	*Commercial*	*Research*
Microprocessor Operation[a]	350 μW [44]	20 μW [40]
Receive 1 bit	200 nJ [47]	12 pJ [41]
Transmit 1 bit	200 nJ [42]	16 pJ [41]
Retain Volatile Memory (VM)—1 bit	100 pW [44]	replaced by NVM
Write 1 bit to NVM	200 nJ [43]	25 pJ [45]
Analog-Digital (A/D) Conversion—1 bit	2 nJ [44]	50 pJ [41]
Sleep	300 nW [44]	5 nW [41]
Digital Signal Processing[a]	200 μW [46]	20 μW[40]
Pin Leakage	100 nW [44]	2.2 nW [48]

[a] Operation is scaled to processor speeds of 500 kHz. Volatile memory (VM) is assumed to be replaced by low-power non-volatile memory (NVM) [68].

It should also be noted that in the context of fatigue monitoring it is important to be able to capture each loading cycling. Many biomechanical structures are only subjected to significant loading cycles (i.e., greater than the fatigue limit) infrequently. During the times between significant loading cycles, it is possible that the sensor would experience periods of brown-outs and black-outs since any on-board rechargeable battery or storage capacitor might loose the charge between these intermittent loading cycles. This motivates the use of non-volatile memory storage, i.e., volatile memory storage would be lost during power black-outs.

The functional specification of a complete self-powered fatigue sensor can therefore be summarized as follows:

1. **Self-powered computation:** Energy to perform sensing and computation on the sensor has to be harvested from the converted mechanical signal.
2. **Non-volatile storage:** All the parameters of the internal state variables (intermediate and final) have to be stored on a non-volatile memory to account for unavailability of power (i.e., black-outs).
3. **Sub-microwatt operation:** All computation and storage functions have to be performed at sub-microwatt power dissipation levels to meet the power budget requirement of 1 μW.

Previous research in our group [49] has shown that it is possible to self-power some basic electronic switching and RF circuits using a 28 μm $\times$ 4 cm^2 polyvinylidene fluoride (PVDF) piezoelectric material under a single trapezoidal pulse of applied strain (approximately 1500 $\mu\varepsilon$ in magnitude and 0.5 seconds in duration). The estimated total energy generated by the loading is approximately 3 nJ. This corresponds to an average operational power level of 3 nW. The piezoelectric generated voltage is approximately 15 V. In this experiment, it would be possible theoretically to increase this energy level by a factor of 100 (i.e., generate 300 nJ) by using a 0.2 mm $\times$ 4 cm^2 lead zirconate titanate PZT piezoelectric material under the same loading conditions. However, bulk PZT is typically damaged under applied tensile loads of 500 $\mu\varepsilon$, which limits its practical application for fatigue monitoring of strains greater than 500 $\mu\varepsilon$. It should be noted that several research groups [50] have developed PZT composites with excellent mechanical-electrical coupling that are also flexible and can sustain strains greater than 1700 $\mu\varepsilon$. At this stage these materials remain expensive, but the price could be reduced with increased demand.

4.4 Fundamentals of Piezoelectric Transduction and Power Delivery

Piezoelectric materials have the unique ability both to generate mechanical movement when a voltage is applied to them, and conversely generate electrical charge when stressed mechanically. Piezoelectric materials have been proposed for a number of medical applications; it is best known for it extensive use in medical ultrasound. Ultrasound relies on an array of piezoelectric elements that are excited by a synchronized voltage source creating the focused ultrasonic wave. The same array is then switched into sensing mode to measure the reflected wave. Piezoelectric implants have been proposed in orthopaedics [51, 52, 53], dentistry [54], audiology [54], cardiology [56], and neurology.

Piezoelectric powered implants were proposed as early as 1969 by Ko [57]. However, it was not until 1984 when Hasler [58] and Cochran et al. 1985 [51] demonstrated the first in-vivo self-powered piezoelectric implant. Hasler [58] showed a micro-implant capable of generating 1 mW of power from stretching of human ribs during breathing. Cochran et al. 1985 [51] showed a piezoelectric implantable internal fracture fixation device that is capable of generating microampere current either through external ultrasonic actuation or through direct loading during walking. It was proposed that the generated current could then be used to simulate bone growth. Subsequently Elvin et al. [37] proposed a fracture healing sensor that was capable of measuring and wirelessly transmitting the increase in bone stiffness during fracture healing. Due to the large loads applied during normal walking, self-powering for orthopedic monitoring was one of the first applications proposed and studied for piezoelectric self powering [37, 51]. Using a nine-channel inductively powered strain wireless sensor, Bergmann et al. (2001) [59] has shown that peak contact forces on a hip implant is approximately 2.5 times body weight even at moderate walking speeds, as shown in Figure 4.3.

4.4.1 Piezoelectric Basics

The direct piezoelectric effect is the ability of certain crystalline materials to generate electric charge from an applied mechanical stress. Consider a piezoelectric material with dimensions $L \times b \times h$ polled through its thickness with electrodes on the top and bottom surfaces (Figure 4.4).

A mechanical force (F) is applied along the materials length.

The generated voltage can be expressed in a number of different ways as shown below:

$$V = \frac{Fg_{31}}{b} = SY^E hg_{31} = \frac{SY^E d_{31} h}{\varepsilon} \tag{4.5}$$

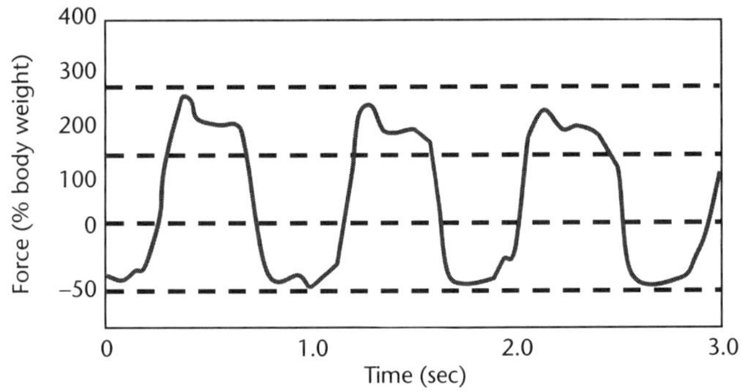

Figure 4.3 Typical loading on the hip during normal walking.

where V is the generated voltage, g_{31} and d_{31} are piezoelectric constants, S is the applied mechanical strain, Y^E is the short circuit elastic modulus and ε is the electrical permittivity. Another important property of piezoelectric materials is their capacitance. The capacitance of a piezoelectric generator is given by

$$C = \frac{LW\varepsilon}{h} \tag{4.6}$$

Two different piezoelectric material classes are commonly used for electric energy harvesting. The first class of material is a ceramic composed of lead zirconate titanate (PZT), the second is a semi-crystalline plastic polyvinylidene fluoride (PVDF). These two materials have very different properties and are typically used for different applications. The mechanical and electrical properties of these two materials are compared in Table 4.3.

To illustrate the difference between the two materials, consider two piezoelectric strips 30 mm long and 12 mm wide. PVDF is typically formed in 20 μm thickness, while PZT is manufactured in thicknesses of 0.1 mm or thicker.

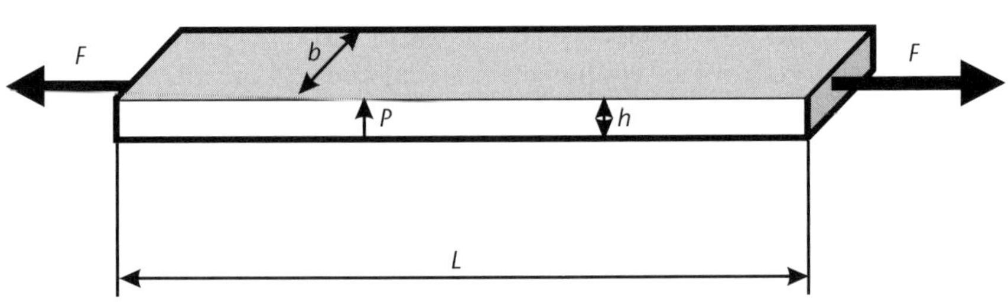

Figure 4.4 Schematic depiction of a piezoelectric material pulled by a force F. The material undergoes an axial strain of S.

Table 4.3 Comparison of Material Properties of Two Commonly Used Piezoelectric Materials

Property	*PVDF*	*PXT-5H*
Young's Modulus Y^E	2×10^9N/m^2	60×10^9N/m^2
Permittivity (ε)	106×10^{-12}F/m	106×10^{-10}F/m
Piezo Strain Constant (d_{31})	23×10^{-12}C/N	110×10^{-12}C/N
Piezo Stress Constant (g_{31})	216×10^{-3}m/C	10×10^{-3}m/C

1. For L = 30 mm, W = 12 mm, T = 28 μm PVDF film: C = 1.36 nF; V = 12×10^{-3} V/$\mu\varepsilon$
2. For L = 30 mm, W = 12 mm, T = 100 μm PZT: C = 38 nF; V = 65 V/$\mu\varepsilon$

Though PZT can generate significantly more voltage than PVDF per unit strain, PZT is a brittle ceramic and thus can fracture at relatively low strains. Furthermore, tensile strains as low as 500 $\mu\varepsilon$ can cause fatigue damage in PZT. On the other hand, PVDF is a flexible plastic that can withstand at least 10,000 $\mu\varepsilon$ of applied tensile strain. PVDF has been extensively used in medical sutures for its excellent flexibility and biocompatibility. The biocompatibility of PZT is unknown. However, since one of the basic elements of PZT is lead, it is unlikely that it will be readily implanted without significant testing and approval by the Food and Drug Administration (FDA). Furthermore, its brittleness could cause particular debris that might be toxic to cells.

4.4.2 Piezoelectric Modeling

Piezoelectric material is typically used in two energy harvesting modalities. The first modality is by attaching the material to a substrate and applying a slowly changing dynamic load. In this modality, the piezoelectric element can be modeled using a simple high-pass filter circuit as shown in Figure 4.5. The piezoelectric voltage generated is given by Equation (4.5). The capacitance is given by Equation (4.6). The nature of the high-pass filter circuit shows that very little voltage is generated for slow loading rates. The adequate matching of both the generated voltage and the capacitance to the applied mechanical load magnitude and frequency content is therefore critical for maximal electrical energy generation. It should be noted that the method of attachment (bond) of the piezoelectric material to its substrate in this modality is critical, and significant voltage loss (a factor as high as two to four) is common.

If the sensor circuit in Figure 4.5 is modeled by a resistor R_L, then for a harmonic loading of the piezoelectric transducer at a frequency f Hz the magnitude of voltage across the sensor is given by

$$V_L(f) = \frac{2\pi f R_L C V}{\left(1 + 4\pi^2 f^2 R_L^2 C^2\right)^{1/2}} \tag{4.7}$$

and the power delivered to the sensor is $P_L = \frac{V_L^2(f)}{R_L}$. The maximum power that can

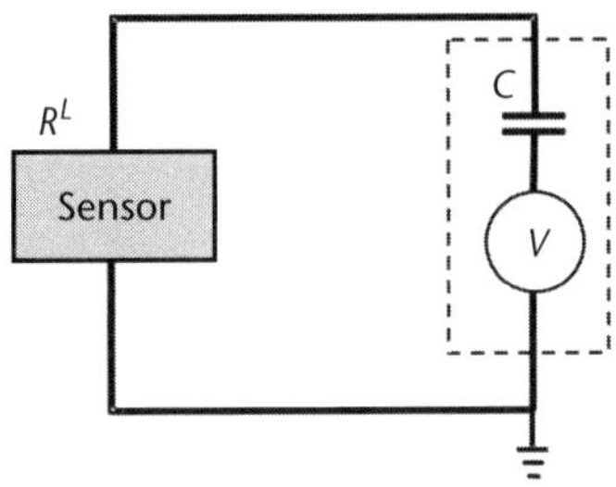

Figure 4.5 Equivalent circuit diagram (the dashed block) for a piezoelectric material under slow dynamic loading. The voltage (V) and capacitance (C) is given by Equations (4.5) and (4.6), respectively.

be delivered at a loading frequency can be obtained by optimizing Equation (4.7) with respect to R_L which can be expressed as the condition

$$\frac{dP_L}{dR_L} = \frac{4\pi^2 f^2 C^2 R_L V}{\left(1+4\pi^2 f^2 R_L^2 C^2\right)} - \frac{16\pi^4 f^4 C^4 R_L^3 V}{\left(1+4\pi^2 f^2 R_L^2 C^2\right)^2} = 0 \tag{4.8}$$

The optimal value of the load resistance R_L is given by

$$R_L = \frac{1}{2\pi f C} \tag{4.9}$$

For a loading frequency of 1 Hz and a transducer capacitance of 10 nF the optimal load according to Equation (4.9) is 15 MΩ. For a 5-V input, this is equivalent to a load current of 300 nA. This simple calculation demonstrates the importance of a fatigue sensor that consumes less than 1 μA current.

The second mode of energy generation is through higher frequency vibration. In this case the piezoelectric material is driven by ambient mechanical vibration. The approximate equivalent circuit for this excitation is given in Figure 4.6 [28, 29]. The two modalities are typically used under different ambient mechanical operating conditions. For example, although relatively large impact accelerations are available during walking, the vibrating generator (Figure 4.6) requires a non-negligible volume to house the vibrating mass. This size constraint might limit the applicability of this modality for implantable applications. However, the significant progress in MEMS piezoelectric harvesters might allow for smaller-scale implantable vibration scavengers.

In general, an energy storage circuit is required to store the generated electrical energy. One typical circuit is shown in Figure 4.7. At low voltage generation levels, the losses through the various circuit elements are significant and need to be minimized.

4.4.3 Orthopaedic Applications

As previously mentioned, the relatively high and repetitive nature of loads applied during walking makes orthopaedics an attractive area for implantable energy har-

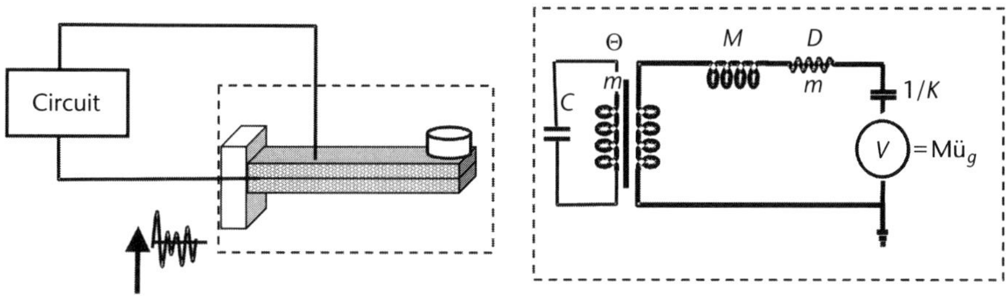

Figure 4.6 Equivalent circuit diagram (the dashed block) for a piezoelectric bimorph cantilever beam under arbitrary dynamic loading. The voltage ($M\ddot{u}_g$) is dependent on the excitation acceleration ($\ddot{u}_g$) and tip mass (M). The mechanical stiffness (K), damping (D), piezoelectric coupling (θ) are a function of the material properties and geometry of the piezoelectric material.

vesters. Two applications are considered. The first is a "smart intramedullary (IM) rod." IM rods are used to fix a fracture in long bones. The rod is driven into the intramedullary canal of the bone, and provides fixation to the bone until the fracture heals. 5% to 10% of these long bone fractures do not heal properly, and there is currently no way of assessing the extent and progress of fracture healing since radiographs only provide a basic visual assessment.

The flexible and low-profile advantages of PVDF film makes it ideal for attaching it to the small radius IM nail. Testing under physiological walking loads produces approximately 1200 $\mu\varepsilon$ on the nail surface, which corresponds to 14.5 volts (open circuit) per step for a 5 cm × 4 cm × 28 μm PVDF film. Using the storage capacitor circuit in Figure 4.7, this corresponds to approximately 0.2 μJ per steps or an average power of 0.16 μW. The generated electrical power can be used to power a simple RF link [35]. The number of steps required to activate the RF link directly indicates the mechanical force carried by the IM rod. As normal healing progresses, the bone carries more mechanical load and thus the number of steps to power the RF link increases. The hip and knee implants are typically much stiffer than IM nails. For example, the mechanical strains at the neck of a hip implant are approximately 200 $\mu\varepsilon$ during normal walking.

This corresponds to 2.4 volts (open circuit) per step for a 5 cm × 4 cm × 28 μm PVDF film. Once again, using the storage capacitor circuit in Figure 4.7, this corresponds to approximately 6 nJ per steps or an average power of 4 nW. For the total hip implant, six times more piezoelectric material is required to produce the same power level as for the IM nail (assuming the same loading magnitude). Figure 4.8

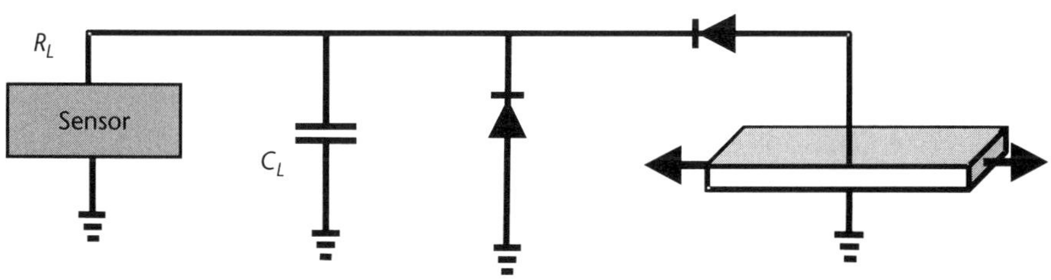

Figure 4.7 A typical piezoelectric generator storage circuit. Charge is collected during each load cycle on the capacitor.

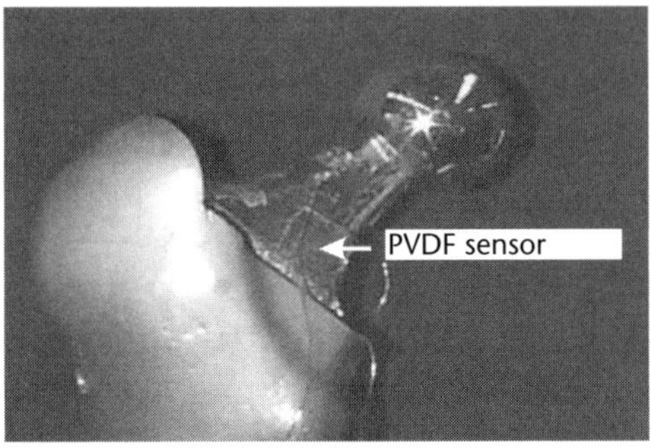

Figure 4.8 Stainless steel hip implant with three layers of 28μ PVDF film. The PVDF film is placed on the frontal and dorsal plane to measure torsional loads during activities such as stair-climbing and rising from a chair. The open circuit voltage generated by the piezoelectric is 2.4 volts.

shows a commercially available stainless steel instrumented total hip implant with an attached three layers of 28 μm PVDF film. This implant is capable of generating 2.4 volts per step when subjected to physiological loading. Platt et al. [52] are working on a self-powered knee implant using PZT. As previously mentioned, the biocompatibility and brittleness of PZT remain issues that have to be addressed. The self-powered total knee implant consists of a 1 cm × 1 cm × 1.8 cm PZT piezoelectric element. This implant is capable of generating approximately 2 mW of power under physiological loading.

4.5 Sub-Microwatt Piezo-Powered VLSI Circuits

The previous sections discussed some of the limitations of self-powering using piezoelectric transduction. Even though the transducer can generate a large open load voltage (> 15 V), its capacitive nature (see Figure 4.6) limits the total current that can be delivered to its load. Typically, this current is in the order of nanoamperes for a loading cycle of 1 Hz or less. The properties of the piezoelectric transducer, however, are attractive for operating analog floating-gate circuits that typically require high voltage for programming. A floating gate is a poly-silicon gate surrounded by an insulator, which in the standard semiconductor fabrication process is silicon-dioxide [60, 61]. Because a floating gate is surrounded by high-quality insulation any electrical charge injected onto this gate is retained for long intervals of time (> 8 years). The principle of operation of an integrated piezoelectric floating-gate sensor is illustrated in Figure 4.9, in which the floating gate is coupled to a p-channel metal-oxide-semiconductor (pMOS) transistor. The electrical energy produced by the piezoelectric transducer is used to inject electrons from the transistor channel onto the floating gate. The repeated accumulation of charge on the floating gate is indicative of the history of mechanical loading and therefore can be used as an integrated platform for sensing, computation, and storage in fatigue monitoring applications. The following sections present an overview of the VLSI circuits based on this principle to implement a fatigue monitoring microsystem.

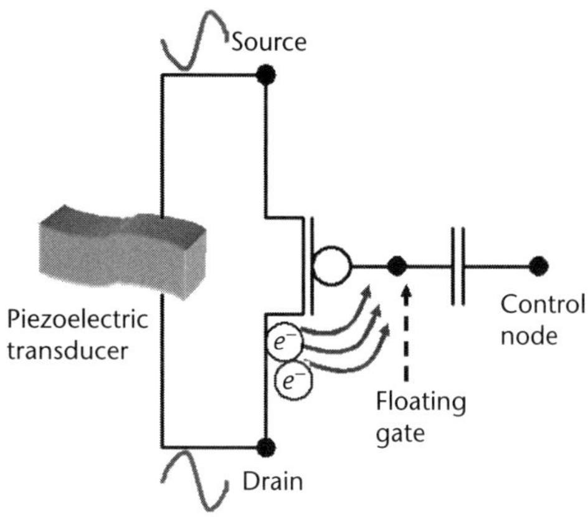

Figure 4.9 Principle of the piezo-powered floating-gate sensor.

4.5.1 Floating-Gate Transistors

In a standard CMOS process, a floating gate is a poly-silicon gate surrounded by silicon-dioxide that acts an insulator. When the floating gate is coupled to a gate of a transistor, as shown in Figure 4.10(a), the cumulative charge stored on the floating gate can be sensed by measuring the transistor's drain current.

The charge on the gate can be modified using either hot electron injection or using tunneling [61]. Hot electron injection in a pMOS transistor occurs when a high-electric field is formed at the drain-to-channel depletion region. Due to this high-electric field, the holes gain significant energy to dislodge electrons by hot-hole impact ionization. The released electrons travel back into the channel region, gaining energy and when their kinetic energy exceeds the silicon and silicon-dioxide (> 3.2 eV) barrier, the electrons are injected into the oxide. As more electrons are added to the floating gate, its potential decreases, which results in an equivalent increase in the drain current through the transistor. Hot-electron injection in a pMOS transistor is a feedback process because an increase in injection onto the floating gate (decrease in gate potential) reinforces the injection process. Thus injection is required to be carefully controlled to be able to perform any useful and sustained computation. Empirically, the injection current has been found to be proportional to the source current through the pMOS cell and drain-to-channel (source) potential and can be expressed as

$$I_{inj} = I_S e^{f(V_{dc})} \tag{4.10}$$

where $f(V_{dc})$ is a smooth function of drain-to-channel potential V_{dc} and I_S is the source current through the pMOS transistor. Figure 4.10(b) shows measured injection characteristics of a pMOS floating-gate transistor when the source-to-drain terminal is subjected to pulses (duration 1 second) of varying voltage amplitude. For each excitation pulse, the pMOS transistor injects a packet of charge on the floating gate that results in an increase in the drain current. Subsequently, a larger packet of charge is injected per pulse as evident from Figure 4.10(b) reiterating the positive

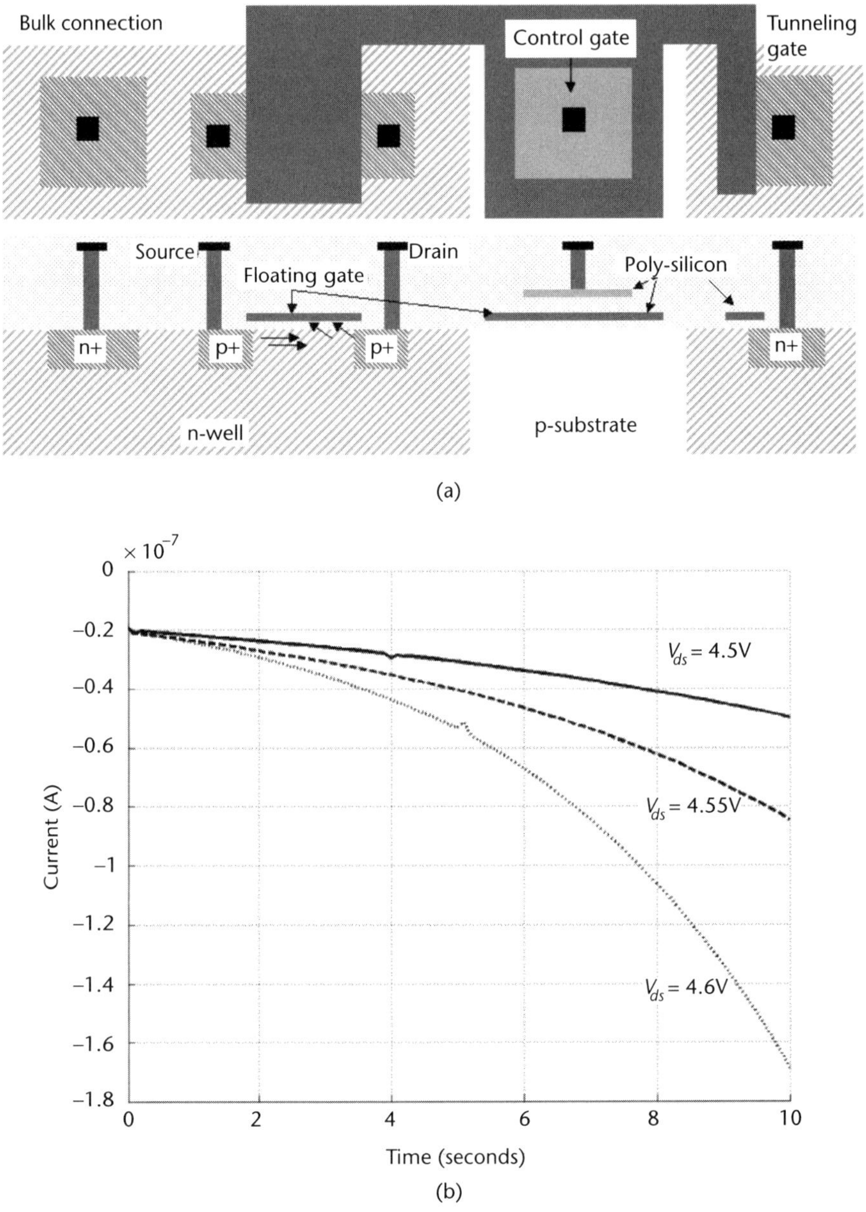

Figure 4.10 (a) Top and cross-sectional view of a floating-gate transistor and (b) the measured drain current when injection pulses of different amplitude are repeatedly applied across the drain-source terminal.

feedback nature of pMOS injection. This mechanism has been used by several researchers to accelerate programming of the floating gate to a pre-determined voltage. It has also been demonstrated that the injection current is practically independent of the floating-gate-to-channel potential, as long as the gate potential is greater than the drain potential, which is naturally satisfied for pMOS transistors operating in weak-inversion. For a pMOS transistor fabricated in a 0.5 μm CMOS process and biased in weak-inversion, drain-to-source voltages greater than 4.2 V have been found to be sufficient for onset of hot-electron injection [34]. It can also be seen from equation (4.10) that the injection efficiency (ratio of injection current to source current) is practically constant over different values of source current [34]. Therefore, compared to digital FLASH programming, analog floating-gate programming can be performed with power dissipation as small as 100 pW during the write cycle. Even though equation (4.10) has been expressed in terms of drain-to-channel potential, different variants of equation (4.10) have been proposed that employ measurable potentials that are the drain, source, and gate potentials. In our study, we have found a simplified empirical model to be sufficient for injection-based circuits and it is expressed as

$$I_{inj} \approx \beta I_S e^{\frac{V_{sd}}{V_{inj}}} \tag{4.11}$$

where β and V_{inj} are bias-dependent parameters. Hot-electron injection is typically a one-way process in which electrons can be added to the floating gate.

Removal of electrons from the floating gate can be achieved either through exposure to ultraviolet (UV) radiation or by use of tunneling. Tunneling is a quantum mechanical phenomenon whereby the electrons, instead of surmounting an energy barrier, propagate through it. A tunneling capacitor as shown in Figure 4.10(a) is coupled to the floating gate and a large potential is applied to initiate tunneling. The magnitude of the tunneling current has been empirically determined as

$$I_{tun} \approx -I_{tun0} e^{-\frac{V_f}{V_{ox}}} \tag{4.12}$$

where I_{tun0} is a pre-exponential current, V_{ox} is the voltage across the oxide, and V_f is a constant that depends on the oxide thickness. In addition to the tunneling capacitor, the floating gate is capacitively coupled to other terminals. A model of a pMOS floating-gate transistor with capacitive elements is shown in Figure 4.11.

The control gate capacitance C_{cg} serves as the dominant capacitance and is used for modulating the drain-to-source current. The tunneling capacitor in Figure 4.11 is denoted by C_{tun}, the parasitic capacitance between the supply voltage and substrate is denoted by C_{dd} and C_{sub} respectively and the overlap capacitance between

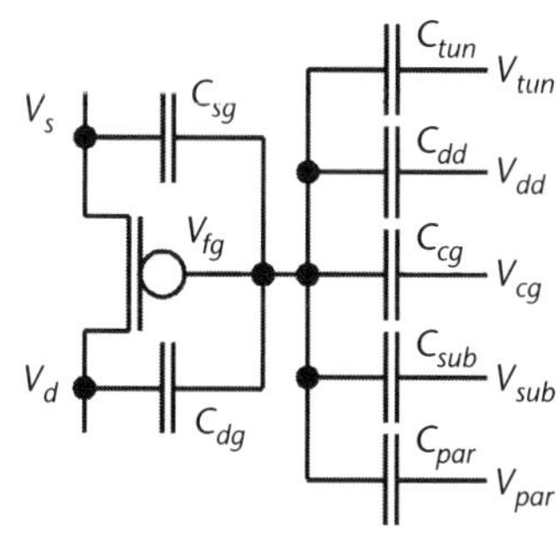

Figure 4.11 Capacitive model of a pMOS floating-gate transistor.

the floating gate to the drain and source terminal is denoted by C_{dg} and C_{sg}. The auxiliary parasitic capacitance to the neighboring buses is denoted by a lumped capacitance C_{par}. All these capacitors play key roles in achieving uniform and matched injection response in an array of floating-gate transistors. Based on the circuit model in Figure 4.11, the voltage on the floating gate V_{fg} can be expressed as

$$V_{fg} = \frac{Q_{fg} + C_{cg}V_{cg} + C_{dd}V_{dd} + C_{sub}V_{sub} + C_{par}V_{par} + C_{dg}V_d + C_{sg}V_s + C_{tun}V_{tun}}{C_T} \tag{4.13}$$

where $C_T = C_{cg} + C_{dd} + C_{sub} + C_{par} + C_{dg} + C_{sg} + C_{tun}$ and Q_{fg} is the residual charge on the floating gate modulated by injection and tunneling. The source-to-drain current through the pMOS transistor when biased in weak-inversion can then be expressed in terms of the floating-gate voltage V_{fg}, drain voltage V_d, and source voltage V_s as

$$I_{ds} = I_o \frac{W}{L} \exp(-\kappa \frac{V_{fg}}{U_T}) \left[\exp(\frac{V_s}{U_T}) - \exp(\frac{V_d}{U_T}) \right] \tag{4.14}$$

where W and L are the width and length of the transistors, κ is the floating gate efficiency, I_o is the specific current, and U_T is the thermal voltage with value 26 mV at room temperature. For $V_{sd} > 3U_T$, equation (4.14) simplifies to

$$I_{ds} = I_o \frac{W}{L} \exp(-\kappa \frac{V_{fg}}{U_T}) \exp(\frac{V_s}{U_T}) \tag{4.15}$$

which is the saturated mode of operation for the pMOS transistor biased in weak-inversion.

4.5.2 Floating-Gate Injector and Its Mathematical Model

The schematic of a single-channel piezo-powered floating-gate sensor is shown in Figure 4.12.

The injection rate of the floating gate transistor Q_1 can be controlled by limiting the source current in equation (4.11) by a constant current reference I_b. Also, as shown later, the drain-to-source voltage can be controlled by inserting diodes between the current reference and the floating-gate transistor. Let V_g denote the voltage of the floating gate at a fixed control gate bias voltage V_B. The total floating-gate capacitance is given by C_T according to equation (4.13). The current reference biases the floating transistor in weak-inversion satisfying the following relationship:

$$I_b = I_o \frac{W}{L} \exp\left(-\kappa \frac{V_g}{U_T}\right) \exp\left(\frac{V_{out}}{U_T}\right) \tag{4.16}$$

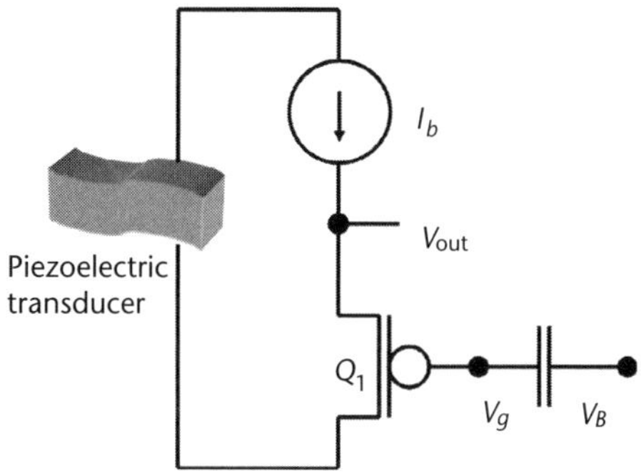

Figure 4.12 Simplified circuit model for piezo-driven floating-gate sensor. From [67] with permission, © IEEE 2007.

Provided that conditions are suitable for hot-electron injection (high-electric field at the drain-to-channel region), the injection current charges the floating gate capacitor according to

$$I_{inj} = -C_T \frac{dV_g}{dt} = \beta I_b \exp\left(\frac{V_{out}}{V_{inj}}\right) \tag{4.17}$$

where we have used the Equation (4.11).

Eliminating the variable V_{out} using equation (4.16) and (4.17), the first-order differential equation is obtained in terms of the gate voltage V_g:

$$C_T \frac{dV_g}{dt} = -\beta \frac{(I_b)^{1+\frac{U_T}{V_{inj}}}}{(I_o \frac{W}{L})^{\frac{U_T}{V_{inj}}}} \exp\left(\kappa \frac{V_g}{V_{inj}}\right) \tag{4.18}$$

which is written in its closed form as

$$V_g(t) = -\frac{1}{K_2} \log\left(K_1 K_2 \int_{\tau \in t} d\tau + \exp\left(-K_2 V_{g0}\right)\right) \tag{4.19}$$

with the values of K_1 and K_2 given by

$$K_1 = \left(\frac{\beta I_b}{C_T}\right)\left(\frac{I_b}{I_o}\frac{W}{L}\right)^{\frac{U_t}{V_{inj}}}$$

$$K_2 = \frac{\kappa}{V_{inj}}$$

V_{g0} in equation (4.19) is the initial floating-gate voltage and t denotes the total duration during which the injector circuit in Figure 4.12 is operational. The output voltage $V_{out}(t)$ can also be expressed in terms of $V_g(t)$ as

$$V_{out}(t) = V_g(t) + K_3 \tag{4.20}$$

with $K_3 = U_T \log\left(\frac{I_b}{I_o}\right)$.

Figure 4.13 shows a typical response of the output voltage $V_{out}(t)$ as a function of injection duration t. The response as shown in Figure 4.12 consists of two distinct regions. The linear region which is characterized by the condition $t << \frac{\exp(-K_2 V_{g0})}{K_1 K_2}$, and by using which equation (4.19) can simplified as

$$V_{out}\left(t\right) = V_{g0} + K_3 - \frac{K_1 K_2}{\exp\left(-K_2 V_{g0}\right)} t \tag{4.21}$$

where the approximation $\log(1 + x) \approx x$ has been used. Thus in the linear region, the change in the output voltage is linear with respect to the injection duration and therefore is suitable for short-term fatigue monitoring (typically less than 100 loading cycles). The other region, which is particularly important for long-term monitoring, is the log-linear region and is characterized by the condition $t >> \frac{\exp(-K_2 V_{g0})}{K_1 K_2}$, which when applied to equation (4.19) leads to

$$V_{out}\left(t\right) = K_3 - \frac{1}{K_2}\log(K_1 K_2) - \frac{1}{K_2}\log(t) \tag{4.22}$$

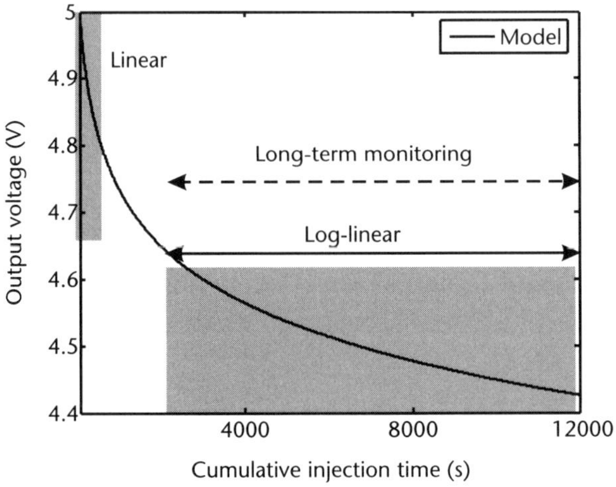

Figure 4.13 Response of a floating-gate injector based on the mathematical model in equation 4.19.

Thus, the change in output voltage is a logarithmic function of time and could be used for long-term event monitoring. The first part in equation (4.22) is an offset term that captures the dependence of the output voltage on the biasing conditions, initial conditions, and ambient temperature.

Figure 4.14(a) and (b) show the output voltage $V_{out}(t)$ response plotted on a logarithmic scale for typical values of parameters K_1,K_2. It can be seen from Figure 4.14(a) that the slope of the log-linear response is a function of K_2 and hence determines the maximum monitoring duration. Using typical parameters obtained from a 0.5 μm CMOS process, we have verified that "log-linear" response can easily last

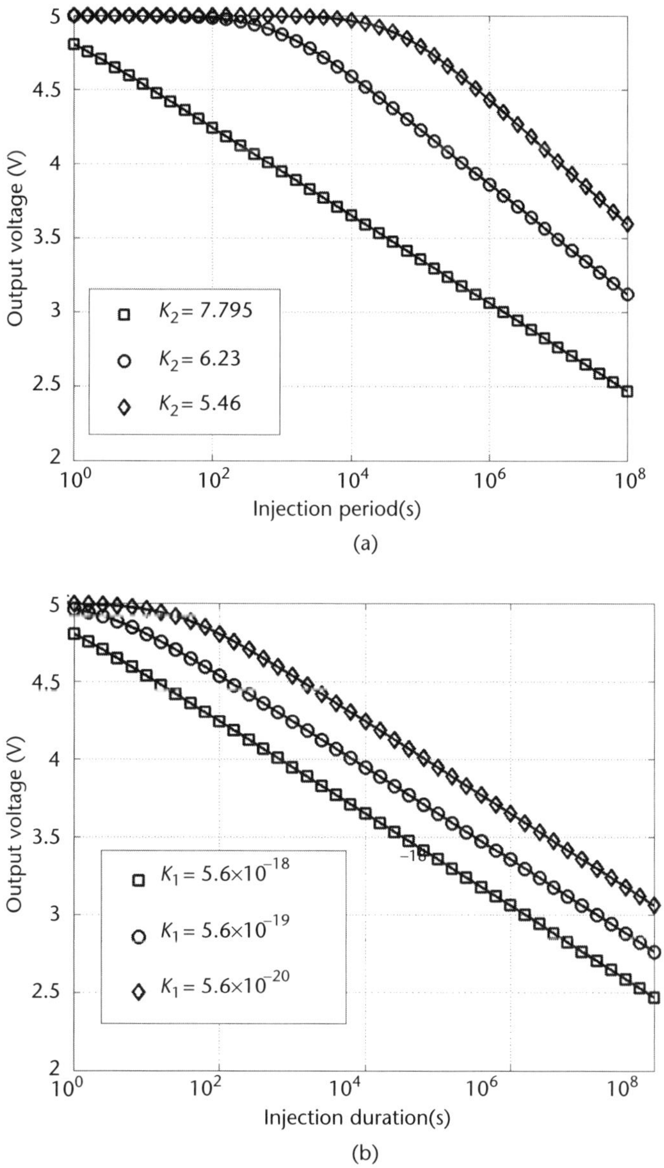

Figure 4.14 Response of the floating-gate injector for different values of (a) parameter K_2 and (b) parameter K_1.

beyond a million injection seconds. The parameter K_1, which is a function of the ambient conditions, only introduces an offset in the log-linear response. This principle will be important in compensating the response of the injector for initialization errors that can be seen when equation (4.22) is expressed in its incremental form as

$$\Delta V_{out}(t) = -\frac{1}{K_2}\log\left(\frac{t}{t_0}\right) \tag{4.23}$$

where $\Delta V_{out}(t)$ is the change in voltage measured with respect to voltage at reference time-instant t_0. Details related to calibration will be discussed in the implementation section of this chapter.

4.5.3 CMOS Current References

The current reference in the schematic shown in Figure 4.12 is important for ensuring stable floating-gate injection. The reference therefore has to establish a bias current that is insensitive to the voltage fluctuation at the output of the piezoelectric transducer. Also the reference should be robust to variations in process and ambient conditions (for example temperature). In the literature most current references fall into either one of the following categories: (a) references whose output is proportional to absolute temperature (PTAT); (b) references whose output is temperature independent. In this section, we first discuss principles behind design of a CMOS PTAT current reference and to illustrate some of its performance limitations [62, 63, 64]. In the next section, a modified circuit is presented that can achieve temperature compensation using floating-gate transistors.

Figure 4.15 shows a schematic of a basic current reference that was first proposed using bipolar transistors [65] and later in its CMOS form [66] as shown in the figure. If the width-to-length ratio $\frac{W}{L}$ of transistors Q_1 and Q_2 be denoted by $\frac{W_1}{L_1}$ and $\frac{W_2}{L_2}$, then $I_{ref} = KI_2$, with $K = \frac{W_1 L_2}{L_1 W_2}$. The current I_{ref} determines the potential drop across

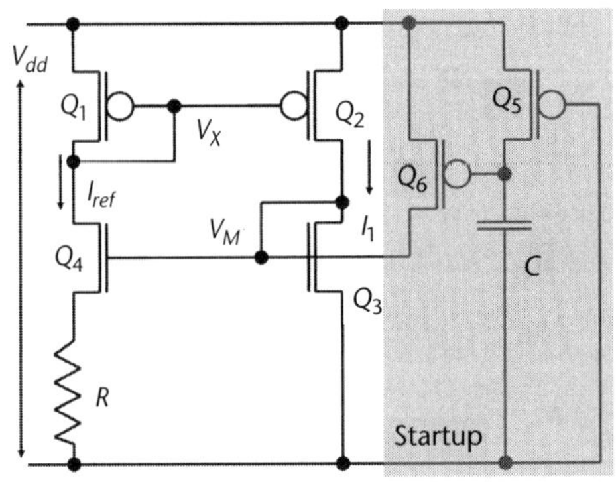

Figure 4.15 Schematic of a CMOS current reference.

the resistor R, which in turn determines the ratio of the currents flowing through the nMOS transistors Q_3 and Q_4. If the transistors are biased in weak-inversion, the current I_{ref} can be calculated as

$$I_{ref} = \frac{U_T}{R} \log K \tag{4.24}$$

which is theoretically independent of the supply voltage and linearly proportional to temperature through U_T.

It can be verified that $I_{ref} = 0$ is also a stable state for the current in the CMOS reference circuit. The schematic in Figure 4.15, therefore, requires a startup circuit that is formed by transistors Q_5 and Q_6. Initially the capacitor C is fully discharged and therefore Q_5 and Q_6 are ON. This ensures that the node V_M is at a sufficiently higher potential than the source of Q_4 during startup. When the equilibrium condition is achieved as determined by the Equation (4.24), the capacitor C charges to the supply voltage, which then turns off the transistors Q_5 and Q_6. Under ideal conditions (perfectly matched transistors), I_{ref} does not depend on supply voltage or threshold voltage, but is monotonic in temperature (approximately PTAT in weak-inversion). In practice, the reference is affected by the supply voltage variation due to finite drain-to-source impedance of transistor Q_2, and also by threshold voltage mismatch between the pMOS pair Q_1,Q_2 and nMOS pair Q_3,Q_4. The sensitivity of the current reference to the supply voltage variations can be reduced by either using long transistors and through cascoding. Stability of the current reference is another design consideration that is important during its start up. By limiting the total capacitance at node V_M, limit-cycle behavior can be avoided.

4.5.4 Floating-Gate Current References

Even though temperature inside the body is well regulated, local heating could arise in some biomechanical implants (knee or hip implants) due to continuous loading conditions or in the case of misalignment. In such cases, temperature compensation could be important to ensure validity of accumulated statistics. The popular approach toward achieving temperature compensation is to use passive and active circuit elements with positive and negative temperature coefficients. Designing temperature-compensated CMOS current references in nanoamperes range poses a challenge due to the inherent exponential dependency between voltage, drain current, and temperature. In many instances, external trimming circuits have to be used to achieve reasonable cancellation.

In this section, a translinear principle using floating-gate transistors has been used to achieve temperature compensation [67]. A schematic of a floating-gate temperature-compensated current reference is shown in Figure 4.16. For the sake of clarity, the startup network is not included in the schematic. If the charge on the floating-gate capacitor C_G is programmed (using injection or tunneling) to Q_f, the relationship between the drain currents through Q_1 and Q_2 can be expressed as

$$K = \frac{I_{ref}}{I_1} = \exp\left(\kappa \frac{Q_f}{C_G U_T}\right) \tag{4.25}$$

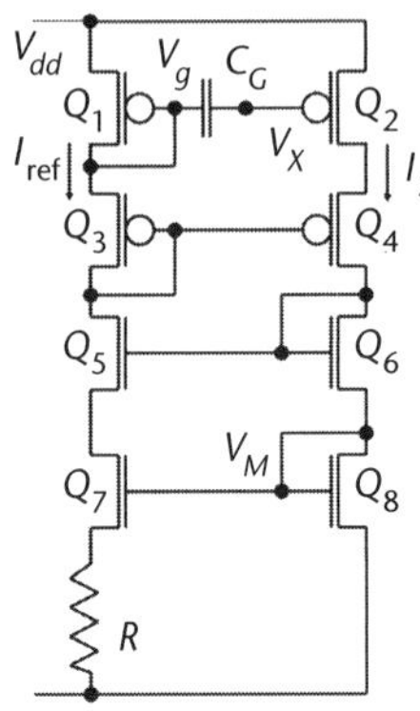

Figure 4.16 Schematic of a floating-gate CMOS current reference.

where κ is the gate efficiency of the pMOS mirrors. Equation (4.25) when inserted into equation (4.24) leads to

$$I_{ref} = \frac{Q_f}{C_{eff} R} \tag{4.26}$$

with $C_{eff} = C_G/\kappa$. It can be seen from equation (4.26), that the reference current is independent of temperature as compared to the PTAT reference given by equation (4.24). The capacitance C_{eff} is a weak function of temperature due to its dependence on depletion capacitance. Also, the resistance R exhibits a positive temperature coefficient and is the limiting factor for the floating-gate current reference. We have validated temperature compensation of the floating-gate reference circuit with less than 2% variation over a 70°C temperature variation. Other than being temperature compensated, the floating-gate reference can be programmed (using injection and tunneling) at fine increments and hence can be used for generating sub-nanoampere currents. Unfortunately, floating-gate transistors exhibit low drain-to-source impedance (due to capacitive coupling between the drain and the floating-gate terminal), which increases the sensitivity of the current reference with respect to the supply voltage variations. Cascoded transistors Q_3–Q_6 have been used in Figure 4.15 to improve the performance of the reference by limiting the voltage variation at the drain of the pMOS current mirrors.

4.6 Design and Calibration of a Complete Floating-Gate Sensor Array

In this section we will describe a complete design of an array of floating-gate injectors and present measured results that will verify the theoretical model proposed in the previous section. A complete sensor will have the piezoelectric transducer outputs directly connected to a full-wave rectifier, implemented using a standard diode bridge. For the prototype presented in this section, an n^+- p-substrate and p^+-n-well diodes were used, which are naturally integrated on electrostatic discharge (ESD) protection pads of the VLSI chip. A storage capacitor is used at the output of the rectifier to filter out unwanted high-frequency components. The size of this capacitor also provides a trade-off between the total hold-time versus the voltage swing at the sensor. For the prototype, an external capacitor (10 nF) was chosen, which is equivalent to a voltage swing of up to 8 V across the rectifier when a 20-V pulse is generated by the piezoelectric transducer. A voltage over-protection and clamping circuitry (consisting of zener diodes) was integrated at the output of the diode bridge to prevent damage due to unwanted piezoelectric surges.

The basic sensor circuit given in Figure 4.12 has been extended to an array by inserting MOS diodes between the current reference and the source of the floating-gate transistor. A schematic implementing a complete floating-gate injector array with an integrated current reference is shown in Figure 4.17. Table 4.4 provides the respective sizes of the transistors, resistors, and capacitors used for this prototype. Eight injectors have been integrated on the chip, even though the schematic in Figure 4.17 shows only three floating gate cells (F1–F3).

A reference current generator circuit is implemented using transistors Q_1–Q_{10} and a resistor R. If the ratio of the pMOS current mirror transistors Q_3,Q_4 is denoted by K, then the magnitude of the reference current is $I_b = \frac{U_T}{R}\log K$, where U_T denotes a thermal voltage (26 mV at room temperature). Transistors Q_1 and Q_2 form a startup circuit for the current reference. The reference current is copied by mirrors Q_{11},Q_{14} and Q_{18}, which drive the floating-gate cells F1–F3. Diode-connected transistors Q_{16}, Q_{20} and Q_{21} are used to control the potential drop between the supply terminal and source of the floating-gate transistors Q_{13},Q_{17}, and Q_{22}. This ensures that each of the floating-gate cells (F1–F3) start injecting at a differential supply potential (V^+–V^-). For an injector circuit consisting of M diodes between the current

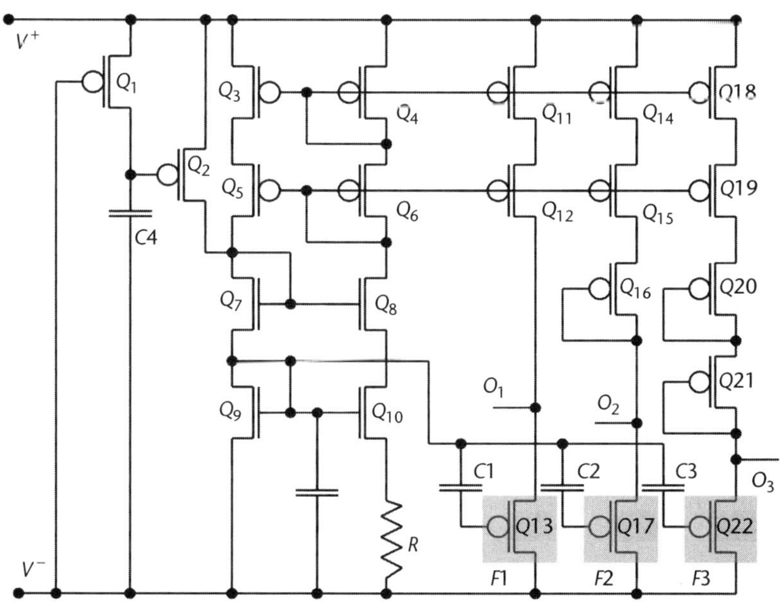

Figure 4.17 Floating-gate reference array.

Table 4.4 Size of the Circuit Elements for the Sensor Circuit

Element	*Size*
Q4,Q5,Q6,Q11,Q12,Q14,Q15,Q18,Q19	30 μm/10 μm
Q16,Q20,Q21	10 μm/10 μm
Q13,Q17,Q22	6 μm/6 μm
Q1,Q2,Q3	60 μm/10 μm
Q7,Q8,Q9,Q10	60 μm/10 μm
C4,C5	1 pF
R	1.5 MΩ

source and the floating-gate transistor, the minimum supply voltage required for onset of injection is

$$V^+ - 2V_{dsat} - MU_T \log\left(\frac{I_b}{I_{d0}}\right) - V_{out_i} = V^- \tag{4.27}$$

where V_{dsat} is the drain-to-source voltage drop for the cascoded current mirrors, I_{d0} is specific current for the pMOS diode transistors, and V_{out_i} is the calibrated floating-gate source voltage for nodes $O_i, i = 1,\dots,8$. For transistors biased in weak-inversion $V_{dsat} \geq 3U_T$, which leads to

$$V^+ - V^- \geq MU_T \log\left(\frac{I_b}{I_{d0}}\right) + V_{out0} + 6U_T \tag{4.28}$$

For $V_{out0} = 5V$, the inequality (4.28) leads to

$$V^+ - V^- \geq 0.6M + 5.15 \tag{4.29}$$

Therefore the minimum amplitude of voltage pulses required to be generated by the piezoelectric transducer is 5.15 V. While interfacing the transducer with the floating-gate sensor array, this minimum supply voltage should be set to be equal to the piezoelectric voltage representing the fatigue limit of the material (see Figure 4.2(a)).

A prototype floating-gate injector array has been fabricated in a standard 0.5 μm CMOS process and its micrograph is shown in Figure 4.18 with its specifications summarized in Table 4.5. Before the prototype is used for monitoring, an equalization procedure is required to initialize the state of the floating-gate injector array. The equalization algorithm is summarized as a flow chart in Figure 4.19. Initially, each of the floating-gate cells (F1–F3) is programmed (using tunneling and injection) to store a fixed amount of charge and hence a fixed floating-gate voltage across F1–F3. These gate voltages are indirectly monitored by measuring drain-to-source voltages across each of the floating-gate cells (O_i, $i = 1,2,\dots,8$). For different supply voltages Vdd_i, $i = 1,2,\dots,8$ each of the cells F1–F8 is programmed till the corresponding output V_{out_i} is set to a fixed potential (5 V for this work). Figure 4.20

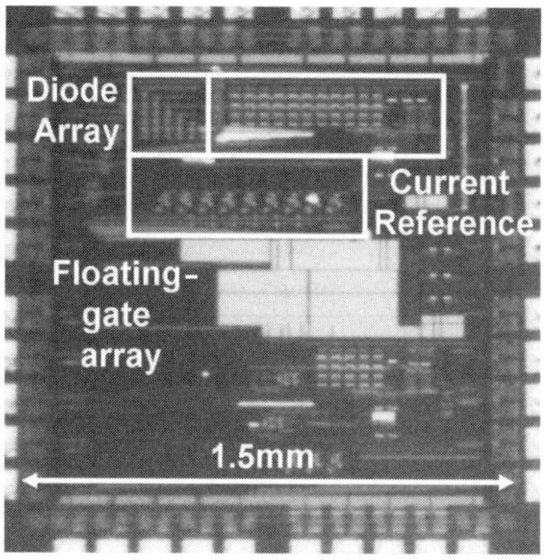

Figure 4.18 Micrograph of the prototype floating-gate sensor.

shows the output voltages O1–O3 corresponding to three cells F1–F3 which were equalized using the algorithm in Figure 4.19.

The result demonstrates that after equalization each of the cells has a different injection threshold (according to equation 4.29), where F3 reaches the injection threshold at 5 V input.

After equalization, the functionality of the prototype was validated by interfacing it with a programmable signal generator that was used to emulate the output of a piezoelectric transducer. In this experiment, voltage pulses (emulating piezoelectric transducer response) with different amplitudes are applied to the prototype. The startup time for the current reference and injection circuitry was measured to be less than 30 ms, which is sufficient for a typical loading cycle (1000 ms). Figures 4.21 to 4.23 show the measured output voltage O1–O3 corresponding to the three injector cells F1–F3, for continuous amplitude voltage pulses of different amplitude (Vdd_1 = 5.3 V, Vdd_2 = 6.1 V, and Vdd_3 = 6.9 V).

It can be seen from Figure 4.21 that only cell F1 injects when pulses of amplitude 5.3 V are applied. Also the response of the injector F1 is log-linear and produces a change in output voltage as a function of duration of injection. The cells F2 and F3 show negligible injection compared to cell F1. Figure 4.22 shows the response of the injector array when voltage pulses with amplitude 6.1 V were applied. Both F1 and F2 inject at an identical rate, whereas cell F3 shows negligible injection. Thus cells F1 and F2 gather statistics of occurrence of events when voltage amplitude exceeds 6.1 V. For pulses with amplitude greater than 6.9 V, all the cells F1–F3

Table 4.5 Summary of Measured Specifications

Parameter	*Value*
Technology	0.5 μm CMOS
Size	1.5 mm × 1.5 mm
Number of Injectors	8
Injection Range	4.2 V–8 V
Maximum Current	160 nA
Startup Time	< 30 ms

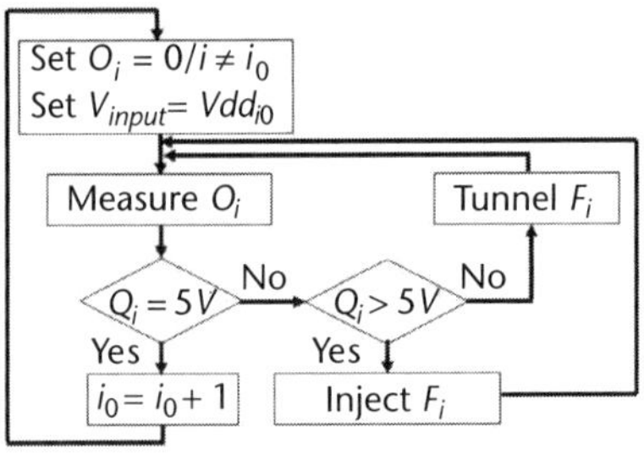

Figure 4.19 Sensor initialization algorithm.

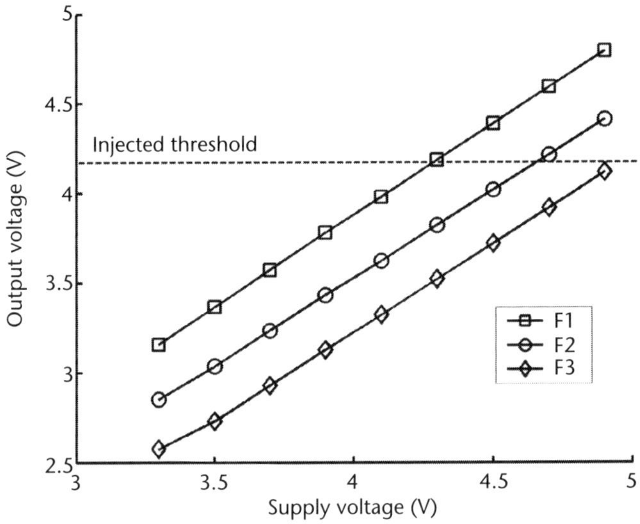

Figure 4.20 Measured output voltages (O1–O3) response vs. input voltage.

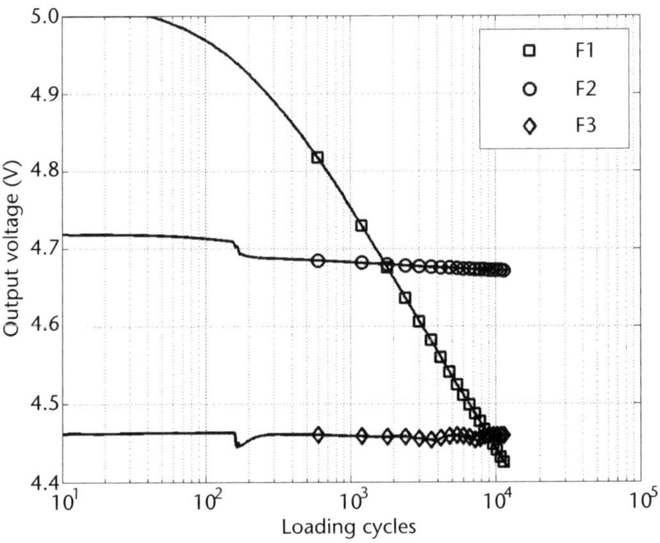

Figure 4.21 Measured source-to-drain voltage response across floating-gate elements at V_{dd} = 5.3 V.

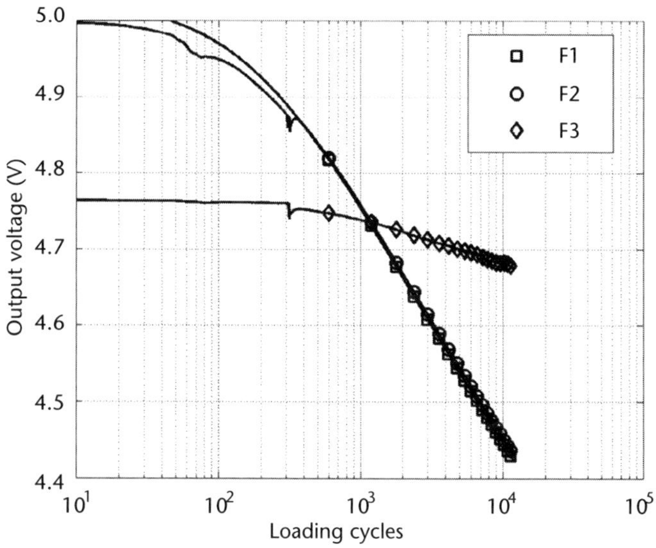

Figure 4.22 Measured source-to-drain voltage response across floating-gate elements at V_{dd} = 6.1 V.

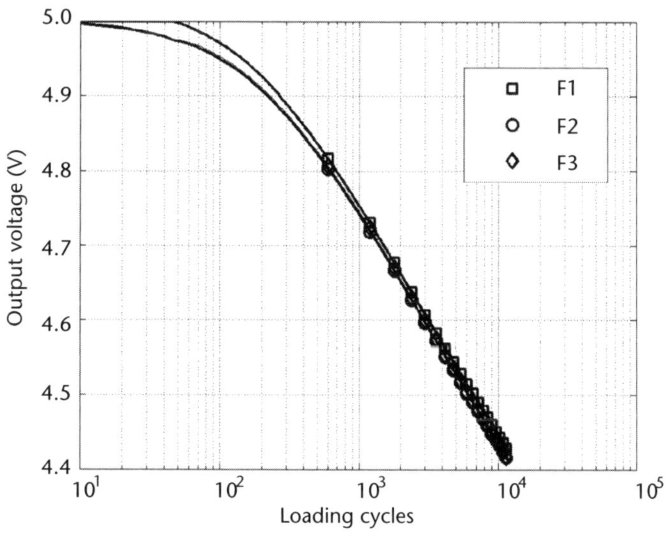

Figure 4.23 Measured source-to-drain voltage response across floating-gate elements at V_{dd} = 6.9 V.

inject at identical rates and the responses show excellent agreement with the mathematical model in equation (4.19). Using the model in equation (4.19), it can be calculated that the total duration that a cell injects before it approaches the threshold (4.2 V) is approximately 70,000 seconds. This period can only be increased beyond 10^8 seconds by decreasing the parameter K2 as was shown in Figure 4.14(a).

The second set of experiments was designed to evaluate the performance of the injector array under variable loading conditions. The floating-gate elements were first initialized using the algorithm described in Figure 4.19. The programmable voltage source was used to generate a periodic arbitrary waveform consisting of three different levels (5.3 V, 6.1 V, and 6.9 V). A sample voltage waveform used for one of the experiments is shown in Figure 4.24, where the duration of the three levels were programmed to be in the ratio of 3:2:1. The measure response from the injector array is also shown in Figure 4.24. The difference in duration of injection translates into an offset in the log-linear response and is evident from the measured results. Figures 4.25 and 4.26 show the response of the injector array for loading cycles with different durations of the voltage levels. It can be seen from the measured results that the array indeed can capture the monotonic relationship of the statistics in the offsets between the curves. The offset, however, also contains information regarding the initial conditions, thus, any error in initializing the injector array will appear as an error in measurement.

A calibration scheme based on equation 4.23 has been applied to compensate for offsets introduced by ambient conditions. It can be seen that equation 4.23 is only a function of parameter K_2 and the reference time instant t_0. For the next set of experiments, the cells F1, F2, and F3 were first calibrated by injecting for a fixed duration (t_0 = 103 cycles), such that the condition $t >> \dfrac{\exp(-K_2 V_{g0})}{K_1 K_2}$ is satisfied. This is shown in Figure 4.26, where it can be seen that at $t_0 = 10^3$ cycles, the errors introduced due to initial conditions are approximately equalized.

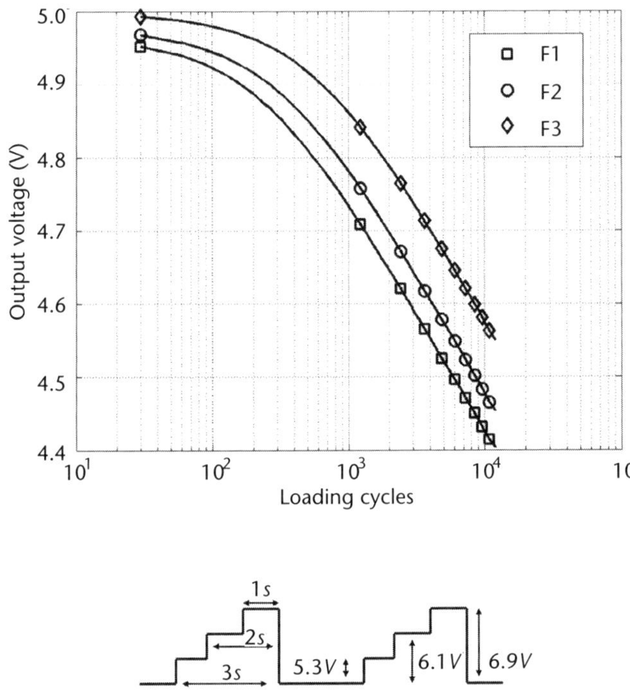

Figure 4.24 Measured output voltage response for the sensor array when subjected to a loading cycle represented by a piezoelectric output with injection duration 3:2:1.

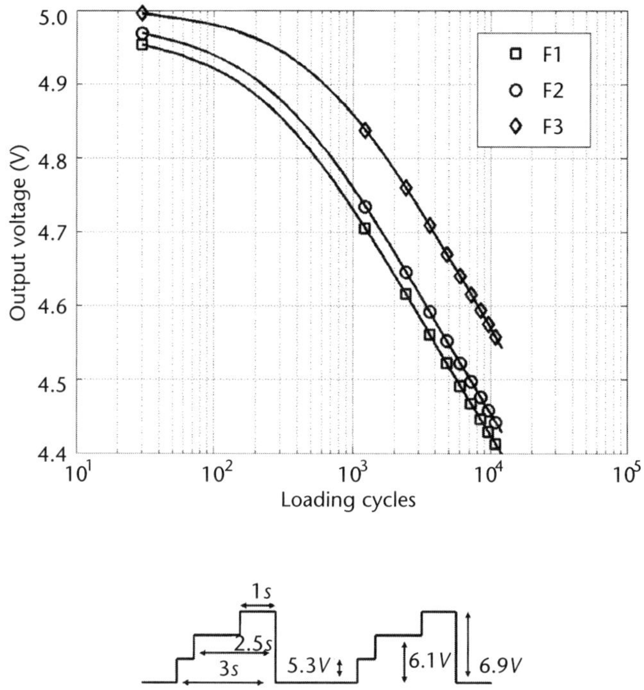

Figure 4.25 Measured output voltage response for the sensor array when subjected to a loading cycle represented by a piezoelectric output with injection duration 3:2.5:1.

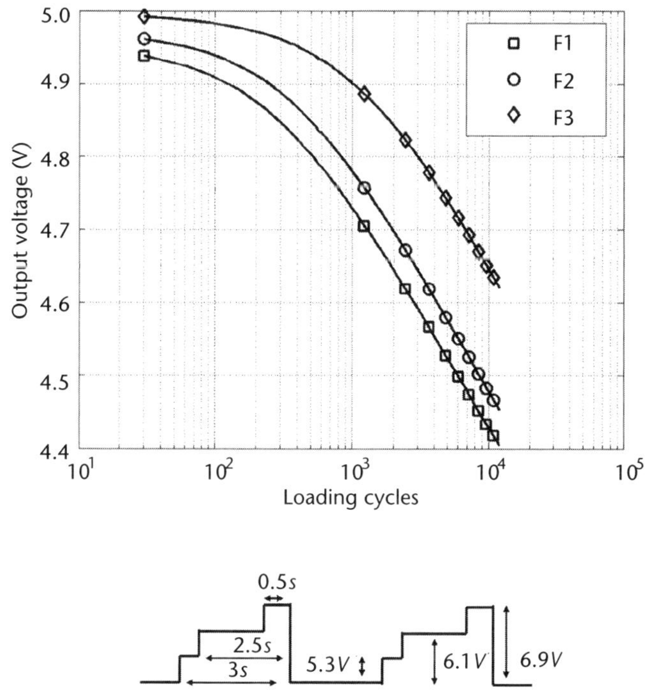

Figure 4.26 Measured output voltage response for the sensor array when subjected to a loading cycle represented by a piezoelectric output with injection duration 3:2.5:0.5.

Subsequently, the cells are subjected to variable loading cycles, whereby each cell injects only for a fraction of the duration. If α denotes the fraction of total injection period, then

$$\Delta V_{out}(t) = -\frac{1}{K_2}\log\left(\frac{t_0 + \alpha\Delta t}{t_0}\right)$$

and the parameter α can be calculated as

$$\alpha = \frac{\exp\left[-K_2\left(V_{out1}(t) - V_{out1}(t_0)\right)\right] - 1}{\exp\left[-K_2\left(V_{out2}(t) - V_{out2}(t_0)\right)\right] - 1}$$

where V_{out1} and V_{out2} are the output voltage for cells F1 and F2. In Figure 4.26, the parameter α is computed to be equal to 0.30 for cell F3 and 0.71 for cell F2, which is close to the ratio 1/3 and 2/3. The sources of error include a mismatch in parameter K2 for the different cells, as well as imperfect startup and shutdown of the injector cells. Figure 4.27 shows a similar result but for a different ratio (3:2.5:1) of loading cycles. It can be seen from Figure 4.26 and Figure 4.28 that the offset between injection response for cells F1 and F3 is identical, whereas the offset between F1 and

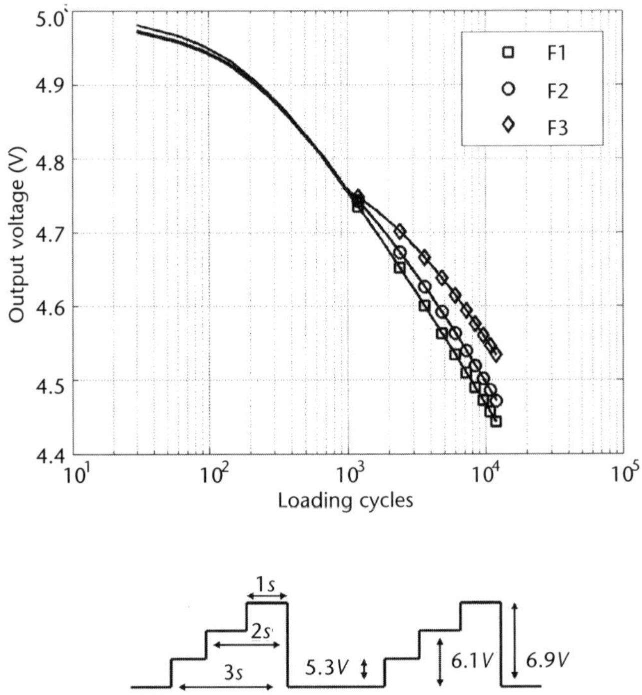

Figure 4.27 Measured output voltage response using the sensor array in which the first 1000 cycles have been used as calibration intervals and the subsequent three level loading cycles with the duration of injection are in the ratio 3:2:1.

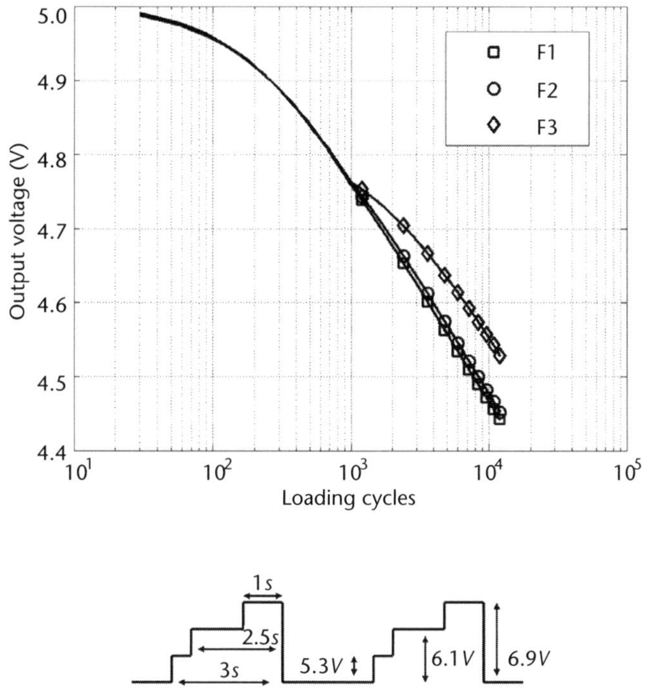

Figure 4.28 Measured output voltage response using the sensor array in which the first 1000 cycles have been used as calibration intervals and the subsequent three level loading cycles with the duration of injection are in the ratio 3:2.5:1.

F2 has been reduced, which is consistent with the statistics of the loading cycle. The nominal power dissipation by the sensor (current reference and floating-gate array) at 5.5 V was determined to be 800 nW. Figure 4.29 plots the current drawn by the sensor at different supply voltages. It can be seen that around 5.5 V the current saturates, indicating that all the cells on the chip are active (but not injecting).

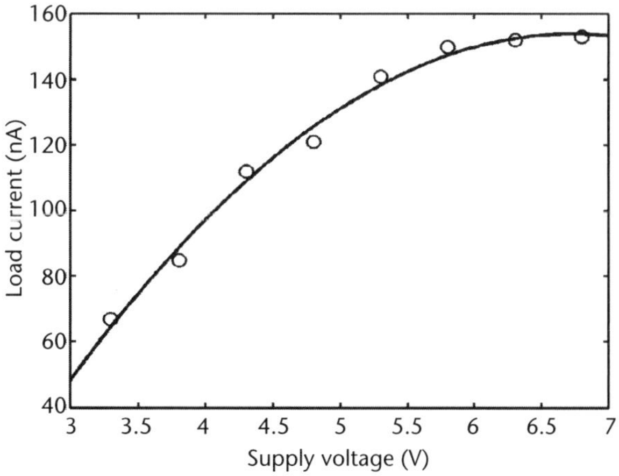

Figure 4.29 Supply current drawn by the sensor at different supply voltages.

4.7 Conclusions

The measurement of the cumulative loading statistics experienced by an implant is essential for prediction of long-term fatigue failure. However, the total power that can be harvested under typical in-vivo strain levels is less than 1 μW. In this chapter, we presented techniques that can be used for designing VLSI circuits that can be used in conjunction with a piezoelectric transducer to facilitate long-term, battery-less fatigue monitoring. The core techniques discussed in this chapter utilize computational paradigms inherent in floating-gate injection. The fundamentals of piezoelectric transduction have been discussed and a complete design of a floating-gate MOS injector array has been presented. A thorough treatment of the calibration and the modeling of the floating-gate injector array have been presented, and also have been illustrated and validated using measured results from a fabricated prototype.

Acknowledgment

This work was supported in part by a research grant from the National Science Foundation (NSF) CMMI-0700632.

References

[1] S. Kurtz et al., "Projections of primary and revision hip and knee arthroplasty in the United States from 2005 to 2030," *J. of Bone and Joint Surgery*, 2007; 89(4):780–785.

[2] Advance Data No.329 [Online]. Available: http://www.cdc.gov/nchs/fastats/pdf/ad329t8.pdf/, Center for Disease Control and Preventation.

[3] T.M Wright and S.B. Goodman, eds., "Implant wear in total joint replacement: Clinical and biological issues, material and design considerations," Rosemont, IL: American Academy of Orthopedic Surgeons, p. 3, Oct 2001.

[4] J.P. Collier et al., "Analysis of the failure of 122 polyethylene inserts from uncemented tibial knee components," *Clin. Orthopaed. Rel. Res.*, vol. 273, pp. 232–242, Dec. 1991.

[5] T.P. Schmalzried and J.J. Callaghan, "Current concepts review: wear in total hip and knee replacements," *J. Bone Joint Surg. A*, vol. 81, no. 1, pp. 115–136, Jan. 1999.

[6] P.S. Walker et al., "Methodology for long-term wear testing of total knee replacements," *Clin. Orthopaed. Rel. Res.*, vol. 372, pp. 290–301, Mar. 2000.

[7] B. Espehaug, O. Fumes, L.I. Havelin, L.B. Engasaeter, and S.E. Vollset, "The type of cement and failure of total hip replacements," *J. Bone Joint Surg. B*, vol. 84, no.6, pp. 832–838, Aug. 2002.

[8] M.A. McGee et al., "Implant retrieval studies of the wear and loosening of prosthetic joints: A review," *Wear*, Volume 241, Number 2, 31 July 2000, pp. 158–165(8).

[9] P.F. Sharkey et al., "Why Are Total Knee Arthroplasties Failing Today?" *Clinical Orthopaedics & Related Research*, 404:7–13, November 2002.

[10] Wikipedia: The free encylcopedia [Available Online] http://en.wikipedia.org.

[11] M. Matsuiski, M. and T. Endo, "Fatigue of metals subjected to varying stress," *Japan Soc. Mech. Engrg*, 1969.

[12] S. Suresh, *Fatigue of Materials*, 2nd edition, Cambridge University Press, 1998.

[13] S.S. Mason, "Fatigue—A complex subject," *Experimental Mechanics*, Vol. 5, No. 7, pp. 193–226, 1965.

[14] S.D. Downing and D.F. Socie, "Simple rainflow counting algorithms," *International Journal of Fatigue*, Volume 4, Issue 1, January, 31–40, 1982.

[15] I. Rychlik, "A new definition of the rainflow cycle counting method," *Int. J. Fatigue*, 119–122, 1987.

[16] ASTME 1049-85, Standard practices for cycle counting in fatigue analysis, ASTM International, 2005.

[17] B.R. Bannister and D.G. Whitehead, *Instrumentation: Transducers and Interfacing*, London, UK: Chapman and Hall, 1991.

[18] J.W. Gardner, *Microsensors: Principles and Applications*, New York: Wiley, 1994.

[19] J. Fraden, *Handbook of Modern Sensors, Physics, Designs and Applications*, Woodbury, NY: AIP, 1997.

[20] K.J. Loh, J.P. Lynch, and N.A. Kotov, "Conformable Single-Walled Carbon Nanotube Thin Film Strain Sensors for Structural Monitoring," *Proceedings of the 5th International Workshop on Structural Health Monitoring*, Stanford, CA, USA, Sept. 12–14, 2005.

[21] I. Kang, M.J Schulz, J.H. Kim, V. Shanov, and D. Shi, "A carbon nanotube strain sensor for structural health monitoring," *Smart Mater. Struct.* 15, 737–748, 2006.

[22] W. Zhang, J. Suhr, and N. Koratkar, "Carbon Nanotube/Polycarbonate Composites as Multifunctional Strain Sensors," *Journal of Nanoscience and Nanotechnology*, vol. 6, No. 4, pp. 960–946, 5 April 2006.

[23] Y. Liu, S. Chakrabartty, D.S. Gkinosatis, A.K. Mohanty, and N. Lajnef, "Multi-walled carbon nanotubes/poly(L-lactide) nanocomposite strain sensor for biomechanical implants," *IEEE Proceedings on Biomedical Circuits and Systems, (BioCAS 2007)*, Montreal, Canada.

[24] J. Sirohi and I. Chopra, "Fundamental understanding of piezoelectric strain sensors," *Journal of Intelligent Material Systems and Structures*, vol. 11, April, pp. 246–257, 2001.

[25] M. Rahimi, H. Shah, G.S. Sukhatme, J. Heideman, and D. Estrin, "Studying the feasibility of energy harvesting in a mobile sensor network," *Proceedings of the 2003 IEEE International Conference on Robotics & Automation*, Taipei, Taiwan, September 14–19, pp. 19–24, 2003.

[26] H.A. Sodano, D.J. Inman, and G. Park, "A review of power harvesting from vibration using piezoelectric materials," *The Shock and Vibration Digest,* vol. 36, No. 3, May, pp. 197–205, 2004.

[27] H.A. Sodano, G. Park, and D.J. Inman, "Estimation of electric charge output for piezoelectric energy harvesting," *Strain*, vol. 40, pp. 49–58, 2004.

[28] S. Roundy, P.K. Wright, and J. Rabaey, "A study of low level vibrations as a power source for wireless sensor nodes," *Computer Communications*, vol. 26, pp. 1131–1144, 2002.

[29] S. Roundy, "On the effectiveness of vibration-based energy harvesting," *Journal of Intelligent Material Systems and Structures*, vol. 16, pp. 809–823, 2005.

[30] B.A. Warneke, K.S.J. Pister, "Exploring the limits of system integration with Smart Dust," *Proceedings of IMECE'02*, New Orleans, Louisiana, 2002.

[31] Wright et al., "Ulnar nerve excursion and strain at the elbow and wrist associated with upper extremity motion," *J. Hand Surg.*, July 2001, 26(4):655–662.

[32] J. Borodkin et al., "The influence of mechanical strain magnitude on bone adaptation to porous coated implants," *IEEE Eng. Medicine Biology Soc. Conf.*, p. 768, 1999.

[33] B.D. Beynnon and B.C. Fleming, "Anterior cruciate ligament strain in-vivo: A review of previous work," *J. Biomech.* 1998;31:519–525.

[34] Pradhan et al., "Superior labral strain during the throwing motion (shoulder strain)," *Am. J. of Sports Medicine*, 2001.

[35] N. Elvin, A. Elvin, and D.H. Choi, "A self-powered damage detection sensor," *The Journal of Strain Analysis for Engineering Design*, vol. 38, no. 2, pp. 115–125, 2003.

[36] C.C. Enger and J.H. Kennedy, "An improved bioelectric generator," *Trans. Am. Soc. Artif. Intern. Organs*, vol. 10, pp. 373–377, Oct. 1964.

[37] N. Elvin, A. Elvin, and M. Spector, "Smart Orthopaedic Implant," US Patent No: 06034296.

[38] B. Otis, Y.H. Chee, R. Lu, N.M. Pletcher, and J.M. Rabaey, "An ultra-low power MEMS-based two-channel transceiver for wireless sensor networks," *IEEE Symp. VLSI Circuits*, June 2004.

[39] S.W. Arms, C.P. Townsend, D.L. Churchill, and N. Phan, "Energy harvesting, wireless, strain sensor for damage tracking of helicopter components," *3rd European Workshop on Structural Health Monitoring*, 2006.

[40] R. Amirtharajah and A. Chandrakasan, "A micropower programmable DSP using approximate signal processing based on distributed arithmetic," *IEEE Journal of Solid-State Circuits*, vol. 39, pp. 337–347, Feb 2004.

[41] PicoRadio: University of California, Berkeley Project.

[42] X-bow: X-Bow Technologies Mica2Dot Wireless sensor Mote.

[43] Micron:-Micron Technology NOR Flash Memory.

[44] Texas Instrument: MSP430 microprocessor.

[45] Cavendish:-Cavendish Kinetics Corp, MEMS memory.

[46] LSI: - LSI Logic Corp—LSI403LC Digital Signal Processor.

[47] Telos:- Moteiv Corporation.

[48] J. Kao, "Subthreshold leakage control techniques for low power digital circuits," Ph.D. Thesis, Massachusetts Institute of Technology, 2001.

[49] N.G. Elvin, A.A. Elvin, and M. Spector, "A self-powered mechanical strain energy sensor." *Smart Materials and Structures*, No. 10, pp. 293–299, 2001.

[50] A.A. Bent and N.W. Hagood, "Piezoelectric fiber composites with interdigitated electrodes," *Journal of Intelligent Material Systems and Structures*, vol. 8:11, pp. 903–919, Nov. 1997.

[51] G.V.B. Cochran, M.W. Johnson, M.P. Kadaba, F. Vosburgh, M.W. Ferguson-Pell, and V.R. Palmeiri, "Piezoelectric internal fixation devices: A new approach to electrical augmentation of osteogenesis," *Journal of Orthopaedic Research*, 3(4):508–513, 1985.

[52] S.R. Platt, S. Farritor, K. Garvin, and H. Haider, "The use of piezoelectric ceramics for electric power generation within orthopedic implants," *Mechatronics, IEEE/ASME Transactions* on 10(4):455–461, 2004.

[53] J.B. Park, A.F. Von Recum, G.H. Kenner, B.J. Kelly, W.W. Coffeen, and M.F. Grether, "Piezoelectric ceramic implants: A feasibility study." *Journal of Biomedical Materials Research*, 14(3):269–277, 1980.

[54] N. Mukherjee, R.D. Roseman, and J.P. Willging, "The piezoelectric cochlear implant: Concept, feasibility, challenges, and issues," *Journal of Biomedical Materials Research*, 53(2):181–187.

[55] J. Snoeck, M. Berkhof, M. Claeys, C. Vrints, J. Bosmans, H. Decoster, and H. Heuten, "External vibration interference of activity based rate responsive pacemakers." *Pacing and Clinical Electrophysiology*, 15(11):1841–1845, 1992.

[56] W.B. Phillips, B.C. Towe, and P.J. Larson, "An ultrasonically-driven piezoelectric neural stimulator," *Engineering in Medicine and Biology Society, Proceedings of the 25th Annual International Conference of the IEEE*, 1983–1986, 2003.

[57] W.H. Ko, "Piezoelectric energy converter for electronic implants," US Patent 3,456,134, 1969.

[58] E. Häsler, L. Stein, and G. Harbauer, "Implantable physiological power supply with PVDF film ferroelectrics," 60, 277–282, 1984.

[59] G. Bergmann, G. Deuretzbacher, M. Heller, F. Graichen, A. Rohlmann, J. Strauss, and G.N. Duda, "Hip contact forces and gait patterns from routine activities." *J. Biomech.*, 34(7):859–871, 2001.

[60] C. Dorio, P. Hasler, B. Minch, and C.A. Mead, "A single-transistor silicon synapse," *IEEE Trans. Electron Devices*, vol. 43 (11), Nov. 1996.

[61] T. Shibata and T. Ohmi, "A functional MOS transistor featuring gate-level weighted sum and threshold operations," *IEEE Transactions on Electron Devices*, vol. 39 (6), pp. 1444–1455, June 1992.

[62] G.A. Rincon-Mora, *Voltage References: From Diodes to Precision High-Order Bandgap Circuits*, New York: John Wiley, 2001.

[63] W.M. Sansen, F. Op't Eynde, and M. Steyaert, "A CMOS temperature-compensated current reference," *IEEE Journal of Solid-State Circuits*, vol. 23, no. 3, pp. 821–824, June 1988.

[64] P.R. Gray, P.J. Hurst, S.H. Lewis, and R.G. Meyer, *Analysis and Design of Analog Integrated Circuits*, 4th Edition: John Wiley, 2001.

[65] R.J. Widlar, "Design techniques for monolithic operational amplifiers," *IEEE Journal of Solid-State Circuits*, vol. SC-4, pp. 184–191, 1969.

[66] E. Vittoz and J. Fellrath, "CMOS analog integrated circuits based on weak inversion operation," *IEEE Journal of Solid-State Circuits*, vol. 12, pp. 224–231, 1977.

[67] N. Lajnef, S. Chakrabartty, N. Elvin, and A. Elvin, "Piezo-Powered Floating Gate Injector for Self-Powered Fatigue Monitoring in Biomechanical Implants," *IEEE Symposium on Circuits and Systems (ISCAS'2007)*, New Orleans, 2007.

[68] M.R. Stan, P.D. Franzon, S.C. Goldstein, J.C. Lach, and M. Ziegler, "Molecular electronics: from devices and interconnect to circuits and architecture," *Proc. IEEE*, vol. 91, 1940–1957, 2003.

CHAPTER 5

CMOS Circuits for Wireless Medical Applications

Chris Siu and Krzysztof Iniewski

5.1 Introduction

Healthcare—the very mention of the word can spark a fierce debate in some countries, and it's not difficult to see why. Modern medical care is expensive, and with rising costs and an aging population, governments have difficult choices on how to allocate expenditures. New technologies may help to ease this burden.

One emerging area is the use of wireless technology in medical devices. Wireless can open up new methods of healthcare delivery that lower cost, reduce patient trauma, and provide other advantages. For example, a company named Given Imaging has commercialized a wireless endoscope [1]. The device is in the form of a capsule that a patient can swallow, and while the capsule travels down the digestive tract, two pictures are taken every second. Each picture is transmitted wirelessly to a vest worn by the patient. This scheme reduces a patient's discomfort compared to an invasive endoscopic procedure.

Since it takes an average of 8 to 12 hours for the capsule to pass through the body, the capsule must contain enough on-board battery power for the entire examination period. Since the wireless transmitter is on at regular intervals, the RF circuitry must be ultra-low power for this to work.

A different example of ultra-low power consumption can be found in the pacemaker. Implanted into a patient to regulate heartbeat, the pacemaker must not only be reliable, but draw minimal power so that battery replacement is infrequent. One representative pacemaker consumes only 4 micro-amps at 2.5 V, and lasts more than 7 years on a single battery [2]. Wireless can open up new ways of preventive care. For example, a pacemaker can send patient health and device operating data to a wireless monitor. The monitor, which may be patient-worn, then relays the data to a base station for further processing, and direct it to the attention of a doctor if necessary. Needless to say, the addition of wireless must not impact the pacemaker's battery life too much.

To facilitate the use of wireless in implanted medical devices, the Federal Communications Commission (FCC) has established the Medical Implant Communications Service (MICS) frequency band. This allows a physician to establish a short-range wireless link between an implanted device and a monitoring tool. Likewise, the FCC has established the Wireless Medical Telemetry Service (WMTS) band to allow communication between a non-implanted medical device and the monitor.

Aside from ultra-low power consumption and reliability, cost is also important for these applications. Full integration of digital and RF circuitry on a single CMOS die had been a holy grail to reduce cost, and over the past decade this has become a reality. Highly integrated System-On-Chips (SOC), with both RF transceiver and complex digital functions on the same die, can be readily acquired on the open market [3, 4]. As wireless usage proliferates, the cost pressures will continue to steer designers to use CMOS. This chapter explores the choices that analog and RF IC designers have to make for ultra-low power designs. The paper begins by reviewing operational requirements in the MICS and WMTS bands. Selection of radio architectures, and the tradeoffs for low-power consumption is discussed next. A RF transceiver architecture suitable for MICS is then proposed. Circuit level implementation of key functions inside the RF transceiver will be examined, including LNA, mixer, transmitter, and frequency synthesis.

5.2 Spectrum Regulations for Medical Use

The MICS band was established to enable short-range wireless communication between an implanted medical device and external equipment. Prior to the existence of MICS in 1999, medical implant devices had to be magnetically coupled to external programmers or readers, requiring the patient to be in close contact with the external equipment. In addition, this form of communication supports a very low data rate, sometimes requiring the patient to sit for 15 minutes [5]. Recognizing the potential benefit of a short-range, high-speed wireless link between implants and external tools, the FCC established MICS in the 402 to 405 MHz frequency range. These frequencies are harmonized with Europe, as implemented in the European Telecommunications Standards Institute (ETSI) standard EN301 839.

Although operation in the MICS band does not require a license, at this time MICS equipment must be operated by a medical professional. Since MICS is intended to connect an implant to external equipment for monitoring, diagnostic, or control purposes, no voice communication is allowed in this band.

To reduce interference between MICS transmitters, a device must perform the equivalent of a Clear Channel Assessment (CCA) before transmitting on a channel. In other words, an MICS device must check that another transmitter is not using the same channel. The exception to this rule is a "medical implant event," when a device must transmit to ensure the safety of the implant patient.

Operation in the MICS band limits the effective isotropic radiated power (EIRP) to 25 microwatts, or –16 dBm. The channel bandwidth is restricted to 300 kHz maximum, hence 10 channels can be implemented in the MICS band.

WMTS was established to enable wireless communication between an externally worn medical device and other equipment. For example, a portable device can measure the heart rate of a patient and transmit the data to a nearby base station. This monitoring can be done without tying the patient to one spot, and may lower cost by allowing remote monitoring of several patients simultaneously.

Prior to establishing WMTS, wireless medical telemetry used certain TV channels, and as a result was subject to interference from broadcasters. In 2000, the FCC allocated three blocks of frequencies to WMTS: 608–614 MHz, 1395–1400 MHz, and 1427–1432 MHz. Similar to MICS, the use of WMTS does not require a license, but WMTS equipment must be operated by medical professionals within a healthcare facility.

Regulation (Part 95.639) stipulates that the maximum field strength allowed for WMTS in the 608 to 614 MHz band is 200 mV/m, measured at 3 meters. For operation in the 1395–1400 MHz and 1427–1432 MHz bands, the maximum field strength is 740 mV/m, measured at 3 meters. This translates into +11 dBm and +22 dBm of transmit power, respectively. Note that compared to MICS, the allowed transmit power is much higher, so telemetry data can be sent over a longer distance. However, the higher transmit power also means higher power consumption. For an externally worn device this may be an acceptable tradeoff, if the device can be recharged regularly.

Since MICS implanted devices pose a severe power constraint on the integrated circuit designer, we will focus on MICS for the remainder of this chapter. Before diving into actual circuits, we need to choose a radio architecture that fits our constraints. Though a quantitative analysis depends on the application, a MICS transceiver will meet these general criteria:

1. Very low power consumption
2. Highly integrated with minimal external components, for small form factor
3. Robust link with low Bit Error Rate (BER)
4. Channel selectivity within the MICS band; rejection of nearby interference

Later in this chapter, we will analyze the requirements of a pacemaker, and apply that to the design of a MICS transceiver.

5.3 Integrated Receiver Architectures

To achieve the objective of low cost and low power, commercial vendors as well as researchers have had to focus on new radio architectures. Although the superheterodyne receiver is a proven architecture with excellent selectivity, its use of external filters and multiple conversion stages increases the cost, power, and form factor.

One big shift by commercial RFIC vendors in the last decade has been to eliminate the external SAW filters by using a direct conversion architecture. Also known as a homodyne or zero-IF radio, the idea is not new, but difficulties with implementation have prevented wider adoption until recently [6]. As shown in Figure 5.1, the mixer simply moves the desired RF channel directly to baseband, eliminating any need for an IF. Channel selection is done by an on-chip low-pass filter before demodulation. The image rejection requirement is not severe since the interferer is the signal itself.

While conceptually simple, in practice, the direct conversion receiver has difficulties with time-varying DC offsets. Since every block has finite port-to-port isolation, the large LO signal driving the mixer can leak to the LNA input, reflect off the antenna, and enter the receive chain again. The mixer translates this LO leakage down to baseband, creating a DC offset. Since the antenna reflection may vary over time, this offset can also be time-varying.

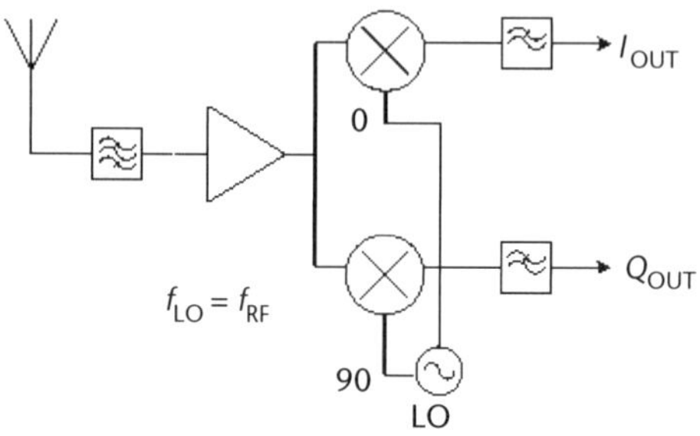

Figure 5.1 Direct conversion receiver.

Another practical issue with direct conversion receivers in CMOS is the flicker noise. With the RF channel translated directly to baseband, the weak signal is susceptible to the low frequency noise attributed to MOS devices. In recent years, design techniques have been developed to make direct conversion more viable. For example, DC offset cancellation is used in the latest 802.11 receivers [6]. Another possibility is to use a DC-free modulation scheme; for example, a 3.3 mW direct conversion receiver was reported using Frequency Shift Keying (FSK) [7].

One architecture that gets around the limitations of the zero-IF radio is the low-IF receiver. Instead of translating the RF directly to baseband, it is converted to a very low IF, a popular choice being an IF equal to half channel spacing; for example, in GSM the channel spacing is 200 kHz, so a low-IF receiver may use a 100 kHz IF [8].

By not placing the signal directly at baseband, the low-IF receiver avoids the DC-offset and flicker noise issues mentioned earlier. Unfortunately, the tradeoff here is image rejection, which is typically dependent upon the on-chip channel filter and I/Q matching. If the IF is equal to half channel spacing, then the image is the adjacent channel.

While both the zero-IF and low-IF receive architecture have been proven to be commercially viable, certain vintage architectures have seen a revival in integrated circuit implementation. Using the super-regenerative architecture, shown in Figure 5.2, researchers have constructed a 5 kbps receiver with an ultra-low power consumption of 450 μW [9].

Invented by Edwin Armstrong in 1922, this architecture uses as few active devices as possible to construct a high-gain RF receiver. The idea is to wrap positive feedback around a device, such that large gain can be achieved in a single stage. In fact, the device becomes an oscillator, and the signal grows exponentially with time. Eventually the oscillator will limit the signal, so it needs to be "reset" or quenched regularly to maintain the receiver sensitivity. As shown in Figure 5.3, the strength of the

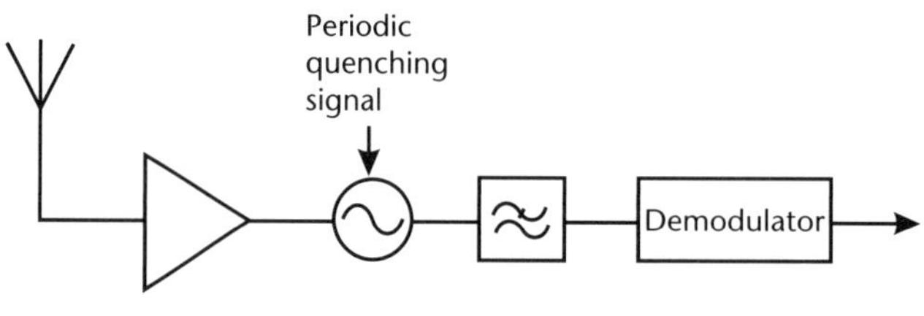

Figure 5.2 Super-regenerative receiver.

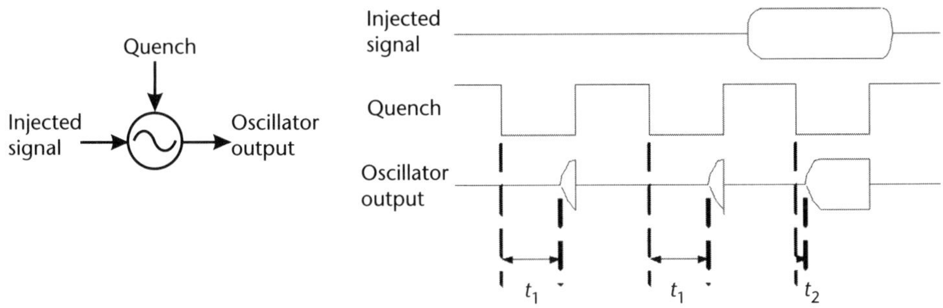

Figure 5.3 Super-regenerative waveforms.

RF input signal modulates the oscillator start-up time, and it is the detection of this envelope delay that allows the super-regenerative receiver to demodulate Amplitude Shift Keying (ASK).

Note that for the architecture in Figure 5.2, no LO generation or phase locked loop (PLL) is required. To enhance selectivity, this receiver uses a Bulk Acoustic Wave (BAW) filter to tune the oscillator. However, since the BAW filter cannot be manufactured with conventional CMOS processing, the receiver and BAW filter are on separate dies. The higher cost and larger size are drawbacks to this approach for MICS.

A more recent approach to the super-regenerative receiver, without using a BAW filter, is to use on-chip digital calibration [10] (Figure 5.4). Though still employing the super-regenerative principle, this architecture uses a PLL for oscillator tuning. Though it loses the original appeal of low device count, in the CMOS age this is not necessarily an issue as long as power consumption is kept low.

The LNA injects the received RF signal into the oscillator tank. After quenching, the oscillator current is set at a level I_{CRIT} at which the negative resistance is not

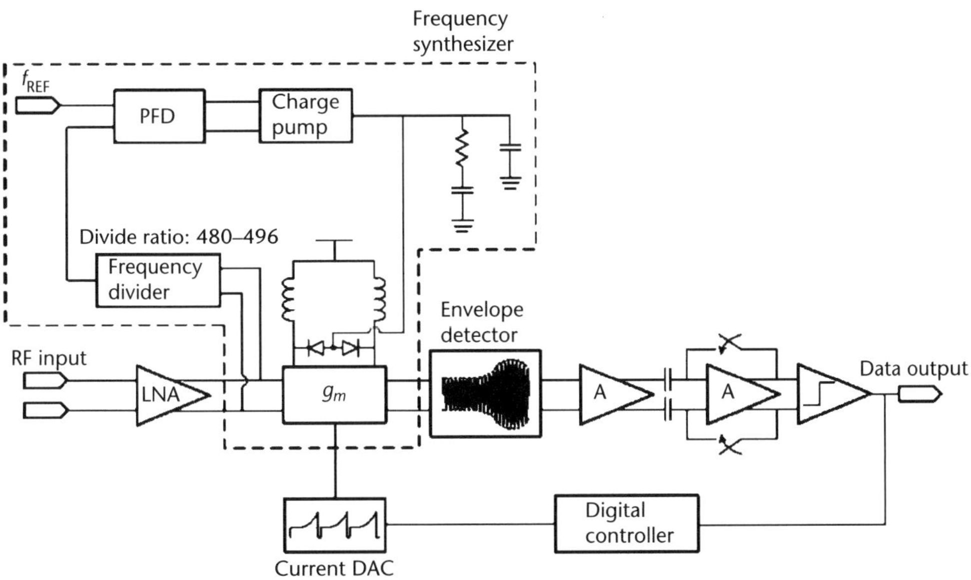

Figure 5.4 Super-regenerative receiver with digital calibration. From [10] with permission.

sufficient for oscillation. Thus the g_m block becomes a Q-enhanced filter, used for improving the receiver selectivity. I_{CRIT} is set by a 9-bit DAC using a successive approximation algorithm. After an interval operating as a filter, the current is increased so that oscillation is possible. The start-up delay is influenced by the filtered signal at the end of the Q-enhancement phase. The oscillation envelope is then detected by subsequent circuitry to produce a demodulated digital signal.

In this receiver, the PLL is used to center the tank frequency on the desired channel. Hence, during the Q-enhancement phase, the filter is centered on the receive channel. Subsequently, when the current is increased above I_{CRIT}, the oscillation frequency is still centered. Overall, this receiver consumes 2.8 mW on a 1.2 V supply, and achieves a 500 kbps data rate at a 500 kHz quench rate.

In summary, we have reviewed several integrated receiver architectures, namely zero-IF, low-IF, and super-regenerative. In the next section we will explore some integrated solutions for the transmitter side.

5.4 Integrated Transmit Architectures

Contemporary standards such as 802.11 use digital modulation to achieve high spectral efficiency. For example, at 54 Mbps WLAN uses 64-QAM modulation on each OFDM sub-carrier, resulting in a transmit waveform with high Peak to Average Ratio (PAR). A linear power amplifier must be used, which often has low-Power Added Efficiency (PAE), resulting in high-power consumption. For example, a direct conversion I/Q transmitter suitable for 802.11 is shown in Figure 5.5.

One step toward more power-efficient drivers is to use constant envelope modulation. Examples of constant envelope schemes include Frequency Shift Keying (FSK) and variants such as Minimum Shift Keying (MSK). Constant envelope transmitters can be driven close to compression, resulting in a higher PAE; this in turn means lower power consumption.

With constant envelope phase modulation, one technique to implement the transmitter is to embed the modulation control within a Phase Locked Loop (PLL). A one-point modulation TX loop is shown below. This architecture yields several benefits. First, it is another step toward lowering power consumption, since this scheme removes the two upconverters in Figure 5.5. Second, the PLL provides inherent filter-

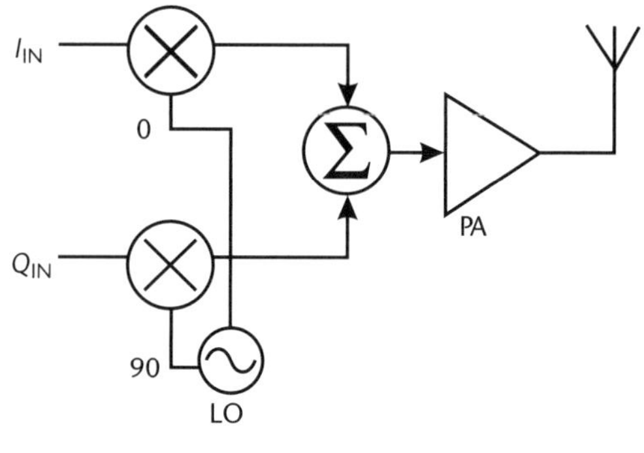

Figure 5.5 Direct conversion transmitter.

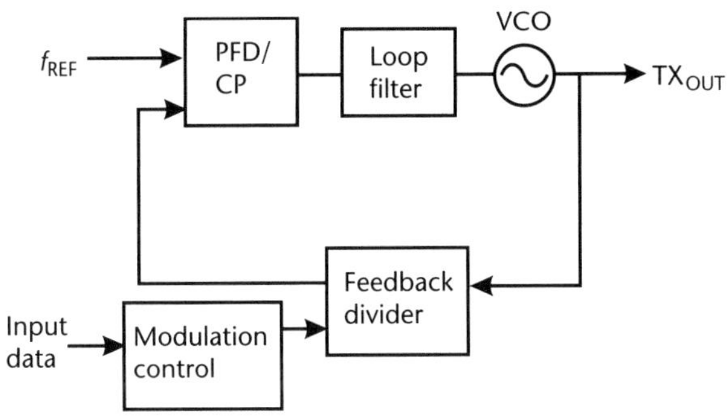

Figure 5.6 Modulation loop using divider control.

ing for the modulated signal. Lastly, for the example below, no digital to analog conversion is needed for the modulation control; the divider ratio can be adjusted entirely in the digital domain.

For the architecture shown in Figure 5.6, since the transfer function from the divider to the PLL output is low-pass, the modulation bandwidth is essentially the same as the loop bandwidth. If the channel bandwidth requirement is greater than the loop bandwidth, then the designer must either increase the latter, or consider VCO modulation.

As shown in Figure 5.7, direct VCO modulation modifies the control voltage via a DAC. Since the transfer function from VCO to PLL output is high-pass, the modulation must concentrate most of its power spectral density outside of the PLL bandwidth. For example, FSK with high modulation index can satisfy this condition.

Another way of realizing a low-power transmitter is to use On-Off Keying (OOK) modulation [9]. With OOK, the transmitter is turned on only when a logic "1" is sent; otherwise the transmitter is turned off. A CMOS OOK transmitter is shown in Figure 5.8.

On average, the transmitter is now consuming half the power of one using constant envelope modulation, at the sacrifice of spectral efficiency and other performance.

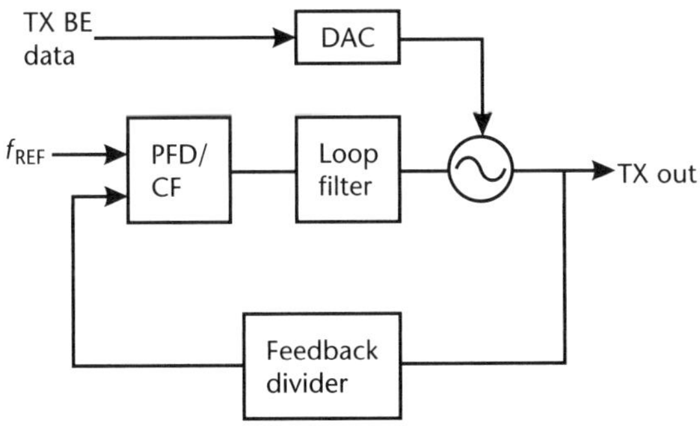

Figure 5.7 Modulation loop using VCO control.

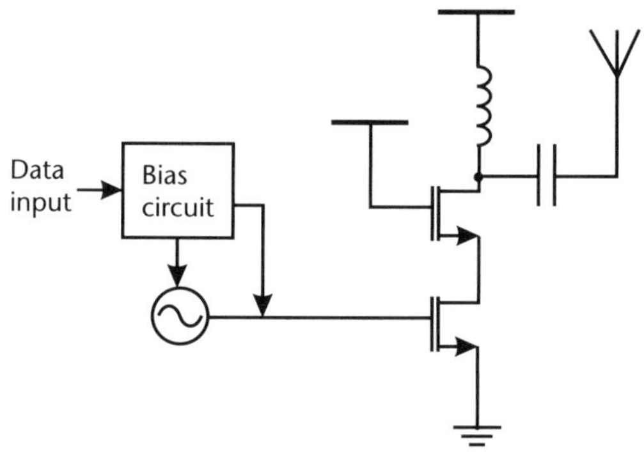

Figure 5.8 Low-power OOK transmitter.

5.5 Radio Architecture Selection

Having reviewed a number of different architectures, what is a good choice for MICS? Recall that while low-power consumption is the key consideration, other factors such as form factor and robustness are also important. For each medical application, there is an acceptable Bit Error Rate (BER) for the link. If in the blind optimization for lowest power, the link budget is insufficient for the stated BER, then re-transmission will be needed. Repeated re-transmission will actually cause the average power consumption to go up.

To help illustrate the point, we will use the requirements of a pacemaker in choosing a radio architecture. Listed below are some of the salient points for this application:

1. Pacemakers typically use a lithium iodide battery; this battery has a high impedance that limits its load current. Open circuit voltage of a lithium iodide battery starts at around 2.8 V, and decays steadily as it is discharged.
2. With a 2.5 A·h capacity and a minimum lifetime of 8 years, the pacemaker must consume less than 35 μA on average. If we budget 80% of the battery capacity for cardiac stimulation, and the other 20% for data communication, that means the MICS transceiver must consume less than 7 μA on average.
3. Operating in the MICS band, the channel spacing is only 300 kHz. If we assume in the future that multiple MICS transceivers are in a Body Area Network, a MICS receiver must have good selectivity to tolerate other transceivers on the body.
4. The MICS transceiver will operate on a low-duty cycle, transmitting only for diagnosis and maintenance. Hence, its sleep mode must have very low leakage current. Also, how we choose to wake the transceiver from sleep mode also has a great impact on overall current consumption.

Given that only 7 μA average is budgeted for the wireless transceiver, we must carefully plan the latency and duty cycle in this design. In other words, the transceiver must be in sleep mode most of the time to conserve power, but it should also sniff the antenna often enough for a wakeup-signal. To illustrate the point, let us assume that 1 second of latency is acceptable. Hence, every second the receiver is powered up for a defined period to sniff the antenna. The tradeoff between duty cycle and the maximum receiver current is shown in Figure 5.9.

Hence, even if the MICS transceiver does nothing but sniff periodically for a wakeup-signal, at 1% duty cycle the receiver can consume no more than 700 μA. Thus, if this design searches for the wakeup-signal on the antenna, we must drive the duty cycle to much less than 1%.

Besides sniffing, the transceiver must of course perform data communication. For the pacemaker application, it is expected that data communication is required during routine check and maintenance, which may be once a month at a doctor's office. Hence the duty cycle for actual data transfer is very low, but the transceiver current should be kept below 5 mA due to the high battery impedance.

In summary, from a power consumption standpoint, the following constraints are set:

1. Sniffing duty cycle is set at 0.1%, with the receiver consuming less than 700 μA during this process. This consumes about 2% of the battery capacity.
2. Data communication is set at 0.05% duty cycle, equivalent to 20 minutes per month. If the transceiver consumes 5 mA during this process, about 7% of the battery capacity is consumed.

With these constraints, the MICS transceiver consumes about 10% of the battery capacity over an 8-year lifetime. Since the maximum output power for MICS is –16 dBm, it can be shown that even for continuous transmission, assuming a moderate efficiency of only 25%, the transmit amplifier will consume about 1.5 mA. Thus FSK modulation is chosen, and the modulation loop architecture shown in Figure 5.6 can be applied, with about 2 mA budgeted for the PLL.

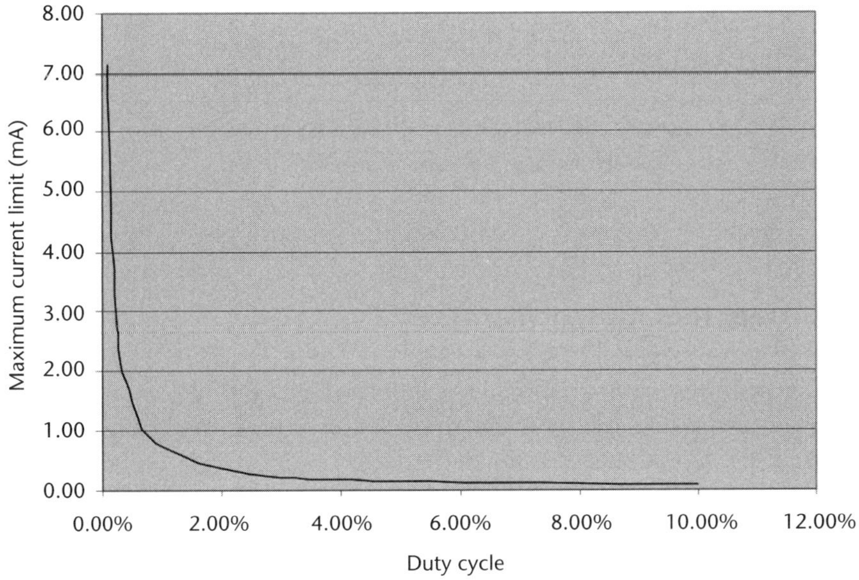

Figure 5.9 Duty cycle and current tradeoff.

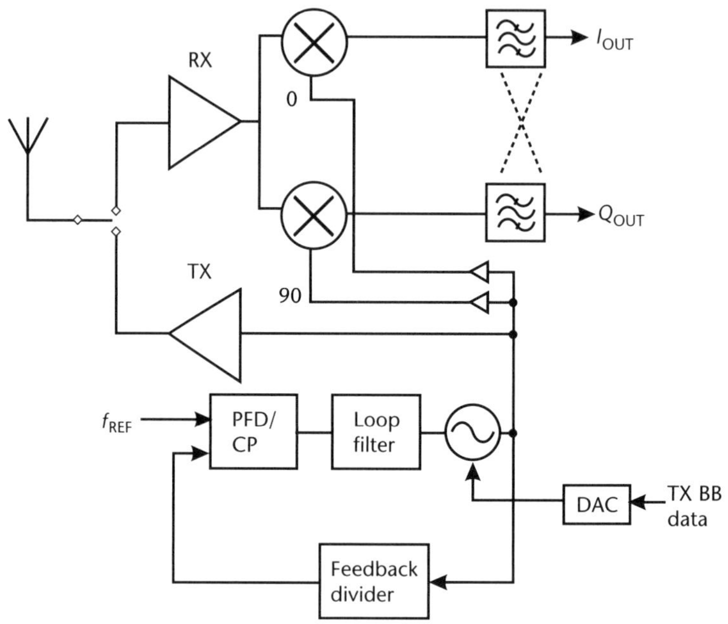

Figure 5.10 MICS radio architecture.

For the receiver, due to the 300 kHz channel spacing, a super-regenerative architecture will have difficulty achieving the channel selectivity without using a BAW filter. For example, if the filter Q is about 500 using Q-enhancement, the adjacent channel rejection is less than 3 dB.

With a PLL already available in the transmitter, we can re-use it in the receiver with a zero-IF or low-IF architecture. Since the channel bandwidth is less than 300 kHz, a zero-IF receiver will be greatly impacted by DC offsets and MOS flicker noise. A low-IF receiver is less susceptible to flicker noise, and provides sufficient image rejection using a polyphase filter.

In summary, the proposed radio architecture as shown Figure 5.10 has the following characteristics:

- Low-power FSK transmitter using a modulation loop
- Low-IF receiver with polyphase filter

In the next section, we will examine various aspects of the system budget.

5.6 System Budget Calculations

The previous section outlined some of the basic parameters of the transmitter, such as output power and efficiency. To get an idea of the required receiver performance, the following constraints are used:

1. A channel bandwidth of 300 kHz
2. Binary FSK modulation. Non-coherent detection is assumed with a bit error rate (BER) target of 1E-3

3. A range of 3 m between transmitter and receiver; at 400 MHz, the path loss is about 35 dB
4. Additional loss of 40 dB is included to account for human body loss, antenna loss, etc.

Regarding the second constraint, a moderate BER is used in order to relax the RF receiver design. Forward error correction such as Reed-Solomon code can be used to drastically lower the BER after the RF front end. With a channel bandwidth of 300 kHz, the thermal noise floor is computed to be

$$N_{TH} = -174 \text{ dBm/Hz} + 10*\log10(300\text{k}) = -119 \text{ dBm}$$

At the maximum range of 3 m, we assume that the transmitter is also at a maximum output of –16 dBm. With the path loss and other losses included, the receiver will detect –91 dBm at the antenna. For non-coherent FSK detection at the stated BER, a SNR of about 12 dB is needed. Using a 3 dB implementation margin for component variations, the required receiver noise figure is about 13 dB.

Note that a cascaded noise figure of 13 dB is not a difficult design problem. The challenge comes about in using the lowest power consumption to meet this requirement, with moderate linearity for interference protection. In the next sections, the transceiver building blocks at the circuit level will be reviewed and discussed.

5.7 Low-Noise Amplifiers

The Low-Noise Amplifier (LNA) often has a dominant impact on the overall noise figure (NF) of a receiver. The LNA must provide enough gain such that the desired signal can overcome the noise of subsequent stages. In the meantime, the LNA must add minimal noise of its own, and be linear enough to withstand incoming interferers.

Although various LNA topologies exist, two widely used topologies are the common-source (CS) and common-gate (CG) LNA with inductive source-degeneration shown in Figure 5.11. The CS LNA has good gain and noise figure, while the CG LNA has the advantage of a broadband input impedance.

The common-source (CS) LNA with inductive degeneration is frequently used in CMOS implementations. The source inductance introduces a real part in Z_{IN}, and the

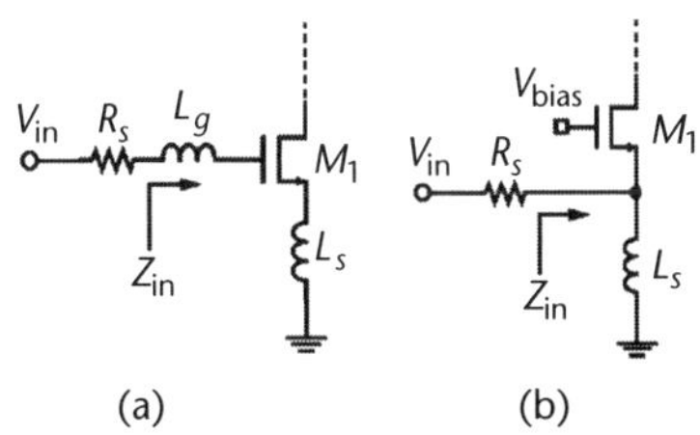

Figure 5.11 (a) Common-source and (b) common-gate LNA.

input matching network creates a series resonance, amplifying the input voltage by the Q of the network. The input impedance of the CS-LNA is given below:

$$Z_{in,CS-LNA} = s(L_g + L_s) + \frac{1}{sC_{gs}} + \omega_T L_S \tag{5.1}$$

The minimum noise figure can be obtained by applying constant-power optimization [11], giving the estimate below:

$$NF_{CS-LNA} = 1 + 1.426\sqrt{\delta\gamma} \cdot \left(\frac{\omega_O}{\omega_T}\right) \tag{5.2}$$

where γ is the channel thermal noise coefficient, with a value of 2/3 for a long channel device in saturation, δ is the gate noise coefficient, ω_o is the nominal operating frequency, and ω_T is the unity gain frequency.

Equation (5.2) shows that if the operating frequency is much below ω_T, then the CS-LNA can provide very good noise figure performance. On other hand, the requirement for high Q matching implies narrowband operation, with sensitivities to process variation and component tolerances.

For the common-gate (CG) LNA, the gate-source and gate-drain capacitances can be resonated out by the LC tank. One advantage of the CG LNA is its broadband input impedance, which is given by

$$Z_{in,CG-LNA} \approx \frac{1}{g_m + g_{mb}} \tag{5.3}$$

where g_{mb} is the backgate transconductance. The noise figure of a CG LNA is shown to be [12]:

$$NF_{CG-LNA} = 1 + \frac{\gamma}{\alpha}\left(\frac{1}{1+\chi}\right) \cdot \left(\frac{r_{DS}}{r_{DS} + R_L}\right) \tag{5.4}$$

where α is the ratio of transconductance to zero bias conductance (g_m/g_{d0}), and χ is the ratio of backgate transconductance (g_{mb}/g_m). The last term in equation 5.4 shows the effect of load resistance and finite output resistance on the NF. As r_{DS} approaches infinity, and assuming $\alpha = 1$ and $\chi = 0$, we get the classical result that the NF of a CG-LNA is $1 + \gamma$, or about 2.2 dB.

To the first order, the noise and gain performance of the CG-LNA is independent of the operation frequency. On the other hand, from equation 5.2, the CS-LNA noise figure has a linear dependence on frequency relative to ω_T. For the MICS application, with a 2.8 V supply, 0.25 μm CMOS would have sufficient performance for 400 MHz operation, since the f_T of a 0.25 μm NMOS device can be close to 30 GHz. Hence the CS-LNA topology is the preferred choice for the MICS receiver.

With modern LNA design techniques, the common-source device geometry can be scaled to move Z_{OPT} close to Z_S. Using these techniques, excellent performance has been shown in a 0.25 μm CMOS 900MHz folded-cascode LNA with 1.35 dB NF and 2 mW power [13].

LNA design using a MOSFET in the subthreshold region has also been explored recently. Experimental work has been done to show that in the subthreshold region, the minimum noise figure remains constant and is independent of drain current [14]. A 3 GHz LNA with 4.5 dB gain, 6.3 dB NF, and 0.16 mW power dissipation was demonstrated on a 0.6 V supply [14].

5.8 Mixers

A mixer has the task of translating an input signal to a different frequency. In the receive path, the frequency translation is downwards to move the RF signal to baseband or IF. To begin, there are two choices a designer can make in implementing a mixer: whether to use a passive or active mixer.

An active mixer has the advantages of high-conversion gain and lower LO drive requirements. In addition, the mixer input presents a light load for the LNA to drive. The most commonly used topology is the Gilbert-cell or double-balanced mixer, as shown in Figure 5.12. In a double-balanced mixer, a signal must be applied at both the RF and LO port to generate an output signal; if a signal is applied only at the RF or LO port, then no output appears.

This topology ideally has zero LO feed-through, but various impairments do cause a finite leakage to appear at the IF output. On the other hand, the single-balanced mixer (Figure 5.13) inherently has a large LO feed-through; even with no RF signal present, driving the LO port will cause an output at the same frequency.

The conversion gain of this mixer is given by

$$A_V = \frac{2}{\pi} g_{m1} \cdot R_L$$

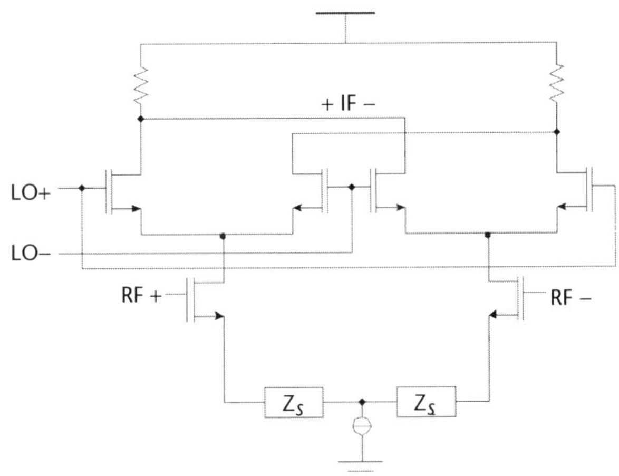

Figure 5.12 Double-balanced mixer.

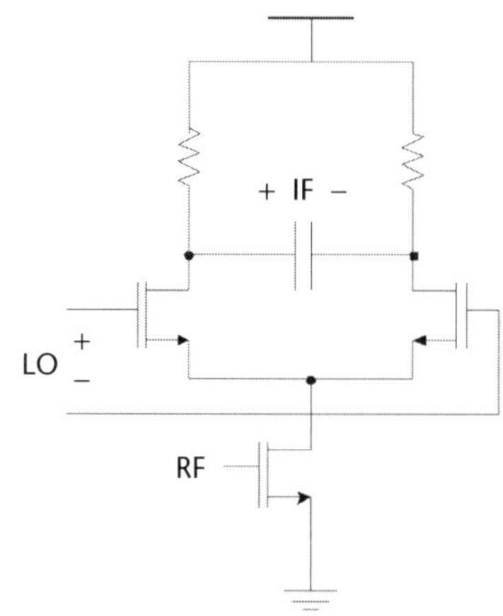

Figure 5.13 Single-balanced mixer.

For a receiver design, the single-balanced mixer is attractive when combined with a single-ended LNA. Moreover, for zero-IF or low-IF architectures, the desired signal is much lower in frequency than the LO feed-through. If the mixer IF port can be terminated in a low impedance for the LO frequencies, most of this LO leakage can be suppressed.

In contrast to an active mixer, the obvious advantage of a passive mixer is that it dissipates no power when processing RF signals. However, this circuit incurs a conversion loss, which impacts the gain budget and noise budget for the receiver. The LNA gain may need to be much higher to reduce the impact of active filter noise that follows the mixer.

An efficient implementation of passive mixers is to use MOSFET as voltage-mode switches. As shown in Figure 5.14, the RF signal can be applied at the source of the NMOS, while a LO signal is driving the gate to modulate the device conduction. The output is taken at the drain, and the shunt capacitors are used to attenuate any high-frequency products and/or feed-through.

The classical view on passive mixers is that since there is no DC current, there is no flicker noise associated. However, recent work [15] has shown that the AC current through the mixer core can still create flicker noise contributions. Compared to an active mixer, though, this flicker noise contribution is still small.

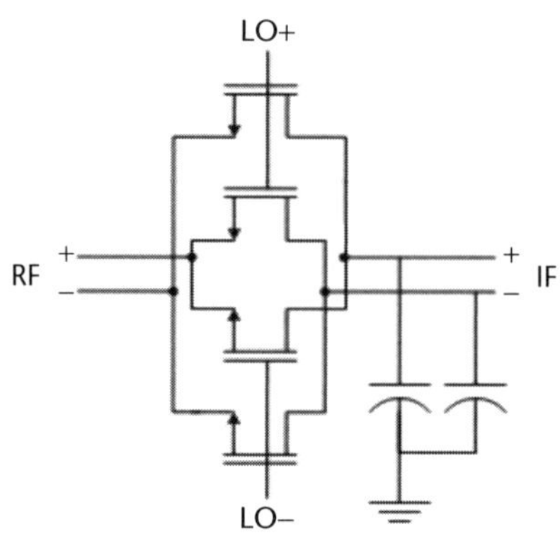

Figure 5.14 CMOS passive mixer.

5.9 Polyphase Filter

Since a non-zero IF frequency was chosen, the image problem exists in this receiver. For on-chip image rejection, a variety of approaches are possible, including the Hartley architecture, Weaver architecture, passive polyphase filter [16], and active polyphase filter [17]. The 90 degree phase shifter required for the Hartley architecture is difficult to implement for low-IF. The extra mixers and PLL required for the Weaver architecture makes it undesirable for an ultra-low power application. Passive polyphase filters, though capable of large image rejection, have limited selectivity [16]. In this section we will consider the design of an active polyphase filter.

To begin, we will review the concept of complex mixing and filtering. Suppose that the input is composed of the desired signal at $\omega_{LO} + \omega_{IF}$ and the image is at $\omega_{LO} - \omega_{IF}$. To translate the desired signal to ω_{IF} while keeping the image separable, we perform a complex mixing operation at ω_{LO} (i.e., multiply the input by the complex exponential $e^{j\omega LOt}$). This mixing operation is illustrated in Figure 5.15.

In practice, the complex mixing is implemented by using two mixers driving by quadrature LO, as shown previously in Figure 5.10. The mixer output consists of the desired signal at $+\omega_{IF}$, and the image at $-\omega_{IF}$. The polyphase filter then passes the desired signal and suppresses the image. However, due to gain and phase mismatches in the I and Q paths, the image rejection ratio (IRR) is finite, as approximated by the equation:

$$IRR_{MAX}(dB) \approx 10 \cdot \log 10\left(\sin^2\left(\frac{\theta}{2}\right) + \left(\frac{\Delta}{2}\right)^2 \right) \tag{5.5}$$

where θ is the phase mismatch, and Δ is the gain mismatch.

A polyphase filter can be implemented by using a low-pass to complex band-pass transformation. Starting with low-pass filters having cutoff at $+\omega_{LP}$, complex

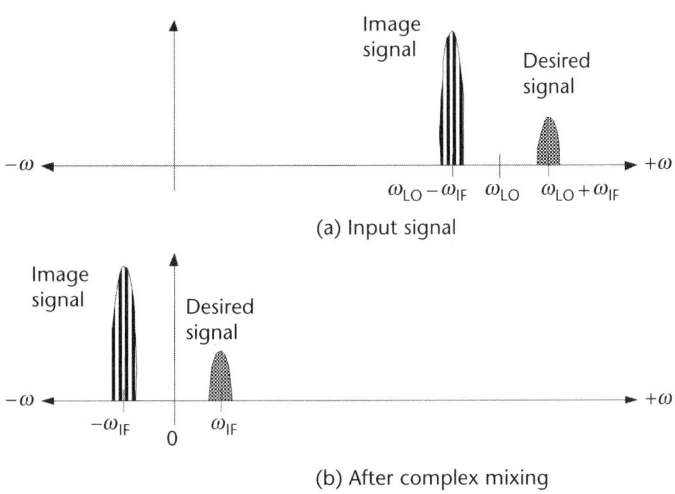

Figure 5.15 Frequency translation by complex mixing.

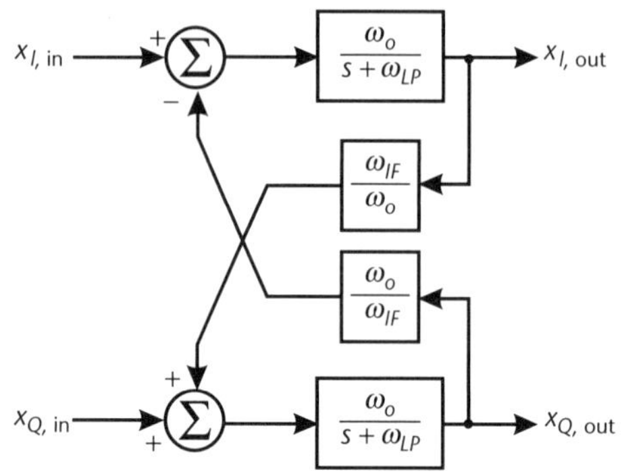

Figure 5.16 Block diagram of polyphase filter.

feedback is applied around them to create a complex bandpass at $+\omega_{IF}$. A block diagram of a single-pole PPF is shown in Figure 5.16.

Circuit-level implementation of this block diagram can vary depending on where gm-C, active RC, or other filter topologies are chosen. One choice for a low-power implementation is to use Nauta transconductors [18] in a gm-C architecture.

The core of the Nauta transconductor is an inverter, with relatively simple common mode control. This structure allows for a good frequency response with low-power consumption.

5.10 Power Amplifier (PA)

In an earlier section, mixer circuit topologies were discussed. For direct conversion transmitters, the mixer translates the baseband signal to RF frequencies. However, since a modulation loop is used in this MICS transmitter, no mixers are needed. Hence, this section will cover the design of a transmit power amplifier (PA) for MICS.

The relatively low-output power requirement of –16 dBm removes many of the design issues associated with an on-chip PA. As noted earlier, for an efficiency of only 25%, the PA will consume no more than 1.5 mA. Nonetheless, it is instructive to review some recent research in low-power amplifiers.

The following characteristics are desirable in a PA: (1) maximum power efficiency when it is switched on, (2) power control to change the output for varying distances, (3) low standby power when idle, and (4) short turn-on time to minimize overhead power dissipation. The choice for PA can be either linear amplifiers (Class A, B, AB) or switched-mode amplifiers (Class E, F). Theoretically, switched-mode power amplifiers have 100% power efficiency if the switch is loss-less.

A Class-E amplifier has been demonstrated in deep-submicron CMOS [19], as shown in Figure 5.17. The gate input to M1 requires a large swing, in order to put the device into either triode or cutoff. The resistance in the triode region degrades the amplifier efficiency, hence a large W/L ratio and/or a large input swing is desired. Note in Figure 5.17 that when the drain voltage is non-zero, the drain current is zero, and vice-versa. Ideally, no power is dissipated across M1 and the efficiency approaches 100%. This work reported efficiencies above 85% operating in the 433 MHz ISM band.

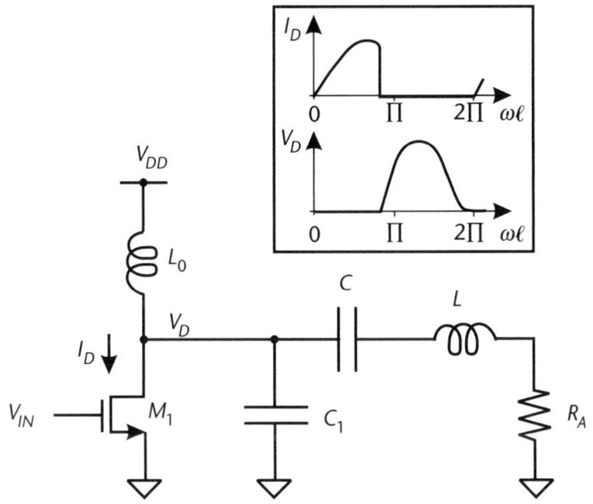

Figure 5.17 Class-E amplifier. From [19] with permission.

A disadvantage of this Class-E topology, aside from the large input requirement, is that the inductor L_0 needs to be fairly large to emulate a current source. At 400 MHz, the inductor size used in [19] is 100 nH, which is a very large value for on-chip integration.

Another transmitter concept uses Film Bulk Acoustic Resonator (FBAR) technology and injection locking to implement a high-efficiency PA [20]. FBAR is used in a reference oscillator at 1.9 GHz; since this technology can provide Q > 1000, a stable RF carrier is generated. The reference oscillator is then used to injection-lock a power oscillator, which outputs 0 dBm at 30% efficiency.

Note that in Figure 5.18, the data control also serves as the power control for the oscillators, hence this transmitter uses On-Off Keying (OOK) for the modulation

Table 5.1 Comparative Summary of Low-Power Amplifier

	[19]	*[20]*	*[21]*
Technology	0.18 μm CMOS process	0.13 μm CMOS process	0.13 μm CMOS process
Topology	Class E	Injection-locked oscillator	Class AB
Frequency (GHz)	0.433	1.9	1.9
Type of results	Simulated	Measured	Measured
Supply Voltage (V)	1.2	N/A	1.2
Output Power (dBm)	0	0	+4
Power added efficiency (%)	87	30	35

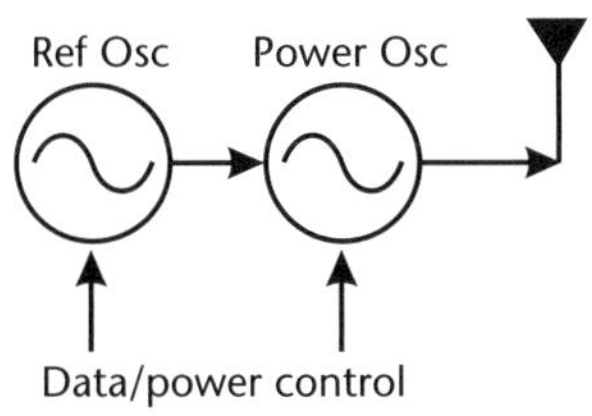

Figure 5.18 Injection locked transmitter. From [20] with permission.

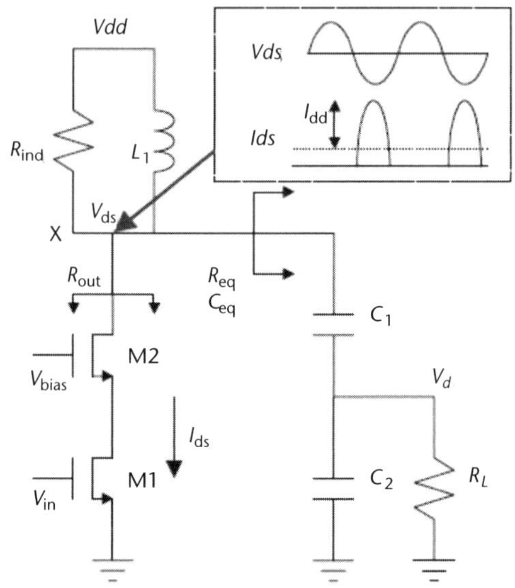

Figure 5.19 Class AB amplifier with capacitive transformer. From [21] with permission.

scheme. A disadvantage of this topology is the use of special process steps (i.e., FBAR) to create an on-chip high-Q passive device.

As noted before, since MICS requires only –16 dBm of output power, a relatively low PA efficiency is still acceptable in the overall budget. For example, a class AB amplifier driven into compression would have moderate efficiency, as shown by the work in [21].

In Figure 5.19, M1 is biased in saturation as a common source amplifier, and M2 serves as a cascode device. A capacitive transformer C_1 and C_2 is used to increase the load resistance, so as to improve the efficiency. Since this paper quoted an on-chip inductor with a Q of only 7, the design uses a bond-wire and external inductor combination for L_1. Overall, an efficiency of 35% is achieved.

5.11 Phase Locked Loop (PLL)

The PLL forms the heart of many radio architectures. Often, the Voltage Controlled Oscillator (VCO) and divider consume the most power within the PLL. For wireless applications, the LC VCO has been the standard workhorse due to its noise advantage over ring oscillators. A typical implementation of a LC VCO is depicted in Figure 5.20.

The phase noise of a VCO is a critical contributor to the radio performance. Though superceded by Hajimiri's recent work [22], Leeson's equation still gives some good first-order insights into factors affecting phase noise.

$$L(f_m) = 10 \cdot \log\left[\frac{FkT}{P_{SIG}} \cdot \frac{1}{2Q^2} \cdot \left(\frac{f_o}{f_m}\right)^2\right] \tag{5.6}$$

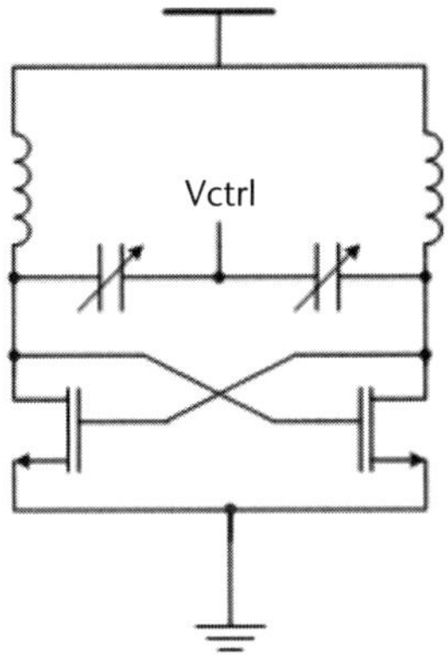

Figure 5.20 LC VCO.

To lower the phase noise, the designer must maximize the Q of the tank. Another way to look at this is for a given bias current, the higher the Q, the larger the voltage swing will be across the tank. This is intuitively satisfying since a larger swing naturally improves the Signal-to-Noise Ratio.

For the radio architecture chosen in this chapter, there are some considerations in choosing the VCO frequency:

1. Generation of quadrature LO for the receiver. This implies at least a 2X frequency in the VCO, meaning an oscillation frequency of about 800 MHz. The use of two coupled 400 MHz LC oscillators [23, 24], while possible, would increase the die area and raise the power consumption.
2. The use of a modulation loop for the transmitter.

A divide-by-2 block following the 800 MHz LC-VCO is used to generate the quadrature LO for the receiver. Modulation is applied at the VCO to generate the FSK transmit signal as shown in Figure 5.21.

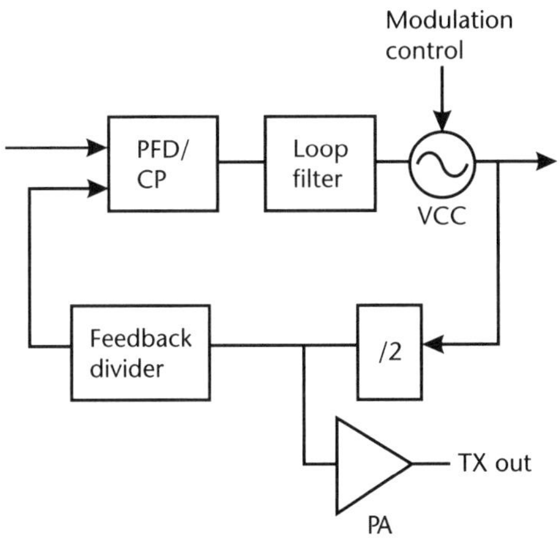

Figure 5.21 PLL block diagram (modulation loop).

5.12 Conclusions

Given the low frequency of 400 MHz for MICS, a low-cost, mature CMOS technology is sufficient to satisfy the RF requirements. It is also noted that while a low-power radio is a necessary condition, it is not sufficient to implement ultra-low-power systems. Power management, co-design of PHY and MAC layers, and use of FEC are also factors to consider in these designs.

As an example, Zarlink has commercialized an ultra-low-power MICS transceiver in 0.18 μm CMOS technology [25]. One unique feature of this chip is how it handles the wake-up feature, using the 2.4 GHz ISM band for the higher transmit power. Since the base station is not as power-constrained as a pacemaker, the base station can transmit at high power in the ISM band to ensure that the MICS receiver can detect the wake-up signal. The Zarlink wake-up receiver consumes only 715 μA when powered on, or an average of 250 nA for a 1.15-second cycle. It also uses OOK modulation to simplify the wake-up receiver circuit, allowing low-power consumption.

References

[1] Vanessa Knivett, "A new tract record," *New Electronics*, June 2004.

[2] Francois Pelletier and Steve Morris, "Doing more with much, much less: ultra-low power design for medical applications," *ECN*, May 15, 2003.

[3] S. Mehta et al., "An 802.11g WLAN SoC," *Proceedings of the International Solid-State Circuits Conference (ISSCC)*, San Francisco, CA, February 2005, pp. 94–95.

[4] H. Darabi et al., "A fully integrated SoC for 802.11b in 0.18μm CMOS," *Proceedings of the International Solid-State Circuits Conference (ISSCC)*, San Francisco, CA, February 2005, pp. 96–97.

[5] http://wireless.fcc.gov/services/personal/medical/implant/about.

[6] Z. Xu et al., "A compact dual-band direct-conversion CMOS transceiver for 802.11a/b/g WLAN," *Proceedings of the International Solid-State Circuits Conference (ISSCC)*, San Francisco, CA, February 2005, pp. 98–99.

[7] T. H. Lin, W. Kaiser, and G. Pottie, "Integrated low-power communication system design for wireless sensor networks," *IEEE Communications Magazine*, December 2004, pp. 142–150.

[8] UAA3535HL Datasheet, Philips Semiconductors, February 2000.

[9] B. Otis, Y. H. Chee, and J. Rabaey, "A 400 μW RX, 1.6mW TX super-regenerative transceiver for wireless sensor networks," *Proceedings of the International Solid-State Circuits Conference (ISSCC)*, San Francisco, CA, February 2005, pp. 396–397.

[10] J.Y. Chen, M.P. Flynn, and J.P. Hayes, "A fully integrated auto-calibrated super-regenerative receiver in 0.13 μm CMOS," *IEEE Journal of Solid-State Circuits*, vol. 42, no. 9, September 2007.

[11] D.K. Shaeffer and T.H. Lee, *The Design and Implementation of Low-Power CMOS Radio Receivers*, Kluwer, Boston, 1999.

[12] X. Guan and A. Hajimiri, "A 24 GHz CMOS front-end," *IEEE Journal of Solid-State Circuits*, vol. 39, no. 2, February 2004.

[13] T.K. Nguyen, C.H. Kim, G.J. Ihm, M.S. Yang, and S.G. Lee, "CMOS low-noise amplifier design optimization techniques," *IEEE Transactions on Microwave Theory and Techniques*, vol. 52, no. 5, pp. 1433–1442, May 2004.

[14] H. Lee and S. Mohammadi, "A 3GHz subthreshold CMOS low noise amplifier," *Proc. RFIC Symposium*, pp. 494–497, June 2006.

[15] D. Leenaerts and B. Redman-White, "1/f noise in passive CMOS mixers for low and zero IF integrated receivers," ESSIRC 2001, pp. 41–66, 2001.

[16] F. Behbahani, Y. Kishigami, J. Leete, and A. Abidi, "CMOS mixers and polyphase filters for large image rejection," *IEEE Journal of Solid-State Circuits*, vol. 36, no. 6, June 2001.

[17] A. Emira and E. Sanchez-Sinencio, "A pseudo differential complex filter for bluetooth with frequency tuning," *IEEE Transactions on Circuits and Systems—II: Analog and Digital Signal Processing*, vol. 50, no. 10, October 2003.

[18] B. Nauta, "A CMOS transconductance-C filter technique for very high frequencies," *IEEE Journal of Solid-State Circuits*, vol. 27, no. 2, February 1992.

[19] D. Aksin, S. Gregori, and F. Maloberti, "High-efficiency power amplifier for wireless sensor networks," *IEEE International Symposium on Circuits and Systems*, 23–26 May 2005, pp. 5898–5901.

[20] Y.H. Chee, A. Niknejad, and J. Rabaey, "An ultra-low power injection locked transmitter for wireless sensor networks," *IEEE Journal of Solid-State Circuits*, vol. 41, no. 8, August 2006.

[21] Y.H. Chee, J. Rabaey, and A. Niknejad, "A class A/B low power amplifier," *Proceedings of the 2004 International Symposium on Circuits and Systems*, vol. 4, 23–26 May, 2004, pp. 409–412.

[22] A. Hajimiri and T. H. Lee, " A general theory of phase noise in electrical oscillators," *IEEE Journal of Solid-State Circuits*, February 1998.

[23] A. Rofougaran, J. Rael, M. Rofougaran, and A. Abidi, "A 900 MHz CMOS LC-oscillator with quadrature outputs," *Proceedings of the International Solid-State Circuits Conference (ISSCC)*, San Francisco, CA, 1996, pp. 392–393.

[24] A. Mirzaei et al., "The quadrature LC oscillator: A complete portrait based on injection locking," *IEEE Journal of Solid-State Circuits*, vol. 42, no. 9, September 2007.

[25] P. Bradley, "RF integrated circuits for medical implants: Meeting the challenge of ultra-low power communication," CMOS Emerging Technology workshop, www.cmoset.com, 2006.

CHAPTER 6

Error-Correcting Codes for In Vivo RF Wireless Links

Sheryl L. Howard and Krzysztof Iniewski

6.1 Introduction

Wireless technology has been extended to implanted medical devices, allowing monitoring of the patient's condition relayed from in vivo devices such as pacemakers, cochlear implants, insulin dispensors, and neuro stimulators. Long battery lifetime of implanted devices is crucial, as replacement is invasive and expensive. Minimizing power, or maximizing power/energy efficiency, in the in vivo wireless link is a top priority, to maximize battery lifetime, reduce tissue heating, and meet regulatory power limitations.

An example of such in vivo wireless technology can be found in the wirelessly controlled pacemaker. Implanted into a patient to regulate their heartbeat, the pacemaker must not only be reliable, but draw minimal power so that battery replacement is infrequent, preferably not required at all. Wireless medical technology can open up new ways of preventive care. For example, a pacemaker can send a patient's health and device operating data to a wireless monitor. The monitor, which could be worn by the patient, then relays the data to a base station, potentially a nearby laptop, for further processing. The monitor could also alert a doctor if the pacemaker data warrants attention. Needless to say, the addition of wireless operation must not impact the pacemaker's battery life too much. Other examples of wirelessly aided in-vivo devices include defibrillators, neuro-stimulators, cochlear implants, and drug infusion/dispensing systems as shown in Figure 6.1.

The Federal Communications Commission (FCC) established the MICS frequency band [1] from 402 to 405 MHz, for short-range (up to 10 m) wireless links between an implanted device and a monitoring tool. This spectrum is shared with the Meteorological Aids Service (METAIDS) for weather balloon transmissions: to prevent interference, MICS systems are specified as indoors-only. These frequencies are harmonized with Europe, as implemented in the European Telecommunications Standards Institute (ETSI) standard EN 301 839 [2]. Although the MICS band is unlicensed at this time, MICS equipment must be operated by a medical professional. Since MICS is intended to connect an implant to external equipment for monitoring, diagnostic, or control purposes, no voice communication is allowed in this band. Operation in the MICS band limits the effective isotropic radiated power (EIRP) to 25 microwatts, or –16 dBm. The channel bandwidth is restricted to 300 kHz maximum.

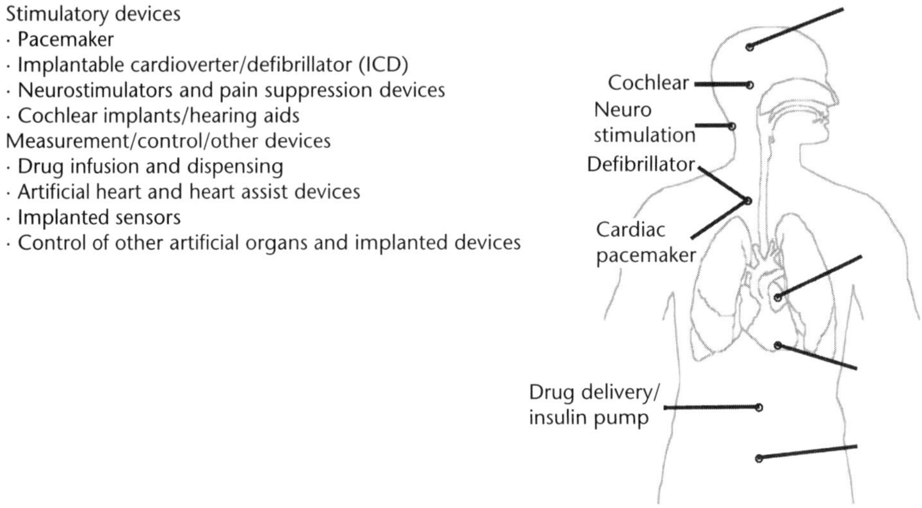

Figure 6.1 Schematic illustration of implantable devices that could utilize RF wireless communication. Courtesy of Zarlink Semiconductor Inc. [20].

The FCC has also established the Wireless Medical Telemetry Service (WMTS) band to allow communication between a non-implanted medical device and the monitor [3]. An implanted medical device would communicate with a monitoring device using MICS, and the monitoring device would then transfer that data to a base station, as shown schematically in Figure 6.2.

The strict limitation on radiated power and the need to minimize dissipated power at the implantable device, to maximize battery life, place enormous challenges on the RF (radio frequency) communication link. This paper explores the use of error-

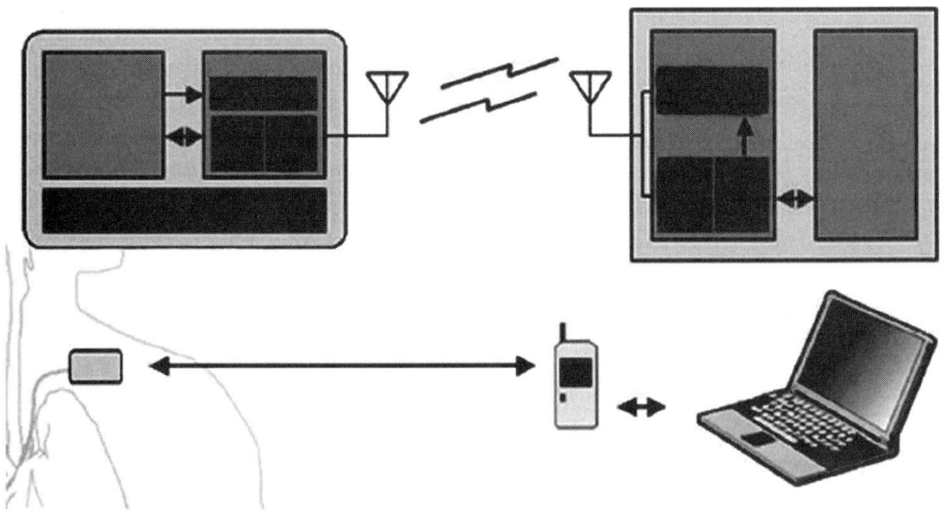

Figure 6.2 Schematic representation of the RF wireless links using MICS for in vivo and WMTS for in vitro communication. Courtesy of Zarlink Semiconductor Inc. [20].

correcting coding (ECC) at the device, to improve the bit error-rate (BER) for RF transmission and reduce the transmit power/energy of the implanted device.

Section 6.2 discusses briefly some of the issues posed by development of a channel model for the human body, and presents a reasonable loss figure for the MICS frequency range based on simulation models. An examination of the minimum power/energy requirements for an uncoded system and coded systems, which incorporate ECC, is presented in section 6.3. A comparison of the energy cost for several different coded systems with respect to an uncoded system for varying distance is shown in section 6.4, and section 6.5 presents our conclusions.

6.2 In Vivo Human Body Channel Modeling

Modeling RF transmission through the human body requires a channel model to characterize the propagation losses involved. The human body is conductive, and thus is a lossy medium. RF waves propagating through the body attenuate with distance, due to heating of conductive tissues. This thermal attenuation depends on the electrical properties of the body tissues, which are tissue- and frequency-dependent. First, we briefly discuss the electrical characteristics of biological tissue as a function of frequency. Following this, some general results regarding propagation of electromagnetic radiation in lossy media are analyzed. Some propagation models that have been presented in the literature for electromagnetic transmission through biological tissue are summarized. Finally, a figure combining all the propagation losses, based on numerical simulations [4] and confirmed by the ITU-R link budget for an MICS system [5], is presented.

The important electrical characteristics that carry information regarding the propagation of electromagnetic waves are the permittivity ϵ (the real part), conductivity σ (alternatively, the imaginary part of the complex permittivity $\epsilon'' = \sigma/\omega$), and permeability μ. In most biological tissues, the permeability is approximately equal to that of free space, (i.e., $\mu \approx \mu_o$). However, the conductivity and permittivity, in general, vary quite significantly from the corresponding free space values and are strong functions of frequency. Qualitatively, the permittivity decreases and the conductivity increases with increasing frequency. In the frequency dependence of these quantities, one also observes regions of rapid change at specific resonance frequencies; these are due to the enabling of specific biological and chemical relaxation mechanisms.

Based on basic laws of physics, the following observations can be made. Wetter materials (e.g., muscle, high water content tissue), are generally more lossy than dry materials (e.g., fat, bone). Signal attenuation depends on the angle of electromagnetic wave with respect to the body; typically it is higher as the direction of incident E becomes parallel to the length of the body. As a result, one can anticipate wide variation in channel loss properties reported in the literature and various methods for modeling the propagation of electromagnetic waves in biological tissue [6–12]. It is important to note that in free space, propagation models have the RF power decreasing at a rate $(1/d)^n$, where $n = 2$, due to path loss; the losses in propagation of electromagnetic radiation through human tissue are mainly due to absorption and dissipation as heat, and do not follow the free space path loss formula.

A model is presented in [6] for propagation loss based on single transmit and receive antennae separated by some given distance d. The antenna is modeled as a simple, elemental oscillating electric dipole. In contrast to many other models, the power absorption in the near-field region as well as the far-field is taken into account. The total received RF power is modeled as a function of the transmitted power as follows:

$$P_R = \frac{\left(P_T - P_{NF} - P_{FF}\right)\lambda^2 G_T G_R}{\left(4\pi d\right)^2} \tag{6.1}$$

where G_T and G_R are the gain of the transmitting and receiving antennae respectively, and P_{NF} and P_{FF} are the power absorbed in the near-field and the far-field regions, respectively; they depend on the characteristics of the antennae and medium (i.e., intrinsic impedence and propagation constant). Note that Equation 6.1 is quite similar in form to the well-known Friis equation for free-space propagation, which is often used to model power loss, except for the additional terms arising from absorption in the near-field and far-field regions. One significant result shown in [6] is that the power absorbed in the near field constitutes a significant portion of the total loss, suggesting that some models that neglect the near-field region may not be applicable to losses in tissue. Unfortunately, the usefulness of Equation 6.1 is limited, as no analytical solutions for P_{NF} and P_{FF} are found.

Lack of an accurate path loss model for the human body steers us toward characterizing the loss based on simulation data. An examination of the path loss from an implanted antenna in the human body radiating at 403 MHz as measured outside the body is presented in [4]. Numerical simulations using the finite-difference time-domain (FDTD) method were performed for electrically equivalent phantom models of the human body models with implanted antenna. FDTD solves Maxwell's equations in space and time for a specified volume and electrical properties using finite difference equations. Four phantom sizes were used, with varying implantation depth. Phantom size resulted in 3 dB difference in loss, and 7 dB change with implantation depth. Different arm and patient orientations were tried; loss varied by 5 dB and 2.5 dB for arm and patient orientation, respectively.

Minimum path loss was 23 dB with a mean path loss of 34 dB. Including the potential loss for arm and patient orientation and size, totalling 10.5 dB, brought the potential maximum path loss to 44.5 dB. The maximum path loss figure found in [4] was 51 dB for a patient in bed, varying position. Adding a 15 dB loss margin to the mean path loss also provides 49 dB body path loss. This compares closely with the ITU-R document SA.1346 [5], which includes a link budget for a MICS system. The uplink (implanted device to monitor or base station) specifies a body loss of –31.5 dB, with an excess loss figure of 15 dB given to cover patient orientation, polarization losses, antenna misalignment and arm movement, resulting in a total loss of 46.5 dB.

The MICS EIRP limitation of 25 μW or –16 dBm is a requirement on power radiated out of the human body, not transmit power from the implanted sensor, which attenuates with travel through the body. Assuming the minimum body path loss of –23 dB, maximum implant power should be 7 dBm, or 5 mW, to avoid exceeding the MICS EIRP limit.

The next section finds the required transmit power and energy for both uncoded and coded systems to achieve a requisite BER, given the body path loss (BPL) figure from this section. An equation for the ratio of minimum required transmit energy per data bit for coded compared to uncoded is then derived. Values for this ratio over the MICS distance range of up to 10 m are calculated for various coded systems in section 6.4 using the maximum BPL of 50 dB.

6.3 Power Dissipation Model for the RF Link with Error-Correcting Codes

For power considerations, the uplink (implant to monitor/base station) is the critical path in this model. The implant sends patient data to the monitor. The monitor contacts the implant infrequently, requesting collected data or operating parameters. Our uplink model consists of an implanted device in the patient, with transceiver including an encoder for a coded system, transmitting to a monitor within the 10 m range of the MICS standard. As the decoder typically consumes 2 to 3 orders of magnitude more power than the encoder, it may not be practical to include a decoder at the implant due to power restrictions. Clearly, inclusion of the decoder at the implant substantially increases power consumption at the implant, and is not necessary, since the monitor is assumed to have substantial available power resources. Thus, we consider an encoder-only scenario at the implant. For the same reasons, the monitor is assumed to contain only the decoder, as the monitor has no need to encode its data request transmissions to the implant.

As low-power consumption is critical for extended battery lifetime at the sensor, and use of ECC enables the implant to transmit with lower power, incorporating the encoder at the implant is a crucial step toward reducing uplink power. The monitor has fewer power limitations and can transmit with higher power, so the implant is able to receive monitor transmissions without requiring coding. Also, the monitor can afford the higher power consumption incurred by the decoder to enable accurate decoding of the implant's low-power transmission.

To determine the power and energy costs at the implant for a coded system requires both the power consumption of the encoder and perhaps the decoder, and the minimum transmit power required to achieve a desired BER at a monitor a distance d from the patient. The uncoded system does not have the extra power cost of the encoder or decoder, but requires higher transmit power to achieve the same BER. The coded system's data throughput $R' = R_c R < F$ due to the (dimensionless) coding rate $R_c < 1$. Using energy per data bit (power divided by data throughput) provides a better measure of comparison between coded and uncoded systems.

The minimum required transmit power $P_{TX,U}$ for an uncoded system to provide SNR_U sufficient to achieve a certain BER is found by adding the body path loss (BPL) figure from section 6.2 to the other sources of noise, such as thermal noise (kTB) and receiver noise figure (RNF). The path loss through the air in the office is modeled as the modified Friis equation, which uses path loss exponent $n > 2$ to emulate obstructions from the line-of-sight free space model. The minimum uncoded transmit power $P_{TX,U}$ and energy per data bit $E_{TX,U}$ are given by [13]

$$P_{TX,U} = kTB\left(\frac{4\pi}{\lambda}\right)^2 d^n 10^{\left(\mathrm{SNR}_U/10+\mathrm{RNF}/10+\mathrm{BPL}/10\right)} \quad [W] \tag{6.2}$$

$$E_{TX,U} = P_{TX,U} / R \quad [J/\mathrm{bit}] \tag{6.3}$$

where d is the distance from the body surface to receiver, n is the path loss exponent (PLE) describing the external environment [14] ($n \approx 3$ for an office environment) [15], and R is the data throughput. The thermal noise is kTB, where k is Boltzmann's constant, T is ambient temperature, and B is transmission bandwidth in Hz. For BPSK modulation, the maximum throughput with the MICS bandwidth limitation is R = 300 kbps. Transmit power has a multiplicative factor of $\eta_u = R/B = 1$, where η_u is the uncoded BPSK spectral efficiency, not shown in Equation 6.3.

For a coded system, the minimum transmit power $P_{TX,c}$ and energy per data bit $E_{TX,c}$ required to achieve the same BER at SNR_c is found as follows: [13]

$$\begin{aligned} P_{TX,c} &= \eta_c kTB\left(\frac{4\pi}{\lambda}\right)^2 d^n 10^{\left(\mathrm{SNR}_c/10+\mathrm{RNF}/10+\mathrm{BPL}/10\right)} \quad [W] \\ E_{TX,c} &= R_c P_{TX,U} / \left(R_c R\right) = E_{TX,U} 10^{\left(-\mathrm{ECC}_{\mathrm{gain}}/10\right)} \quad [J/\mathrm{bit}] \end{aligned} \tag{6.4}$$

where $\eta_c = R_c R/B = R_c$ is the coded spectral efficiency, R_c is the code rate and the coding gain $\mathrm{ECC}_{\mathrm{gain}} = \mathrm{SNR}_U - \mathrm{SNR}_c$. Use of ECC lowers the required minimum transmit power with respect to an uncoded system.

The coded system has the additional power cost of the encoder at the implant as well. The total minimum required energy per data bit of the coded system with respect to an uncoded system includes encoder energy per data bit $P_{\mathrm{enc}}/(R_c R)$ as

$$\begin{aligned} E_{\mathrm{total}} &= E_{TX,c} + P_{\mathrm{enc}} / \left(R_c R\right) \quad [J/\mathrm{bit}] \\ &= E_{TX,U} 10^{-\mathrm{ECC}_{\mathrm{gain}}/10} + P_{\mathrm{enc}} / \left(R_c R\right) \end{aligned} \tag{6.5}$$

A ratio of the coded system's minimum required energy per bit to the uncoded system's minimum required energy per bit is then found as

$$\frac{E_c}{E_{TX,U}} = \frac{E_{TX,U} 10^{\left(\mathrm{SNR}_c - \mathrm{SNR}_U\right)/10}}{E_{TX,U}} + \frac{P_{\mathrm{enc}}}{R_c R E_{TX,U}} \tag{6.6}$$

$$= 10^{\left(\mathrm{SNR}_c - \mathrm{SNR}_U\right)/10} + \frac{P_{\mathrm{enc}}}{R_c R E_{TX,U}} \tag{6.7}$$

$$= 10^{-\mathrm{ECC}_{\mathrm{gain}}/10} + P_{\mathrm{enc}} / \left(R_c P_{TX,U}\right) \tag{6.8}$$

Clearly, if Equation 6.8 < 1, the coded system is more energy efficient!

Equation 6.8 has two terms. The constant term $10^{-ECC_{gain}/10}$ is dependent on the coding gain. The second term, $P_{enc}/(R_c P_{TX,U})$, decreases as the transmit power of the uncoded system, $P_{TX,U}$, increases; thus the second term goes to zero as d approaches ∞. Asymptotically, Equation 6.8 depends only on the coding gain as d becomes very large. In other words, for very large d, the stronger coding systems are the most energy-efficient solution. However, the MICS scenario is short-range only, for distances up to 10 m. The question becomes, is there a distance within that 10 m range beyond which a coded system is more energy-efficient than an uncoded system? Will a coded system save energy over most of that range despite the extra power cost of the encoder (and possibly decoder), or would an uncoded system actually consume less energy?

The next section examines these questions using Equation 6.8 and power consumption figures for some encoder and decoder implementations of several types of error-correcting codes. An uplink model with only an encoder at the implant is used.

6.4 Encoder Implementations and Power Savings for ECC

We now examine several encoder implementations. The block codes include a (255, 223) Reed-Solomon (RS) encoder [16], and the (8, 4) and (16, 11) extended Hamming codes (EHC). A rate 1/2 constraint length 7 convolutional code (CC) and a rate 1/3 turbo code [17] composed of two component rate 1/2 constraint length 3 convolutional codes with an interleaver size of 40 bits are also shown. A $(16, 11)^2$ turbo product code composed of component (16, 11) extended Hamming codes and a rate 1/2 convolutional low-density parity-check code (LDPC-CC) [18] with 128 processors complete our code selection.

Table 6.1 lists power estimates obtained from Synopsis for all encoders except the Reed-Solomon encoder, which lists actual power consumption figures. The maximum throughput that the MICS channel can support for BPSK modulation is 300

Table 6.1 Different Encoder Implementations: Static and Dynamic Power Estimates, and Required SNR for BER = 10^{-6} at Receiver

Encoder Type	*Process Size in nm*	*Supply Voltage* V_{dd}	*Freq. in MHz*	P_{static} *in μW*	P_{dyn} *in μW*	P_{enc} *in μW*	*SNR at BER =* 10^{-6} *in dB*
Uncoded	—	—	—	—	—	—	10.4
(255,223) RS [16]	350	0.5 V	30	2000	2150	4150	6.5
R 1/2 CC	90	0.9 V	100	3.4	13.6	17	5.2
(8,4) EHC	90	0.9 V	100	2.8	13.1	15.9	8.3
(16,11) EHC	90	0.9 V	100	7	29.3	36.3	7.3
$(16,11)^2$ TPC	90	0.9 V	100	1261	1053	2314	3.8
R 1/3 turbo	90	0.9 V	100	18.9	186	205	5.1
R 1/2 LDPC-CC	90	0.9 V	100	1060	271	1331	3.2

kbps; the encoders operate at high speed for short amounts of time, and then the transmitter transmits BPSK symbols at a maximum symbol rate of 300 kbps. For constant channel transmission, the encoders are on only 0.3% of the time at most. Typically, medical implants do not need to relay data constantly, and thus the encoders would actually operate for a smaller percentage of the time.

Both static and dynamic power figures are given in Table 6.1, as well as the total power consumption of the encoder, P_{enc}. Encoder power consumption was approximated using an industry-standard 90-nm CMOS process with dual-threshold standard cells and an operating voltage of 0.9 V, for all but the Reed-Solomon encoder, which used a 0.35 μm, ultra-low-power 0.5 V CMOS process.

Table 6.1 also lists, for each coded system, the required SNR at the receiver to provide a BER of 10^{-6}, assuming BPSK modulation over an AWGN channel with zero-mean Gaussian noise of variance $N_0/2$. SNR is defined as SNR = 10 $\log_{10}(E_b/N_0)$, where E_b is the energy per bit. In determining the BER at a specific SNR for the coded systems, the following decoders were assumed: the Hamming, turbo product and turbo decoders use *maximum a posteriori* (MAP) decoding, while convolutional decoding uses a soft-decision Viterbi decoder, and the LDPC-CC decoder uses sum-product decoding.

Results for the ratio of coded to uncoded minimum required transmit energy per bit (Equation 6.8) to achieve a receiver BER = 10^{-6} vs. distance d between patient implant and monitor for various codes, using the power estimates from Table 6.1, are shown in Figure 6.3. The uplink model includes only the encoder in the implanted device. The encoders are clocked at 100 MHz, but channel transmission rate is limited by the bandwidth constraint to 300 kpbs, so the encoders operate at most 0.3% of the time. SNR values are as per Table 6.1. Table 6.2 lists the parameter values used in evaluating (6.8).

The dashed horizontal black line shown in Figure 6.3 emphasizes where a coded system consumes the same amount of energy as an uncoded system for a given distance, that is, when $E_c/E_{TX,U}$ = 1. This line is the boundary below which a coded system is more energy-efficient than an uncoded system.

The most energy-efficient system choice depends on the distance between the patient and the monitor. Below 50 cm, all of the encoded systems show a ratio of coded to uncoded transmit energy $E_c/E_{TX,U} > 1$. An uncoded system consumes less energy than any of the considered encoded systems at d ″ 50 cm, and is the most energy-efficient choice. Between 50 cm and 4 m, the rate 1/2 convolutional code displays the lowest value for the ratio $E_c/E_{TX,U}$ of 0.3, and is the most energy-efficient choice in this region from 0.5 to 4 m. Note that the convolutional code reaches its asymptotic performance, which depends only on the coding gain, by 2 m. This region is marked as Region I on Figure 6.3. The vertical dot-dashed line at d = 4 m differenti ates Region I from Region II, where different codes provide the best energy efficiency.

Above 4 m, the stronger codes with their greater coding gain begin to assert themselves. The rate 1/2 LDPC-CC provides a ratio $E_c/E_{TX,U}$ = 0.2, or 5 times as energy-efficient as an uncoded system, and 1.5 times as energy-efficient as the convolutional-coded system. The $(16, 11)^2$ turbo product code is nearly as energy-efficient as the rate 1/2 LDPC-CC, with a ratio $E_c/E_{TX,U}$ = 0.23. This region above 4 m is denoted as Region II in Figure 6.3.

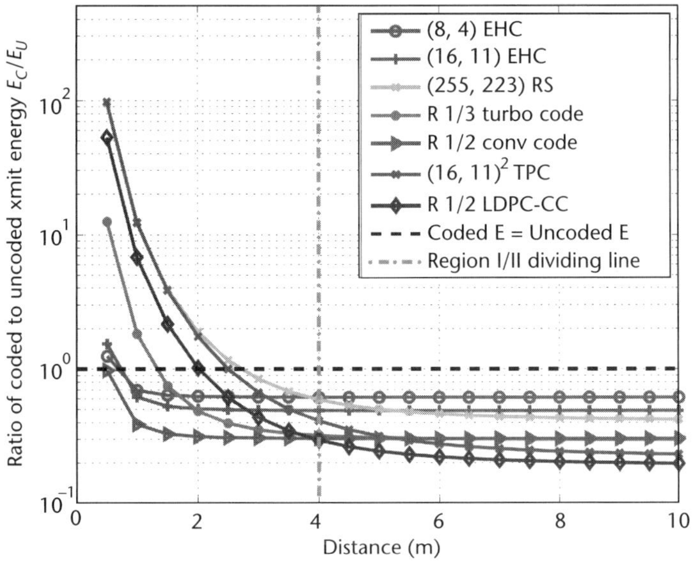

Figure 6.3 Ratio of coded to uncoded minimum required transmit energy per bit vs. distance between implant and monitor for the MICS encoder-only implant scenario, using different codes.

Table 6.2 Parameters Used in Transmit Power Calculations

T, K°	*B*, *kHz*	*RNF*, *dB*	*BPL*, *dB*	*f*, *MHz*	*PLE* n
300	300	5 [19]	50	403	3

6.5 Conclusions

This paper examined the effect of coding on the energy usage of an in-vivo wireless link consisting of a implanted medical device communicating with an external monitor according to the MICS requirements. An uplink model in which the implanted device contains only an encoder, and the external monitor is assumed to have substantial power resources and thus does not require coding of its own transmitted data to save energy, is considered. An equation for the ratio of required minimum transmit energy per bit for a coded versus an uncoded system for a specified receiver BER was derived. This ratio was shown to depend asymptotically on only the coding gain; however, for shorter distances, the encoder power consumption certainly plays a significant part.

Power estimates for various encoder implementations were given. Results for the ratio of required minimum transmit energy per bit for coded versus uncoded systems were found over a distance *d* ranging from 50 cm to 10 m for each encoder, to determine which coding system was the most energy efficient at what distance.

The most energy-efficient system depends on distance between patient and receiver. Below 50 cm, an uncoded system is more energy efficient than any of the coding systems considered here. Between 50 cm and 4 m, a rate 1/2 convolutional code provided the best energy efficiency. Above 4 m, the coding gain of the stronger codes prevailed, and the rate 1/2 LDPC-CC offered the best energy efficiency, with the $(16, 11)^2$ product code providing nearly as good energy efficiency.

Over the entire range of *d*, the convolutional code offers the best performance of the codes considered. The rate 1/2 convolutional code provides the best energy efficiency from 0.5 to 4 m. In this range, the stronger codes are not nearly as energy efficient as the convolutional code, and below 2 m, they are even less energy efficient than an uncoded system. Above 4 m, the convolutional code is nearly, though not quite, as energy efficient as the more complex LDPC-CC and $(16, 11)^2$ turbo product code. The overall energy efficiency of the convolutional code, considering the entire 10 m range of the MICS scenario, is the best, especially if we consider that in the 1-m to 2-m range, the stronger codes are 2 to 50 times less energy efficient than the convolutional code.

Acknowledgments

Many thanks to Amirhossein Alimohammed and Tyler Brandon Lee for their help with the Synopsis power estimates of the encoders, to Ramkrishna Swamy for the LDPC-CC encoder power estimate, and to Dr. Christian Schlegel of the iCORE High Capacity Digital Communications Laboratory, and Dr. Bruce Cockburn of the VLSI Laboratory, at the University of Alberta.

References

[1] *FCC Rules and Regulations*, "MICS Band Plan," Part 95, Jan. 2003. See also 47 CFR 95.601–95.673 Subpart E, Federal Communications Commission, 1999.

[2] ETSI EN 301 839-1 "Electromagnetic compatibility and radio spectrum matters (ERM); Radio equipment in the frequency range 402 MHz to 405 MHz for ultra low power active medical implants and accessories; Part 1: Technical characteristics, including electromagnetic compatibility requirements, and test methods," *European Telecommunications Standards Institute*, 2002.

[3] *FCC Rules and Regulations*, "WMTS Band Plan," Part 95, Jan. 2003. See also 47 CFR 95.601–95.673 Subpart H, Federal Communications Commission, 1999.

[4] A.J. Johansson, *Wireless Communication with Medical Implants: Antennas and Propagation*, Ph.D. thesis, Lund University, Sweden, June 2004.

[5] International Telecommunication Union, *Recommendation ITU-R SA.1346*, 1998.

[6] S.K.S. Gupta, S. Lalwani, Y. Prakash, E. Elsharawy, and L. Schwiebert, "Towards a propagation model for wireless biomedical applications," *IEEE Intl. Conf. Communications (ICC) 2003*, pp. 1993–1997.

[7] T. Zasowski et al., "Propagation effects in UWB body area networks," *ICU 2005: IEEE International Conference on Ultra-Wideband*, Sept. 2005.

[8] T. Zasowski et al., "UWB for noninvasive wireless body area networks: channel measurement and results," *IEEE Conference on Ultra-Wideband Systems and Technologies*, Nov. 2003, pp. 285–289.

[9] J. Ryckaert et al., "Channel model for wireless communication around human body," *Electronics Letters*, vol. 40, no. 9, April 2004.

[10] M.G. Sanchez et al., "Human operator effect on wide-band radio channel characteristics," *IEEE Transactions on Antennas and Propagation*, vol. 45, no. 8, pp. 1318–1320, Aug. 1997.

[11] H. Junker et al., "Wireless networks in context aware wearable systems," *EWSN 2004: 1st European Workshop on Wireless Sensor Networks*, Jan. 2004, pp. 37–40.

[12] A. Ylisaukko-oja, E. Vildjiounaite, and J. Mantyjarvi, "Five-point acceleration sensing wireless body area network—design and practical experiences," *ISWC 2003: Proceedings of the Eighth International Symposium on Wearable Computers*, Oct.–Nov. 2004, vol. 1, pp. 184–185.

[13] S. Howard, K. Iniewski, and C. Schlegel, "Error control coding in low-power wireless sensor networks: When is ECC energy-efficient?," *EURASIP Journal of Wireless Communications and Networking, Special Issue: CMOS RF Circuits for Wireless Applications*, Vol. 2006, Article ID 74812, pp. 1–14.

[14] H. Hasheni, "The indoor propagation channel," *Proc. of IEEE*, vol. 81, pp. 943–968, July 2004.

[15] S.Y. Seidel and T.S. Rappaport, "Path loss prediction in multifloored buildings at 914 MHz," *IEE Electronics Letters*, vol. 27, no. 15, pp. 1384–1387, July 1991.

[16] J. Gambles, L. Miles, J. Hass, W. Smith, and S. Whitaker, "An ultra-low-power, radiation-tolerant reed solomon encoder for space applications," *IEEE Custom Integrated Circuits Conf. (CICC) 2003*, pp. 631–634, May 2003.

[17] C. Berrou, A. Glavieux, and P. Thitimajshima, "Near Shannon limit error-correcting coding and decoding: Turbo codes," *Proc. IEEE Int'l Conf. Comm. (ICC) 1993*, pp. 1064–1070.

[18] S. Bates and R. Swamy, "Parallel encoders for low-density parity-check convolutional codes," *Proc. IEEE Intl. Sym. Circuits and Systems (ISCAS) 2006*, May 2006.

[19] T. Lee, *The Design of CMOS Radio-Frequency Integrated Circuits*, 2nd edition, Cambridge University Press, 2004.

[20] P. Bradley, Zarlink Semiconductor, "RF integrated circuits for medical implants: Meeting the challenges of ultra low-power communication," *2006 CMOS Emerging Technologies Workshop*, July 2006, www.cmoset.com/2006slides.html.

CHAPTER 7

Microneedles: A Solid-State Interface with the Human Body

Boris Stoeber

7.1 Introduction

Microneedles are small mechanical structures that can act as an interface between a microsystem and an organism such as the human body. Microneedles typically have a length in the range L = 50–1500 μm and a width on the order W = 10–250 μm (Figure 7.1). The hollow microneedles have a lumen diameter in the range D = 8–200 μm. The following discussion will focus on hollow needle structures; lancet-like solid structures that are also often referred to as microneedles will only briefly be described.

Research on microneedles started in the early 1990s [1], and this field has been progressively growing. In most cases, microneedles have been designed as a means to provide an artificial pathway across the protective skin barrier. The main application of microneedles is to serve as a minimally invasive interface with the body, either for drug delivery into the skin or for sensing of biological signals or compounds inside the body.

7.1.1 The Structure of the Skin

Figure 7.2 shows a schematic cross-section of the human skin. The epidermis is typically 100 μm thick and forms the outermost layer of the skin. Only very few nerve endings are located in the epidermis [2, 3] so that only little or no sensation of pain may be associated with epidermal insertion of microneedles. The stratum corneum is the outermost layer of the epidermis and protects the body from the environment. The stratum corneum essentially consists of flat dead skin cells that are tightly packed together; the stratum corneum renews itself about once per month. In most locations of the upper human body, the stratum corneum is approximately 20 μm thick, however, it also forms the calices that can be substantially thicker, for example on the palms of the hands. The dermis is located underneath the epidermis and contains the nerve endings as well as blood vessels. The thickness of the dermis varies between 0.6 mm and 3 mm. The subcutaneous fat layer is situated underneath the dermis.

Drug injection through microneedles into the interstitial fluid of the epidermis relies on the drug diffusing into the capillary bed of the dermis. Here, the drug is

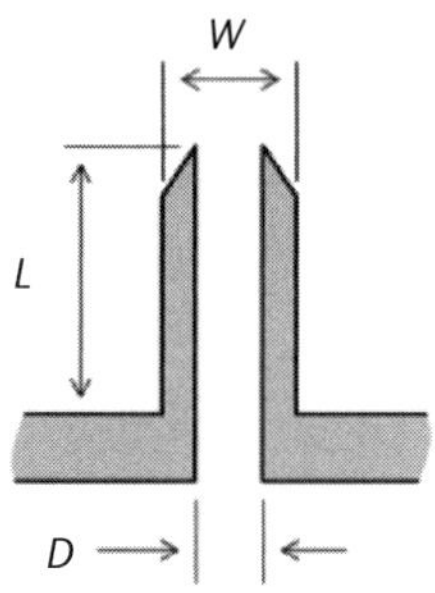

Figure 7.1 Schematic representation of a microneedle of length L, width W, and lumen diameter D.

absorbed into the bloodstream and is then transported through the body. The interstitial fluid of the epidermis also contains many molecules of biological interest such as glucose. Microneedles therefore offer minimally invasive access to a site for sensing of these compounds in the body.

The fact that the skin consists of a very flexible tissue with the stratum corneum as the protective layer has several implications for the mechanics of penetration of the stratum corneum by microneedles. The needle shaft might therefore need to be longer than the intended penetration depth because of skin deformation during insertion. A needle array that is too dense will rather press the skin uniformly down through the bed-of-nails effect instead of penetrating the stratum corneum.

Carefully designed, microneedles are the ideal instrument to penetrate the stratum corneum while reaching no further than into the epidermis. Such an injection avoids contact with the blood vessels of the dermis, thus minimizing the risk of infections. In addition, this allows minimizing the stimulation of the nerve endings, which are located deeper in the skin.

7.1.2 Categories of Microneedles and Probes

Microneedles and probes can be categorized according to the geometry of their design. Here, we will consider hollow structures as needles [1, 6–27] and solid structures as probes [4, 5, 28–35]. Both needles and probes can also be divided into in-

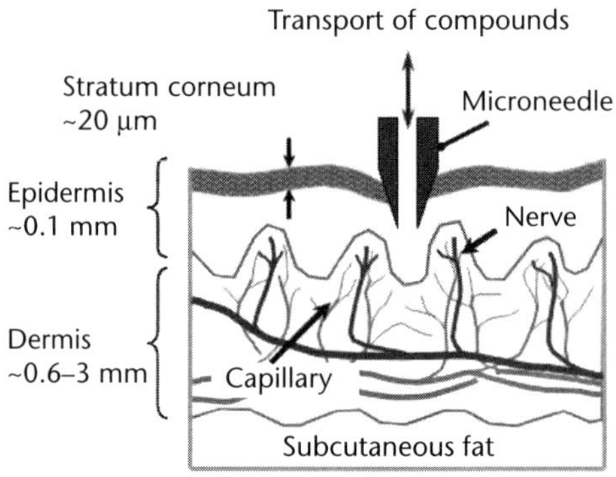

Figure 7.2 The structure of the skin.

plane [1, 6, 12–18, 28, 29] and out-of-plane [4–11, 19–27, 30–35] designs according to the orientation of their shafts in relation to the substrate. Figure 7.3 gives an overview of these four categories.

Solid in-plane probes are typically used as electrodes for sensing applications [29], sometimes combined with channels for drug delivery [14, 15, 18], while solid out-of-plane probes are also used for biopotential measurements [30] and to record neural signals [4, 36]. In addition, some solid out-of-plane probes have simply been used as mechanical puncture devices to perforate the stratum corneum in order to increase the skin permeability for certain compounds; this concept has been demonstrated *in vitro* for calcein by Henry et al. [5]. In some cases, solid needles have been made from biodegradable materials containing compounds that can be slowly released into the skin after needle insertion [33, 34, 37].

The most common application for hollow microneedles is injection or sampling of compounds. In-plane designs are more amenable to monolithic integration with electronics, while out-of-plane designs allow arrangement in high-density arrays and/or in large arrays, where the needles or probes can be packed closely together and/or interfaced with a wide area. Injection of compounds into the skin is limited by the absorbance of the tissue. It is expected that injection of compounds into the skin over a large surface area allows delivery of larger amounts, while avoiding early saturation of the skin with fluid, so that out-of-plane microneedles can provide a significant advantage for drug delivery applications compared to in-plane designs. Likewise, transport of compounds out of the skin for measurement applications can occur at a higher rate through a larger number of needles such as in an array of out-of-plane microneedles. This makes out-of-plane needles a very attractive design solution for transferring compounds across the skin barrier. The following discussion will therefore focus on hollow out-of-plane designs.

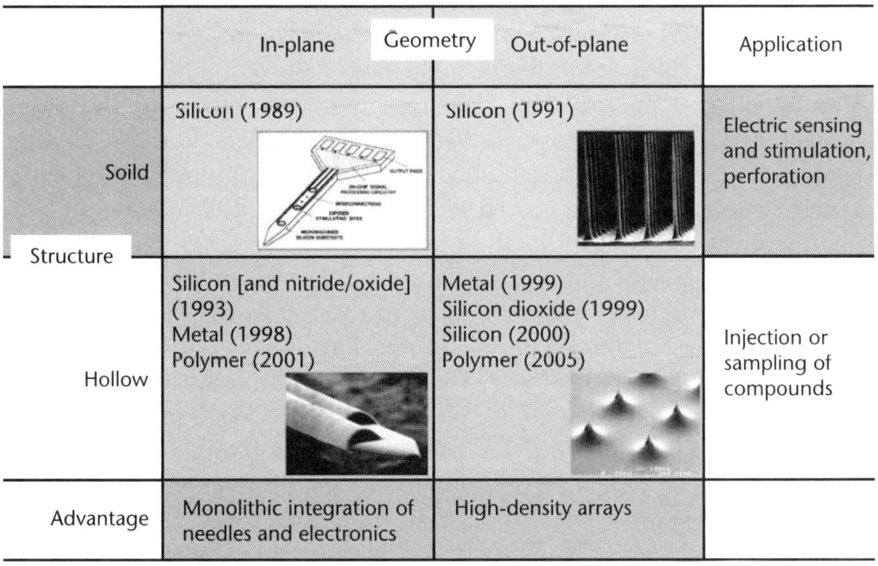

Figure 7.3 The four major microneedle categories: solid in-plane [29], solid out-of-plane [4], hollow in-plane [18], hollow out-of-plane [10].

7.2 Fabrication Methods for Hollow Out-of-Plane Microneedles

Microneedles are typically fabricated using microelectromechanical system (MEMS) technology, which has been derived from integrated circuit (IC) fabrication technology. MEMS fabrication features special processes that allow forming mechanical structures, while pattern transfer is commonly based on photolithography methods [38]. Several microfabrication processes have been reported to form out-of plane microneedles. In particular, hollow microneedles have been formed from a large variety of materials including silicon, silicon nitride, silicon dioxide, metal, and polymers. Out of these, silicon dioxide structures have not been demonstrated at lengths above 30 μm [39], which would be necessary to guarantee penetration of the stratum corneum; since the stratum corneum is located on top of soft deformable skin layers as described above, longer needles than the thickness of the stratum corneum are required to pierce through it.

The following description of fabrication methods for out-of-plane microneedles will therefore focus on metal, silicon and polymers as needle materials. These methods also include the formation of needles with blind holes as lumens. This means that the lumens do not provide a continuous pathway across the substrate, which would be necessary for the transport of compounds through the needles. However, these methods are included because they might be further developed in the future to form truly hollow microneedles.

7.2.1 Fabrication of Metal Microneedles

Several methods have been reported for the fabrication of metal microneedles using electroplating of a metal layer onto a sacrificial structure and subsequently dissolving all or part of this support to release the needles. Kim et al. [8] employed SU-8, a photocurable polymer (by MicroChem Corp.) that was exposed in two steps as shown in Figure 7.4.

A first 200 μm thick SU-8 layer was spun onto a glass substrate and exposed through the substrate to define a backing. A second 200 μm thick SU-8 layer was spun on top of the first one. This layer was exposed through the glass and the first layer of SU-8 to define tapered 30–50 μm thick pillars. Both SU-8 layers were developed in one step, after which only the exposed regions of SU-8 remained. The polymer structure was then coated with a seed layer of chromium and copper for the subsequent nickel electroplating process. After electroplating, an additional SU-8 layer was deposited onto the structure, soft-baked, and then mechanically polished; this allowed removing the metal from the top of the posts of the exposed SU-8 structure in order to open the needle tips. Finally, this last, unexposed SU-8 layer was removed using SU-8 developer. The double layer of cross-linked SU-8 used as a mold was then removed using O_2/SF_6 plasma. Typical needles made with this process had lengths of 200 or 400 μm, diameters of 60 to 200 μm, and wall thicknesses of 10 or 20 μm.

A different process for fabrication of metal microneedles that uses a 500 μm thick Mylar sheet as sacrificial mold material was presented by Davis et al. [9]. The authors used an excimer laser to sequentially drill individual holes through the sheet, one for each needle. An approximately 200 μm wide beam was moved in a circular pattern,

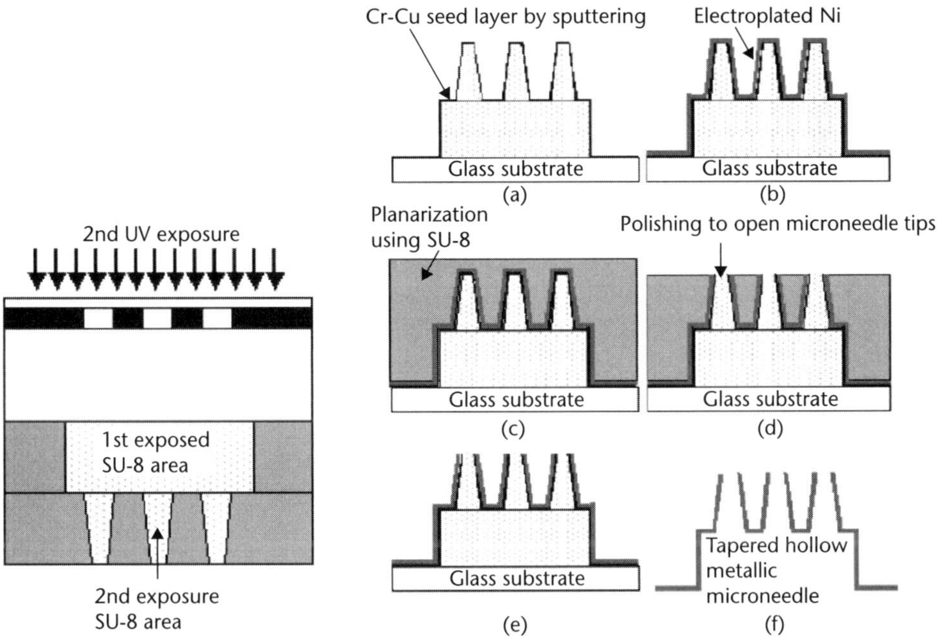

Figure 7.4 Microneedle fabrication through electroplating a polymer mold made from a photocurable polymer (SU-8). From [8] with permission.

where the center of the circle always received laser energy. This led to a deeper drill depth in the center, forming a tapered hole as shown in Figure 7.5. A seed layer of 35 nm titanium, 650 nm copper, and 35 nm titanium was then sputter deposited onto the side of the Mylar sheet that had the wider openings as well as inside the holes. Nickel was then deposited through electroplating at a rate of 10 μm per hour. Finally, the Mylar sheet was dissolved in a caustic solution within 20 minutes. Arrays of needles were fabricated using this method with typical needle diameters of 50 to 400 μm, lengths of 50 to 1000 μm, and wall thicknesses of 2 to 20 μm.

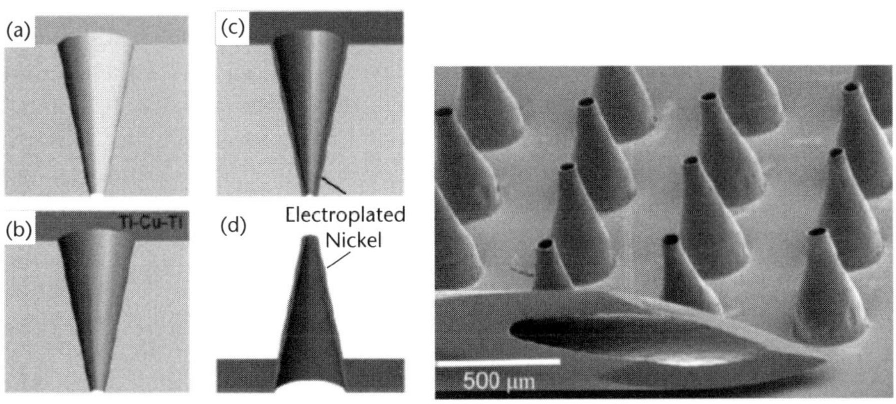

Figure 7.5 Microneedle fabrication through electroplating of a polymer mold made by laser machining of a Mylar sheet (left); an array of hollow metal needles (right) shown next to a 27-gauge hypodermic needle. From [9] with permission, © IEEE 2005.

Shikida et al. fabricated hollow metal needle arrays by dicing of a silicon substrate, anisotropic wet etching and metal deposition [27]. For this purpose, a silicon wafer was coated with a silicon dioxide layer on both sides. The backside silicon dioxide layer was patterned through photolithography and etching, while a dicing saw was used on the frontside to cut 60 μm wide 300 μm deep perpendicular grooves at a pitch of around 250 μm. An anisotropic silicon etch reduced the width of the silicon pillars on the frontside to hourglass shapes. After deposition of a protective chromium and gold layer onto the top of the pillars and onto their sidewalls with positive angles, an additional silicon etch removed the unprotected upper parts of the pillars. After electroplating 5 to 10 μm nickel onto the metal seed layer, a longer, anisotropic silicon etch opened the needle lumens from the front and the back of the substrate. The geometry of the final needles was therefore defined by the orientation of the crystal planes of the silicon.

Kobayashi et al. demonstrated individual needles formed by depositing platinum on to a sacrificial aluminum wire [7]. This process is not well-suited for the fabrication of large arrays of needles.

While the SU-8 process by Kim et al. seems to involve a manageable effort and allows batch fabrication, the sequential fabrication step of laser machining the sacrificial Mylar sheet by Davis et al. occurs to be very time intensive. However, this process provides a higher flexibility for defining the needle shape compared to the sacrificial silicon process by Shikida et al.

7.2.2 Fabrication of Silicon Microneedles

All fabrication methods for hollow out-of-plane silicon microneedles described below employ deep reactive ion etching (DRIE) to form the needle lumens, and most of these methods also use DRIE to define the outer shapes of the needles.

Stoeber and Liepmann used DRIE to etch 40 μm wide circular channels through a 500 μm thick wafer from its backside. The etch was stopped on a silicon dioxide layer on the frontside of the wafer without breaking through the substrate [11, 10]. This allowed photolithographic mask definition on the frontside for subsequent etching of the outer shape of the needles. Underetching of circular masks with diameters of 425 μm, which were centered around the lumen holes, occurred using isotropic etching techniques, while the sidewalls of the needle lumens were protected by a silicon nitride passivation layer. The etch masks stayed attached to the passivation layer inside the needle lumens during the isotropic etch step. The silicon dioxide and silicon nitride thin films were then removed in hydrofluoric acid. Arrays of such needles were formed with a wide needle base and a slender tip with the same diameter as the needle lumen of 40 μm and a typical length of 200 μm (see Figure 7.6a). Needles with a pointed tip as shown in Figure 7.6b could be achieved through simply moving the centers of the circular masks for the isotropic etch and the centers of the needle lumens relative to each other by 5 to 20 μm.

Gardeniers et al. also used a 2-mask process to fabricate silicon microneedles [20]. A first DRIE step from the wafer frontside with an etch depth corresponding to the needle length formed the thin needle lumen openings inscribed into crescent-shaped trenches as shown in Figure 7.7. Wider lumen openings were then etched from the backside using DRIE until they connected with the frontside lumens. A

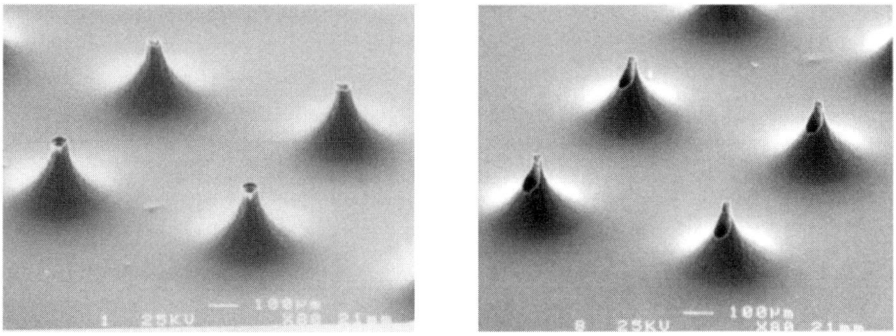

(a) (b)

Figure 7.6 (a) Silicon microneedles, fabricated through a combination of DRIE and isotropic etch steps. (b) Moving the centers of the masks for the frontside etch and for the backside etch relative to another leads to pointed needles. From [46] with permission.

silicon nitride passivation layer was deposited onto the entire substrate including the walls of all cavities, and this layer was then only removed from the horizontal surface of the wafer frontside. An anisotropic KOH etch into the substrate from the frontside stopped on the inclined {111} planes inside the nitride walls of the crescent-shaped trenches as shown in Figure 7.7b. Finally, the nitride layer was removed in hydrofluoric acid. Figure 7.7c shows typical needles with a height of 350 μm, a base width of 250 μm, and a lumen diameter of 70 μm.

In order to protect the needle lumen from potential clogging during needle insertion into tissue, Griss and Stemme developed a fabrication method for side-opened needles with a protective cap [19]. First, the authors etched the needle lumen from the wafer backside and stopped this etch about 75 μm before the frontside. Silicon oxide was then deposited inside the lumen and on the front and backside of the wafer. A cross-shaped mask was then formed on the frontside, centered with the lumen, as shown in Figure 7.8a. A sequence of four etch steps (isotropic-DRIE-isotropic-DRIE) led to pointed side-opened needles, while the connection with the lumen from the frontside was achieved during the second isotropic etch, which also removed silicon from the outer sidewalls of the needle shafts by etching horizontally. Figure 7.8b shows the finished microneedles after removal of the oxide layer. This process was later slightly modified by the authors to form more slender needles.

Mukerjee et al. also formed silicon microneedles with a slightly off-centered lumen to achieve a sharp needle tip [21]. In a two-mask etch, a 30 μm wide lumen opening and a flat flow channel were etched into the backside of the wafer as shown in Figure 7.9. The needle lumens were then connected to the wafer frontside through a third DRIE step forming a 10 μm wide lumen on the wafer frontside. A Pyrex glass wafer with appropriate access holes was then anodically bonded to the wafer backside. The frontside was then machined with a dicing saw to cut a large number of parallel and perpendicular lanes into the substrate, leaving silicon columns around the lumen openings. Individual chips were then etched in the silicon etchant HNA, while alternating between agitated and quiescent etch phases until the sharp slender needles shown in Figure 7.9b were formed, as previously demonstrated for solid needles by Campbell et al. [4].

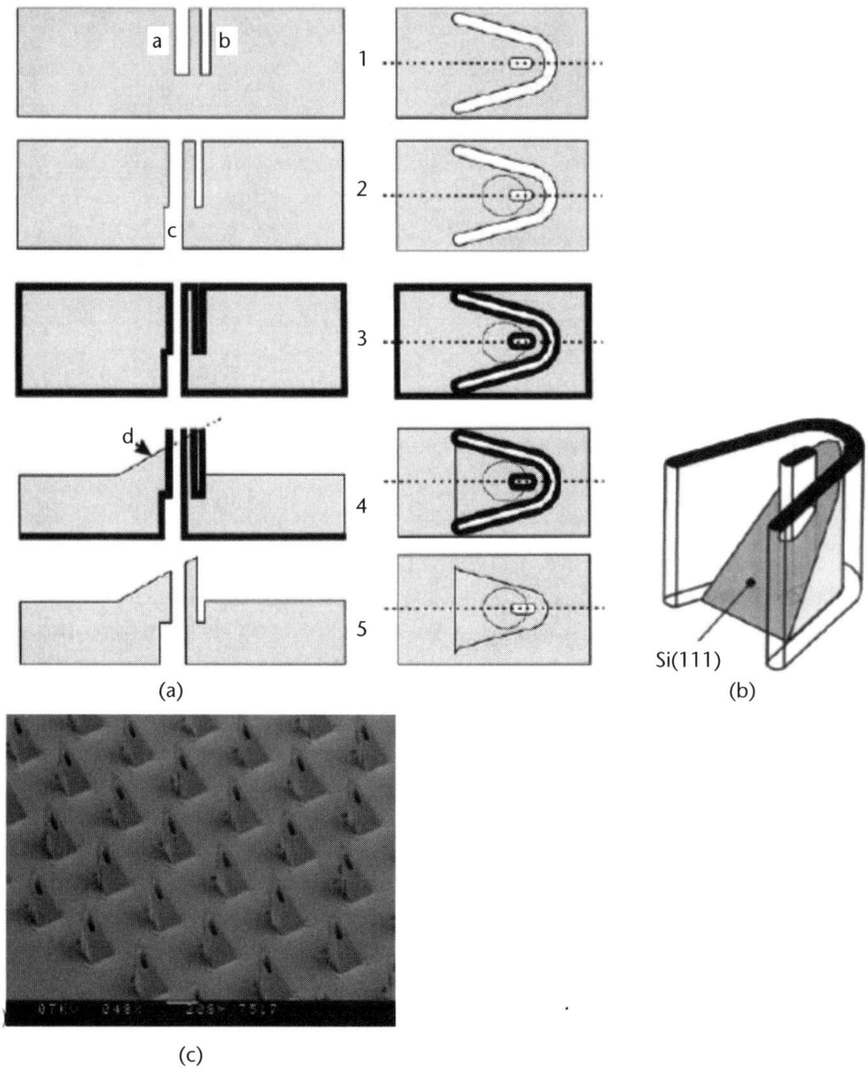

Figure 7.7 (a) Fabrication process for silicon microneedles, using a combination of DRIE and an anisotropic KOH etch step, cross-sections on the left, top views on the right, (b) schematic of needle during fabrication, (c) SEM of fabricated needles. From [20] with permission.

The described silicon microneedle types are adequate for different applications. However, since all of these needle fabrication processes require one or several DRIE steps, these fabrication processes are considered relatively expensive.

7.2.3 Fabrication of Polymer Microneedles

All arrays of hollow polymer microneedles presented to date require deep x-ray exposure. Moon et al. used double deep x-ray exposure through a mask consisting of triangular opaque regions, each of these regions having one clear hole [22]. First, a 750–1,200 μm thick layer of polymethylmethacrylate (PMMA) was exposed to

(a)

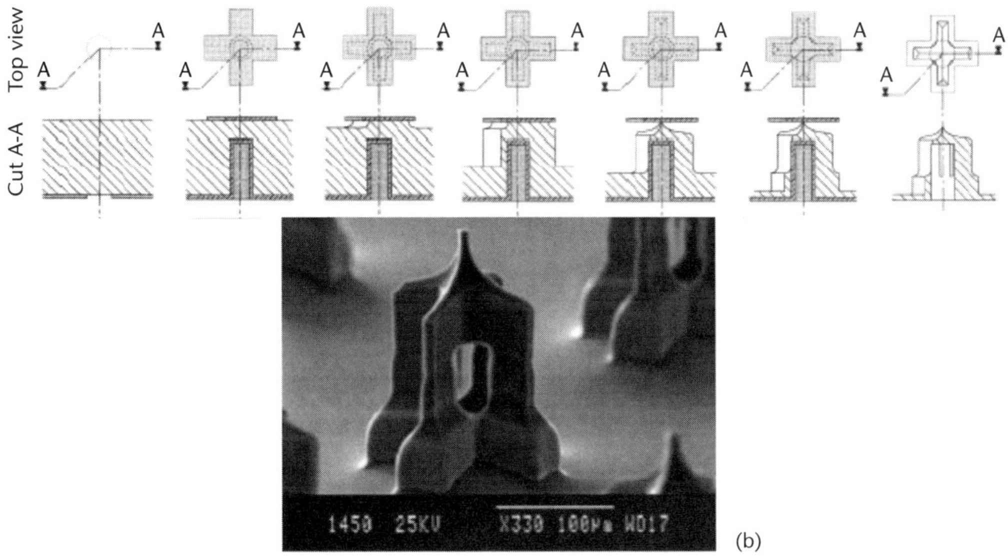

(b)

Figure 7.8 (a) Fabrication process for side-open silicon microneedles, using a combination of DRIE and isotropic etch steps, (b) SEM of fabricated needles. From [19] with permission.

deep x-rays vertically through the mask. PMMA is a positive photoresist so that its exposed areas are removed during developing. The clear holes in the mask defined the needle lumens during the first exposure, while the opaque triangles outlined the needles. A second exposure of the PMMA occurred through the same mask at an angle, typically 20°. Each opaque triangular mask feature now protected a corner of the previously unexposed area, which was protected by a neighboring triangle during the first exposure as shown in Figure 7.10. After developing, the unexposed 3-dimensional regions formed the needles. However, even though the needles were hollow, their lumens were blind holes, terminated by the flat substrate, on which the needles were located.

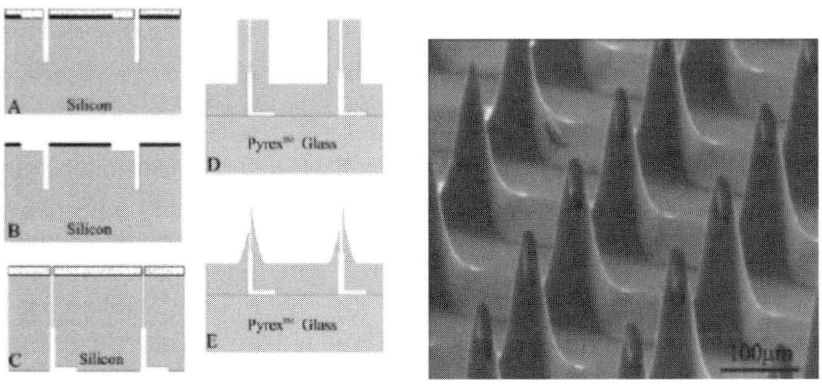

(a) (b)

Figure 7.9 (a) Fabrication process for silicon microneedles with integrated glass channels, (b) SEM of fabricated needles. From [21] with permission.

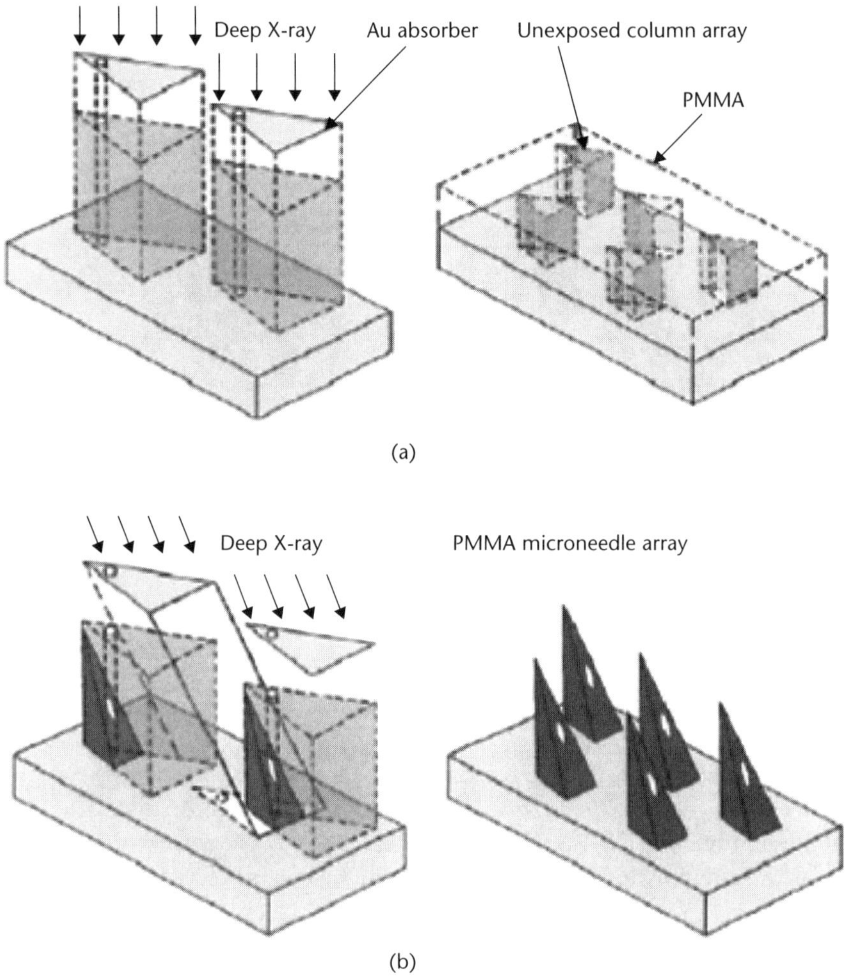

Figure 7.10 Fabrication process for hot embossed polymer microneedles: (a) vertical deep x-ray exposure, (b) subsequent inclined deep x-ray exposure. From [22] with permission.

Pérennès et al. also used a double deep x-ray exposure of PMMA [23]. A 2.7 mm thick sheet of PMMA was exposed through a sawtooth mask pattern to achieve several flat PMMA devices with one straight edge and one sawtooth-shaped edge. These devices were then flipped by 90° to stand on their straight edge, and the saw teeth were aligned. Liquid PMMA was used to bond the pieces together and to bond them to a conductive substrate. The authors then used a mask similar to the one used by Moon et al. [22] with opaque triangular regions, each of which had a clear circle. The second deep x-ray exposure occurred from the top of the sawtooth pattern after alignment of the second mask to the first pattern [23]. The development of PMMA in the lumens occurred at a slower rate than in the bulk around the needles. The development process could therefore be terminated when the needles were generated, while the lumens were not entirely formed yet. Subsequently, a thick layer of nickel was electroplated to the conductive substrate, but not to the electrically insulating PMMA, followed by completion of the development of the lumens. The resulting structure was a master for the subsequent molding process shown in Figure 7.11. A

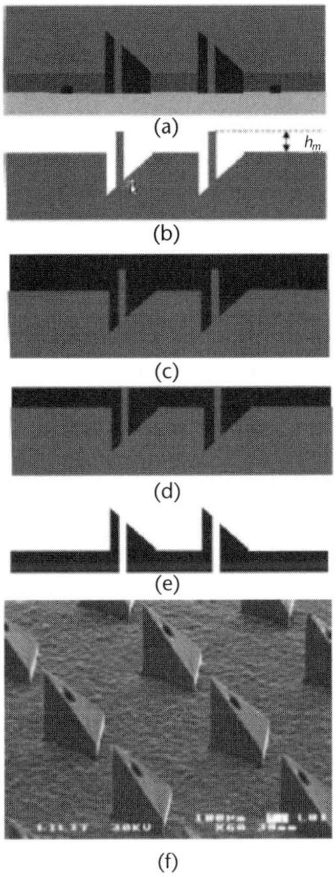

Figure 7.11 Microneedle replication process steps: (a) casting of polymer or second metal plating on top of the original master consisting of a substrate, PMMA and electroplated metal; (b) release of the mold from the master; (c) casting of needle polymer material; (d) lapping of polymer to open up the lumens; (e) release of polymer needle array from the mold; (f) array of replicated microneedles. From [23] with permission.

liquid polyvinyl alcohol (PVA) solution was then cast on top of the master in order to form an intermediate mold, which was then removed from the master. Pillars on this intermediate mold corresponded to the needle lumens of the master (Figure 7.11b). The final polymer was then deposited on this mold and lapped down to the pillars, the placeholders for the lumens of the final structure (Figure 7.11c, d). The needle array was finally released from the mold (Figure 7.11e); Figure 7.11f shows an array of replicated needles with a typical length of 400 μm.

Khumpuang et al. also used multiple deep x-ray exposures of PMMA to fabricate arrays of hollow microneedles [26]. The authors used their "plane pattern to cross-section transfer method," in which a deep x-ray image was projected onto a small section of the substrate through a mask. The substrate was then moved at constant velocity so that the exposure time of a location and thus the exposure energy corresponded to the total length of the mask window in the substrate displacement direction at that location. The exposure dose of the substrate is therefore identical in displacement direction. After exposing the entire substrate, it was rotated by 90°, and the exposure procedure was repeated. The exposure energy at a location determined the depth at which enough energy was received to remove the PMMA during development. The authors applied this method to form out-of-plane microneedles. A final exposure step generated straight lumens through each needle. The fabricated needles had a blind lumen that was terminated on the substrate surface as for Moon et al. [22]. The authors also fabricated a nickel mold (deposition of 400 μm nickel in one week) from their PMMA master. It is possible that in the future such a mold may be used for needle replication [40].

Huang and Fu [24] formed hollow microneedles through backside exposure of SU-8 through a glass substrate. The lumen regions were masked off by local metallization of the substrate, while the proper distance of the photolithography mask from the substrate defined the taper angle of the cross-linked polymer. Before spin casting the SU-8 layer on the glass substrate, the authors spin-cast a thin layer of poly(methydisiloxane) (PDMS) on the substrate and etched through the layer using reactive ion etching through a metal hard mask to form holes through the PDMS to the substrate at the locations of the lumens. The final devices featured tube-like SU-8 structures on a very flexible PDMS membrane.

Polymers could be an attractive inexpensive alternative to silicon or metal needles. However, the needles fabricated by Moon et al. and by Khumpuang et al. do not allow forming a through-hole for a needle lumen. In addition, these processes as well as the process proposed by Pérennès involve deep x-ray exposure, which is expensive; only Pérennès et al. [23] demonstrated the use of PMMA patterned with deep x-rays as a reusable master to form a mold for an array of hollow out-of-plane microneedles, a promising process that will require further development. The needle process proposed by Huang and Fu is less expensive; however, the microneedles formed with their method do not seem to have an adequate geometry for epidermal insertion.

7.2.4 Further Fabrication Methods for Microneedles

Ovsiamikov et al. [25] formed hollow out-of-plane microneedles from organically modified ceramic (Ormocer ®) hybrid materials. Two photon polymerization of this material was achieved by three dimensional scanning of the focal point of a femtosecond laser. Needles with a base diameter between 150 μm and 300 μm and a length of 800 μm were formed on a glass substrate. Even though the needles were hollow, their lumen ended on the surface of the glass substrate.

7.3 Applications for Microneedles

As mentioned above, the main application areas for arrays of hollow out-of-plane microneedles are transport of compounds into the body across the skin barrier, as well as sampling of compounds from the body for sensing applications. These applications will be discussed further.

7.3.1 Drug Delivery Through Microneedles

Solid microneedles have been successfully used to puncture the skin [5, 41] and large arrays of small sharp needle structures ("microenhancer arrays") have been used as abrasive devices [42] on the stratum corneum to generate pathways across the skin barrier for topically applied drugs; similarly, the Macroflux ® microprojection array patch consisting of a large number of 330 μm long metal spikes has been successfully demonstrated for increased protein antigen absorption by hairless guinea pigs through their skin [43]. These studies demonstrate that the skin can be used as an effective pathway for drug delivery—provided the stratum corneum barrier can be overcome. Solid biodegradable polymer needles containing drugs were inserted into the skin in order for the drugs to diffuse slowly out of the biodegradable polymer needles into the skin [33, 34, 37]. In contrast to these solid needles, hollow needles allow more control over drug delivery such as a variable delivery rate over time, for example in response to a biomedical signal or event; a possible implementation of microneedle-based drug delivery could include integrated pumping and dosage systems.

Furthermore, it has been shown that shallow intradermal injection of vaccines with small stainless steel needles into humans is effective [44, 45]; in particular, intrademal delivery of the anthrax recombinant protective antigen vaccine and intrademal delivery of influenza vaccines have been shown to be at least as effective as intramuscular delivery.

Sivamani et al. demonstrated the first clinical test with hollow microneedles on humans [46]. These clinical trials investigated the effectiveness of drug delivery through the microneedles described by Stoeber et al. [10] using methyl nicotinate as a sample drug. Methyl nicotinate is a vascodilator; the widening of blood vessels led to an increased blood flow velocity. The blood flow in the capillaries of the patients' skin was monitored using a Laser Doppler Perfusion Monitor, which recorded the blood flow velocity as a function of time. The treatments were carried out on the volar forearm of each one of eleven volunteers; the drug was applied topically, or it was injected through either pointed or symmetric microneedles.

Two metrics were used to quantify the effectiveness of these four treatments: the time to reach one half, three quarters or the full maximum blood flow velocity, and the ratio of maximum blood flow velocity and baseline flow velocity. The body reacted faster after injection through symmetric microneedles, followed by the reaction speed for injection through pointed microneedles. The response time for topical application was about ten times as long as for injection through symmetric microneedles. The blood flow velocity increase by a factor of eight for injection through pointed needles, while the increase in blood flow velocity for topical application and for injection through symmetric needles was determined as around 2.5 fold. In addition, all volunteers reported they felt pressure during injection, but no pain.

Teo et al. investigated the delivery of insulin into diabetic rats using dense arrays of silicon needle tubes [47]. The straight tubes had an outer diameter of 150 μm and a center-to-center distance of 300 μm. The blood glucose concentration of the animals dropped after injection of insulin through hypodermic needles, but not after treatment using the microtube arrays. Two possible explanations were given: the tubes have either not been sharp enough or the array was too dense, leading to the bed-of-nails effect, thus pressing the skin down uniformly, or both explanations applied.

Davis et al. previously demonstrated successful delivery of insulin into diabetic hairless rats [9] through metal microneedles. The authors used an array of 4×4

microneedles with a 600 μm center-to-center distance; the needles had a 300 μm wide base and a 75 μm wide tip. This needle array had more favorable dimensions than the tube array by Teo et al.

Nordquist et al. demonstrated insulin delivery through silicon microneedles into diabetic rats [48]. Intradermal insulin infusion through hollow microneedles was successful and comparable to subcutaneous delivery, while intravenous infusion led to a faster increase in blood insulin concentration and a faster drop in plasma glucose concentration.

Wang et al. used a single needle formed from glass capillary tubing using drawn glass techniques [49]. The hollow needle had a blunt tip and needed to be retracted after insertion 1,200 μm deep into cadaver skin before significant fluid delivery could occur. This limitation may have been caused by the blunt tip geometry that compressed the tissue rather than piercing into it.

7.3.2 Biosensing Using Microneedles

While many research groups have demonstrated intradermal drug delivery through hollow microneedles, only very few results have been reported on sensing of biological compounds in the body through microneedles, where the compounds are transported through the needle lumen to a sensing site outside the body, which avoids electronics inside the body. Measurements have previously been performed inside the body using probes. All reported sensing concepts involving hollow microneedles seem to focus on the measurement of the glucose concentration in the interstitial fluid of the skin.

Even though the epidermis contains a large amount of interstitial fluid, this interstitial fluid is not easy to extract. Wang et al. used pulled glass capillaries to penetrate 700 to 1500 μm deep below the skin surface of hairless rats as well as humans to extract interstitial fluid [50]. A suction pressure of about ½ atmosphere was applied over several minutes to extract a few μL of interstitial fluid. However, the authors reported a good correlation of the glucose concentration in the interstitial fluid and in the blood of the test subjects. The large effort required to extract interstitial fluid from the skin indicates that it is not easy to remove; the interstitial fluid might be held inside the cellular matrix of the epidermis.

Alternatively, Mukerjee et al. have demonstrated extraction of interstitial fluid from the epidermis through microneedles using capillary forces [21]. Mukerjee inserted arrays of 400 μm long silicon microneedles into an earlobe. The backside of the silicon substrate was bonded to a glass chip to form shallow channels. Capillary forces transported the interstitial fluid along the 30 μm wide needle lumens and into the 15 μm deep and 60 μm wide channels on the backside of the chip. The fluid then reached a reservoir with a small amount of glucose-sensing test strip material. This material changed color after the fluid reached it, indicating the presence of glucose. This process of capillary extraction of interstitial fluid from the earlobe took approximately 20 minutes. This extraction mechanism can only be applied once for a device, as it relies on wetting of a dry surface. For sensing applications that require a fast response or a continuous operation, it might therefore not be advisable to extract interstitial fluid from the body.

In a different approach, Zimmermann et al. proposed glucose transport from the interstitial fluid through microneedles to a sensing region through diffusion [51]. This principle relies on a continuous liquid path from the body into the microsystem. The time for glucose diffusion along the needle lumens was estimated to correspond to a time lag of the sensor response of about 2 minutes, while the enzymatic electrochemical glucose sensing [52] inside the microsystem was considered to occur instantaneously. The glucose-sensing concept proposed by Zimmermann et al. allows continuous minimally invasive glucose monitoring of diabetics, and it requires an array of out-of-plane microneedles.

7.4 Conclusions and Outlook

7.4.1 The State of the Art of Microneedle Research

The field of microneedles is a very active area of research as documented by the rapidly increasing number of related publications in scientific journals over the past few years. A large variety of processes have been developed to fabricate arrays of hollow out-of-plane microneedles. The majority of the needle materials were silicon, silicon dioxide, metal, and polymers. However, none of the fabrication methods demonstrated to date is suitable for high-volume production at low cost.

Clinical trials have been carried out to demonstrate that epidermal drug delivery through microneedles is highly effective. In addition, these trials confirmed that drug injection through microneedles can be painless. While microneedles have been used for various drug injection experiments, their application to biomedical sensing has been limited. However, a number of microneedle-based glucose sensor concepts have been reported.

7.4.2 Future Research Directions

The high potential of microneedles for various biomedical applications has been demonstrated by many research groups as previously outlined. However, when microneedles are used as minimally invasive interface components with the body, the biocompatibility of the needle materials needs to be guaranteed. This is especially important for applications that require long-term needle contact with the body. Even though biocompatibility has been demonstrated for some of the materials mentioned above, especially the biocompatibility of silicon is still under debate. Future microneedles could be directly made from biocompatible materials, or fabricated needles could be encapsulated in a thin layer of a biocompatible polymer. For this purpose, the development of specific biocompatible surface coatings would be necessary.

As mentioned above, current microneedle fabrication methods are expensive. In order to make microneedles a more accessible and cost-effective alternative to conventional needles, new fabrication methods need to be developed. New processes for polymer microneedles will most likely achieve this goal; however, no adequate solution has been proposed yet.

Past and current research on microneedles still takes an empirical approach to the design of the needle shape, following the general guidelines that slender needles with a sharp tip and sufficient needle-to-needle spacing will allow penetrating the stratum corneum. However, no precise design criteria have been developed so far. A first step in that direction would be a comprehensive description of the skin mechanics including the elastic properties and especially the failure modes of the stratum corneum. Such a description will require a broad experimental study, coupled with mechanics simulations in order to develop a complete mechanical skin model.

A different challenge with high potential for future applications is the integration of microneedles with CMOS for sensing applications. Most probably, this will be realized in a different way than through direct monolithic integration of needles and CMOS, especially if the needle material is not silicon. Hybrid integration would also avoid a size and cost mismatch between these two technologies. While the size of a microneedle chip will need to be large to allow sampling a sufficient amount of compounds to achieve a sufficiently large signal, CMOS processing cost might make a smaller size of the CMOS chip a necessary constraint. On the other hand, bringing the CMOS sensor closer to the detection site will potentially reduce the noise and therefore increase the signal-to-noise ratio. This might then allow reducing the sample volume, and hence the required number of needles. Only a careful, application-specific investigation of this problem will tell how large the sizes of the needle array and sensor have to be to acquire a useful signal from the body.

The combination of microneedles and CMOS will enable various attractive applications. The integration of several different sensors with a microneedle chip would lead to largely increased functionality. It would therefore be possible to include several biosensors with one needle array, where either all sensors have access to the entire sample volume, or sensors are matched with individual needles for separate parallel sensing.

More advanced sensing concepts should also include self-calibration and self-diagnostic functionality to increase the robustness of microneedle-based biosensors. Self-calibration could account for the loss of enzyme activity of an electrochemical sensor and therefore increase the accuracy of the reading and possibly the operation time.

A fully integrated microneedle device will include microfluidic networks with additional features including the supply of reference fluids, or cleaning solutions to increase the lifetime and accuracy of the device. Sufficiently elaborate fluidic control will also allow combining sensing and drug delivery capability with the final goal of a complete feedback-controlled drug delivery system.

References

[1] L. Lin, A.P. Pisano, and R.S. Muller, "IC-processed micro needles," *Int. Conference on Sensors and Actuators, Transducers'93, Technical Digest*, pp. 237–240, June 1993.

[2] O. Johansson et al., "Intraepidermal nerves in human skin: PGP 9.5 immunohistochemistry with special reference to the nerve density in skin from different body regions," *Journal of the peripheral nervous system: JPNS*, vol. 4, pp. 43–52, 1999.

[3] M. Nolano et al., "Quantification of myelinated endings and mechanoreceptors in human digital skin," *Annals of Neurology*, vol. 54, pp. 197–205, 2003.

[4] P.K. Campbell et al., "A silicon-based, three-dimensional neural interface: manufacturing processes for an intracortical electrode array," *IEEE Transactions on Biomedical Engineering*, vol. 38, pp. 758–768, 1991.

[5] S. Henry et al., "Microfabricated microneedles: A novel approach to transdermal drug delivery," *Journal of Pharmaceutical Sciences*, vol. 87, pp. 922–925, August 1998.

[6] Zahn et al., "Microfabricated polysilicon microneedles for minimally invasive biomedical devices," *Biomedical Microdevices*, vol. 2, pp. 295–303, December 2000.

[7] K. Kobayashi and H. Suzuki, "A sampling mechanism employing the phase transition of a gel and its application to a micro analysis system imitating a mosquito," *Sensors and Actuators B-Chemical*, vol. 80, pp. 1–8, November 2001.

[8] K. Kim et al., "A tapered hollow metallic microneedle array using backside exposure of SU-8," *Journal of Micromechanics and Microengineering*, vol. 14, pp. 597–603, April 2004.

[9] S.P. Davis et al., "Hollow metal microneedles for insulin delivery to diabetic rats," *IEEE Transactions on Biomedical Engineering*, vol. 52, pp. 909–915, May 2005.

[10] B. Stoeber and D. Liepmann, "Arrays of hollow out-of-plane microneedles for drug delivery," *Journal of Microelectromechanical Systems*, vol. 14, pp. 472–479, June 2005.

[11] B. Stoeber and D. Liepmann, "Fluid injection through out-of-plane microneedles," *1st Annual International Conference On Microtechnologies in Medicine and Biology, 2000*, pp. 224–228, 2000.

[12] F. Sammoura et al., "Polymeric microneedle fabrication using a microinjection molding technique," *Microsystem Technologies*, vol. 13, pp. 517–522, March 2007.

[13] E.R. Parker et al., "Bulk micromachined titanium microneedles," *Journal of Microelectromechanical Systems*, vol. 16, pp. 289–295, April 2007.

[14] D. Ziegler, T. Suzuki, and S. Takeuchi, "Fabrication of flexible neural probes with built-in microfluidic channels by thermal bonding of Parylene," *Journal of Microelectromechanical Systems*, vol. 15, pp. 1477–1482, December 2006.

[15] D.P. Papageorgiou et al., "A shuttered neural probe with on-chip flowmeters for chronic in vivo drug delivery," *Journal of Microelectromechanical Systems*, vol. 15, pp. 1025–1033, August 2006.

[16] J.M. Lippmann, E.J. Geiger, and A.P. Pisano, "Polymer investment molding: Method for fabricating hollow, microscale parts," *Sensors and Actuators A-Physical*, vol. 134, pp. 2–10, February 2007.

[17] S. Chandrasekaran, J.D. Brazzle, and A.B. Frazier, "Surface micromachined metallic microneedles," *Journal of Microelectromechanical Systems*, vol. 12, pp. 281–288, June 2003.

[18] J.K. Chen et al., "A multichannel neural probe for selective chemical delivery at the cellular level," *IEEE Transactions on Biomedical Engineering*, vol. 44, pp. 760–769, August 1997.

[19] P. Griss and G. Stemme, "Side-opened out-of-plane microneedles for microfluidic transdermal liquid transfer," *Journal of Microelectromechanical Systems*, vol. 12, pp. 296–301, June 2003.

[20] H. Gardeniers et al., "Silicon micromachined hollow microneedles for transdermal liquid transport," *Journal of Microelectromechanical Systems*, vol. 12, pp. 855–862, December 2003.

[21] E. Mukerjee et al., "Microneedle array for transdermal biological fluid extraction and in situ analysis," *Sensors and Actuators A-Physical*, vol. 114, pp. 267–275, September 2004.

[22] S.J. Moon et al., "Fabrication of microneedle array using LIGA and hot embossing process," *Microsystem Technologies*, vol. 11, pp. 311–318, April 2005.

[23] F. Pérennès et al., "Sharp beveled tip hollow microneedle arrays fabricated by LIGA and 3D soft lithography with polyvinyl alcohol," *Journal of Micromechanics and Microengineering*, vol. 16, pp. 473–479, March 2006.

[24] H. Huang and C. Fu, "Different fabrication methods of out-of-plane polymer hollow needle arrays and their variations," *Journal of Micromechanics and Microengineering*, vol. 17, pp. 393–402, February 2007.

[25] A. Ovsianikov et al., "Two photon polymerization of polymer-ceramic hybrid materials for transdermal drug delivery," *International Journal of Applied Ceramic Technology*, vol. 4, pp. 22–29, 2007.

[26] S. Khumpuang et al., "Microneedle fabrication using the plane pattern to cross-section transfer method," *Smart Materials & Structures*, vol. 15, pp. 600–606, April 2006.

[27] M. Shikida, T. Hasada, and K. Sato, "Fabrication of a hollow needle structure by dicing, wet etching and metal deposition," *Journal of Micromechanics and Microengineering*, vol. 16, pp. 2230–2239, October 2006.

[28] K. Wise, J. Angell, and A. Starr, "An integrated-circuit approach to extracellular microelectrodes," *IEEE Transactions on Biomedical Engineering*, vol. BME-17, pp. 238–247, 1970.

[29] D. Anderson et al., "Batch-fabricated Thin-film Electrodes for Stimulation of the Central Auditory-system," *IEEE Transactions on Biomedical Engineering*, vol. 36, pp. 693–704, July 1989.

[30] P. Griss et al., "Micromachined electrodes for biopotential measurements," *Journal of Microelectromechanical Systems*, vol. 10, pp. 10–16, March 2001.

[31] T. Kawano et al., "Fabrication and properties of ultrasmall Si wire arrays with circuits by vapor-liquid-solid growth," *Sensors and Actuators A-Physical*, vol. 97–8, pp. 709–715, April 2002.

[32] N. Wilke and A. Morrissey, "Silicon microneedle formation using modified mask designs based on convex corner undercut," *Journal of Micromechanics and Microengineering*, vol. 17, pp. 238–244, February 2007.

[33] J. Park et al., "Polymer particle-based micromolding to fabricate novel microstructures," *Biomedical Microdevices*, vol. 9, pp. 223–234, April 2007.

[34] J. Park et al., "Tapered conical polymer microneedles fabricated using an integrated lens technique for transdermal drug delivery," *IEEE Transactions on Biomedical Engineering*, vol. 54, pp. 903–913, May 2007.

[35] J. Ji et al., "Microfabricated microneedle with porous tip for drug delivery," *Journal of Micromechanics and Microengineering*, vol. 16, pp. 958–964, May 2006.

[36] L.R. Hochberg et al., "Neuronal ensemble control of prosthetic devices by a human with tetraplegia," *Nature*, vol. 442, pp. 164–171, July 2006.

[37] Y. Ito et al., "Feasibility of microneedles for percutaneous absorption of insulin," *European Journal of Pharmaceutical Sciences*, vol. 29, pp. 82–88, September 2006.

[38] M.J. Madou, *Fundamentals of Microfabrication: The Science of Miniaturization.* CRC Press, 2002.

[39] K. Chun et al., "Fabrication of array of hollow microcapillaries used for injection of genetic materials into animal/plant cells," *Japanese Journal of Applied Physics Part 2—Letters*, vol. 38, pp. L279–L281, March 1999.

[40] S. Khumpuang et al., "Geometrical strengthening and tip-sharpening of a microneedle array fabricated by X-ray lithography," *Microsystem Technologies*, vol. 13, pp. 209–214, February 2007.

[41] F. Chabri et al., "Microfabricated silicon microneedles for nonviral cutaneous gene delivery," *British Journal of Dermatology*, vol. 150, pp. 869–877, May 2004.

[42] J.A. Mikszta et al., "Improved genetic immunization via micromechanical disruption of skin-barrier function and targeted epidermal delivery," *Nature Medicine*, vol. 8, pp. 415–419, April 2002.

[43] J.A. Matriano et al., "Macroflux ® microprojection array patch technology: A new and efficient approach for intracutaneous immunization," *Pharmaceutical Research*, vol. 19, pp. 63–70, 2002.

[44] J.A. Mikszta et al., "Microneedle-based intradermal delivery of the anthrax recombinant protective antigen vaccine," *Infection and Immunity*, vol. 74, pp. 6806–6810, December 2006.

[45] J.B. Alarcon et al., "Preclinical evaluation of microneedle technology for intradermal delivery of influenza vaccines," *Clinical and Vaccine Immunology*, vol. 14, pp. 375–381, April 2007.

[46] R.K. Sivamani, B. Stoeber, G.C. Wu, H. Zhai, D. Liepmann, and H. Maibach, "Clinical microneedle injection of methyl nicotinate: stratum corneum penetration," *Skin Research and Technology*, vol. 11, pp. 152–156, May 2005.

[47] A.L. Teo et al., "Transdermal microneedles for drug delivery applications," *Materials Science and Engineering B-Solid State Materials for Advanced Technology*, vol. 132, pp. 151–154, July 2006.

[48] L. Nordquist et al., "Novel microneedle patches for active insulin delivery are efficient in maintaining glycaemic control: An initial comparison with subcutaneous administration," *Pharmaceutical Research*, vol. 24, pp. 1381–1388, July 2007.

[49] P.M. Wang et al., "Precise microinjection into skin using hollow microneedles," *Journal of Investigative Dermatology*, vol. 126, pp. 1080–1087, May 2006.

[50] P.M. Wang, M. Cornwell, and M.R. Prausnitz, "Minimally invasive extraction of dermal interstitial fluid for glucose monitoring using microneedles," February 2005.

[51] S. Zimmermann, D. Fienbork, B. Stoeber, A.W. Flounders, and D. Liepmann, "A microneedle-based glucose monitor: fabricated on a wafer-level using in-device enzyme immobilization," *TRANSDUCERS, Solid-State Sensors, Actuators and Microsystems, 12th International Conference on, 2003*, vol. 1, pp. 99–102, 2003.

[52] M.J.C. Lambrechts and W.M.C. Sansen, *Biosensors: Microelectrochemical Devices*. CRC Press, 1992.

CHAPTER 8

Integrated Circuits for Neural Interfacing: Neuroelectrical Recording

Reid R. Harrison

8.1 Introduction to Neural Recording

Monitoring the electrical potentials produced by living neurons can provide a wealth of information in both scientific and clinical contexts. The development of micromachined multi-electrode arrays in the 1980s and 1990s revolutionized modern neuroscience, permitting scientists and clinicians to monitor the simultaneous activity of many neurons in localized regions of the brain [1–4]. One example of this technology, shown in Figure 8.1, is the Utah Electrode Array. This 10×10 array of platinum-tipped silicon electrodes measures 4 mm × 4 mm × 1.5 mm [4]. Dense multi-electrode arrays are now readily available from multiple commercial sources, but these devices must be connected to external instrumentation via relatively bulky wire bundles and transcutaneous connectors.

In an effort to create fully implantable neural recording devices with wireless power and data transfer, MEMS electrode arrays are being combined with integrated CMOS electronics [5–8]. The miniaturization of these highly-parallel recording systems presents several significant circuit design challenges. The weak neural signals must be amplified and digitized, and this information must be relayed out of the body using a wireless telemetry link to avoid any path for infection. Multi-channel neural recording systems potentially produce large quantities of continuously streaming data that must be transmitted. Yet the power dissipation of small implanted devices must be strictly limited to prevent excessive tissue heating that can kill nearby cells [9, 10]. A good understanding of circuit design trade-offs is essential to meet the severe power, size, and bandwidth constraints inherent in this application.

Implantable neural recording devices have great promise for advancing the understanding of brain function by allowing scientists to observe and manipulate neural activity during normal animal behavior [11]. Clinical applications for this technology include monitoring and diagnosis of epileptic seizures and prosthetic control for the severely disabled. Recent work in the field of neuroprosthetics has demonstrated that rats [12], monkeys [13–15], and paralyzed humans [16, 17] can learn to control robotic arms or computer cursors by thoughts if multiple neural signals from motor regions of the cerebral cortex are used for control.

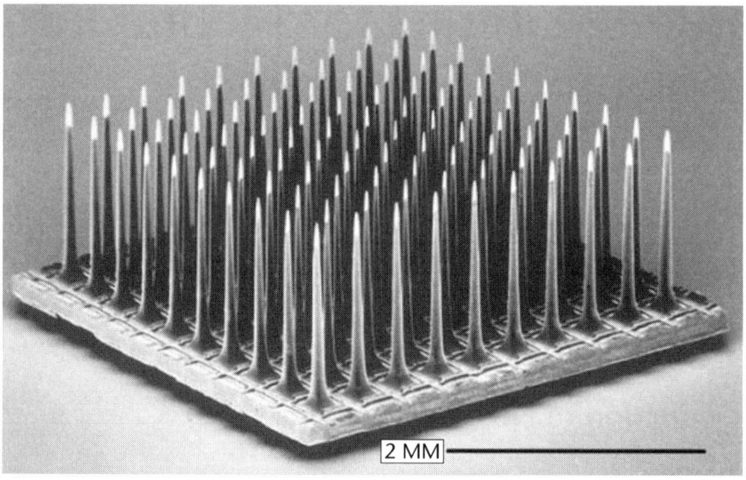

Figure 8.1 SEM photograph of silicon-based Utah Electrode Array [4]. The 100-electrode array measures 4 mm × 4 mm × 1.5 mm.

8.2 The Nature of Neural Signals

Electrically active cells such as neurons produce internal voltage changes on the order of 100 mV relative to the extracellular fluid [18]. While brief intracellular recordings are possible using individually guided microelectrodes, chronic recordings using multi-electrode arrays make use of the smaller extracellular potentials several microns from the cell. The contact between metal electrode tip and extracellular fluid creates an electrical double layer so the electrode-tissue interface behaves primarily as a capacitance for small voltages [19, 20]. The capacitance of the interface depends on electrode area and surface roughness; values between 150 pF–1.5 nF are common in recording electrodes. A typical trace from an extracellular neural recording is shown in Figure 8.2. This waveform was recorded from the motor cortex of an awake cat using a Utah Electrode Array that was implanted approximately three months prior [21].

The features present in typical extracellular neural recordings are visible in Figure 8.2. The amplitude of the signal is on the order of 100 μV, and rapid neural action potentials or "spikes" from a nearby neuron are present (at t = 100 ms, 140 ms, and 180 ms). Neural spikes often appear biphasic in extracellular recordings, and usually have durations of 0.3 to 1.0 ms. Neurons rarely fire more rapidly than 100 spikes per second (though rapid bursts of several spikes are possible), with firing rates around 10 Hz somewhat typical in cerebral cortex. Spikes are "digital" events; neurons produce spikes of nearly identical amplitude and duration, and information is encoded only in the timing of spikes [18].

Also present are low-frequency (<200 Hz) oscillations known as local field potentials (LFPs). Local field potentials arise from the synchronous activity of many neurons in one region of the brain. These neurons are too distant from the electrode for their individual action potentials to be resolved, but the "crowd noise" of many neighboring cells creates a large signal that is easily detected [22]. The LFP is the internal correlate of the EEG signal measured on the scalp (after much attenuation

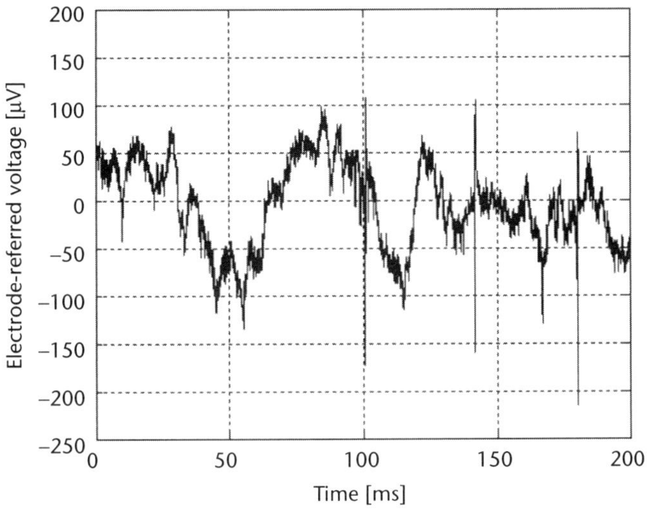

Figure 8.2 Neural recording from cat motor cortex using Utah Electrode Array and integrated CMOS amplifier. Both spikes and LFPs are visible. From [21] with permission, © IEEE 2007.

and spatial blurring). The energy of LFP signals in primate pre-motor and motor cortex have been shown to correlate with specific arm movement reach parameters such as direction, distance, and speed, and thus may be useful in neuroprosthetic applications [23–27]. Figure 8.3 shows the onset of pronounced beta waves (10–15 Hz) in cat motor cortex [21]. LFPs are a robust signal. In some experiments using electrode arrays, scar tissue forms around microelectrode tips. This scar tissue tends to attenuate spike signals from nearby neurons, but LFP signals are less affected [28].

In many applications, it is desirable to separate LFP and spike signals so they may be analyzed separately. This is easily accomplished by linear filtering since LFPs

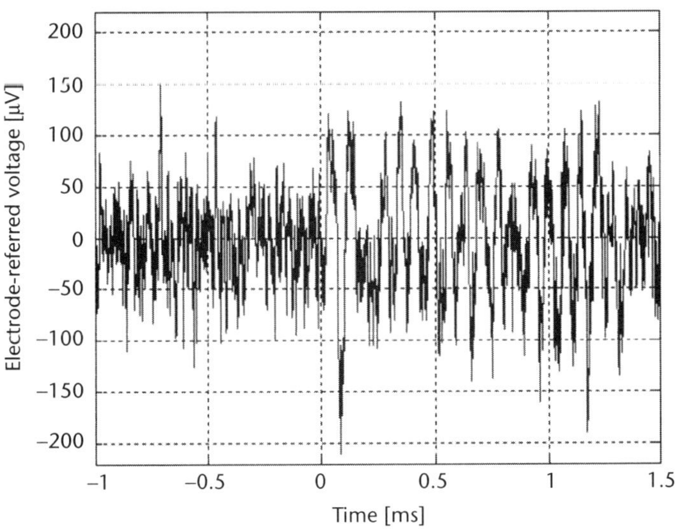

Figure 8.3 Neural recording from cat motor cortex showing spontaneous onset of 10–15 Hz beta activity in the local field potential at t = 0. Note that the time scale is much longer than in Figure 8.2. From [21] with permission, © IEEE 2007.

occupy frequencies from approximately 10 to 200 Hz, while spikes have energy concentrated in the 300 Hz to 5 kHz range. Figure 8.4 shows a neural signal that has been high-pass filtered at 300 Hz, isolating the spikes [21]. Here, a nearby neuron producing relatively large spikes fires twice between 35 and 40 ms, while a more distant neuron fires three spikes between 3 and 12 ms. When multi-electrode arrays are placed in the brain, it is common for some electrodes to detect spikes from 2 to 4 distinct neurons, while other electrodes may see no resolvable spikes. Figure 8.5 shows 51 time-aligned spikes recorded from cat auditory cortex using a Utah Electrode Array. (This data was gathered by the wireless system described in [8].) Three distinct waveform shapes are visible, corresponding to three nearby neurons with different distances and/or orientations with respect to the electrode tip.

8.3 Neural Signal Amplification

8.3.1 Design Requirements

Due to the small amplitude of neural signals recorded extracellularly and the high impedance of the electrode-tissue interface, amplification must be performed before these signals can be digitized or analyzed in any way. An integrated front-end amplifier for neural signals must:

1. have sufficiently low input-referred noise to resolve spikes as small as 30 μV in amplitude;
2. have sufficient dynamic range to convey spikes or LFPs as large as ±1 to 2 mV in amplitude;
3. have much higher input impedance than the electrode-tissue interface and have negligible dc input current;

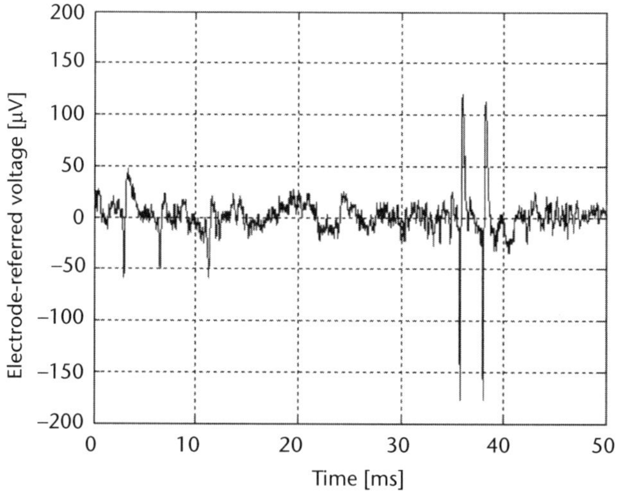

Figure 8.4 Large and small spikes observed in cat motor cortex. A one-pole high-pass filter at 300 Hz was applied to the signal to remove LFPs. From [21] with permission, © IEEE 2007.

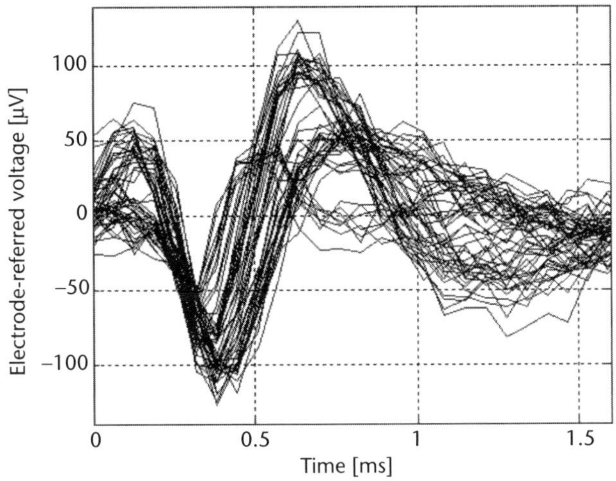

Figure 8.5 Time-aligned spikes recorded from cat auditory cortex using Utah Electrode Array, integrated amplifier, and wireless telemetry [8]. Three distinct neurons are visible.

4. amplify signals in the frequency bands of interest (roughly 300 Hz to 5 kHz for spikes and 10 Hz to 200 Hz for local field potentials);
5. block dc offsets present at the electrode-tissue interface to prevent saturation of the amplifier; and
6. consume little silicon area, and use few or no off-chip components to minimize size.

In addition to these requirements, the amplifier should have a high common-mode rejection ratio (CMRR) to minimize interference from 50/60 Hz power line noise, and a high power-supply rejection ratio (PSRR) if power supply noise is significant (e.g., from ac inductive power links). Arrays of amplifiers should have low crosstalk between channels.

To reduce pickup of 50/60 Hz noise, microphonics, and other capacitively- and inductively-coupled interferers, the distance between electrode and amplifier should be minimized. Additionally, tethering forces introduced by wires cause problems for electrodes inserted into the soft, pliable brain tissue. Thus, the amplifiers are ideally attached directly to the electrodes very near the recording site. This proximity of the electronics to living tissue imposes strict limits on the amount of power that can be dissipated by the circuitry; if cells are exposed to elevated temperatures for extended periods of time, they will die [9, 10]. Thus, we add another requirement for neural signal amplifiers: operation at low power levels to minimize tissue heating.

The precise limits to power dissipation in implanted devices can be difficult to establish. Most devices are designed to limit the chronic heating of surrounding tissue to less than 1°C. Thus, the size and shape of a device determine its power limits; smaller devices can dissipate less power safely. While heat conduction in the body can be simulated with some accuracy, convection from blood flow cannot be modeled accurately and thus experimental validation is required. Preliminary experiments have shown that an implanted cortical 100-electrode array with integrated electronics measuring roughly 6 mm × 6 mm × 2 mm can safely dissipate approximately 10 mW of power [29, 30]. This power limit poses a challenge for high-channel-count recording systems since each electrode requires a dedicated low-noise amplifier. A rough order-of-magnitude analysis of multi-channel neural recording devices presents a sobering picture for circuit designers: with modern MEMS arrays providing approximately 100 electrodes and a power dissipation limit of 10 mW, each channel must consume less than 100 μW, and this does not even include shared resources on a chip such as A/D conversion, power regulation, control, and telemetry circuits.

8.3.2 Circuit Architecture and Design Techniques

Figure 8.6 shows the schematic of a neural signal amplifier that was first described in [32]. The amplifier is based around an operational transconductance amplifier (OTA) that produces a current proportional to the differential voltage applied to its inputs, where G_m is the constant of proportionality. A capacitive feedback network consisting of C_1 and C_2 capacitors sets the mid-band gain of the amplifier. (C_{in} models the input capacitance of the OTA, as well as any bottom-plate capacitance from C_1 and C_2.) The input is capacitively coupled through C_1, so any dc offset from the electrode-tissue interface is removed. C_1 should be made much smaller than the electrode impedance to minimize signal attenuation.

The R_2 elements shown in the feedback loop represent lossy elements that set the low-frequency amplifier cutoff; they may be implemented using real resistors, but the MOS-bipolar element used in [32] provides an area-efficient means of creating a small-signal resistance of $>10^{12}$ Ω for low-frequency operation (i.e., LFPs). The long-time constant associated with this pole can cause the amplifier to recover slowly from large transients, so the M_{FS} transistors can act as switches to implement a "fast settle" function.

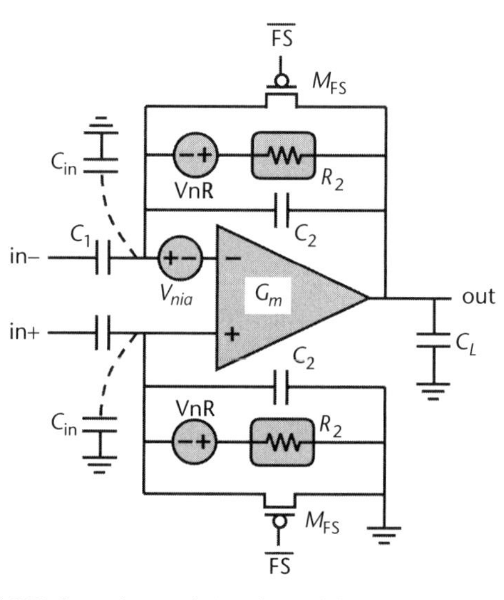

Figure 8.6 Schematic of OTA-based neural signal amplifier with capacitive feedback.

Figure 8.7(a) shows a gain vs. frequency plot for the neural amplifier in Figure 8.6. The approximate transfer function is given by

$$\begin{aligned}\frac{v_{\text{out}}}{v_{\text{in+}} - v_{\text{in-}}} &= \frac{C_1}{C_2} \cdot \frac{1 - sC_2/G_m}{\left(\dfrac{1}{sR_2C_2} + 1\right)\left(s\dfrac{C_LC_1}{G_mC_2} + 1\right)} \\ &= A_M \frac{1 - s/(2\pi f_z)}{\left(\dfrac{2\pi f_L}{s} + 1\right)\left(\dfrac{s}{2\pi f_H} + 1\right)}\end{aligned} \tag{8.1}$$

The mid-band gain A_M is set by the capacitance ratio C_1/C_2, and the gain is flat between the lower and upper cutoff frequencies f_L and f_H. The lower cutoff frequency is determined by the product of R_2 and C_2, while the upper cutoff is determined by the load capacitance C_L, the OTA transconductance G_m, and the mid-band gain. Capacitive feedthrough introduces a right-half-plane zero at f_z. This zero can be pushed to very high frequencies (higher than secondary poles due to parasitic capacitances in the OTA) by setting

$$C_2 << \sqrt{C_1C_L} \tag{8.2}$$

so that it has little practical effect on amplifier operation.

The thermal noise sources in the neural amplifier are shown in Figure 8.6 as voltage sources v_{nia} and v_{nR}. The source v_{nia} models the input-referred voltage noise of the OTA. (If MOSFETs are used as input devices then the current noise is negligible at low frequencies.) The two v_{nR} sources model the thermal noise (or Johnson noise) contributed by the resistive R_2 elements in the feedback loop. If both v_{nia} and v_{nR} are taken to be white (i.e., ignoring $1/f$ noise), their contributions to the total amplifier output noise are shown in Figure 8.7(b). The OTA contributes noise primarily between f_L and f_H. Below a particular frequency, the noise contribution from v_{nR} will dominate; we denote this frequency f_{corner}. If R_2 is implemented as a real resistor so that its noise spectral density is

$$v_{nR}^2(f) = 4kTR_2 \tag{8.3}$$

and $C_1 > C_2$, C_{in}, then f_{corner} is approximately

$$f_{\text{corner}} \approx \sqrt{\frac{3C_L}{2C_1} f_L f_H} \tag{8.4}$$

(A similar result is obtained for the MOS-bipolar element used as R_2 in [32].) To minimize the noise contribution from the R_2 elements, we should ensure that f_{corner}

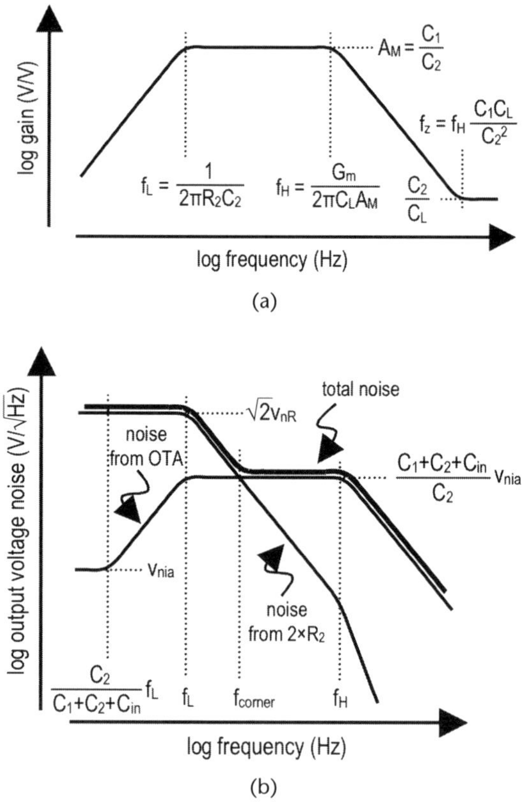

Figure 8.7 (a) Log-log plot of gain vs. frequency for the neural amplifier shown in Figure 8.6. (b) Log-log plot of neural amplifier output noise vs. frequency.

$<< f_H$. For resistive R_2 elements, this can be accomplished by designing the amplifier so that

$$\frac{C_L}{C_1} << \frac{2}{3}\frac{f_H}{f_L} \tag{8.5}$$

In practical circuits, the $1/f$ noise from the OTA may dominate the noise contributed by the R_2 elements. However, if multi-transistor, amplifier-based circuits are used as R_2 feedback elements, the increased thermal noise from these circuits may masquerade as increased $1/f$ noise as shown in Figure 8.7(b).

If the noise contribution from R_2 is negligible (i.e., $f_{corner} << f_H$) and $C_1 >> C_2$, C_{in}, then the output rms noise voltage of the neural amplifier in Figure 8.6 is dominated by the noise from the OTA. Thus, the design of the OTA is crucial to minimize the overall noise of the neural amplifier. We use a cascoded current-mirror OTA as shown in Figure 8.8, but other topologies such as a folded cascode amplifier would work as well.

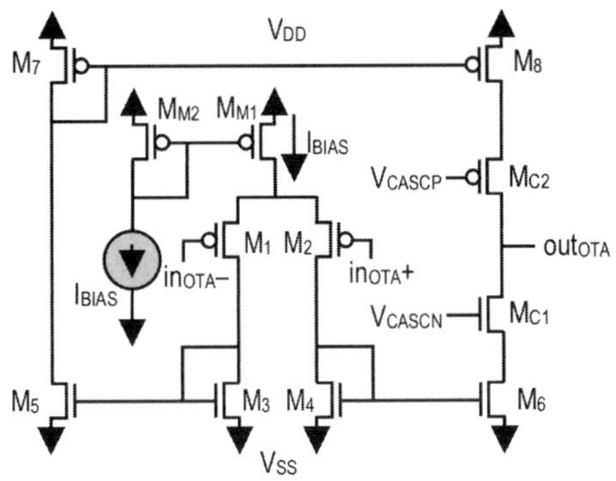

Figure 8.8 Schematic of operational transconductance amplifier (OTA) used in the neural amplifier shown in Figure 8.6.

The input-referred thermal noise spectral density of this OTA is given by

$$v_{nia}^2(f) = \frac{16kT}{3g_{m1}}\left(1 + 2\frac{g_{m3}}{g_{m1}} + \frac{g_{m7}}{g_{m1}}\right) \tag{8.6}$$

where g_{m1} is the transconductance of the input devices M_1 and M_2, g_{m3} represents the transconductance of the nMOS current mirror devices M_3–M_6, and g_{m7} represents the transconductance of the pMOS current mirror devices M_7 and M_8. The biasing transistors (M_{M1} and M_{M2}) and the cascode transistors (M_{C1} and M_{C2}) contribute negligible noise. As described in [32], the input-referred noise of this OTA can be minimized by ensuring that $g_{m1} >> g_{m3}$, g_{m7}. This is accomplished by sizing the transistors so that M_1 and M_2 operate in weak inversion where the ratio of device transconductance to drain current (g_m/I_D) is maximum and M_3–M_8 operate deep in strong inversion where g_m/I_D is greatly reduced [33–36].

Perhaps the most critical tradeoff in neural amplifier design is that between power dissipation and input-referred noise. A dimensionless figure of merit that captures the essence of this tradeoff clearly is the noise efficiency factor (NEF), first proposed in [31]:

$$\text{NEF} \equiv V_{ni,\text{rms}}\sqrt{\frac{2I_{\text{tot}}}{\pi \cdot U_T \cdot 4kT \cdot \text{BW}}} \tag{8.7}$$

where I_{tot} is the total amplifier supply current, U_T is the thermal voltage kT/q, BW is the amplifier bandwidth, and $V_{ni,\text{rms}}$ is the amplifier's input-referred rms voltage noise. An amplifier with noise contributed only by the thermal noise of a single ideal bipolar transistor has an NEF = 1; all physical circuits have NEF > 1. In [32], we demonstrated that the NEF of CMOS neural amplifiers is minimized by selectively operating transistors in weak or strong inversion as described above.

Note that NEF does not directly account for power dissipation since supply voltage is not present in the expression. However, in modern IC amplifiers, supply voltage only varies by a factor of perhaps five (e.g., 1 V to 5 V), while supply current can vary by many orders of magnitude (e.g., 1 nA to 1 A). So NEF is closely correlated with power consumption. In weak inversion, transconductance is linearly proportional to bias current [33–36], so from Equation (8.6) we can see that noise spectral density is inversely proportional to bias current.

8.3.3 Noise vs. Layout Area

The rms input-referred noise of the neural amplifier in Figure 8.6 is given as

$$\overline{v_{ni}^2} = \left(\frac{C_1 + C_2 + C_{in}}{C_1}\right)^2 \frac{16kT}{3g_{m1}}\left(1 + 2\frac{g_{m3}}{g_{m1}} + \frac{g_{m7}}{g_{m1}}\right)\Delta f \tag{8.8}$$

If the amplifier is designed so that $C_1 >> C_2$, C_{in} and $g_{m1} >> g_{m3}$, g_{m7}, the input-referred noise is minimized to

$$\overline{v_{ni}^2} \approx \frac{16kT}{3g_{m1}}\Delta f \tag{8.9}$$

The equivalent brick-wall bandwidth (Δf) of the amplifier (which has one dominant pole) is given by $(\pi/2) \times f_H$ if $f_H >> f_L$ [37]:

$$\Delta f = f_H \cdot \frac{\pi}{2} = \frac{1}{2\pi} \cdot \frac{G_m C_2}{C_L C_1} \cdot \frac{\pi}{2} = \frac{G_m}{4C_L A_M} \tag{8.10}$$

Therefore, the total rms noise referred to the input of the amplifier is found to be

$$V_{ni,\text{rms}} \approx \sqrt{\frac{4kT}{3C_L A_M}} \tag{8.11}$$

From this expression, it is clear that the total amplifier noise integrated across its bandwidth is only a function of temperature, load capacitance C_L, and closed-loop gain A_M. Temperature will be nearly constant in implanted applications, and A_M must be limited to be significantly less than the (poorly controlled) open-loop gain of the amplifier if we want the gain to be well controlled by the ratio of C_1 to C_2. Thus, Equation (8.11) demonstrates a clear tradeoff between input-referred noise and silicon area, which is often dominated by capacitors.

Since C_2 is usually made as small as possible while staying above parasitic capacitances, A_M is set by sizing C_1. If the area of the amplifier is dominated by capacitors, then the layout area will be proportional to $C_L + 2C_1 + 2C_2$. We can write an expression for amplifier area as

$$\text{Area} = \frac{C_L + 2C_1 + 2C_2}{C'} = \frac{C_L + 2(A_M + 1)C_2}{C'} \tag{8.12}$$

where C' is the capacitance per unit area of linear capacitors (typically around 1 fF/μm^2 in modern CMOS processes). Solving Equation (8.11) for C_L, and substituting into Equation (8.12), we derive an expression for amplifier area as a function of input-referred noise, mid-band gain, and C_2:

$$\text{Area} = \frac{4}{3} \frac{kT}{V_{ni,\text{rms}}^2 A_M C'} + 2(A_M + 1)\frac{C_2}{C'} \tag{8.13}$$

For varying mid-band gain, Equation (8.13) has a minimum at

$$A_{\text{Mopt}} = \frac{1}{V_{ni,\text{rms}}} \sqrt{\frac{2}{3} \cdot \frac{kT}{C_2}} \tag{8.14}$$

Taking C_2 = 200 fF as a practical lower limit (to stay above stray parasitic capacitances) and $V_{ni,\text{rms}}$ = 2 μV$_{\text{rms}}$, an optimum gain of 60 is found. If the input-referred noise specification is raised to 5 μV$_{\text{rms}}$, the optimum gain to minimize layout area is 24.

Thankfully, these values of A_M fall in a practical range. A gain of perhaps 10 or more is desirable to boost the signal above the input-referred noise of successive circuits. A gain of greater than 100 or so is difficult to achieve with high accuracy unless the open-loop gain of the amplifier is extremely high and a large C_1/C_2 ratio is used.

The data from Figures 8.2 to 8.4 were obtained using a commercial RHA1016 integrated neural amplifier (Intan Technologies, LLC, Salt Lake City, UT) developed using the techniques described here. This amplifier uses a fully-differential design throughout to improve common-mode noise rejection, and has an input-referred noise of 2 μV$_{\text{rms}}$ [21]. The data from Figure 8.5 was obtained using a 100-channel neural recording system with an integrated ADC and wireless RF telemetry [8]. Figure 8.9 shows a photograph of this chip, which measures 4.7 mm × 5.9 mm after fabrication in a 0.5-μm 2-poly, 3-metal CMOS process. Each amplifier fits into

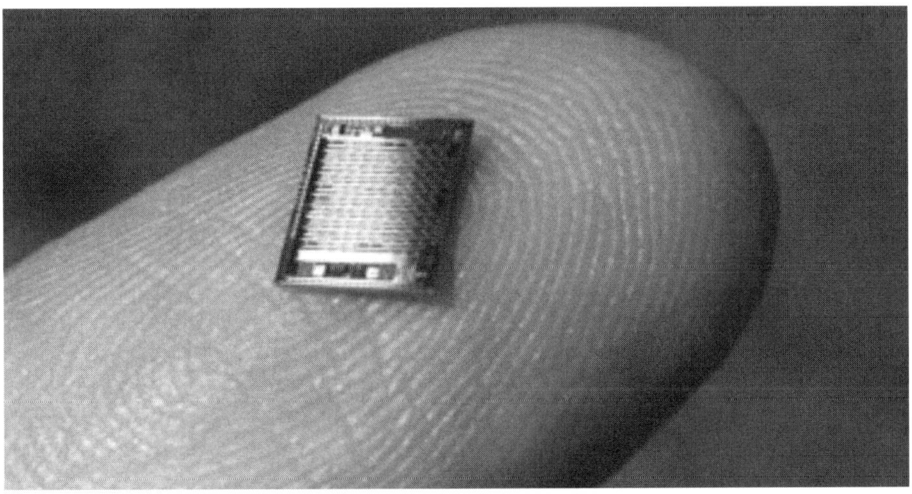

Figure 8.9 Photograph of 100-channel neural recording integrated circuit. The chip measures 4.7 mm × 5.9 mm and includes an ADC, spike detectors, and a wireless RF telemetry system [8].

a layout area of 400 μm × 400 μm so that it may be flip-chip bonded to the back of a Utah Electrode Array for complete integration. The amplifiers on this chip were designed for an input-referred noise of 5 μV_{rms} to reduce the required layout area. Since the layout area of neural amplifiers is typically dominated by capacitance and C' for linear capacitors does not scale dramatically in deep submicron processes, moving to smaller processes results in modest area savings.

References

[1] J. Pine, "Recording action potentials from cultured neurons with extracellular microcircuit electrodes," *J. Neurosci. Methods*, vol. 2, pp. 19–31, 1980.

[2] A.C. Hoogerwerf and K.D. Wise, "A three-dimensional microelectrode array for chronic neural recording," *IEEE Trans. Biomed. Eng.*, vol. 41, pp. 1136–1146, Dec. 1994.

[3] A.L. Owens, T.J. Denison, H. Versnel, M. Rebbert, M. Peckerar, and S.A. Shamma, "Multi-electrode array for measuring evoked potentials from the surface of ferret primary auditory cortex," *J. Neurosci. Methods*, vol. 58, pp. 209–220, 1995.

[4] C.T. Nordhausen, E.M. Maynard, and R.A. Normann, "Single unit recording capabilities of a 100 microelectrode array," *Brain Research*, vol. 726, pp. 129–140, 1996.

[5] K. Najafi and K.D. Wise, "An implantable multielectrode array with on-chip signal processing," *IEEE J. Solid-State Cir.*, vol. 21, pp. 1035–1044, Dec. 1986.

[6] K.D. Wise, D.J. Anderson, J.F. Hetke, D.R. Kipke, and K. Najafi, "Wireless implantable microsystems: high-density electronic interfaces to the nervous system," *Proc. IEEE*, vol. 92, pp. 76–97, Jan. 2004.

[7] R.H. Olsson III and K.D. Wise, "A three-dimensional neural recording microsystem with implantable data compression circuitry," *IEEE J. Solid-State Cir.*, vol. 40, pp. 2796–2804, Dec. 2005.

[8] R.R. Harrison, P.T. Watkins, R.J. Kier, R.O. Lovejoy, D.J. Black, B. Greger, and F. Solzbacher, "A low-power integrated circuit for a wireless 100-electrode neural recording system," *IEEE J. Solid-State Cir.*, vol. 42, pp. 123–133, January 2007.

[9] T.M. Seese, H. Harasaki, G.M. Saidel, and C.R. Davies, "Characterization of tissue morphology, angiogenesis, and temperature in the adaptive response of muscle tissue to chronic heating," *Lab. Investigation*, vol. 78(12), pp. 1553–1562, 1998.

[10] J.C. LaManna, K.A. McCracken, M. Patil, and O.J. Prohaska, "Stimulus-activated changes in brain tissue temperature in the anesthetized rat," *Metabolic Brain Disease*, vol. 4, pp. 225–237, 1989.

[11] A. Jackson, J. Mavoori, and E.E. Fetz, "Long-term motor cortex plasticity induced by an electronic neural implant," *Nature*, vol. 444, pp. 56–60, 2006.

[12] J.K. Chapin, K.A. Moxon, R.S. Markowitz, and M.A.L. Nicolelis, "Real-time control of a robot arm using simultaneously recorded neurons in the motor cortex," *Nature Neurosci.*, vol. 2, pp. 664–670, 1999.

[13] J. Wessberg, C.R. Stambaugh, J.D. Kralik, P.D. Beck, M. Laubach, J.K. Chapin, J. Kim, S.J. Biggs, M.A. Srinivasan, and M.A.L. Nicolelis, "Real-time prediction of hand trajectory by ensembles of cortical neurons in primates," *Nature*, vol. 408, pp. 361–365, 2000.

[14] M.D. Serruya, N.G. Hatsopoulos, L. Paninski, M.R. Fellows, and J.P. Donoghue, "Instant neural control of a movement signal," *Nature*, vol. 416, pp. 141–142, 2002.

[15] D.M. Taylor, S.I.H. Tillery, and A.B. Schwartz, "Direct cortical control of 3-D neuroprosthetic devices," *Science*, vol. 296, pp. 1829–1832, 2002.

[16] P.R. Kennedy, R.A.E. Bakay, M.M. Moore, K. Adams, and J. Goldthwaite, "Direct control of a computer from the human central nervous system," *IEEE Trans. Rehab. Eng.*, vol. 8, pp. 198–202, June 2000.

[17] L.R. Hochberg, M.D. Serruya, G.M. Friehs, J.A. Mukand, M. Saleh, A.H. Caplan, A. Branner, D. Chen, R.D. Penn, and J.P. Donoghue, "Neuronal ensemble control of prosthetic devices by a human with tetraplegia," *Nature*, vol. 442, pp. 164–171, 2006.

[18] E.R. Kandel, J.H. Schwartz, and T.M. Jessell, *Principles of Neural Science*, 4th ed. Boston, MA: McGraw-Hill, 2000.

[19] R.C. Gesteland, B. Howland, J.Y. Lettvin, and W.H. Pitts, "Comments on microelectrodes," *Proc. IRE*, vol. 47, pp. 1856–1862, 1959.

[20] C.D. Ferris, *Introduction to Bioinstrumentation.* Clifton, NJ: Humana, 1978.

[21] R.R. Harrison, "A versatile integrated circuit for the acquisition of biopotentials," In: *Proc. IEEE Custom Integrated Circuits Conf. (CICC)*, San Jose, CA, 2007.

[22] A.C. Metting van Rijn, A. Peper, and C.A. Grimbergen, "High-quality recording of bioelectric events," *Med. Biol. Eng. Comput.*, vol. 29, pp. 1035–1044, 1986.

[23] V.N. Murthy and E.E. Fetz, "Coherent 25- to 35-Hz oscillations in the sensorimotor cortex of awake behaving monkeys," *Proc. Natl. Acad. Sci. USA*, vol. 89, pp. 5670–5674, 1992.

[24] J.P. Donoghue, J.N. Sanes, N.G. Hatsopoulos, and G. Gaal, "Neural discharge and local field potential oscillations in primate motor cortex during voluntary movements," *J. Neurophysiol.*, vol. 79, pp. 159–173, 1998.

[25] K.V. Shenoy, M.M. Churchland, G. Santhanam, B.M. Yu, and S.I. Ryu, "Influence of movement speed on plan activity in monkey pre-motor cortex and implications for high-performance neural prosthetic system design," In: *Proc. 2003 Intl. Conf. of the IEEE Eng. in Medicine and Biology Soc.*, pp. 1897–1900, Cancún, Mexico, 2003.

[26] C. Mehring, J. Rickert, E. Vaadia, S. Cardoso de Oliveira, A. Aertsen, and S. Rotter, "Inference of hand movements from local field potentials in monkey motor cortex," *Nature Neurosci.*, vol. 6, pp. 1253-1254, 2003.

[27] H. Scherberger, M.R. Jarvis, and R.A. Andersen, "Cortical local field potential encodes movement intentions in the posterior parietal cortex," *Neuron*, vol. 46, pp. 347–354, 2005.

[28] B. Pesaran, J.S. Pezaris, M. Sahani, P.P. Mitra, and R.A. Andersen, "Temporal structure in neuronal activity during working memory in macaque parietal cortex," *Nature Neurosci.*, vol. 5, pp. 805–811, 2002.

[29] S. Kim, R.A. Normann, R. Harrison, and F. Solzbacher, "Preliminary study of thermal impacts of a microelectrode array implanted in the brain," In: *Proc. 2006 Intl. Conf. of the IEEE Eng. in Medicine and Biology Soc.*, pp. 2986–2989, New York, NY, 2006.

[30] S. Kim, P. Tathireddy, R. Normann, and F. Solzbacher, "*In vitro* and *in vivo* study of temperature increases in the brain due to a neural implant," In: *Proc. 3rd Intl. IEEE EMBS Conf. on Neural Engineering*, Kohala Coast, HI, 2007.

[31] M.S.J. Steyaert, W.M.C. Sansen, and C. Zhongyuan, "A micro-power low-noise monolithic instrumentation amplifier for medical purposes," *IEEE J. Solid-State Cir.*, vol. 22, pp. 1163–1168, Dec. 1987.

[32] R.R. Harrison and C. Charles, "A low-power low-noise CMOS amplifier for neural recording applications," *IEEE J. Solid-State Cir.*, vol. 38, pp. 958–965, June 2003.

[33] E.A. Vittoz and J. Fellrath, "CMOS analog integrated circuits based on weak inversion operation," *IEEE J. Solid-State Cir.*, vol. 12, pp. 224–231, June 1977.

[34] C. Mead, *Analog VLSI and Neural Systems*, Reading, MA: Addison-Wesley, 1989.

[35] C.C. Enz, F. Krummenacher, and E.A. Vittoz, "An analytical MOS transistor model valid in all regions of operation and dedicated to low-voltage and low-current applications," *Analog Integrat. Circuits Signal Process.*, vol. 8, pp. 83–114, 1995.

[36] Y. Tsividis, *Operation and Modeling of the MOS Transistor*, 2nd ed. Boston, MA: McGraw-Hill, 1998.

[37] D.A. Johns and K. Martin, *Analog Integrated Circuit Design*, New York, NY: John Wiley & Sons, 1997.

CHAPTER 9

Integrated Circuits for Neural Interfacing: Neurochemical Recording

Pedram Mohseni

9.1 Introduction to Neurochemical Recording

Rapid long-distance communication in the nervous system occurs via action potentials conducted along the neuronal axon to the synapse. In the extracellular cleft of this junction between two neurons, however, communication is mediated through the release and uptake of neurotransmitters [1, 2]. Elicited from the pre-synaptic neuron by the action potential, released neurotransmitter diffuses towards the post-synaptic neuron and binds to specific protein receptors as illustrated in Figure 9.1, eliciting a change in the physiological status of the target neuron that ultimately determines the probability of whether a new action potential will be generated.

Abnormal variations of physiological levels of neurotransmitters within the brain have been linked to several neurological disorders such as Alzheimer's and Parkinson's disease, and epilepsy [3]. Many neuroactive substances, such as therapeutic drugs (e.g., Zoloft) and drugs of abuse (e.g., cocaine) act by changing neurotransmitter levels at synapses, or by mimicking the actions of neurotransmitters at post-synaptic receptors. Moreover, much of the plasticity of the nervous system, which underlies learning and memory, is due to modifications of chemical synapses. Many of the biogenic aminergic systems, such as those that release dopamine or serotonin, provide outputs to large regions of the brain that affect mood, learning, and cognition [4]. Hence, understanding brain function on a fundamental level requires measurements of both electrical and chemical activity for a more holistic image of neural signal pathways.

9.2 Chemical Monitoring

The field of neurochemical monitoring is dominated by microdialysis and voltammetry, although other approaches including optical probes and imaging techniques such as functional magnetic resonance imaging, positron emission tomography, and single photon emission computerized tomography have been used as well [5, 6]. Microdialysis and voltammetry exhibit distinct monitoring strengths [7, 8]. Because a sample is physically removed from the brain by the probe, microdialysis can be coupled to exquisitely sensitive and selective analytical techniques like chromatography, electrophoresis, florescence detection, and mass spectrometry.

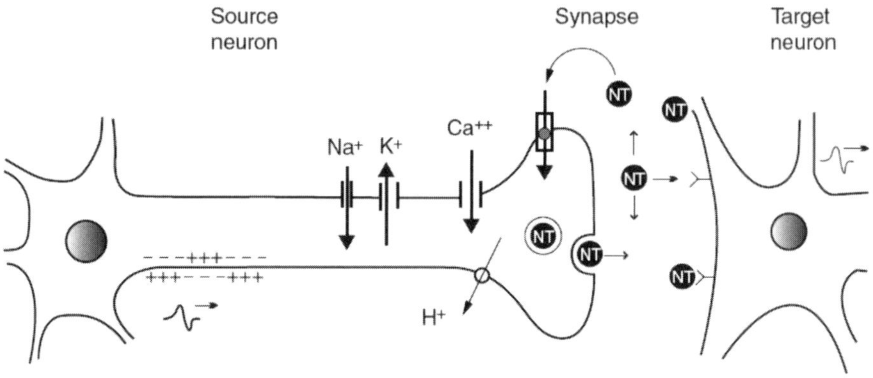

Figure 9.1 Neuronal signaling. From [11] with permission.

In contrast, voltammetry, which detects neurotransmitters electrochemically directly in the brain, excels at rapid measurements at small probes. Electrochemistry involves bi-directional charge transfer between an electrode and a sample in solid or liquid phase, with the applied electrode potential providing energy for an electron transfer (i.e., a chemical reaction) to occur [9]. The chemical reactions occur at the electrode's surface or very short distances away within the probed sample volume, and the resulting charge transfer or current, which is proportional to the concentration of the electroactive neurotransmitter, is measured. Several important neurotransmitters, including dopamine, norepinephrine, serotonin, histamine, and nitric oxide, are electroactive and thus amenable to electrochemical detection [10]. Voltammetry can also be incorporated into wireless devices [11]. These attributes make voltammetry the best choice for chemical measurements.

The three most commonly used voltammetric methods in the modern era are amperometry [12], high-speed chronoamperometry [13], and fast-scan cyclic voltammetry (FSCV) [14]. Although all monitor analyte with sub-second temporal resolution at a carbon-fiber microelectrode (CFM), performance differences have driven distinct applications in cell biology and neurobiology [15]. FSCV offers the greatest specificity, because a chemical signature called a cyclic voltammogram is recorded to identify the detected species, and hence is recognized as the best choice for monitoring endogenous neurotransmitters in behaving animals.

FSCV at a CFM for dopamine is illustrated in Figure 9.2. The potential (E) of the CFM is linearly scanned every 100 ms by a triangle wave between a resting potential of –400 mV and a peak voltage of 1 V at a typical scan rate of 300 V/s, resulting in a scan duration of ~9.3 ms (Panel A). During the positive sweep, dopamine is oxidized to dopamine-ortho-quinone (DOQ), which is reduced back to dopamine during the negative sweep. The middle plot in Panel B shows a recording obtained using a CFM implanted in the striatum of an anesthetized rat during a single triangular voltage scan (top plot in Panel B). The black line depicts the measured *background* current in the absence of dopamine, whereas the red line shows the measured total current at the same CFM when electrical stimulation was applied to the dopamine axons traversing the medial forebrain bundle (MFB) in order to evoke dopamine

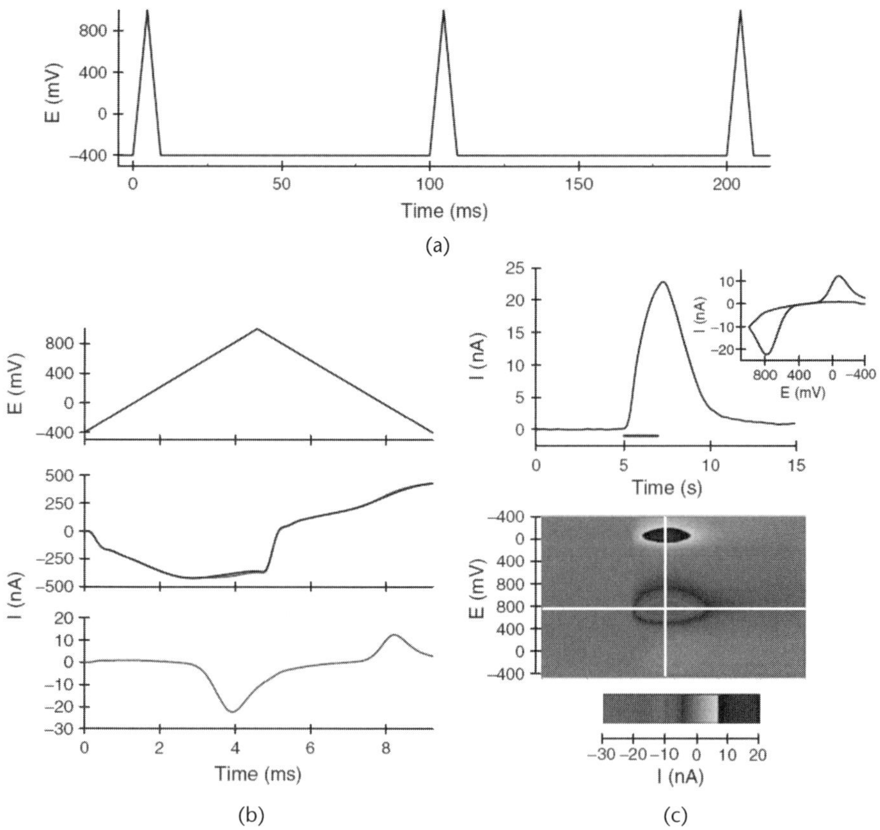

Figure 9.2 Fast-scan cyclic voltammetry at a carbon-fiber microelectrode. (a) Timing protocol for the 10-Hz FSCV scanning waveform. (b) Measured current during a single scan. (c) Voltammetric recordings of transient dopamine release in the striatum of an anesthetized rat evoked by electrical stimulation of the dopaminergic fibers. From [11].

release throughout the forebrain. Since background current is stable, it can be subtracted from the total current in order to reveal the faradaic oxidation-reduction (redox) current, resulting from dopamine oxidation into a quinone and reduction of the electroformed quinone back to dopamine (bottom plot in Panel B).

Redox currents, when plotted against voltage, create the background-subtracted voltammogram, which is used as a chemical signature to uniquely identify the analyte as shown in Panel C (INSET) where the peaks indicate dopamine. Successive background-subtracted voltammograms can be plotted versus time in a color plot with the x, y, z axes corresponding to time, applied voltage, and measured current, respectively (bottom plot in Panel C). Dynamic information, indicative of the temporal pattern of extracellular concentration variation, is obtained by plotting dopamine current measured in each scan at dopamine oxidation voltage versus time as shown by the top plot in Panel C, corresponding to the horizontal white line in the color plot (i.e., applied potential of ~750 mV). The cyclic voltammogram shown in Panel C (INSET) is obtained by recording the current at ~7 s versus the applied potential, corresponding to the vertical white line in the color plot.

9.3 Sensor and Circuit Technologies

9.3.1 Neurochemical Sensing Probes

For electrochemical detection of neurotransmitters, researchers have previously used gold electrodes, carbon-fiber microelectrodes, and microfabricated, screen-printed, polymer-modified carbon sensor arrays [16, 17]. Carbon-fiber microelectrodes (CFMs) are conventional neurochemical sensing probes that enable highly sensitive direct detection of oxidizable species released from single cells and vesicles [17]. These electrodes are typically fabricated by aspirating a single carbon fiber (5–10 μm in diameter) into a borosilicate glass capillary tube and pulling the capillary to a taper using a standard pipette puller. The exposed carbon fiber is then cut to a desirable length (typically 100–250 μm) under a microscope. A stainless steel lead wire is then inserted into the open end of the capillary and secured to the carbon fiber and glass capillary by molten bismuth or graphite powder.

Conductive diamond has emerged as a potentially superior electrode biomaterial. It is chemically and mechanically robust with a low baseline current, allowing long-term use and greater sensitivity for detecting lower analyte concentrations. The investigation of new chemistries is also possible due to diamond's wide-potential window of water stability. In addition, diamond's predictable surface chemistry discourages adsorption and oxygen reduction [18].

These electrodes are fabricated by selectively depositing heavily conductive, boron-doped, polycrystalline diamond onto individual polished tips of tungsten microelectrodes using standard hot-filament chemical vapor deposition (CVD) as shown in Figure 9.3.

Each tungsten microelectrode substrate is fabricated by pre-sealing a tungsten microwire (25 μm in diameter) into a pulled quartz capillary, and then beveling at a 45° angle to form a coarsely polished elliptical disk. Polycrystalline diamond is selectively deposited for up to 3 hours in a standard methane/hydrogen/trimethylboron

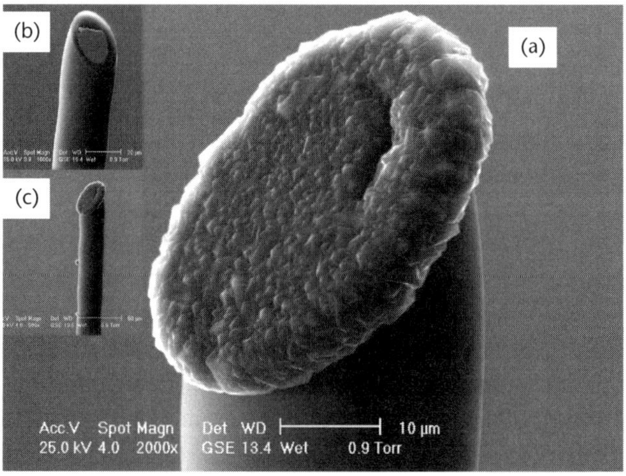

Figure 9.3 SEM images of (a, c) selective diamond deposition on a (b) tungsten microelectrode; final tip diameter is 35 μm. Negligible diamond growth is observed on the walls of the quartz insulating capillary. From [23] with permission, © IEEE 2008.

CVD environment at 20 Torr [18, 19]. The novel needle-like geometry of these diamond micro-needle electrodes mimics that of commercially available carbon- and metal-based microelectrodes. Hence, it enables implantation with minimal tissue damage and, when used in fast-scan mode, permits kinetic studies that are not confounded by mass transfer considerations. Using the diamond electrodes *in vitro*, biogenic amines have been electrochemically measured at millisecond time scales, e.g., serotonin in the vicinity of individual identified nerve cells in a marine mollusk *Aplysia californica* [20].

9.3.2 Neurochemical Sensing Interface Circuitry

One prominent challenge in designing integrated interface electronics for electrochemical-based neurochemistry is the wide range of input currents that can be encountered in a neurophysiological application. Such currents could be as large as hundreds of nA while current resolution levels of a few pA might be required at the same time. Given that the physiological levels of neurotransmitter concentrations typically do not change rapidly with time, delta-sigma (ΔΣ) front-end architectures that enable a trade-off between conversion speed and resolution are quite amenable to sensing the low-frequency current signals that result from an electrochemical transduction. Single- and multi-channel integrated interface circuits for *amperometric* electrochemical biosensors have been previously reported in [21–27], with some employing a first-order ΔΣ modulator (ΔΣM) front-end architecture.

As stated previously, FSCV is another electrochemical technique that not only provides measurements on the same time scale (~100 ms) as that of neurotransmission, thus making real-time monitoring of chemical dynamics possible, but also offers the greatest specificity in a complex biological matrix *in vivo*, because a chemical signature (cyclic voltammogram) is recorded to identify the detected species. However, integrated circuits supporting FSCV need to have much faster conversion speed and much larger dynamic range compared to their amperometric counterparts.

Figure 9.4 shows the architecture of a wireless monitoring system comprising an implantable integrated transmitter chip as well as external receiver electronics that is described in [28]. The chip can support both FSCV and amperometry when configured for neurochemistry. On the transmitter side, a reconfigurable third-order ΔΣM is interfaced with the sensing electrode, and can measure either electric currents proportional to extracellular concentration variations of neurotransmitter levels or electrophysiological voltages. The digital output bit-stream of the ΔΣM is wirelessly sent to the outside world using a back-end RF-FSK transmitter after on-chip Manchester encoding. In neurochemical sensing mode, an on-chip arbitrary waveform generator applies the FSCV scanning waveform to a standard chloridized silver wire (Ag/AgCl) used as the reference electrode. Since physiological concentrations of various neurotransmitters are on the order of nanomolar, very small currents are typically involved in electrochemical detection of neurotransmitters. As a result, the ohmic drop across the reference electrode would be negligible. Therefore, a two-electrode electro-analysis setup without a counter electrode can be employed.

As shown in Figure 9.5, the core recording module is a continuous-time third-order ΔΣM with a single-bit quantizer that occupies 850 μm × 180 μm in silicon area and dissipates ~28 μA from a 2.5-V supply when clocked at ~680 kHz. It is designed

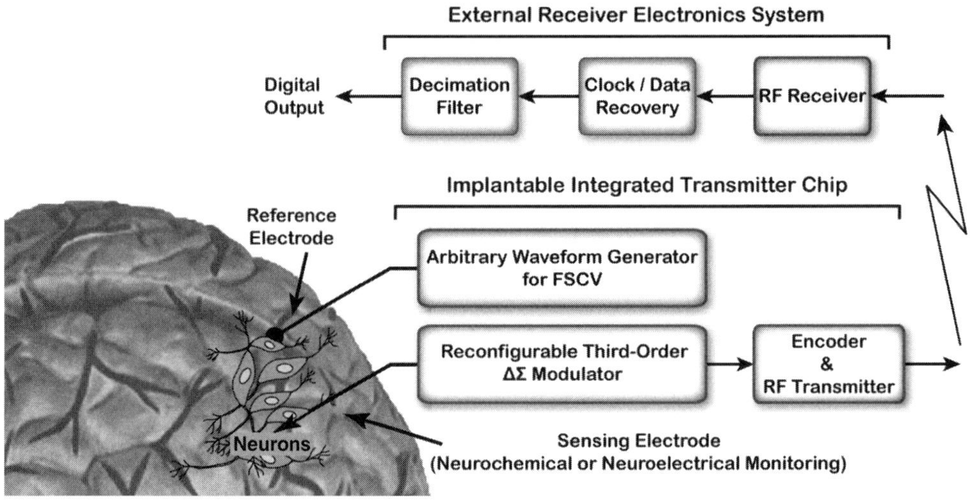

Figure 9.4 Architecture of the single-channel integrated circuit for wireless monitoring of chemical or electrical neural activity. The chip can support both amperometry and FSCV when configured for neurochemistry. From [28] with permission, © IEEE 2008.

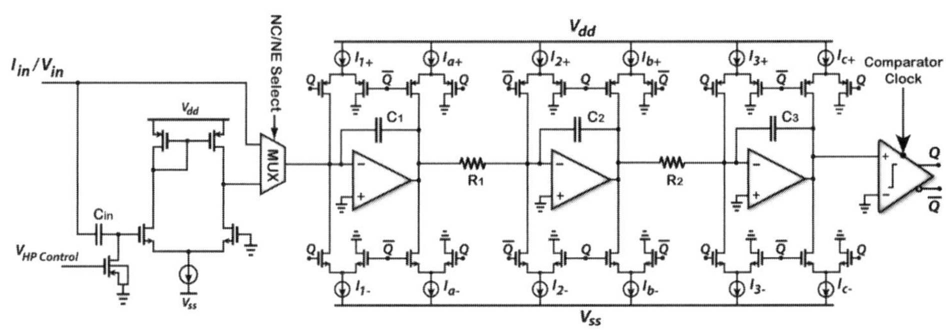

Figure 9.5 Circuit schematic of the core sensing module, comprised of a current-input third-order ΔΣM with single-bit quantization as well as a front-end voltage-to-current (V/I) converter with dc baseline stabilization. From [28] with permission, © IEEE 2008.

to be stable in the targeted input range of ±750 nA required for neurochemical sensing using FSCV, and reliably converts very small currents directly into digital data with no need for current amplification that can be inherently noisy, nonlinear and thus unsuitable for very-low-current sensing applications.

While I_1, I_2, and I_3 are the main feedback current source pairs for addition/subtraction in the ΔΣM, additional sets of current source pairs (I_a, I_b, and I_c) are also employed to relax the bandwidth and slew rate requirements of the integrating amplifiers, allowing a current consumption of only 4.4 μA per amplifier.

The recording channel can also be configured for electrophysiological studies using an ac-coupled open-loop transconductance (G_m) block that converts the μV-range neuroelectrical input voltages to currents manageable by the ΔΣM for further processing. The G_m block occupies a silicon area of 100 μm × 180 μm, draws ~3.6 μA, and incorporates a 4-pF on-chip capacitor (C_{in}) and a subthreshold PMOS transistor for dc baseline stabilization [29, 30].

The arbitrary waveform generator in Figure 9.4 consists of a timing controller, a 128 × 8-bit memory, an 8-bit charge-redistribution DAC and an analog output buffer, incorporating a class AB output with rail-to-rail I/O capability to generate the FSCV waveform with a programmable scan rate of 100–500 V/s typically used in neurochemistry [14]. The FSCV waveform generator, including the memory, occupies an active area of 1758 μm × 600 μm, and can drive capacitive loads in a wide range of 0–100 nF.

A prototype integrated circuit was fabricated using the AMI 0.5 μm 2P/3M n-well standard CMOS process. Figure 9.6 shows a microphotograph of the 2.7 × 2.9-mm^2 chip containing 16 data channels. The top plot in Figure 9.7 depicts the measured frequency spectrum of the digital data bit-stream at the $\Delta\Sigma$M output in neurochemical sensing mode for a 1-kHz, 10-nA$_{pp}$ sinusoidal input current.

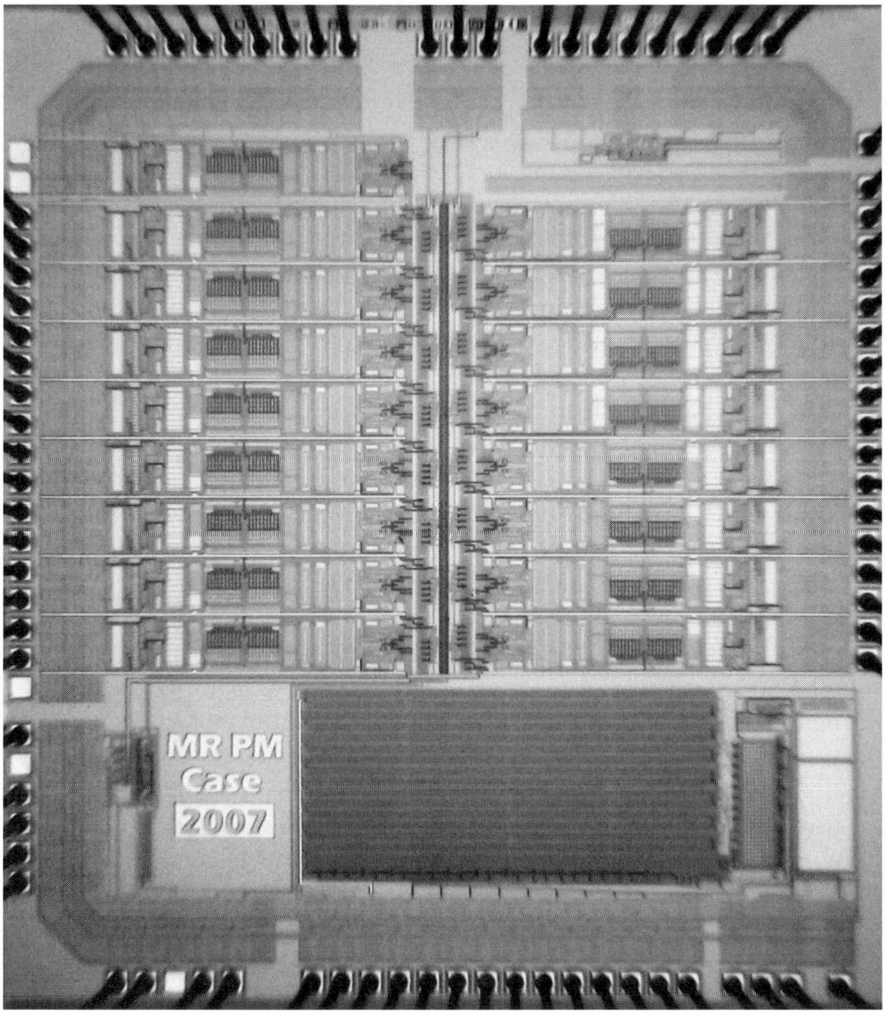

Figure 9.6 Microphotograph of the chip fabricated in AMI 0.5 μm 2P/3M n-well CMOS process. From [28] with permission, © IEEE 2008.

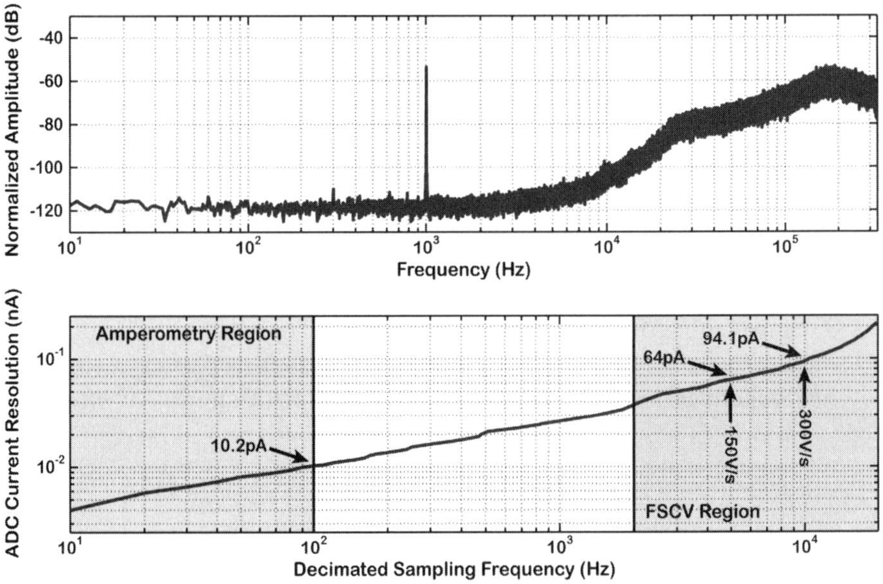

Figure 9.7 Measured frequency spectrum of the ΔΣM digital output for a 1-kHz, 10-nA_{pp} sinusoidal input current (top) and the resulting measured ADC current resolution versus the decimated sampling frequency for amperometry and FSCV modalities of neurochemical sensing (bottom). From [28] with permission, © IEEE 2008.

The resulting current resolution as a function of the decimated sampling frequency (i.e., twice the decimation filter bandwidth) for amperometry (up to 100 Hz) and FSCV at various scan rates is also shown in the bottom plot. The peak-to-peak voltage variation in the FSCV scanning waveform is taken to be 1.5 V and 100 data points are sampled during its time duration. As can be seen, by setting the decimation filter bandwidth to 50 Hz in software, a current resolution of 10.2 pA is achieved in amperometry. Setting the decimation filter bandwidth to 5 kHz instead allows one to achieve a current resolution of 94.1 pA in 300-V/s FSCV. Software implementation of the decimation filter on the receiver side provides flexibility for dynamic trade-off between data conversion speed and required resolution at the expense of elevated data rates in wireless transmission.

A similar chip that employed a second-order ΔΣM front-end architecture and wireless RF telemetry was designed, fabricated in the same CMOS process, and tested with an anesthetized rat, which is a workhorse preparation for studying dopamine neurotransmission and will assess how devices operate *in vivo* under well-defined conditions [31].

Considerable research interest in the field of neurobiology has been directed towards dopamine. Although relatively few in number in the human brain, dopaminergic neurons play important roles in the functions of cognition, motor control, and motivation, and when dysfunctional, are intimately involved in the neuropathologies of schizophrenia, Parkinson's disease, and drug addiction [32]. At the post-synaptic level, dopamine regulates synaptic plasticity, the cellular manifestation of learning, and memory [33]. Although great strides have occurred in our understanding of dopamine neurobiology and neuropathology over the five decades since its identification as a neurotransmitter, how dopamine precisely acts at the cellular level to mediate behavior remains incompletely understood. Hence, development of instrumentation supporting chemical and electrical recording for mechanistic studies of dopamine function in freely behaving animals is an important technological goal.

Acute biological experiments were performed on urethane-anesthetized adult male Sprague-Dawley rats in accordance with NIH guidelines. A twisted bipolar stimulating electrode was implanted in the MFB and a CFM in the caudate-putamen (dorsal striatum), a rich dopamine-innervated region of the forebrain implicated in the control of movement. Biphasic current pulses (±300 μA, 60 Hz, 4-ms pulse width) were applied for two seconds (a total of 120 pulses) to the dopamine axons traversing the MFB in order to evoke dopamine release [34]. The CFM, whose position was optimized in the caudate-putamen to sense the electrically evoked dopamine release, was externally interfaced with the fabricated CMOS chip. FSCV measurements were conducted at a scan rate of 300 V/s and a frequency of 3.3 Hz. Figure 9.8 shows the wirelessly measured background-subtracted cyclic voltammogram of dopamine recorded in the rat brain.

The peak current at ~650 mV during the forward sweep corresponds to dopamine oxidation, whereas the peak current at nearly –180 mV in the reverse sweep corresponds to reduction of the electroformed quinone back to dopamine. Figure 9.9 depicts the wirelessly measured transient dopamine release in the rat caudate-putamen following electrical stimulation of its MFB for two seconds at 60 Hz as indicated by the black bar underneath the trace. Peak dopamine concentration was estimated to be ~1.5 μM, and data agreed favorably with recordings collected by a hardwired FSCV system in the same animal at the same CFM (not shown)

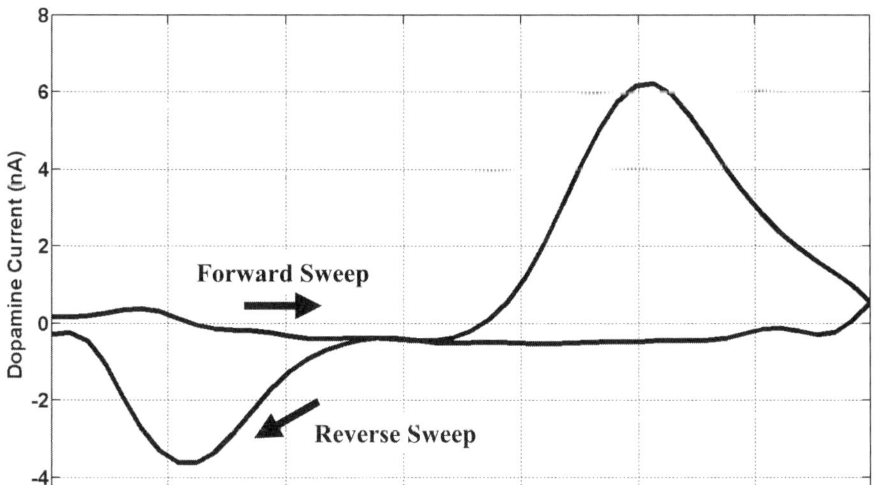

Figure 9.8 Background-subtracted cyclic voltammogram of dopamine measured wirelessly in the rat caudate-putamen. The peak current at ~650 mV during the forward sweep corresponds to dopamine oxidation, whereas the peak current at nearly –180 mV in the reverse sweep corresponds to reduction of the electroformed quinone back to dopamine. From [31] with permission, © IEEE 2008.

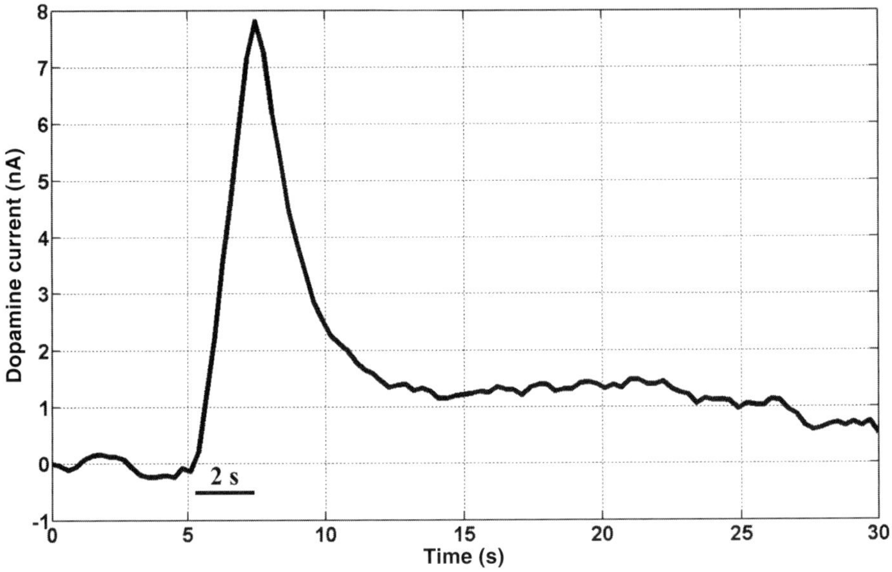

Figure 9.9 Transient dopamine release measured wirelessly in the rat caudate-putamen after two seconds of 60-Hz stimulation applied to the rat medial forebrain bundle as indicated by the black bar underneath the trace. From [31] with permission, © IEEE 2008.

References

[1] M.J. Zigmond, F.E. Bloom, S.C. Landis, J.L. Roberts, and L.R. Squire (1999) *Fundamental Neuroscience*. San Diego: Academic Press.

[2] E.R. Kandel, J.H. Schwartz, and T.M. Jessell (2000) *Principles of Neural Science*. New York: McGraw-Hill.

[3] M. Glass and M. Dragunov, "Neurochemical and morphological changes associated with human epilepsy," *Brain Res. Revs.*, vol. 21, no. 1, pp. 29–41, 1995.

[4] M.E. Hasselmo, J. Hay, M. Ilyn, and A. Gorchetchnikov, "Neuromodulation, theta rhythm and rat spatial navigation," *Neural Networks*, vol. 15, pp. 689–707, 2002.

[5] I. Baranowska and M. Zydron (2002) Liquid chromatography in the analysis of neurotransmitters and alkaloids. *J Chromatogr Sci* 40: 224–228.

[6] R. Schlosser (2000) Detection of neurotransmitter interactions with PET and SPECT by pharmacological challenge paradigms. *Nervenarzt* 71: 9–18.

[7] P.E.M. Phillips and R.M. Wightman (2003) Critical guidelines for validation of the selectivity of *in vivo* chemical microsensors. *Trends Anal Chem* 22: 509–514.

[8] C.J. Watson, B.J. Venton, and R.T. Kennedy (2006) *In vivo* measurements of neurotransmitters by microdialysis sampling. *Anal Chem* 78: 1391–1399.

[9] A. Hierlemann (2005) *Integrated Chemical Microsensor Systems in CMOS Technology*. New York: Springer, pp. 59–84.

[10] L.M. Borland and A.C. Michael (2007) *An introduction to electrochemical methods in neuroscience*. In: Electrochemical methods for neuroscience (Michael AC, Borland LM, eds), pp. 1–15. Boca Raton: CRC Press.

[11] P.A. Garris, P.G. Greco, S.G. Sandberg, G. Howes, S. Pongmayteegul, B.A. Heidenreich, J.M. Casto, R. Ensman, J. Poehlman, A. Alexander, and G.V. Rebec (2006) *In vivo voltam-*

metry with telemetry. In: Electrochemical methods for neuroscience (Michael AC, Borland LM, eds), pp. 233–259. Boca Raton: CRC Press.

[12] F. Gonon (1995) *Monitoring dopamine and noradrenaline release in central and peripheral nervous systems with treated and untreated carbon-fiber electrodes*. In: Neuromethods: Voltammetric methods in brain systems (Boulton A, Baker G, Adams RN, eds), pp. 153–177. Totowa, New Jersey: Humana Press Inc.

[13] G.A. Gerhardt (1995) *Rapid chronocoulometric measurements of norepinephrine overflow and clearance in CNS tissues*. In: Neuromethods: Voltammetric methods in brain systems (Boulton A, Baker G, Adams RN, eds), pp. 117–151. Totowa, New Jersey: Humana Press Inc.

[14] P.A. Garris and R.M. Wightman (1995) *Regional differences in dopamine release, uptake, and diffusion measured by fast-scan cyclic voltammetry*. In: Neuromethods: Voltammetric methods in brain systems (Boulton A, Baker G, Adams RN, eds), pp. 179–220. Totowa, New Jersey: Humana Press Inc.

[15] S.G. Sandberg and P.A. Garris (2007) *Neurochemistry of addiction: monitoring essential neurotransmitter of addiction*. In: Novel approaches to addiction (Kuhn CM, Koob GF, eds), In Press. Boca Raton: CRC Press.

[16] M. Naware, N.V. Thakor, R.N. Orth, K. Murari, and P.A. Passeraub, "Design and microfabrication of a polymer-modified carbon sensor array for the measurement of neurotransmitter signals," in *Proc. 25th Annu. Int. IEEE Eng. Med. Biol. Conf. (EMBC'03)*, pp. 1952–1955, Cancun, Mexico, 2003.

[17] P.S. Cahill, Q.D. Walker, J.M. Finnegan, G.E. Mickelson, and R.M. Wightman, "Microelectrodes for the measurement of catecholamines in biological systems," *Anal. Chem.*, vol. 68, pp. 3180–3186, 1996.

[18] H. B. Martin, A. Argoitia, J. C. Angus, and U. Landau, "Voltammetry studies of single-crystal and polycrystalline diamond electrodes," *J. Electrochem. Soc.*, vol. 146, pp. 2959–2964, 1999.

[19] S. Xie, G. Shafer, C.G. Wilson, and H.B. Martin, "*In vitro* adenosine detection with a diamond-based sensor," *Diam. Rel. Mater.*, vol. 15, pp. 225–228, 2006.

[20] J.M. Halpern, S. Xie, G.P. Sutton, B.T. Higashikubo, C.A. Chestek, H.J. Chiel, and H.B. Martin, "Diamond electrodes for neurodynamic studies in *Aplysia californica*," *Diam. Rel. Mater.*, vol. 15, pp. 183–187, 2006.

[21] H.S. Narula and J.G. Harris, "VLSI potentiostat for amperometric measurements for electrolytic reactions," in *Proc. IEEE Int. Symp. Circuits and Systems (ISCAS'04)*, pp. 457–460, Vancouver, Canada, May 23–26, 2004.

[22] J. Zhang, N. Trombly, and A. Mason, "A low-noise readout circuit for integrated electrochemical biosensor arrays," in *Proc. IEEE Sensors Conf.*, pp. 36–39, Vienna, Austria, October 24–27, 2004.

[23] M. Roham, J.M. Halpern, H.B. Martin, H.J. Chiel, and P. Mohseni, "Wireless amperometric neurochemical monitoring using an integrated telemetry circuit," *IEEE Trans. Biomed. Eng.*, 2008, In Press.

[24] R. Genov, M. Stanacevic, M. Naware, G. Cauwenberghs, and N.V. Thakor, "16-channel integrated potentiostat for distributed neurochemical sensing," *IEEE Trans. Circuits and Systems-I*, vol. 53, no. 11, pp. 2371–2376, November 2006.

[25] M. Stanacevic, K. Murari, A. Rege, G. Cauwenberghs, and N. Thakor, "VLSI potentiostat array with oversampling gain modulation for wide-range neurotransmitter sensing," *IEEE Trans. Biomed. Circuits and Systems*, vol. 1, no. 1, pp. 63–72, March 2007.

[26] K. Murari, M. Stanacevic, G. Cauwenberghs, and N.V. Thakor, "Integrated potentiostat for neurotransmitter sensing," *IEEE Eng. Med. Biol. Magazine*, vol. 24, no. 6, pp. 23–29, November/December 2005.

[27] A. Gore, S. Chakrabartty, S. Pal, and E. Alocilja, "A multichannel femtoampere-sensitivity conductometric array for biosensing applications," in *Proc. IEEE Eng. Med. Biol. Conf. (EMBC'06)*, New York City, NY, August 30–September 3, 2006.

[28] M. Roham and P. Mohseni, "A reconfigurable IC for wireless monitoring of chemical or electrical neural activity," in *Proc. IEEE Int. Symp. Circuits and Systems (ISCAS'08)*, Seattle, WA, May 18–21, 2008, In Press.

[29] P. Mohseni and K. Najafi, "A fully integrated neural recording amplifier with DC input stabilization," *IEEE Trans. Biomed. Eng.*, vol. 51, no. 5, pp. 832–837, May 2004.

[30] R.R. Harrison, P.T. Watkins, R.J. Kier, R.O. Lovejoy, D.J. Black, B. Greger, and F. Solzbacher, "A low-power integrated circuit for a wireless 100-electrode neural recording system," *IEEE J. Solid State Circuits*, vol. 42, no. 1, pp. 123–133, January 2007.

[31] M. Roham, D.P. Daberkow, E.S. Ramsson, D.P. Covey, S. Pakdeeronachit, P.A. Garris, and P. Mohseni, "A wireless IC for wide-range neurochemical monitoring using amperometry and fast-scan cyclic voltammetry," *IEEE Trans. Biomed. Circuits and Systems*, vol. 2, no. 1, pp. 3–9, March 2008, In Press.

[32] M. Le Moal and H. Simon, "Mesocorticolimbic dopaminergic network: functional and regulatory roles," *Physiol. Rev.*, vol. 71, pp. 155–234, 1991.

[33] J.N. Reynolds and J.R. Wickens, "Dopamine-dependent plasticity of cortico-striatal synapses," *Neural Networks*, vol. 15, pp. 507–521, 2002.

[34] B.P. Bergstrom and P.A. Garris, "Passive stabilization of striatal extracellular dopamine across the lesion spectrum encompassing the pre-symptomatic phase of Parkinson's disease: A voltammetric study in the 6-OHDA-lesioned rat," *J. Neurochemistry*, vol. 87, pp. 1224–1236, 2003.

CHAPTER 10

Integrated Circuits for Neural Interfacing: Neural Stimulation

Maysam Ghovanloo

10.1 Introduction to Neural Stimulation

Electrical stimulation of the excitable tissue such as muscle fibers and neurons is probably the most prevalent function that is performed by today's biomedical implantable devices. The term that is often used for this type of intervention in medical literature is *neuromodulation*, which denotes controlled electrical or chemical stimulation of the central or peripheral nervous system [1–3]. Figure 10.1 shows four functional categories in which stimulation may be applied in order to (a) cause a mechanical contraction in muscles to reanimate a paralyzed limb or eliminate atrophy in functional neuromuscular stimulation (FNS) [4–6]; (b) synchronize and readjust the rhythm of a repetitive physiological activity such as the heartbeat in cardiac rhythm management or stomach pace [7–9]; (c) disrupt ailing flow of information or malicious neural activity in the central nervous system, such as in deep brain stimulation (DBS) to treat Parkinson's disease or spinal cord stimulation (SCS) for pain management [10–12]; and (d) transfer and apply artificially acquired sensory information to the central or peripheral nervous system to substitute a damaged or lost sensory modality such as in auditory or visual prostheses [13–16].

In addition, there are quite a few newer applications for neural stimulation that are still in various stages of research and clinical trial, such as bladder control for treatment of incontinence [17], use of DBS in psychotherapy [18], and brain-machine interfacing for computer access and environment control [19].

Even though the physiological basis and clinical therapeutic effects of the aforementioned applications of electrical stimulation are quite different, from the circuits and systems design point of view, there are a few similarities among these implantable stimulating systems, which can help designers of this emerging technology take advantage of the prior knowledge in this field and apply it in their new designs. There are also a certain set of rules and requirements that govern all these applications, especially in terms of efficacy of stimulation and safety, which need to be carefully considered in human applications. In this chapter, I intend to describe some of these common principles in design and development of implantable microstimulation systems, particularly for neural interfacing and neuromodulation applications.

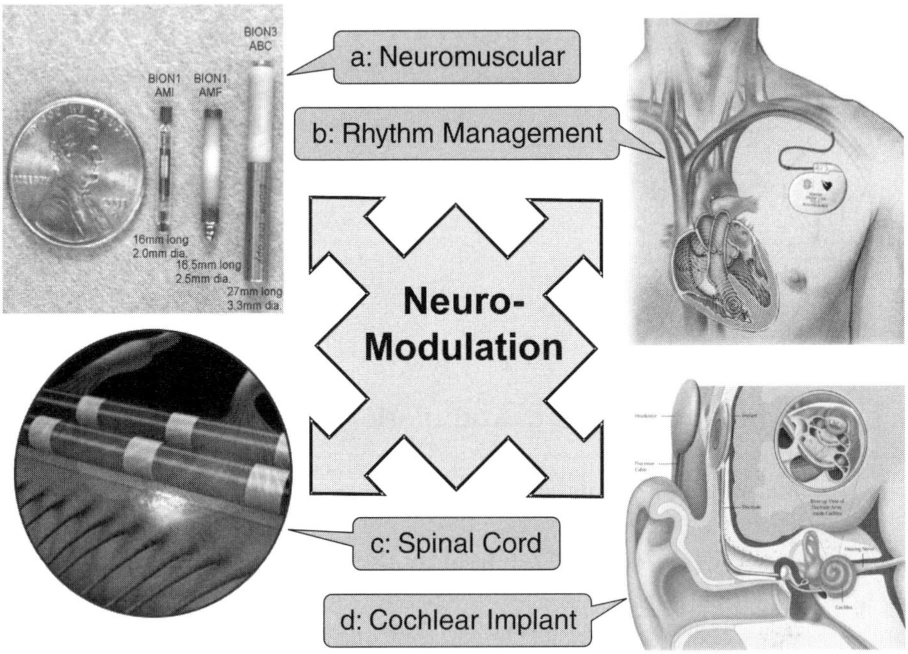

Figure 10.1 Functional categories of biomedical stimulation for (a) causing mechanical contractions in muscles to reanimate a paralyzed limb or eliminate atrophy in functional neuromuscular stimulation (FNS) [4]; (b) synchronizing and readjusting the rhythm of a repetitive physiological activity such as the heartbeat in cardiac rhythm management or stomach pace; (c) disrupting ailing flow of information or malicious neural activity in the central nervous system, such as in deep brain stimulation (DBS) to treat Parkinson's disease or spinal cord stimulation (SCS) for pain management [8], and (d) transferring and applying artificially acquired sensory information to the central or peripheral nervous system to substitute a damaged or lost sensory modality such as in auditory or visual prostheses [16].

10.2 Electrode Configuration and Tissue Volume Conductor

Stimulation requires at least a pair of electrodes, a positive anode and a negative cathode, as well as a stimulus generator, all of which are often implanted in the patient's body. The excitable tissue of interest, which could be the retina, cochlea, or a certain region of the brain or spinal cord, closes the current loop between the two electrodes, and the neurons that are close enough to the active electrodes to pass their stimulation threshold level (see Section 10.4) get activated by initiating an electrophysiological response called an *action potential* [20–22]. In most cases, only one of the electrodes of small surface area, called the *active* or *working electrode*, is placed within the targeted neural tissue. The other electrode, known as the *counter electrode*, is a much larger titanium or platinum metal can, which also forms the body of the implanted device package and hermetically seals the stimulus generator circuitry [23, 24]. In this type of stimulation, which is called *monopolar*, tissue excitation only takes place around the working electrode that is much smaller and therefore creates a much larger stimulus current density compared to the counter electrode. In monopolar stimulation, the stimulus current propagates through a relatively large volume of the tissue since the counter electrode is large and far from the active electrode site. Hence this type of stimulation is omnidirectional and less spatially specific.

On the other hand, there are cases in which two, three, or even four small nearby electrodes are simultaneously activated with different polarities and amplitude levels to limit the stimulus current distribution and the resulting tissue excitation to a highly confined volume of the tissue. These stimulation configurations, which have more specificity compared to monopolar, are known as *bipolar*, *tripolar*, or *quadripolar* stimulation [25]. By steering current among multiple electrodes, it is possible to create virtual stimulating sites by generating high potential gradients in areas between the active sites where there is physically no electrode. However, a more effective way of stimulating different regions of the targeted tissue is to implant a large array of 8, 16, or more electrodes, depending on the application, and steer current among them. The stimulus generator in this case is equipped with multiplexers and connects the pulse generator circuitry to the desired electrode(s) that are otherwise open-circuit [26]. The downside of increasing the number of electrodes is the increased complexity of implant microassembly and interconnects, volume of the device, and risk of damage to the surrounding neural tissue during implantation [27]. Up until now the only viable solution for developing neuroprosthetic devices with a large number of stimulating sites has been using high-density microelectrode arrays made of silicon or biocompatible polymers, such as those described in [28–30]. The stimulus generator in such systems can be designed with a stand-alone modular architecture to be scalable depending on the application and the patient's requirements [31].

10.3 Electrode-Electrolyte Interface

Stimulating circuits need to drive small metal electrodes placed within the excitable tissue and surrounded by physiological medium such as extracellular fluids, where charge transfer takes place by flow of ions including sodium, potassium, and chlorine as opposed to electrons. When a metal electrode is inserted in a solution, a capacitor forms all around its exposed areas, which is known as the *double-layer capacitor*. One plate of this capacitor, on the metallic side (electrode), utilizes electrons for charge transfer and the other plate, on the solution side (electrolyte), utilizes ions. Depending on the stimulation pulse amplitude, duration, and materials involved, two types of reactions can take place at the electrode-electrolyte interface [23]: (1) *non-Faradaic* reactions, in which no electrons transfer between the electrode and electrolyte. These reactions only result in redistribution of charged chemical species in the electrolyte as a result of the stimulation pulse and therefore, both electrode and electrolyte remain neutral. The double-layer capacitor in this case can be modeled as a simple linear capacitor. (2) *Faradaic* reactions, in which electrons are transferred between the electrode and electrolyte, resulting in reduction or oxidation of chemical species in the electrolyte. It should be noted that a combination of both reactions can take place at the stimulating site, depending on the stimulus parameters, electrode characteristics, and tissue conditions [23, 24].

Unlike the former solely capacitive mechanism, Faradaic charge injection forms chemical products in the solution that cannot be recovered upon reversing the direction of the current if they diffuse away from the electrode [23]. Hence, Faradaic reactions are divided into *reversible* and *irreversible* reactions. Irreversible Faradaic reactions result in a net change in the chemistry of the environment that leads to variations in the pH of the electrolyte and potentially create chemical species that are damaging to the surrounding tissue as well as the electrode. Thus, an important principle in long-term electrical stimulation is that irreversible Faradaic reactions should be avoided at all costs [32]. This would impose a higher limit over the density of charge that can be injected through an electrode, which depends on the electrode material and its surface roughness. Another practical implication of this principle from a circuit's point of view is that all of the charge that is injected into the tissue in one phase of stimulation has to be recovered afterwards, preferably before the beginning of the next pulse. This requirement, which is generally known as *charge balancing*, is a safety measure that avoids charge accumulation in the tissue and has to be incorporated in all stimulating circuits [33].

Considering the aforementioned reactions, the circuit shown in Figure 10.2 has been proposed to model the metal electrode-electrolyte interface [23, 34]. C_{DL} represents the double layer capacitor that is considered linear in this simplified model. Depending on the type of metal used and the way its surface is treated, C_{DL} value is on the order of 10–20 μF/cm^2 of real electrode surface area, which is its geometric area multiplied by its surface roughness factor. Z_F represents the leakage current and charge transfer between the electrode and electrolyte as a result of Faradaic reactions. Z_F is a complicated highly nonlinear time-varying component that has been the subject of numerous modeling efforts [34–36]. However, it can be neglected where non-Faradaic reactions are quite dominant, such as when the electrodes are made of noble metals such as gold or platinum and the stimulus amplitude and duration are low. Φ is a DC equilibrium interfacial potential, also known as *half-cell potential*, which depends on the type of electrode and concentration of ions in the electrolyte. Φ gradually changes with time and temperature; however, it can be neglected in simple models if both working and counter electrodes are made of the same type of metal. Finally, R_S represents the electrolyte and tissue resistance between the two electrodes, which is also known as *access* or *spreading resistance*. The equivalent model shown in Figure 10.2 is important from the circuit design perspective, because it represents the type and characteristics of the load that should be driven by the stimulus generating circuitry. The impedance of the series interconnect between the stimulus generator and the exposed electrode site can also be added to this model, which is nontrivial in high-density micromachined electrode arrays, where narrow thin metal or polysilicon lines are used for this purpose [29, 30].

10.4 Efficacy of Neural Stimulation

Regardless of what type of stimulus generation circuitry is used, the key parameters affecting the efficacy of neural stimulation in the order of importance are the location of the electrodes within the neural tissue, amplitude, pulse width, waveform,

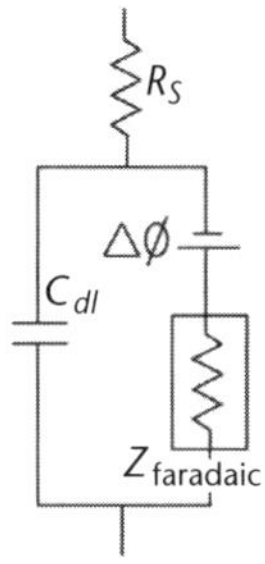

Figure 10.2 Electrical circuit model for electrode-electrolyte interface. C_{dl}: Double layer capacitor, R_S: Access resistance, Z_f: Faradaic impedance, Φ: half-cell potential. Source: [23].

and frequency of the stimulus pulses [37]. In general, it is fair to say that tailoring the spatial extent of the effective field of stimulation in the tissue volume conductor such that only the desired neural ensemble is stimulated and not the neighboring neuronal structures is the key objective in neural stimulation [38]. For example, in DBS, which is widely accepted for treatment of severe Parkinson's disease and several other movement disorders, four cylindrical electrodes (1.5 mm in height, 1.27 mm in diameter, and 6 mm^2 in electrode area) that are equally spaced along the same lead, are placed in the subthalamic nucleus (STN), which is a deep structure in the brain about the size of an almond [39]. Even though statistical data from the human brain atlases provides the average coordinates of the STN target, individual variability of this region from one patient to another requires neurosurgeons to take a few extra steps including magnetic resonance imaging (MRI), neural signal microrecording, and intraoperative neural stimulation to more precisely target the real patient's STN structure [10]. Nonetheless, DBS surgery only takes care of the electrodes placements and their fine positioning. About two weeks after the surgery, the patient should undergo the DBS programming phase for 3 to 5 weeks, during which period a therapist adjusts the amplitude, pulse width, waveform, and frequency of the stimulus pulses by receiving feedback from the patient and closely observing the DBS symptoms [40]. Too little stimulation in this phase renders the therapy to be ineffective, while too much stimulation results in undesired side effects and symptoms such as involuntary limb movements, mood changes, and speech problems. After the initial programming phase, the only control that the DBS patients have over their stimulator is turning it on and off using a simple magnetic switch. There are other types of stimulators, however, such as SCS or cochlear implants that, through a wireless patient programmer, provide the patient with limited control over some stimulation parameters within a safe range that is predefined by the doctor based on their desired level of pain relief or hearing loudness, respectively [12].

It is also desired to improve the efficacy of stimulation by maximizing the volume of the tissue activated (VTA) per stimulation pulse, while injecting the minimum possible amount of charge. This would improve the stimulator safety by minimizing the charge injection density on the active electrodes, thus reducing the risk of irreversible Faradaic reactions, as well as limiting heat generation and extending the battery lifetime by reducing the implant power consumption.

By and large, the following principles govern neural stimulation [21, 37]: (1) a uniform DC electric field is not effective, (2) neurons that are farther away from the electrode are less likely to be stimulated (*strength-distance relationship*), (3) axons are stimulated at lower stimulation thresholds than nerve cell bodies, (4) larger axons respond to lower stimulus amplitudes, (5) an electric field applied parallel to the nerve fiber is more effective than a perpendicular field, and (6) axons with branching processes will be more easily activated than those without branching.

Stimulus amplitude and duration, which control the total amount of charge injected per stimulation phase, strongly affect the stimulation threshold of the neural tissue. This is known as the *strength-duration relationship* and is usually depicted by the Weiss equation

$$I_{th} = I_{rh}\left(1 + \frac{T_{ch}}{PW}\right) \tag{10.1}$$

where I_{th} is the stimulus threshold current required to excite neural elements, I_{rh} is known as the *rheobase current*, defined as the minimum current needed to excite neural elements with a pulse of infinite duration, PW is the stimulus pulse width, and T_{ch} is known as the *chronaxie*, which is defined as the threshold pulse width when the stimulus amplitude is equal to two times I_{rh}. Figure 10.3 is a graphical representation

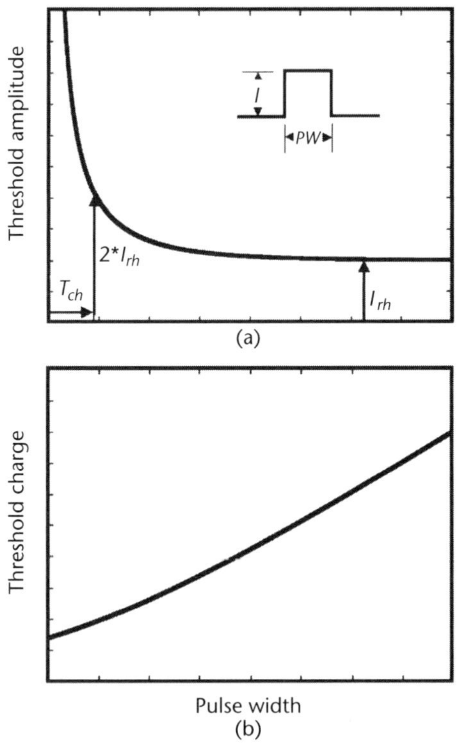

Figure 10.3 (a) The strength-duration curve: threshold amplitude as a function of stimulus duration. (b) The charge-duration curve: describes the threshold charge for stimulation as a function of stimulus duration. Source: [21].

of Equation (10.1), which also shows the minimum required charge, $Q_{th} = I_{rh} \times (PW + T_{ch})$, for tissue excitation *vs.* stimulus pulse width [21, 37].

These curves imply that narrow sharp pulses at high amplitude levels are more charge-efficient than the longer and low amplitude pulses. However, they require higher voltage and current levels, which increase the stimulus generator power consumption (see Section 10.6). Further, they result in higher charge injection densities at the stimulation site and may cause irreversible reactions. Therefore, there is a delicate balance between the neurophysiologic requirements of the clinical application, limitations of the stimulus generator, electrode characteristics, and various parameters of the stimulus waveform, a multitude of which should be considered in implementation of a safe and efficacious neural stimulation mechanism [41]. Figure 10.4 shows a variety of stimulus waveforms that are often used in neural stimulation [32].

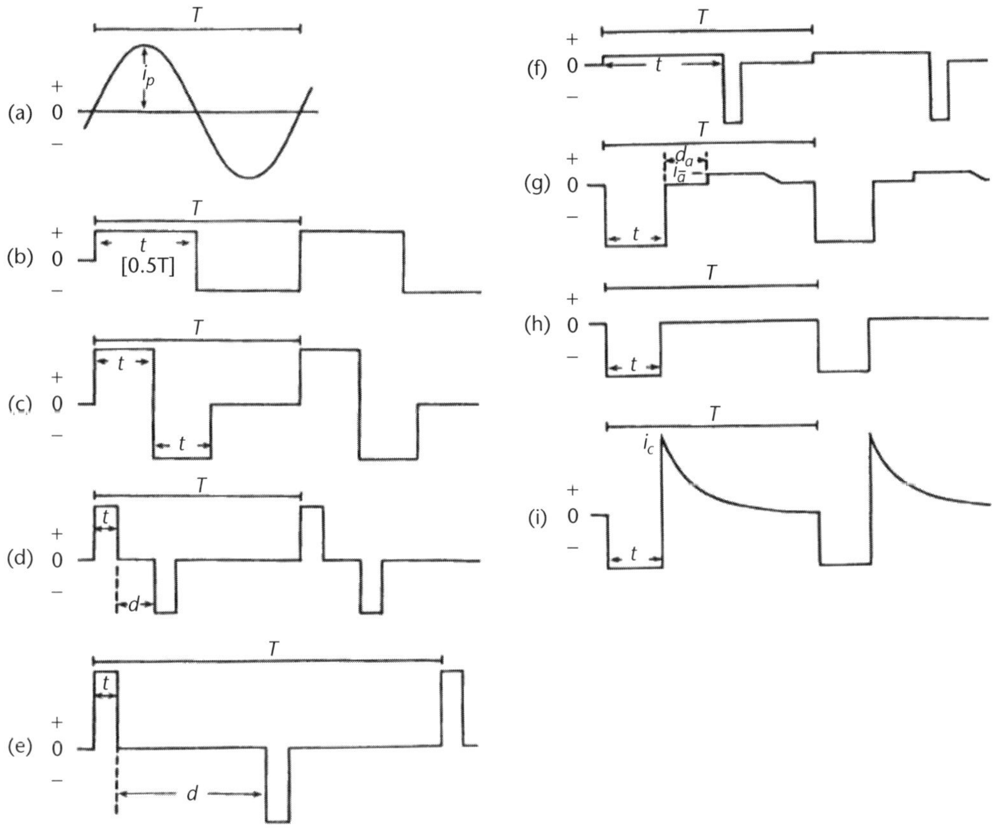

Figure 10.4 Current waveforms often used in neural stimulation: (a) sinusoidal; (b) square wave, pulsatile either unilateral or bidirectional; (c) charge-balanced, symmetrical biphasic; (d) charge-balanced, biphasic with interphase delay; (e) charge-balanced, alternating bidirectional; (f) charged-balanced, asymmetric biphasic; (g) anapol; (h) monophasic; (i) monophasic, capacitively coupled. Parameters: T: stimulus period; t: pulse duration; iP: peak current in sinusoidal waveform; da: delay before anodization phase of Anapol waveform; ia: anodization current following Anapol stimulus waveform; iC: current due to capacitive discharge in monophasic capacitively-coupled waveform. Source: [32].

10.5 Stimulus Generator Architecture

Even though the applications of implantable stimulators are quite different, these differences mostly affect the electrodes size, configuration, and location as well as the stimulus patterns, frequency, and waveforms. On the other hand, the architecture of the stimulus generators and the circuitry behind them are quite similar. After all, these circuits are responsible for delivering electricity in a safe, highly efficient, programmable, and precisely controlled fashion from an implanted or external energy storage in the form of a battery to the excitable tissue.

Figure 10.5 shows the block diagram of a generic stimulus generating system. In this diagram, those components that reside outside the patient's body are enclosed in a dashed box, and those blocks that could potentially be integrated on one or more application-specific integrated circuit (ASIC) are shaded in gray. The energy source could be an implanted high energy density primary or rechargeable battery, which may also stay outside of the body in the case of inductively-powered devices [42]. This is often dictated by the overall stimulator power consumption and the designated anatomical location of the implanted device in the human body.

Pacemakers and implantable cardioverter defibrillators (ICD) for instance, use a primary battery inside the stimulus generator implantable metallic can, which lasts for more than a decade [7]. This is mainly because the number of channels and rate of stimulation in pacemakers are relatively low, and there is enough space in the chest area for implanting a device the size of a matchbox. Cochlear implants, on the other hand, need to drive up to 30 stimulating electrodes with thousands of pulses per second [13]. They should also be small enough to be implanted into the temporal bone, which is the bone next to the ears. Therefore, due to high power consumption and extreme size constraints, cochlear implants are often inductively powered across the skin through a pair of loosely coupled coils (L_t and L_r in Figure 10.4) that constitute a transformer [43, 44]. Both coils are often tuned with capacitors to form LC reso-

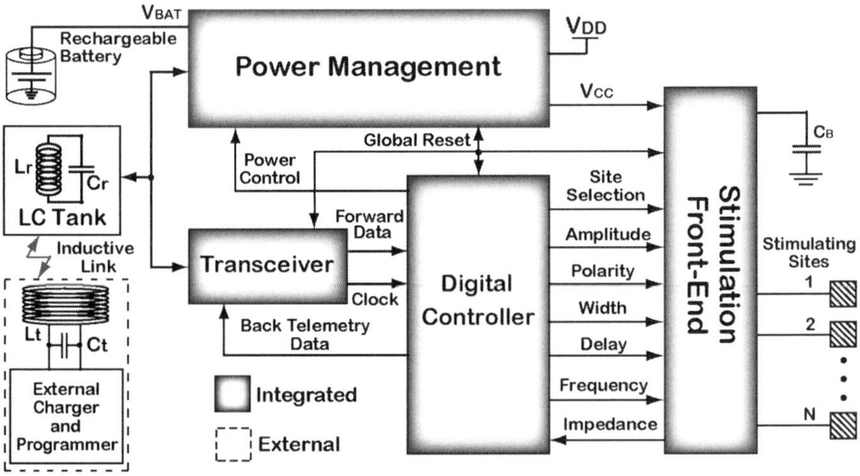

Figure 10.5 Block diagram of a generic stimulus generating system, demonstrating the external and implantable units as well as the integrated blocks within the implantable unit. Source: [53] with permission, © IEEE 2006.

nance tank circuits at the power carrier frequency to improve power transmission efficiency. The energy source, in this case, is a rechargeable battery within the external unit, which also houses the microphone, speech processor, charger, and power/data transmitter circuitry [45].

The power management block includes a rectifier, DC-DC converter, voltage regulator, and power-on reset (POR) [46, 47]. This block often has at least two DC voltage outputs. V_{DD} is a constant low voltage, usually below the battery level, V_{BAT}, which supplies the internal blocks such as digital controller and data transceiver. V_{CC}, on the other hand, is a variable DC voltage that can be externally programmed depending on the required stimulus amplitude levels and electrode impedances. V_{CC}, which can be as high as 20 V, often supplies the stimulation front-end (SFE) only [7, 48, 49]. The POR circuit has a safety role, and is in charge of ensuring all internal supplies have been stabilized before releasing the global reset to eliminate any risk of metastability especially in digital blocks.

The digital controller block is basically an ultra-low-power dedicated microcontroller, whose most important function is spatiotemporal control of stimulus pulses by selecting the proper stimulating sites to be activated, and timing the delivery of stimulus pulses based on a pre-programmed (in DBS) or real-time externally-controlled (in cochlear implant) stimulation strategy [26]. The controller block needs to be either constantly (cochlear) or occasionally (DBS, ICD, and SCS) in touch with the external programmer unit to receive the stimulus commands and parameter adjustments, and also send the results of self-check procedures and overall status of the implant. More advanced stimulators are also equipped with recording capability to report the measured electrode impedance levels as well as neural or cardiac response after stimulation. The former is a safety measure to monitor the overall health of the electrodes in the long run and indicate any possible leakage or breakage [31]. The latter would help physicians to fine-tune the stimulus parameters or even change the electrode positions if necessary [21, 50].

The transceiver block is responsible for establishing a wireless bidirectional communication link between the implanted and external units for the aforementioned information exchange. The forward data into the body has been traditionally transferred through the inductive link by modulating the power carrier that is responsible for energizing the implant or recharging its internal battery [44]. The back telemetry can also take place through the same power transfer inductive link using a method known as *load shift keying* (LSK), which is quite popular in passive radio frequency identification (RFID) systems [51]. More recently, however, in order to improve the wireless link bandwidth in both directions for high performance neuroprostheses, such as retinal implants, researchers have started using multiple individual carrier signals for power transfer, forward data transfer, and back telemetry functions [52].

10.6 Stimulation Front-End Circuits

The key block in the stimulus generator architecture of Figure 10.5 is the stimulation front-end, which is the interface between the digital control block and the electrode array. This block contains a few mixed-mode circuits such as digital-to-analog converters (DAC), analog multiplexers, high voltage compliance current sources and current sinks, precision current mirrors, impedance measurement circuits, and charge integrators [26, 48, 49]. The main challenge in design of the SFE is that the ASIC designer should deal with a delicate, highly nonlinear, time variant, dynamic living load that can even react to stimulation conditions as explained in Section 10.4. In addition, the SFE circuit should guaranty both the safety of the electrodes as well as their surrounding tissue. The load can be driven by voltage, current, or charge, each of which has its own advantages and limitations [53]. Regardless of how the load is driven, the SFE designer should not allow any charge accumulation inside the tissue, as it can cause irreversible Faradic reactions, as mentioned in Section 10.3, with detrimental consequences [33]. Hence, numerous researchers have tried to address the important issue of charge balancing in their SFE ASIC designs [7, 26, 48, 49, 54, 55].

In conventional multichannel stimulators, depending on the type of stimulation, described in Section 10.2, the SFE circuitry selects either one active electrode and the grounded metallic pulse generator package (monopolar) or a pair of nearby identical active electrodes (bipolar), and controls either the voltage or the current between them, while all other inactive electrodes are at high impedance. In voltage-controlled stimulation (VCS), shown in Figure 10.6(a), a voltage source, which could be a large capacitor charged to the programmed level, V, is connected between the active sites.

The current passing through the tissue in this case depends on Z, which is the RC load seen between a pair of electrodes, shown in Figure 10.2, and the tissue in between. Therefore, this method is only applicable when the range of variations in Z over time or from one active electrode to another is small and well known. The VCS-SFE circuitry has little control over the stimulus current, except for clamping it within safe electrode charge injection limits in order to eliminate irreversible Faradic reactions. The efficiency of the VCS-SFE is high when the stimulus voltage is close to V_{BAT}. However, it degrades when higher or lower voltages are needed. Several versions of the VCS-SFE have been described in [7, 56, 57].

In current-controlled stimulation (CCS), shown in Figure 10.6(b), the stimulus current level is defined by the physician and the CCS-SFE circuitry automatically controls the voltage across the two active electrodes such that the desired current, I, passes through the tissue regardless of Z. This method is preferred for microstimulation with micromachined (MEMS) electrodes, in which Z variations are notable from site to site or over time [28–30]. If Z becomes too large, however, the voltage required to pass I through Z would go beyond the maximum permissible CCS-SFE voltage, known as the *voltage compliance*, which is close to V_{CC}. In this case, the current source saturates before I reaches the designated level [58]. In general, VCS circuits are simpler and more power efficient than CCS. CCS, however, is safer and provides better control over the amount of charge injected into the tissue according to $Q_{CS} = I \times T_P$, where Q_{CS} is the injected charge and T_P is the stimulus pulse duration [41].

More recently, a new stimulation method has been proposed based on charge injection using switched capacitors (SC) in order to combine the power efficiency of the VCS with the safety and controllability of the CCS [53]. The SC-SFE, shown in Figure 10.6(c), involves charging an array of relatively small capacitors, C, up to V, and discharging a designated number of them, n, into the excitable tissue during each stimulation phase to achieve $Q_{CS} = nC \times V$. Therefore, Q_{SC} can be controlled by either n or V depending on the tissue requirements or stimulation parameters such as Z.

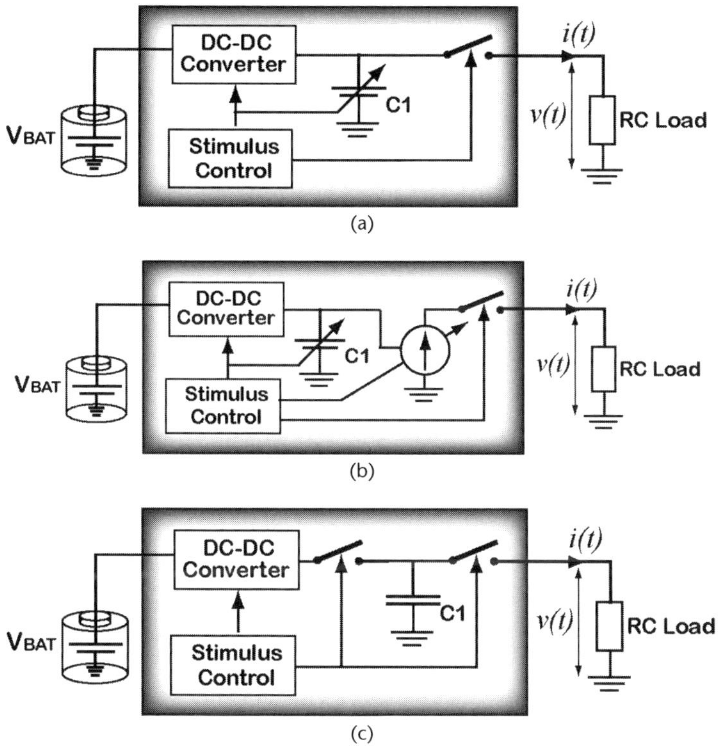

Figure 10.6 Simplified block diagram of the three major stimulation front-end (SFE) circuits: (a) voltage-controlled stimulation, (b) current-controlled stimulation, (c) switched-capacitor based stimulation. Source: [41] with permission, © 2007.

The maximum capacitor discharge current is also controllable by a current source in series with the main current path [53]. The actual amount of injected charge over each stimulation phase can be measured, by integrating the stimulus current, and used for charge balancing. Figure 10.7 shows a simulated train of exponentially decaying

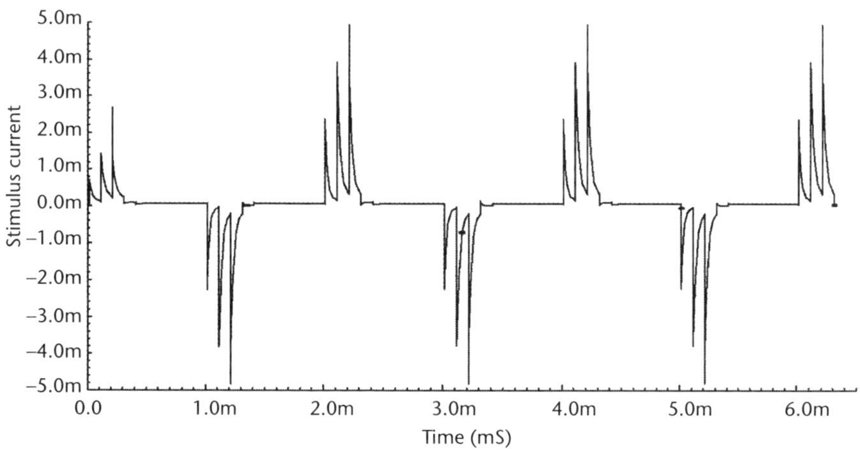

Figure 10.7 A simulated train of exponentially decaying stimulus waveforms generated by a switched-capacitor based stimulation front-end (SC-SFE) circuit, which spectrum contains both high and low frequency components. Source: [53] with permission, © IEEE 2006.

stimulus waveforms generated by the SC-SFE, which could potentially be more efficacious than the common square-shaped stimulus pulses in some applications, such as DBS, due to being comprised of both high and low frequency components [59, 60].

References

[1] R.J. Andrews, "Neuromodulation I. Techniques—deep brain stimulation, vagus nerve stimulation, and transcranial magnetic stimulation," *Ann. N.Y. Acad. Sci.*, no. 993, pp. 1–13, 2003.

[2] R.J. Andrews, "Neuromodulation I. Applications—epilepsy, nerve regeneration, neurotrophins," *Ann. N.Y. Acad. Sci.*, no. 993, pp. 14–24, 2003.

[3] P.R. Troyk and N.N. Donaldson, "Implantable FES stimulation systems: What is needed?," *Neuromodulation*, vol. 4, no. 4, pp. 196–204, 2001.

[4] G.E. Loeb, F.J.R. "RF-powered BIONs™ for stimulation and sensing," Richmond, J. Singh, R.A. Peck, W. Tan, Q. Zou, and N. Sachs, *Proc. IEEE 26th Eng. in Med. and Biol. Conf.*, pp. 4182–4185, Sept. 2004.

[5] G.E. Loeb and R. Davoodi, "The functional reanimation of paralyzed limbs," *IEEE Eng. Med. Biol. Mag.*, vol. 24, no. 5. pp. 45–51, Sept. 2005.

[6] P.H. Peckham and J.S. Knutson, "Functional electrical stimulation for neuromuscular applications," *Annual Review of Biomedical Engineering*, no. 7, pp. 327–360, 2005.

[7] L.S.Y. Wong, S. Hossain, A. Ta, J. Edvinsson, D.H. Rivas, and H. Naas, "A very low-power CMOS mixed-signal IC for implantable pacemaker applications," *IEEE J. Solid-State Circuits*, vol. 39, no. 12, pp. 2446–2456, Dec. 2004.

[8] Boston Scientific, ICD (Defibrillator) Implantation, [Online]. Available: http://www.controlyourpain.com/printables/PrecPlusSalesSheet.pdf.

[9] J. Chen and P.J. Pasricha, "Gastrointestinal electrical stimulation," U.S. Patent 6826428, Nov. 13, 2004.

[10] A.L. Benabid, "Deep brain stimulation for Parkinson's disease," *Current Opinion Neurobiology*, vol. 13, pp. 696–706, 2003.

[11] A.L. Benabid et al. "Therapeutic electrical stimulation of the central nervous system," *C.R. Biologies*, vol. 328, pp. 178–186, 2005.

[12] Boston Scientific, Precision Plus SCS system, [Online]. Available: http://www.bostonscientific.com/procedure/ProcedureLanding.bsci/,,/navRelId/1000.1002/id/10000951/seo.serve.

[13] P.C. Loizou, "Mimicking the human ear," *IEEE Signal Processing Magazine*, pp. 101–130, Sept. 1998.

[14] Advanced Bionics, Treatments for Hearing Loss, [Online]. Available: http://www.bionicear.com/Your_Journey_to_Hearing/Adults/Learning/Treatments_forHearing_Loss.cfm?langid=1.

[15] J.D. Weiland and M.S. Humayun, "A biomimetic retinal stimulating array," *IEEE Engineering in Medicine and Biology Magazine*, vol. 24, No. 5, pp. 14–21, Sept. 2005.

[16] M. Ortmanns, A. Rocke, M. Gehrke, and H.J. Tiedtke, "A 232-channel epiretinal stimulator ASIC," *J. Solid-State Circuits*, vol. 42, no. 12, pp. 2946–2959, Dec. 2007.

[17] S.M. Boyer, M. Sawan, S. Abdel-Gawad, S. Robin, and M.M. Alhilali, "Implantable selective stimulator to improve bladder voiding: design and chronic experiment in dogs," *IEEE Trans. Rehab. Eng.*, vol. 8, no. 4, pp. 789–797, Dec. 2000.

[18] S.K. Moore, "Psychiatry's shocking new tools," *IEEE Spectrum*, vol. 43, no. 3, pp. 24–31, Mar. 2006.

[19] L.R. Hochberg and J.P. Donoghue, "Sensors for brain computer interfaces," *IEEE Eng. in Med. and Biol. Magazine*, vol. 25, pp. 32–38, Sept. 2006.

[20] F. Rattay, "Analysis of the electrical excitation of CNS neurons," *IEEE Trans. on Bio. Eng.*, vol. 45, no. 6, pp. 766–772, June 1998.

[21] A.M. Kuncel and W.M. Grill, "Selection of stimulus parameters for deep brain stimulation," *Clinical Neurophysiology*, vol. 115, pp. 2431–2441, July 2004.

[22] C.R. Butson and C.C. McIntyre, "Role of electrode design on the volume of tissue activated during deep brain stimulation," *J. Neural Engineering*, vol. 3, pp. 1–8, 2006.

[23] D.R. Merrill, M. Bikson, and J.G.R. Jefferys, "Electrical stimulation of excitable tissue: Design of efficacious and safe protocols," *J. Neurosci. Meth.*, vol. 141, pp. 171–198, Feb. 2005.

[24] X. Beebe and T. L. Rose, "Charge injection limits of activated iridium oxide electrode with 0.2 ms pulses in bicarbonate buffered saline," *IEEE Trans. Biomed. Eng.*, vol. 35, pp. 494–496, June 1988.

[25] C.N. Jolly, F.A. Spelman, and B.M. Clopton, "Quadrupolar stimulation for cochlear prostheses: modeling and experimental data," *IEEE Trans. on Bio. Eng.*, vol. 43, no. 8, pp. 857–865, Aug. 1996.

[26] M. Ghovanloo and K. Najafi, "A modular 32-site wireless neural stimulation microsystem," *IEEE Journal on Solid-State Circuits*, vol. 39, no. 12, pp. 2457–2466, Dec. 2004.

[27] M. Sivaprakasam, W. Liu, G. Wang, J.D. Weiland, and M.S. Humayun, "Architecture tradeoffs in high-density microstimulators for retinal prosthesis," *IEEE Trans. on Circuits and Systems I*, vol. 52, no. 12, pp. 2629–2641, Dec. 2005.

[28] E.M. Maynard, C.T. Nordhausen, and R. A. Normann, "The Utah intracortical electrode array: A recording structure for potential brain-computer interfaces," *Electroencephalography Clin. Neurophysiol.*, vol. 102, no. 3, pp. 228–239, 1997.

[29] P.J. Rousche, D.S. Pellinen, D.P. Pivin, Jr., J.C. Williams, R.J. Vetter, and D.R. Kipke, "Flexible polyimide-based intracortical electrode arrays with bioactive capability," *IEEE Trans. Biomed. Eng.*, vol. 48, no. 3, pp. 361–371, Mar. 2001.

[30] K.D. Wise, "Silicon microsystems for neuroscience and neural prostheses," *IEEE Eng. Med. and Bio. Magazine*, vol. 24, pp. 22–29, Oct. 2005.

[31] M. Ghovanloo and K. Najafi, "A wireless implantable multichannel microstimulating system-on-a-chip with modular architecture," *IEEE Trans. on Neural Sys. Rehab. Eng.*, vol. 15, no. 3, pp. 449–457, Sept. 2007.

[32] L.S. Roblee and T.L. Rose, "Electrochemical guidelines for selection of protools and electrode materials for neural stimulation," in *Neural Prostheses: Fundamental Studies*, W.F. Agnew and D.B. McCreery, Eds. Englewood Cliffs, N.J.: Prentice Hall, 1990, ch. 2.

[33] W.F. Agnew, D.B. McCreery, L.A. Bullara, and T.G.H. Yuen, "Effects of prolonged electrical stimulation of peripheral nerves," in *Neural Prostheses: Fundamental Studies*, W.F. Agnew and D.B. McCreery, Eds. Englewood Cliffs, N.J.: Prentice Hall, 1990, ch. 6.

[34] D.A. Robinson, "The electrical properties of metal microelectrodes," *Proccedings of IEEE*, vol. 56, no. 6, June 1968.

[35] J.D. Weiland and D.J. Anderson, "Chronic neural stimulation with thin-film, iridium oxide electrodes," *IEEE Trans. on Biomed. Eng.*, vol. 47, no. 7, pp. 911–918, July 2000.

[36] L. A. Geddes, "Historical evolution of circuit models for the electrodeelectrolyte interface," *Ann. Biomed. Eng.*, vol. 25, pp. 1–14, 1997.

[37] R.L. Testerman, M.T. Rise, and P.H. Stypulkowski, "Electrical stimulation as therapy for neurological disorders: The basicas of implantable neurological stimulators," *IEEE Eng. in Med. and Biol. Magazine*, vol. 25, pp. 74–78, Sept. 2006.

[38] C.R. Butson and C.C. McIntyre, "Role of electrode design on the volume of tissue activated during deep brain stimulation," *J. Neural Eng.*, vol. 3, pp. 1–8, 2006.

[39] E.R. Kandel, *Principles of Neural Science*, 4th Ed. New York: McGraw-Hill, 2000.

[40] CNI Thompson Center for Restorative Neurosurgery, "Subthalamic nucleus deep brain stimulation for advanced parkinson's disease: patient education," [Online]. Available: http://www.thecni.org/thompsoncenter/stndbs-kumar.pdf.

[41] J. Simpson and M. Ghovanloo, "An experimental study of voltage, current, and charge controlled stimulation front-end circuitry," *Proc. IEEE Intl. Symp. on Circuits and Systems*, pp. 325–328, May 2007.

[42] W.H. Ko, S.P. Liang, and C.D.F. Fung, "Design of radio-frequency powered coils for implant instruments," *Med. Biol. Eng. Comput.*, 15, pp. 634–640, 1977.

[43] M.W. Baker and R. Sarpeshkar, "Feedback analysis and design of RF power links for low-power bionic systems," *IEEE Trans. Biomed. Cir. and Sys.*, vol. 1, no. 1, pp. 28–38, March 2007.

[44] M. Ghovanloo and G. Lazzi, (April 14, 2006) "Transcutaneous magnetic coupling of power and data," In *Wiley Encyclopedia of Biomedical Engineering* (Metin Akay, ed.), Hoboken: John Wiley & Sons, Inc. [Online] http://www.mrw.interscience.wiley.com/ebe/articles/ebs1372/bibliography-fs.html.

[45] F.A. Spelman, "The past, present and future of cochlear prostheses," *IEEE Engineering in Medicine and Biology Magazine*, vol. 18, no. 3, pp. 27–33, May 1999.

[46] M. Ghovanloo and K. Najafi, "Fully integrated wide-band high-current rectifiers for wireless biomedical implants," *IEEE Journal of Solid-State Circuits*, vol. 39, no. 11, pp. 1976–1984, Nov. 2004.

[47] A.M. Sodagar, K. Najafi, K.D. Wise, and M. Ghovanloo, "Fully-integrated CMOS power regulator for telemetry-powered implantable biomedical microsystems," *Proc. of the IEEE Custom Integrated Circuits Conf.*, Sept. 2006.

[48] Y.T. Wong, N. Dommel, P. Preston, L.E. Hallum, T. Lehmann, N.H. Lovell, and G.J. Suaning, "Retinal neurostimulator for a multifocal vision prosthesis," *IEEE Trans. on Neural Sys. Rehab. Eng.*, vol. 15, no. 3, pp. 425–434, Sept. 2007.

[49] Maurits Ortmanns, André Rocke, *Member, IEEE*, Marcus Gehrke, and Hans-Jüergen Tiedtke, "A 232-channel epiretinal stimulator ASIC," *IEEE Journal on Solid-State Circuits*, vol. 39, no. 12, pp. 2457–2466, Dec. 2004.

[50] Powerhouse Museum, Cochlear Implants: The Future, [Online]. Available: http://www.powerhousemuseum.com/hsc/cochlear/cochlear_future.htm.

[51] K. Finkenzeller, "RFID-Handbook," 2nd Ed. Hoboken, NJ: Wiley, 2003.

[52] M. Ghovanloo and S. Atluri, "A wideband power-efficient inductive wireless link for implantable microelectronic devices using multiple carriers," *IEEE Trans on Cir. and Sys. I*, vol. 54, no. 10, pp. 2211–2221, Oct. 2007.

[53] M. Ghovanloo, "Switched-capacitor based implantable low-power wireless microstimulating systems," *IEEE Intl. Symp. on Circuits and Systems*, pp. 2197–2200, May 2006.

[54] J.F. Patrick, P.M. Seligman, D.K. Money, and J.A. Kuzma, "Engineering," in *Cochlear Prostheses*. Edinburgh, U.K.: Churchill-Livingstone, 1990.

[55] X. Liu, A. Demosthenous, and N. Donaldson, "A stimulator output stage with capacitor reduction and failure-checking techniques," in *Proc. IEEE ISCAS*, 2006, pp. 641–644.

[56] S.K. Kelly and J. Wyatt, "A power-efficient voltage-based neural tissue stimulator with energy recovery," *IEEE Digest Intl. Solid-State Cir. Conf.*, pp. 228–524, Feb. 2004.

[57] M. Schwarz and M. Maschmann, "Area saving stimulator cells for multielectrode arrays featuring adaptive waveform generation and monitoring," *Proc. IEEE Eng. in Med. Biol. Conf.*, vol. 2, pp. 4314–4317, 2004.

[58] M. Ghovanloo and K. Najafi, "A compact large voltage compliance high output impedance programmable current source for biomedical implantable microstimulators," *IEEE Trans. on Biomed. Eng.*, vol. 52, no. 1, pp. 97–105, Jan. 2005.

[59] J. Gimsa, B. Habel, U. Schreiber et al., "Choosing electrodes for deep brain stimulation experiments—electrochemical considerations," *J. Neuroscience Methods*, vol. 142, pp. 251–265, Mar. 2005.

[60] W.M. Grill and J.T. Mortimer, "The effect of stimulus pulse width duration on selectivity of neural stimulation," *IEEE Trans. Biomed. Eng.*, vol. 43, no. 2, pp. 161–166, Feb. 1996.

CHAPTER 11

Circuits for Implantable Neural Recording and Stimulation

Andreas Demosthenous, Iasonas F. Triantis, and Xiao Liu

11.1 Introduction

Diseases or injuries that affect the nervous system can result in some of the most devastating medical conditions. This is evident in the spinal cord injury paradigm, in which damage to the central nervous system results in loss of motor function in various parts of the body, mainly those located below the area of injury [1]. Currently, conventional medicine does not offer any method for curing the damage and fully restoring function. Therapy is focused on rehabilitation, which involves training and exercise to assist patients to get used to their new condition and to re-establish some daily routine, although full independence is usually not achievable. On top of the functional problems, treatment sometimes involves solutions that are unpleasant and can even introduce social difficulties.

Neuroprostheses may assist in partial restoration of function and mobility using functional electrical stimulation (FES), which involves the process of passing pulses of electrical current into the muscle tissue of interest or into nerves, which cause the activation of the muscle. Implantable stimulators were introduced in 1959 with the development of the heart pacemaker and the first FES systems reported in the early sixties. Since then such systems have developed to fully implantable devices, using RF links for the power supply and for the transmission of control signals [2]. Closed-loop systems are the main focus of FES research nowadays. In such systems, the idea is to record naturally occurring nerve signals (i.e., electroneurogram; ENG) for control inputs or feedback to implantable stimulators [3].

This chapter provides an introductory overview of recent advances in circuits and methods for nerve recording and stimulation. The chapter begins with an introduction of how the action potential in nerves is generated and proceeds to discuss the common types of electrodes for peripheral nerve recording and stimulation with particular emphasis on cuff electrodes. Next, the lumped-impedance model of the tripolar cuff for ENG recordings is discussed along with tripolar amplifier configurations used to suppress interference from other bio-potentials such as muscle interference. Following this, the chapter focuses on bioamplifier circuits and on stimulator output stage circuits. Features such as low-noise, high common-mode rejection ratio (CMRR) and electrode offset removal are key requirements for bioamplifiers, whereas miniaturization and safety are important issues in recent developments in implantable neural stimulators for FES systems. Some circuit design techniques to address these requirements, suitable for implantable microsystems, are discussed.

11.2 Neurophysiology and the Action Potential

Neurons are specialized, nonspherical cells consisting of a cell body (soma), many short dendritic processes, and one longer protrusion called the axon. The voltage difference between the extracellular fluid and the inside of the neuron is the membrane potential, which is called the "resting potential" when the neuron is in a state of readiness to fire. The resting potential, with typical values around –70 mV across the membrane (with the internal being more negative), is established by the sodium-potassium pump maintained by a concentration gradient and an electrical gradient. The membrane potential of a neuron whose dendrites are connected to other neurons is affected by the inputs resulting from the signals of the connecting synapses. There are two main types of synapses, the inhibitory and the excitatory. The inhibitory synapses result in inhibitory postsynaptic potentials, which cause hyperpolarization of the neuron, decreasing its membrane potential by allowing into the neuron negative ions, e.g., chloride (Cl^-), making it less likely to fire. The excitatory synapses result in excitatory postsynaptic potentials that cause depolarization of the neuron, increasing its membrane potential by allowing into the neuron positive ions, e.g., sodium (Na^+), thus making it more likely to fire [4].

The summation of inputs to the dendrites of the neuron may result in the generation of the "action potential," an electrical pulse occurring when the membrane potential reaches the firing threshold (typically –60 mV). Sodium (Na^+) and potassium (K^+) ions are allowed to enter or to exit the cell by their respective ion channels (gates). Sodium channels are voltage activated and therefore, as the membrane potential becomes less negative, the channels open to allow sodium ions into the neuron. Once the firing potential is reached, the neuron fires an action potential, which results from a great and rapid inflow of Na^+ ions and is then followed by an outflow of K^+ ions leading to rebalancing of the membrane potential. The inflow of Na^+ depolarizes the adjoining part of the membrane causing it to follow the same procedure and therefore the action potential propagates as a wave along the axon, when the axon is not myelinated.

The electrical operation of a small segment of an unmyelinated nerve fiber is illustrated in Figure 11.1. The segment has length Δx and the extracellular and intracellular media are considered purely resistive [5], with resistivities ρ_e and ρ_i, respectively, defining the resistance of the external and the internal paths of the transmembrane current i_{AC}. The external and internal potentials are v_e and v_i respectively and are shown in the figure as functions of distance x along the fiber segment. The membrane representation includes capacitance C_m (in μF per unit area), which depends on the area of the membrane under consideration, and the conductances g_{Na}, and g_K (in mS per unit area) corresponding to the Na^+ and the K^+ channels as defined by the Hodgkin-Huxley equations [6]. The conductance g_L, which is usually neglected, corresponds to leakage currents from ions other than Na^+ or K^+ (e.g., Cl^-) [5]. This model allows the electrical analysis of the action potential.

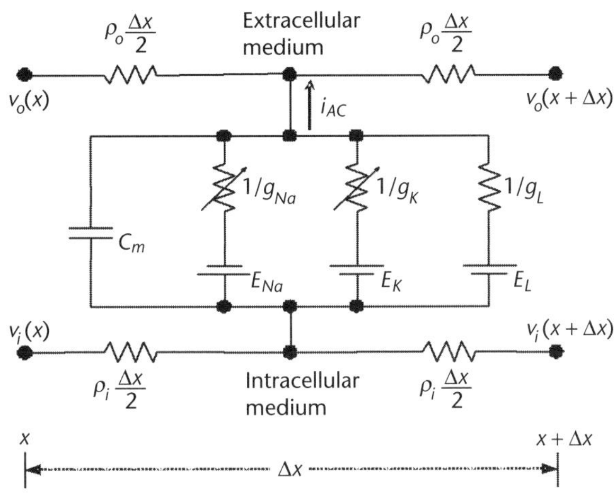

Figure 11.1 Equivalent circuit diagram of a part of an unmyelinated nerve fiber with length Δx [5].

Figure 11.2(a) illustrates the charge distribution along the membrane of an unmyelinated fiber. As the action potential propagates along the nerve, the membrane of the segment of the fiber that is active (labeled "active region" in the figure) is depolarized (polarity reversed), the membrane before the active region has repolarized while the one after is still in the resting state. The polarity differences of the adjacent regions cause closed path (solenoidal) ionic current flow, as shown in Figure 11.2(a). The currents flowing toward the region after the active membrane region cause the

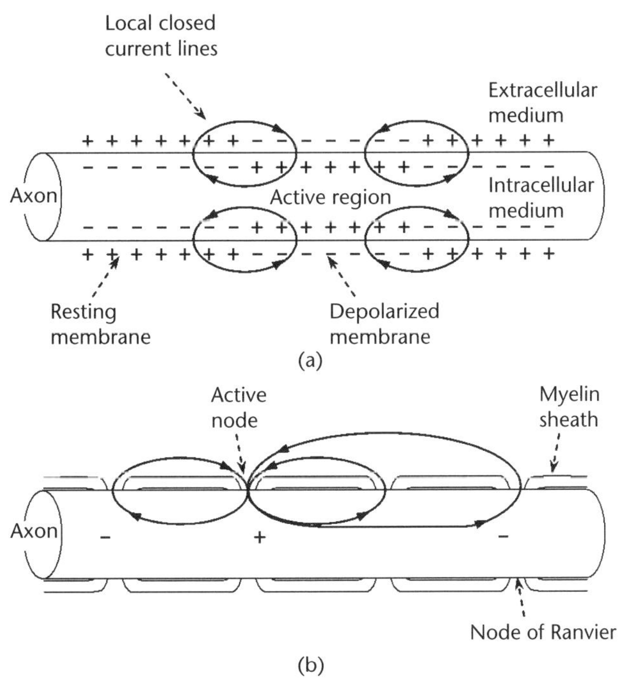

Figure 11.2 Neuron conduction: (a) Unmyelinated fiber, (b) Myelinated fiber [5].

membrane there to depolarize and to become active as well. However, the currents flowing towards the region before the active one cannot re-excite the membrane, as this is in the refractory state, during which no stimulus can excite the membrane. As a result, the action potential propagates along the fiber in a self-excitatory manner (i.e., membrane excitation occurs and propagates on its own, without the need for extra stimulus being applied), without being attenuated [5].

When the axon is myelinated the action potential is conducted in two ways. Ion exchange is used in the "nodes of Ranvier" and cable properties [7] describe conduction in the myelinated sections. Conduction in an activated nerve fiber is achieved again via solenoidal currents, as in the unmyelinated fibers, however the current loops flow between the nodes (Figure 11.2(b)), where almost all ion channels are concentrated. This method provides faster and less energy consuming pulse propagation. However, the pulse amplitude decreases under the myelin sheath, and if not amplified, it is difficult to reach the end of the axon. The nodes of Ranvier serve in reinstating ion exchange with the extracellular fluid, thus amplifying the action potential by restoring the pulse's amplitude to its initial value. This type of conduction, which occurs by the alternation between ion exchange and cable conduction is called saltatory conduction and is much faster than the conduction that takes place in the unmyelinated neurons, where conduction is based on ion exchange only. The amplitude of the action potential (approximately 30 mV) and the length of the myelin sections (approximately 1 to 2 mm) ensure that the amplitude of the signal does not fall below the firing threshold, as this would stop the ion exchange from being reinstated at the node of Ranvier [4, 8].

It is also possible to artificially trigger an action potential by electrical neural stimulation. Local extracellular application of a short current pulse can trigger an action potential travelling in both directions from the stimulation site (Figure 11.3). The stimulation may be excitatory (depolarizing) or inhibitory (hyperpolarizing). A technique called *anodal blocking* can be used for generating unidirectional propagating action potentials, allowing restoration of function without the need for rhisotomy (nerve root cutting) of sensory pathways that may be intact after an injury. This allows pain avoidance and prevention of sensation during stimulation [9]. Biological tissue can also be stimulated by means of electromagnetic induction (magnetic stimulation [10]). Though non-invasive, the large size, heavy weight, high cost, and the requirement of high rate of magnetic field change, greatly limit the applications of magnetic stimulation.

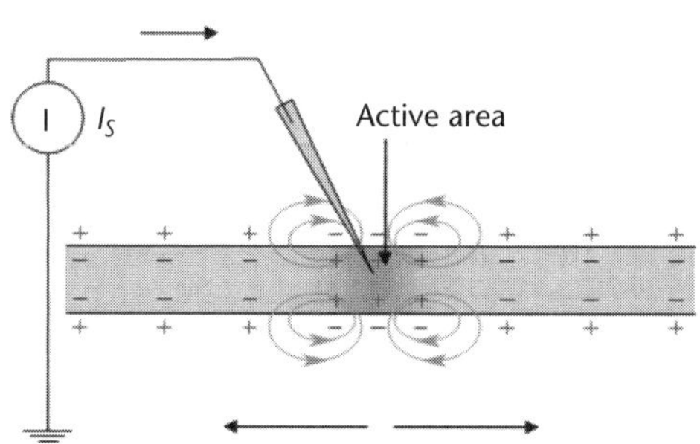

Figure 11.3 Stimulation applied to a nerve fiber using a needle electrode (from [10]).

11.3 Electrodes

In order to interface with peripheral nerves for recording or stimulation, it is possible to penetrate the nerve, using *intrafascicular* electrodes or *cuff electrodes* that encircle the nerve. Intrafascicular electrodes, similar to the microelectrodes used in the central nervous system, are implanted to penetrate the nerve tissue itself and hence provide better electrical access to deep fascicles (distinct groups of nerve fibers) inside a nerve but being invasive, they can cause damage. Various designs of microneedles have been produced to provide one-, two-, and three-dimensional electrode matrices, using micromachining technology on silicon and glass substrates [11, 12]. The electrodes themselves are either the tips of the needles (in 2D or 3D arrays), or form arrays of contacts on silicon or glass needles (in 1D arrangements). They are commonly made of platinum, stainless steel, indium, or platinum-iridium. All these materials can be made biocompatible with stable electrochemical properties (e.g., corrosion stability).

The one- and two-dimensional arrays are more commonly used in brain implants (Figure 11.4(a)), with the latter consisting of a matrix of equal-length needles whose tips are the electrodes. When groups of needles on such an array have their lengths varied gradually by a constant offset, i.e., the array is slanted, these structures are called three-dimensional (Figure 11.4(b)) because such penetrating structures offer the best fascicle selectivity in peripheral nerve interfaces. Penetrating electrodes for stimulation require a lower stimulus amplitude than electrodes that encircle the nerve and when used for recording tend to produce a relatively large neural signal (in the region of 50–500 μV); however, the likelihood of irreversible tissue damage during insertion of the electrode and its subsequent movement is high, which is the main reason why intrafascicular electrodes (for both recording and stimulation) can only be implanted for limited periods, or acutely.

For chronic peripheral nerve recording and stimulation, the use of cuff electrodes is the preferred method [13]. Cuff electrodes are placed on the inside of a tubular cuff wrapped around a nerve and do not penetrate the nerve itself. They have been in use since the mid-seventies [14]. Cuff electrodes typically contain between 2 and 10 electrodes. In the case of nerve recording, cuff electrodes when made tripolar (i.e., containing 3 electrodes) can suppress interference from other bio-potentials, the dominant one being the muscle signal or electromyogram (EMG). Typical cuffs consist

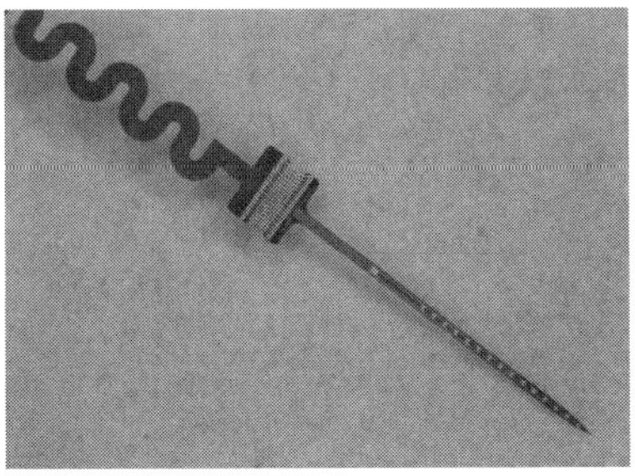

(a)

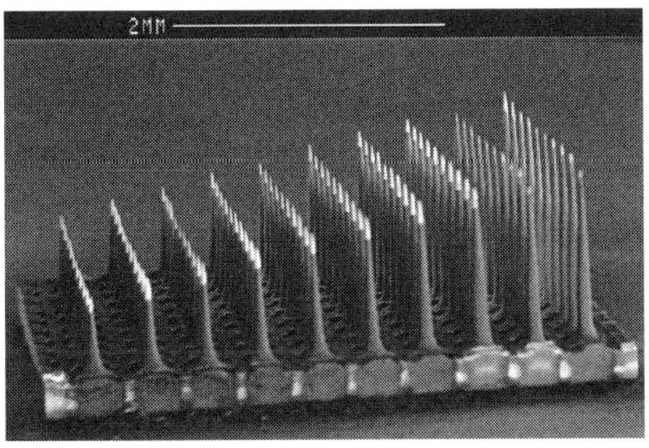

(b)

Figure 11.4 (a) Implantable recording/stimulation 1D micro-electrode (Michigan neuro probe). (b) Slanted needle array electrode (University of Utah, USA).

of insulating tubes made from biocompatible flexible insulating materials such as silicone rubber, polytetrafluoroethylene or polyimide [12, 13], with ring electrodes made of platinum-iridium or stainless steel attached to the inside wall, covering most of the circumference but leaving a gap for a longitudinal opening so that the nerve may be inserted into the cuff (Figure 11.5(a)). Naples et al. [15] introduced the "spiral cuff" (Figure 11.5(b)) which curls up to fit the nerve tightly but is still able to expand if the nerve swells, perhaps due to inflammation. A cuff made by dip-coating a mandrel and pre-formed platinum electrodes was presented in [16], in which the cuff closure mechanism was implemented using interdigitating cubes (Figure 11.5(c)). Typically, the slit along the tube is glued or covered by a silicone flap attached to the cuff [17] (Figure 11.5(a)). It is important for the cuff to insulate the whole circumference of the nerve, as this ensures that the flow of ions in the extrafascicullar fluid remains within the cuff when action potentials propagate the nerve. In this way, extracellular ion currents create potential differences inside the cuff as the action potential moves across its length, which can be measured by the ring electrodes placed inside it.

To avoid compression neuropathy (nerve damage due to compression), the cuff diameter has to be at least 20% larger than that of the nerve bundle and its length must be at least ten times larger than its inner diameter [18]. In addition, the cuff length must be equal or larger than the distance between the nodes of Ranvier and at least ten times larger than its inner diameter. Increasing the length significantly reduces interference as the impedance inside the cuff increases; however, there are limitations depending on the location of implantation. The optimum cuff length was shown experimentally in [14] and [18] to be between 20 and 30 mm, with the neural signal amplitude decreasing when the length is smaller than 15 mm. The amplitude of the signal was also shown in [19] to decrease with the square of the cuff diameter for diameters up to 4 mm, indicating that the effectiveness of cuff electrodes improves for tighter-fitting cuffs, as shown experimentally in [18, 20] where single-fiber action potentials ranging from 3 μV to 20 μV were recorded using cuffs with inner diameters of 2.6 mm and 0.3 mm, respectively. A special type of cuff electrodes is the so-called book electrodes (Figure 11.6(a)). These are most commonly used in the spinal canal for nerve root stimulation [12]. In addition to cuff electrodes, helical electrodes (Figure 11.6(b)) are used to apply stimulus pulses to nerves [21].

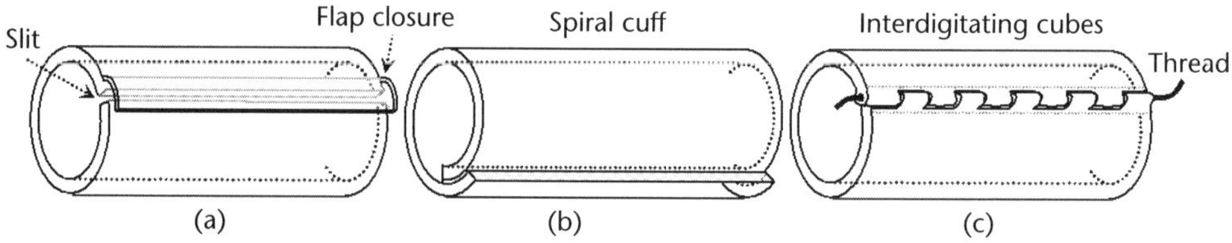

Figure 11.5 Three different types of cuff closure: (a) slit along the tube covered by silicone flap [17], (b) "spiral cuff" [15], (c) closure mechanism using interdigitating cubes and thread through them [16].

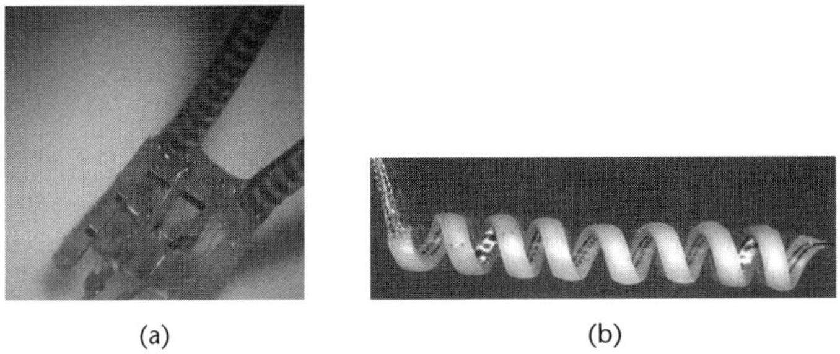

Figure 11.6 (a) A book electrode used for nerve root stimulation (manufactured by Finetech Medical Ltd, UK). (b) Huntington helical electrode used to apply stimulus pulses to nerves [21].

11.4 The Tripolar Cuff Model and Tripolar Amplifier Configurations

Interference signals, as for example EMG from muscles in the vicinity of the recording cuff, cause ionic currents to flow through the tissue inside the cuff. The EMG amplitude is in the order of a few millivolts, sometimes three orders of magnitude larger than the microvolt ENG detected by cuff electrodes, and the spectra of the two signals overlap [22]. The muscle's field lines and the respective isopotential lines are distorted by the cuff (Figure 11.7(a)). As the medium inside the cuff is only resistive, there are no significant phase variations to the interfering potentials across the electrodes and ideally the potential varies *linearly* with distance across the length of the cuff (Figure 11.7(b)) [23]. The cuff linearization property can be exploited by tripolar amplifier arrangements to suppress EMG breakthrough [21].

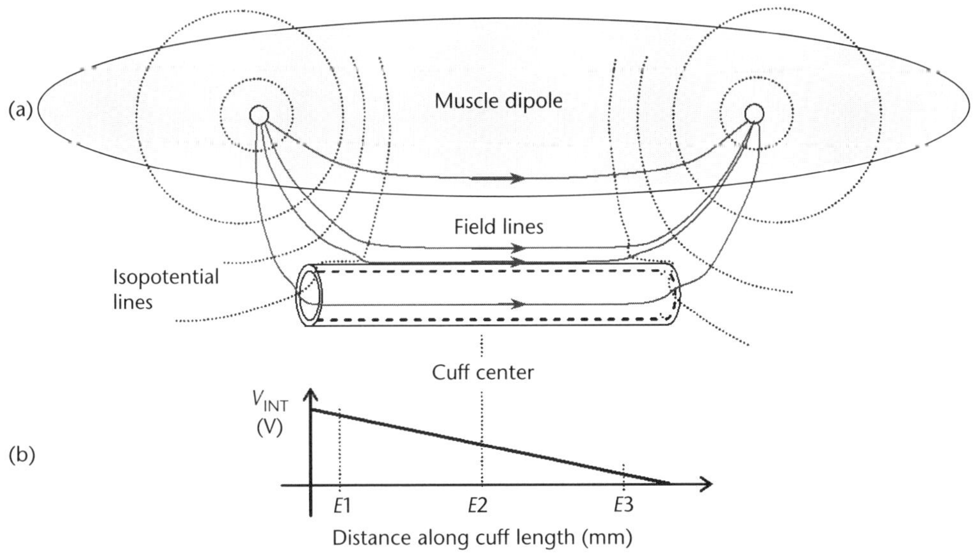

Figure 11.7 (a) The perturbation of the muscle dipole field by the cuff, similar to the effects described in [13]. (b) The cuff linearizes the EMG field (V_{INT}) inside it [23]. *L* is the cuff length and *E*1, *E*2 and *E*3 are electrode positions (assuming a tripolar cuff).

Various studies [8, 22] have proposed close approximations of circuit models for the tripolar recording cuff, similar to that in Figure 11.8(a), illustrating the equivalent signal sources, the interface impedances of the cuff and the internal potential gradients of the ENG and interference sources due to its linearizing property. This schematic diagram allows an analysis of the voltages appearing between the electrodes in terms of the currents of the nerve and muscle sources and the tissue and electrode impedances. The electrode impedances are Z_{e1}, Z_{e2}, and Z_{e3}, whereas the tissue impedance outside the cuff is Z_o and inside it is separated into Z_{t1} and Z_{t2} between the middle and each of the end electrodes. The current source I_{INT} produces the interference signal from its field outside and inside the cuff. The interfering voltages across electrode points AB and BC appear as anti-phase, while the respective ENG signals appear in-phase. Typical cuff circuit model values are: Z_o = 200 Ω, $Z_{t1,2}$ = 2.5 kΩ, $Z_{e1,2,3}$ = 1 kΩ, I_{INT} = 1 μA [21]. This model can be used for the analysis of tripolar amplifier configurations [8].

In practice, some EMG interference is apparent at the ENG amplifier output even when tripolar cuffs are used. This breakthrough of EMG has been attributed by Rahal [8] mainly to (a) manufacturing tolerance on electrode position, and (b) impedance irregularities in the tissue inside the cuff. Another factor that has been

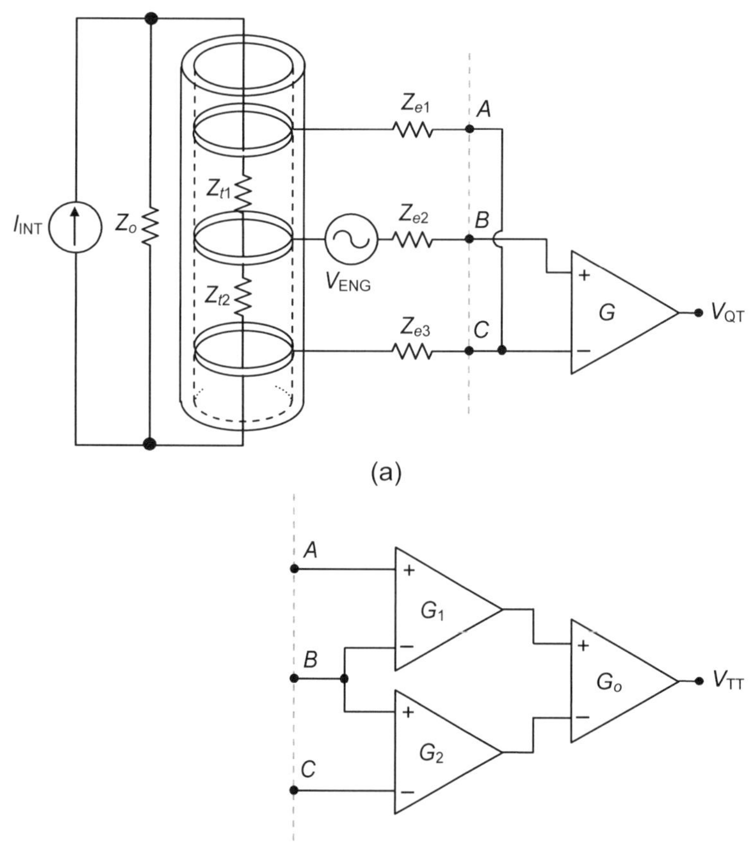

Figure 11.8 Tripolar ENG amplifier configurations: (a) the QT connected to a tripolar cuff (cuff lumped model is shown), (b) the TT. V_{ENG} is the ENG source. Nodes A, B and C are circuit nodes.

reported to cause the deviation of the cuff behavior from its ideal model is (c) "end-effects." The end-effect phenomenon was initially shown by Rahal [24] to reduce the linearity of the interference field inside the cuff due to its finite length. Triantis [25] found that the effect is related to the proximity and orientation of the external source relative to the cuff. All these factors contribute to what has been termed *cuff imbalance* since a perfectly symmetrical (or balanced) cuff would be immune to external fields. The first cause of imbalance can be reduced by good fabrication technique, the other two are unavoidable. The ENG is not affected by imbalance [21].

The tripolar amplifier configuration used by Stein et al. [14] is shown in Figure 11.8(a). It is referred to as the quasi-tripole (QT) because the outer electrodes are connected together and this changes the field. This is advantageous because it has a "screening effect" [14]: the two end electrodes are shorted together, and some EMG current flows through the wire, reducing the potential gradient inside the cuff and therefore the interference. The QT is attractive because only one differential amplifier is required but has the disadvantage that there is no way to adjust the balance to remove interference. However, a modified version of the QT was recently suggested by Pachnis et al. [26] where they have added a parallel RC network in series with the outer electrodes to balance the electrode impedances, which enables some removal of myoelectric interference.

The true-tripole (TT) introduced by Pflaum et al. [27] and shown in Figure 11.8(b) has several advantages compared to the QT: (a) As every electrode is connected to an input of the differential amplifiers, which presents a high impedance load, the TT is insensitive to the electrode interface impedance. This reduces phase differences due to the electrode capacitance. (b) It gives higher ENG amplitude (approximately double) and thus by tuning the gain can potentially improve the signal-to-interference ratio (SIR). (c) By varying the gain of the two first stage differential amplifiers to equalize the EMG in the two sides, the EMG can be cancelled in the second stage. This adjustment can be made automatic leading to the adaptive-tripole (AT) [21] shown in Figure 11.9. In this arrangement, the input amplifiers have variable gain controlled by the differential feedback signals V_a and $-V_a$. The

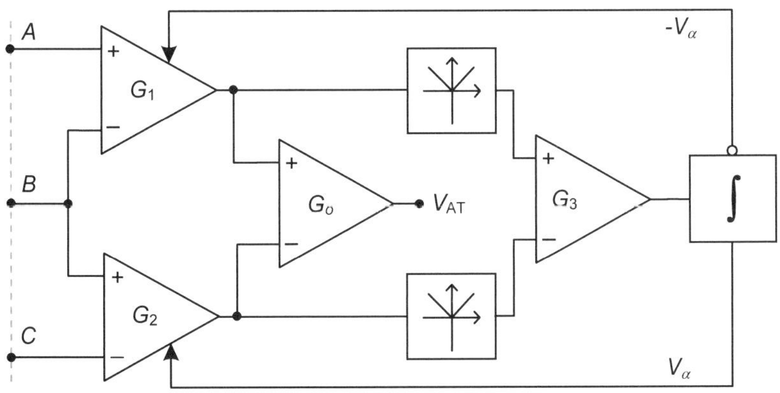

Figure 11.9 The AT circuitry [21], [28]. Gains of G_1 and G_2 are controlled by feedback signals V_a and $-V_a$, equalizing interfering EMG signals in the two measuring channels, which are then eliminated at the output. The input stage is preceded by low-noise preamplifiers, not shown here.

control stage performs a comparison of the amplitudes from the two channels by first rectifying the signals and then amplifying the difference of their absolute values, using amplifier G_3. The output of G_3 is applied to a long-time constant integrator, which produces the feedback signals V_a and $-V_a$. The variable-gain amplifiers counterbalance the cuff imbalance by equalizing the amplitudes of the composite signal at the outputs of the two channels that are applied to summing amplifier G_o, similar to the TT. As a result, the equal and anti-phase interfering signals from the two channels are eliminated and in-phase ENG signals are added and amplified. An integrated realization of the AT using BiCMOS technology was presented in [28], which demonstrated up to 300 times greater SIR in the presence of cuff imbalance, compared to both the TT and the QT.

11.5 Bioamplifier Circuits

Biopotential signals are low-frequency and low-amplitude signals. For example, the ENG signal recorded using tripolar cuff electrodes is typically in the order of 1 μV r.m.s. with a broad, flat power spectral density centered at about 1–2 kHz, with most power concentrated between 300 Hz and 5 kHz [22]. Even recording neural activity with penetrating electrodes, the recorded neural action potentials often have amplitudes of only a few tens of microvolt. Hence, amplifiers for weak bioelectrical signals must have low-noise performance and ideally dissipate little power so that battery life is prolonged, especially in systems intended for chronic implantation. In addition, most designs are required to reject (DC) electrode offsets due to electrochemical effects at the electrode-tissue interface, or common-mode interference (hence the need for high CMRR). Various methods have been developed to address these issues. These may be classified into clock-based and continuous-time techniques.

11.5.1 Clock-Based Techniques

Different clock-based approaches have been described to improve the performance of low-noise amplifiers. Noise reduction based on physical effects (bias switching), chopper modulation, and autozeroing are amongst these techniques. These techniques aim at the reduction of flicker noise, also known as $1/f$-noise, but do not improve on the white noise.

11.5.1.1 Bias Switching

This technique aims at reducing the $1/f$-noise of a MOS transistor by cyclically increasing and decreasing its gate bias so that the device alternates between inversion and accumulation (Figure 11.10) [29].

The transistor noise is modulated by the switching wave where the switching operation can be represented as a multiplication of the noise current with the switching signal $m(t)$. Using a square wave with 50% duty cycle as switching signal, $m(t)$ is approximated by its Fourier representation:

$$m(t) = \frac{1}{2} + \frac{2}{\pi}\sin(\omega_{sw}t) + \frac{2}{3\pi}\sin(3\omega_{sw}t) + \frac{2}{5\pi}\sin(5\omega_{sw}t) + \cdots \quad (11.1)$$

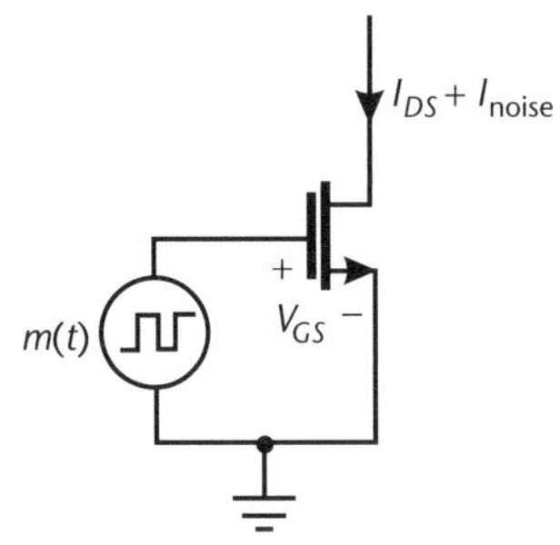

Figure 11.10 Cycling of MOSFET gate bias between inversion and accumulation to reduce 1/*f*-noise [29].

where ω_{sw} is the switching frequency. If ω_{sw} is chosen sufficiently high, the baseband noise reduces by half and any modulation effects represented by the sine terms in Equation (11.1) remain outside the bandwidth of interest and can be removed by filtering. Note also that the baseband signal of interest is modulated so that the signal-to-noise ratio (SNR) remains unchanged. However, the reduction of 1/*f*-noise achieved by switching is reported to be in excess of the effect expected from modulation theory [29]. It is instead explained by physical mechanisms, mainly a reduction in the time between carrier trapping and release due to cycling [30]. The maximum SNR improvement thus achieved is around 30% [29]. Hence, bias switching may improve noise performance at low frequencies, but requires a high-speed clock applied to the gate or bulk of the transistor with potential problems due to charge feedthrough and additional noise originating from the driver circuit. Applying the clock to the back-gate further introduces distortion due to the bulk-effect. Bias-switching may therefore be impractical for the design of very low-noise front-ends.

11.5.1.2 Chopper Technique

The chopper technique is also an approach based on signal modulation. Before amplification, the amplifier input signal is modulated by a wave of frequency ω_{sw} (f_{chop}) much higher than the baseband frequencies of interest. The up-converted signal is then amplified and bandpass filtered. The modulated signal spectrum is located at frequencies higher than the 1/*f*-noise corner, so that the amplifier noise floor alone determines the SNR. After amplification, the signal is converted back to the baseband by multiplication with the same modulation waveform used for up-conversion [31]. Finally, low-pass filtering restores the desired signal. Although this technique reduces 1/*f*-noise and output offset voltages (DC), the noise performance is ultimately limited by the noise floor of the amplifier. Furthermore, non-idealities may lead to signal distortion. Such non-idealities include the amplifier bandwidth, which must be at least twice the modulation frequency to satisfy the Nyquist criterion. It should be noted that the chopper technique enables the design of amplifiers with high CMRR performance.

Various integrated bioamplifiers employing the chopper technique have been described for both implanted and surface electrodes [32–35]. The design in [35] employs an AC-coupled chopping technique to reject both electrode offsets and achieve low-noise performance. The concept of this technique is shown in Figure 11.11.

The system consists of a feedforward stage and a feedback stage. To suppress the 1/*f*-noise of the IA, the feedforward stage employs an input chopper, a current-feedback instrumentation amplifier (IA), and an output chopper. To eliminate the electrode offset, the feedback stage employs a low-pass operational transconductance (OTA) stage followed by a chopper stage. The operation of the circuit is as follows [35]: The input differential electrode offset ($V_{\text{offset, elec}}$) is modulated by the input chopper and it appears across resistor R_1. By action of the current-feedback, the current through R_1 is copied to R_2 and defines the output voltage after demodulation by the output chopper. The low-pass OTA stage with transconductance G_m filters the DC component of the output and converts it into current. The OTA output current is in turn modulated by the proceeding chopper stage. At steady state, the current supplied by the OTA is $V_{\text{offset, elec}}/R_1$. Hence, no current is supplied by the IA and the current passing through R_2 is zero so the output (V_{out}) is zero.

11.5.1.3 Autozeroing

The principle of the autozero technique is illustrated in Figure 11.12.

During sampling phase φ_1, the amplifier is configured as a unity gain buffer and the input noise is sampled. During the amplification phase φ_2, the noise sample is subtracted from the instantaneous amplifier input noise. As the sampling frequency is chosen higher than the 1/*f*-noise frequency, the sample is highly correlated to the instantaneous noise, so that the low-frequency noise cancels. A detailed analysis of the autozero amplifier is complex and can be found in [36]. A major drawback of the autozero technique is that high frequency white noise is undersampled and folded back into the baseband where it increases the noise floor.

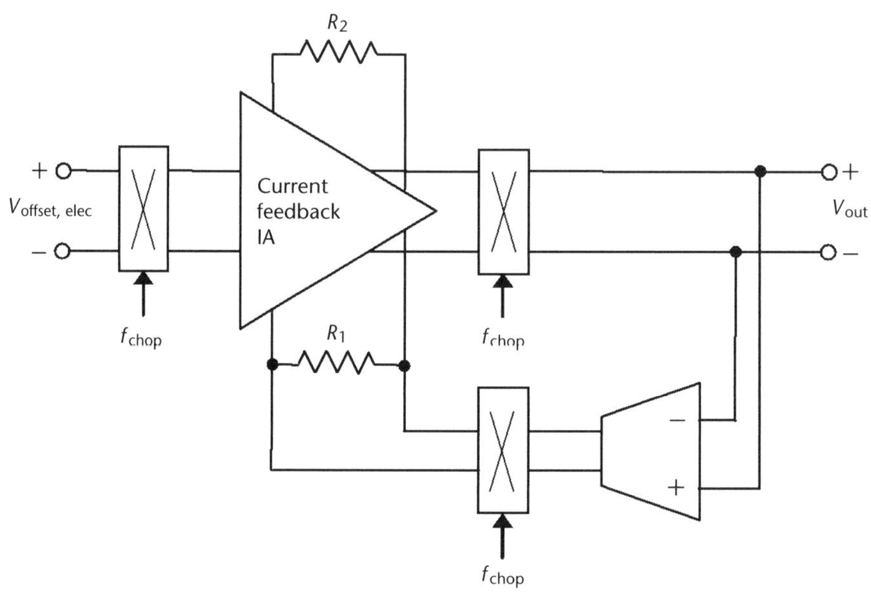

Figure 11.11 Concept of the AC-coupled chopper IA described in [35].

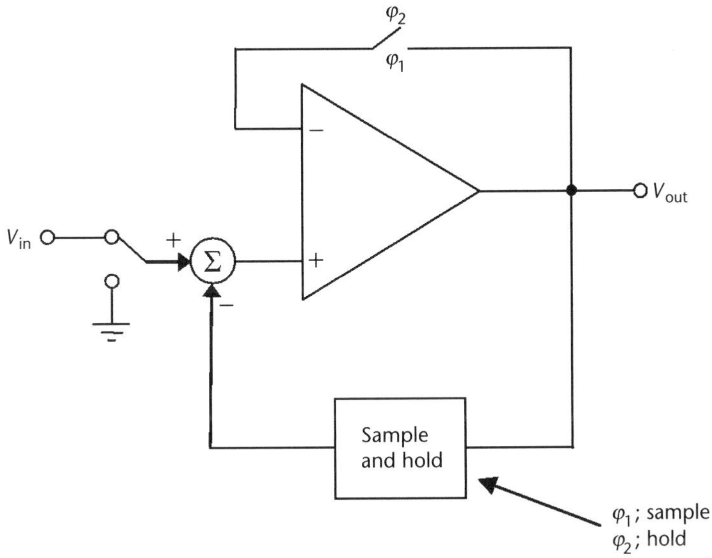

Figure 11.12 The autozero amplifier concept.

11.5.2 Continuous-Time Techniques

The noise reduction techniques described above require a clock generation circuitry and hence suffer from potential problems associated with high-frequency interference and clock-feedthrough. To overcome this limitation, the use of non clock-based techniques has been exploited for the design of bioamplifiers. A popular example circuit is the AC-coupled bioamplifier shown in Figure 11.13 [37], which is particularly suitable for use with penetrating electrodes.

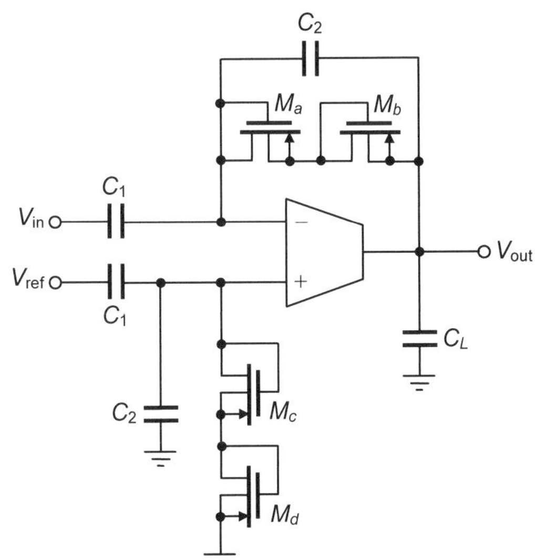

Figure 11.13 An AC-coupled bioamplifier circuit employing pseudoresistors [37].

The circuit is built around a single-stage OTA. The ratio of capacitors C_1 and C_2 sets the mid-band gain. Transistors M_a–M_d implement pseudoresistors with an extremely large incremental resistance (>10^{12} Ω). This allows the cut-off of the input high-pass filters (i.e., AC-coupled stage) to be set to the millihertz region. Assuming that C_1, $C_L > C_2$, the amplifier bandwidth may be approximated by $(G_mC_2) / (C_1C_L)$ where G_m is OTA transconductance and C_L is the load capacitance. To reduce the effect of 1/*f*-noise, the OTA input transistors are made pMOS devices with large gate areas.

Electrode offset removal may also be implemented by means of active feedback loops. An example bioamplifier topology with active feedback for DC rejection is shown in Figure 11.14 [38]. The circuit consists of a low-noise OTA (OTA1) with an active feedback circuit implemented by a second OTA (OTA2) configured as a Miller integrator. The integrator's time-constant is set by capacitor C_1 and the MOS pseudoresistor implemented by M_a and M_b. The mid-band gain of the bioamplifier is the same as the gain of OTA1 and its low-pass cut-off can be set by the dominant pole of OTA1. The common-mode voltage is set by voltage V_{ref}.

A very low-noise bioamplifier for tripolar cuff electrodes was described in [28, 39] using BiCMOS technology. As shown in Figure 11.15, this circuit consists of a simple BiCMOS OTA (Q_1, Q_2, M_1, and M_2) terminated in the load resistor R_1, followed by a first-order bandpass filter, which restricts the bandwidth to about 100 Hz to 10 kHz. The upper cut-off frequency is obtained by the combination of resistor R_2 and capacitor C_1, while the lower cut-off frequency is obtained by capacitor C_2 with the series combination of transistors M_6 and M_7, the latter transistor pair forming a high value (~20 MΩ) grounded linear active resistor [40]. In addition to eliminating low frequencies below the ENG pass-band, the high-pass section of the bandpass filter also removes some of the low-frequency flicker noise voltage tail and ensures a DC offset-free amplifier output. The DC bias voltages of M_6 and M_7 are provided by the diode-connected transistors M_8 and M_9, respectively, which are in turn biased by the DC current sources I_{b2} and I_{b3}. Circuitry is also included to cancel the base currents of Q_1 and Q_2. This is very important, as significant current flowing into the tissue cannot be permitted. Essentially, Q_3 generates a replica of the base currents of Q_1 and Q_2, which is fed into the pMOS current mirror M_3–M_5

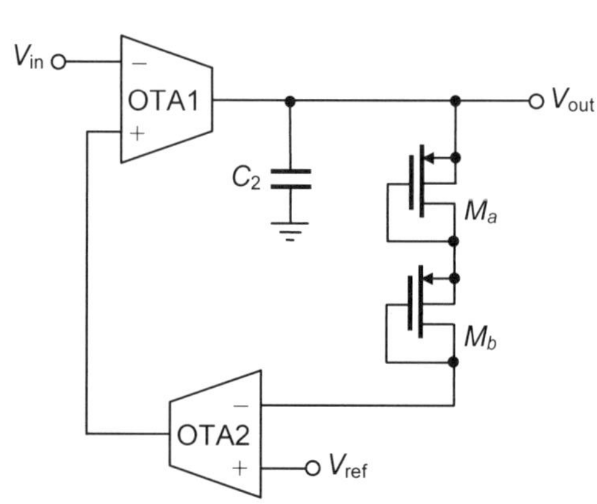

Figure 11.14 A bioamplifier circuit with active DC rejection [38].

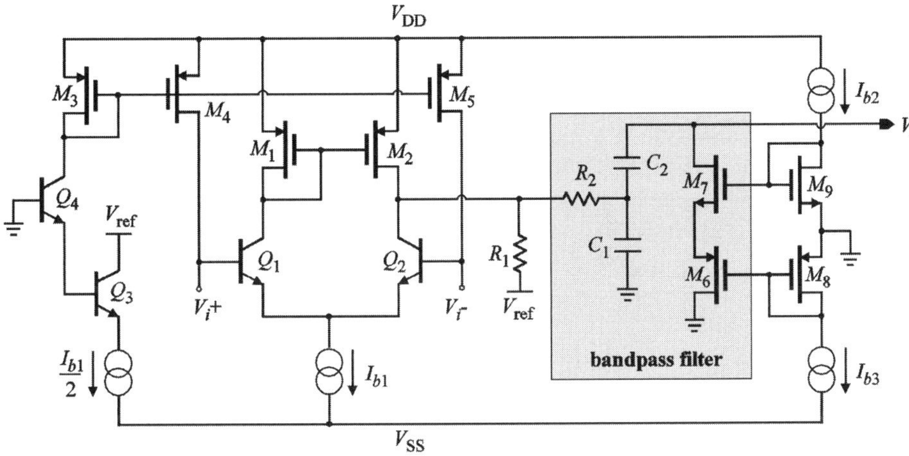

Figure 11.15 A BiCMOS bioamplifier for tripolar cuff electrode recording [28].

whose outputs feed the bases of Q_1 and Q_2, respectively. The base of Q_4 is connected to ground to ensure that the emitter voltage of Q_3 is at the appropriate level. Furthermore, the collector of Q_3 is connected to V_{ref} to mimic as far as possible the DC conditions of Q_1 and Q_2. This bioamplifier was reported to achieve a measured input-referred r.m.s. noise voltage of only 290 nV (noise bandwidth of 1 Hz–15 kHz). A variant of this bioamplifier in CMOS technology utilizing lateral bipolar devices for Q_1 and Q_2 was described in [41]. However, for the same target noise specification, the use of lateral pnp bipolar devices (available in CMOS technology) results in a considerable increase in silicon area compared to using standard npn bipolar devices in BiCMOS technology.

For biomedical front-ends requiring high CMRR performance and accurate gain setting, the use of an IA (rather than an OTA) is desirable. An IA may be constructed using the classic three-opamp topology [42]. However, the CMRR of the three-opamp IA depends on the matching of the resistors and the need for low output impedance amplifiers can increase power consumption. Another technique for IA design is to employ switched-capacitor circuits [43] but the fold-over of noise above Nyquist frequency can be a major limitation. Another IA topology is the *current-feedback* (or current balancing) technique [44, 45]. In a current-feedback IA, the gain is accurately set by the ratio of two resistors and the CMRR does not rely on the matching of resistors. Figure 11.16 shows an example of a MOS-based current-feedback IA with a bandpass response (the circuit is a modification of the bipolar design described in [44]).

The circuit consists of two stages: an input transconductance stage and an output transimpedance stage. The use of active current-feedback in the transconductance stage serves to exactly balance the drain currents of M_1 and M_2 (provided that the current-feedback gain is sufficiently large). A direct consequence of this is that the input differential voltage V_{in} (across the gates of M_1 and M_2) is forced across resistor R_1 and, hence, the input stage is essentially a unity-gain buffer. To enhance the CMRR performance, the mirror transistors M_5 and M_6 should be cascoded. The output transimpedance stage converts the differential feedback currents of the input stage

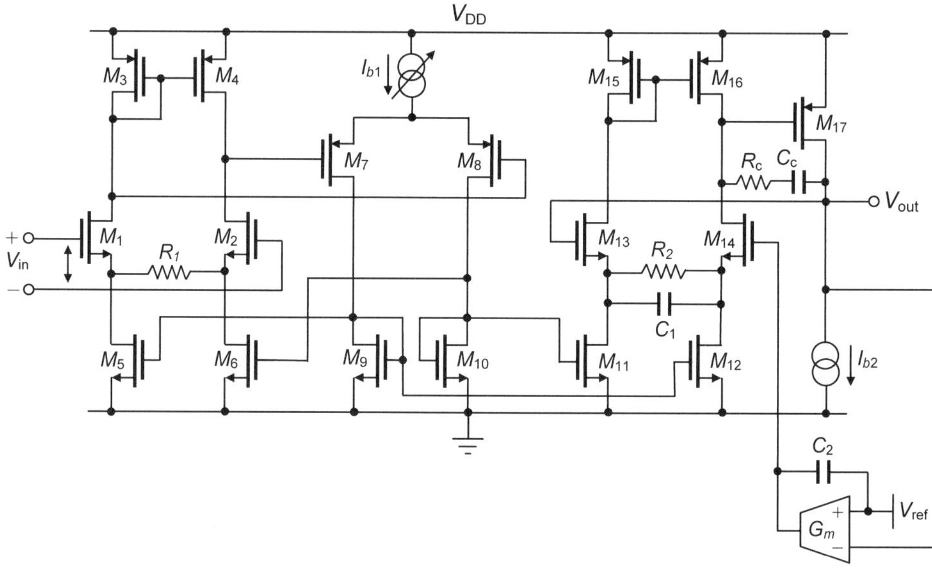

Figure 11.16 A CMOS current-feedback bandpass IA.

into a single-ended output voltage V_{out} (which also appears across resistor R_2). Ignoring source resistance effects in the input transistors and assuming that the feedback gains of the input and output stages are large (>60 dB), the IA gain may be calculated by the ratio of R_2/R_1. This IA features a bandpass response, with the high cut-off frequency (dominant pole) given by

$$f_H = \frac{1}{2\pi R_2 C_1} \tag{11.2}$$

The addition of the first-order high-pass G_m-C filter in the transimpedance stage creates the desired lower cut-off frequency, given by

$$f_L = \frac{G_m}{2\pi C_2} \tag{11.3}$$

The main contributors to the noise floor of this IA topology after the input devices M_1 and M_2, are the mirror devices M_3 and M_4, followed by the load devices M_5 and M_6. It can be shown that the input-referred noise voltage due to R_1 is heavily attenuated by the current-feedback gain.

11.6 Stimulation and Circuits

As mentioned earlier, electrical pulses applied to nerves can trigger action potentials. At least two electrodes are required in order to produce current flow; the electrodes can be arranged in either a monopolar or bipolar configuration. In both cases, the active electrode is placed near the peripheral nerve to be stimulated. In monopolar stimulation, the indifferent electrode is placed away from the active electrode. In bipolar stimulation, the reference electrode is placed near the active electrode. The remaining sections of this chapter focus on the stimulator output stage design that is the circuitry that drives the stimulating electrodes. The chapter ends with a review of stimulator current generator circuits.

11.6.1 Modes of Stimulation

There are two distinct modes for stimulation: current-mode and voltage-mode as shown in Figure 11.17.

Current-mode stimulation (Figure 11.17(a)) is widely used in implantable stimulators for FES applications. The current amplitude is directly controlled by a digital-to-analogue converter (DAC) and it is not affected by changes in the load (tissue-electrode impedance). Therefore, the quantity of charge delivered per stimulus pulse is easily controlled. Active current sources are used to supply the stimulus current to the load. The current source requires additional headroom over the maximum voltage appearing at its output node.

In voltage-mode stimulation (Figure 11.17(b)), the stimulator output is a voltage, and therefore the magnitude of the current delivered to the tissue is dependent on the inter-electrode impedance. Thus, it is difficult to control the exact amount of charge supplied to the load because of impedance variations. In [46], the stimulator drives the electrodes with a sequence of voltage steps, charging the electrode metal-fluid capacitance. This applies a voltage waveform that is an approximation of the waveform that would appear at the electrode if a current pulse was applied. Since the charge is delivered to the electrode directly from intermediate voltage supplies (the capacitors), it avoids the substantial unnecessary power in the current sources of its current-mode counterpart, as well as providing large voltage compliance. It is believed that voltage-mode stimulus is more effective than the common square-shaped stimulus pulses due to its being comprised of both high and low frequency components at the output spectrum [47]. However, this method requires large capacitors (which act as voltage sources) that are difficult to be implemented on-chip. Kelly et al. [46] used five 1 μF capacitors for a 15-electrode stimulation system, which would

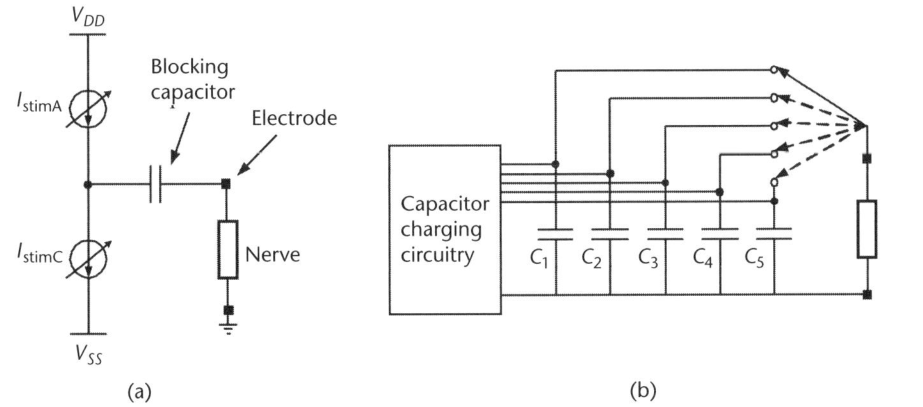

(a) (b)

Figure 11.17 Stimulation circuit. (a) current-mode, (b) voltage-mode.

increase for more electrodes. It is also difficult to achieve fine resolution compared to current-mode stimulation since voltage-mode is an approximate method of producing a current pulse and increasing the resolution needs more capacitors.

11.6.2 Types of Stimulation Waveforms

Most common stimulus waveforms are either monophasic or biphasic, as depicted in Figure 11.18.

A monophasic stimulus consists of a repeating unidirectional cathodic pulse; this type of stimulus is common in surface electrode stimulation. A biphasic waveform consists of a repeating current pulse that has a cathodic (negative) phase followed by an anodic (positive) phase. The cathodic phase depolarizes nearby axons and triggers the action potential. The succeeding anodic phase reverses the potentially damaging electrochemical processes that can occur at the electrode-tissue interphase during the cathodic phase by (ideally) neutralizing the charge accumulated in the cathodic phase, allowing stimulation without tissue damage. The application of charge-balanced waveforms is very important especially for implanted electrodes. Usually the stimulus for the cathodic phase is square, supplied by active circuits, while the stimulus for the anodic phase could be either square or exponentially decaying. The square secondary phase is also known as active discharging and the exponentially decaying phase as passive discharging.

11.6.3 Stimulator Failure Protection Techniques

Safe electrical stimulation of neural tissue is typically achieved using charge-balanced biphasic current pulses to reduce the generation of DC current and the production of harmful electrochemical products, such as gases, toxic oxychlorides, corrosion products, and associated pH changes. Studies have shown that a 2 μA DC current leads to auditory nerve damage [48]. Charge imbalance can be caused by many reasons including: (i) semiconductor failure, (ii) leakage currents due to crosstalk between adjacent stimulating channels, and (iii) cable failure.

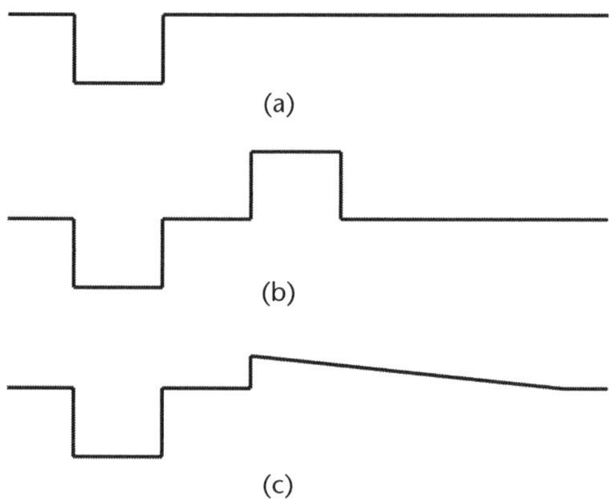

Figure 11.18 Common stimulus shapes. (a) monophasic, (b) biphasic; both active phases, (c) biphasic; active cathodic and passive anodic phases.

11.6.3.1 Semiconductor Failure Induced Charge Imbalance and Solutions

Various mechanisms of semiconductor failure in stimulators either implanted or under accelerated tests have been reported. These include short-circuit due to moisture penetration into the glass seal of the silicon package [49], gate-oxide breakdown [50], and change of device parameters after implantation, for example, due to ionizing radiation [51]. The moisture-caused short-circuit should be addressed by more reliable packaging techniques and this is an active research area especially for implant micro-packaging. Semiconductor failure due to breakdown of gate-oxide in CMOS integrated circuits is not rare. The gate-oxide of a transistor is distributed in three regions: GD (between gate-and-drain), GB (between gate-and-substrate), GS (between gate-and-source). When charge build-up at the gate is large enough and has no other leakage path to substrate, a current flows through the connected transistor gate-oxide causing breakdown [52]. Breakdown in the region GD causes a gate-oxide short between gate-and-drain; so do the other regions. Semiconductor failures are potentially harmful because they could generate prolonged DC current to the electrode and tissue.

Charge imbalance can be corrected by shorting the output of the stimulator between current pulses, or coupling the output of the stimulator through an appropriate *blocking capacitor*. The blocking capacitor is preferable to the electrode shorting because it not only provides better correction of DC level [53], but also serves as a barrier to any prolonged DC current [54] in the event of semiconductor failure. Given the "allow-AC," "block-DC" characteristic of capacitors, the blocking capacitor limits the maximum net charge that can be passed to the tissue to $Q_{max} = CV$, where C is the capacitance of the blocking capacitor and V is the power supply voltage. Thus, by careful choosing of the capacitance value (Q_{max} should be below the safety limit of the electrode and neural tissue), the blocking capacitor serves as a barrier for harmful prolonged DC current.

Another approach that is similar to the blocking capacitor method is to use electrodes made of porous tantalum or iridium oxide because an electrode is able to work as a "capacitor-electrode" [55]. Other methods of protection that do not utilize blocking capacitors include continuous monitoring of the electrode-tissue impedance [56], electrode voltage [57], or the stimulus current level [58]. The recorded values are continuously compared with a pre-defined reference, which when exceeded, inhibits the stimulator output stage to prevent nerve damage. The advantage of this approach is volume saving because the monitoring circuit can be integrated with the stimulator output stage circuit. However, the monitoring circuit increases the stimulator output stage complexity, which itself may increase the likelihood of semiconductor failure.

11.6.3.2 Inter-Channel Crosstalk Induced Charge Imbalance

Figure 11.19 shows a three-channel stimulator output stage. Each stimulating channel includes a blocking capacitor (C_1–C_3) for safety reasons as discussed above.

Due to their large size (μF), these blocking capacitors are implemented as off-chip surface mount components. The configuration of common voltage at all electrode anodes reduces the wire count between the anodes and the integrated chip, while the required contact pads for the integrated chip are also minimized [59].

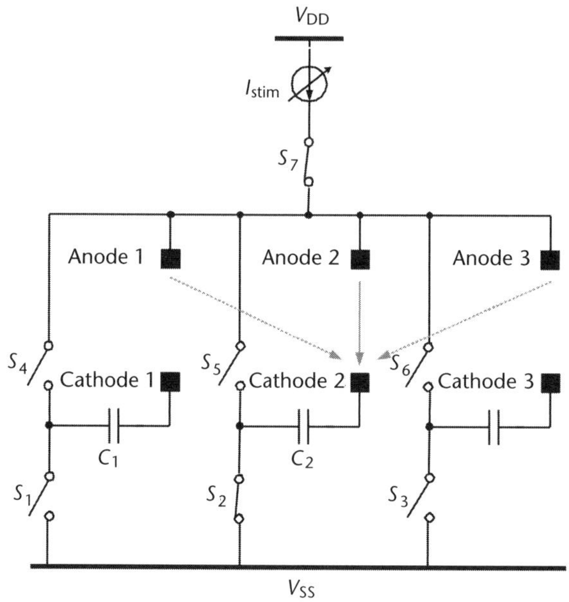

Figure 11.19 An illustration of leakage current from adjacent channels.

However, this configuration introduces a problem of leakage current between adjacent channels. For example, assume that channel 2 is activated for stimulation. Switches S_7 and S_2 are closed and the stimulus current (I_{stim}) flows from anode-2 to cathode-2. However, the voltage difference between adjacent anodes and cathode-2 will cause leakage current from other anodes to cathode-2. If the blocking capacitor is not present and the accumulated net charge is not corrected, once the net charge through adjacent anodes exceeds the safety limit that the electrode can tolerate, it will electrolyte the anode-tissue interface.

11.6.3.3 Cable-Failure Induced Charge Imbalance

Usually, several wires are packed into an implantable cable. Each wire is used to deliver stimulus current, power supply, data stream or clock information, depending on the application. If the insulation fails on only one wire in the cable, it will still be safe because there is no applied potential (voltage difference) between the exposed part of the broken wire and the internal body. Hence, there will be no pathway for the current to flow from the exposed part of the broken wire in a single-wire failure. However, if two wires or more are exposed in a failure, current will flow between the exposed parts because of the voltage difference between them, causing electrolysis. This would be a severe safety hazard for the tissue near the exposed area. In order to ensure fail-safe operation, the current between the wire exposures has to be charge balanced. If the average voltage of each wire is identical, there may be a current from one exposed wire to another at a certain time. But shortly, there will be a current in the reversed direction that neutralizes the net charge. Thus, it will not cause harm to nearby tissue.

A method to achieve charge balance was proposed in [60] employing Manchester non-return-to-zero (Manchester NRZ) encoding for the data signal in each wire.

The average voltage of the Manchester NRZ output is half the supply voltage, independent of the original input signal. As an example, Figure 11.20 shows the Manchester NRZ code for data streams of 0001110110 and 1011100010. Figure 11.20 also shows the current, I_{fail}, flowing from wire-1 to wire-2 in a cable failure that involves both wire-1 and wire-2.

As shown in the figure, I_{fail} is a bidirectional current in which the positive charge is balanced by the negative charge, maintaining the tissue near the failure site in safe condition. For safety reasons, an AC signal is also applied to the power-line. For simplicity, a differential clock signal with the same DC level as that in the data wires may be employed. A rectifier and a regulator can be configured at the end of the power wire to extract a stable DC voltage.

11.6.4 Stimulator Output Stage Configurations Utilizing Blocking Capacitors

Figure 11.21 shows three commonly used stimulator output stage configurations each employing a blocking capacitor: (a) dual supplies with both active phases, (b) single supply with both active phases, and (c) single supply with active cathodic phase and passive anodic phase.

For the configuration in Figure 11.21(a) [61], an electrode common to all stimulating channels is always connected to a reference voltage (V_{common}), usually the midpoint of the two supply voltages. The programmable current sink I_{stimC} and current source I_{stimA} generate the cathodic and anodic currents, respectively. These currents are driven through the load, Z, representing the nerve-electrode impedance, by the control of switches S_1 and S_2. When only a single supply is available (Figure 11.21(b)), the anodic and cathodic currents are generated from a single current sink (I_{stim}) by reversing the current paths by switches S_2 [62, 63]. Both configurations in Figures 11.21(a) and 11.21(b) are (ideally) designed to be charge-balanced to avoid charge accumulation. However, achieving exactly zero net charge after each stimulation cycle is not possible due to mismatch or timing errors and leakage from adjacent stimulus sites [61]. Therefore, it is important to include switch S_3 to periodically

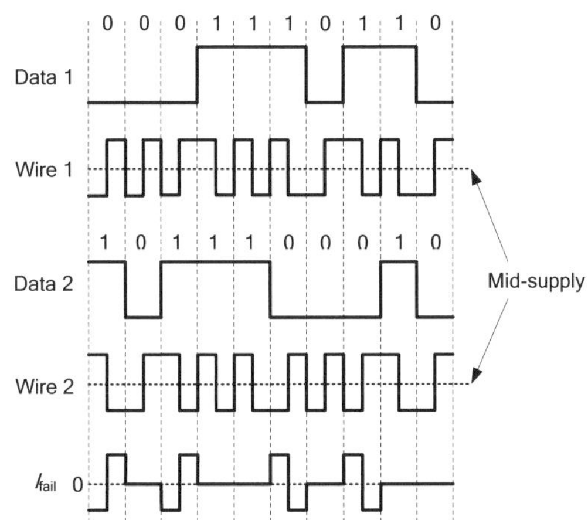

Figure 11.20 Manchester NRZ coded signal in the cable [60].

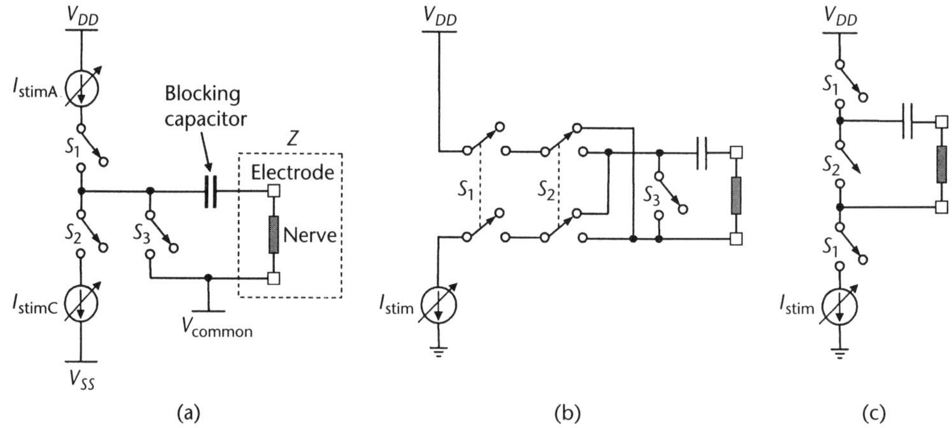

Figure 11.21 Conventional stimulator output stage configurations. (a) Dual supplies with active cathodic and active anodic phases. (b) Single supply with active cathodic and active anodic phases. (c) Single supply with active cathodic phase and passive anodic phase.

remove the residual charge by providing an extra passive discharge phase in which the voltage on the blocking capacitor drives current through the electrodes to fully discharge them. Given the necessity for the third phase in the circuits of Figures 11.21(a) and 11.21(b), some designers use the passive discharge phase as the main anodic phase [9], as shown in the circuit of Figure 11.21(c). It should be noted that the use of capacitive electrodes may also drive the passive discharge phase. However, blocking capacitors may still be considered necessary to ensure that direct current cannot flow in the event of semiconductor failure [54] because the break-down voltage or leakage current of these electrodes may be inadequate or too uncertain.

The configurations in Figure 11.21(b) and 11.21(c) require two leads for each stimulation channel, while the configuration in Figure 11.21(a) requires only $N + 1$ leads in total for N stimulation channels. Using two leads per stimulation site doubles the number of contact pads in the stimulator output stage chip, increasing chip area. For an available area, using one lead per stimulation site maximizes the number of stimulation sites that the chip can drive.

11.6.5 Method to Reduce the Blocking Capacitor Value

The value of the blocking capacitor depends on the requirement for a specific stimulation. For example, to recover partial leg movements, stimulus currents of about 1 mA intensity and 1 ms pulse-width, are required. To calculate the required capacitance, the following elementary equation may be used:

$$C = I_{stim}\frac{\Delta t}{\Delta V} \tag{11.4}$$

where I_{stim} is the stimulus current amplitude, Δt is the stimulus current pulse-width, and ΔV is the voltage across the blocking capacitor. For the above numerical example, to limit the capacitor voltage drop, to say 1 V, a 1 μF capacitor is required.

Clearly, such a large capacitor is impractical to implement on silicon due to large area and cost requirements, thus the use of off-chip surface mount capacitors (Figure 11.22). The blocking capacitor value may be reduced at the expense of a larger voltage drop across it, but this will result in a higher supply voltage.

From Equation (11.4), with constant I_{stim} and ΔV, the capacitor value is proportional to the time the stimulus current flows through it. Thus, shorter charging periods lead to a smaller blocking capacitor. For example, if the 1 mA stimulus current consists of a train of 50 ns pulses (i.e., the charging time is limited to 50 ns), only a 50 pF capacitor is required for 1 V drop across it. The idea behind this high-frequency current-switching technique [64] is illustrated by the timing waveforms in Figure 23. As shown in the plot, the biphasic stimulus current I_{stim} may be generated by the summation of the 4 sub-currents $I_{source1}$, $I_{source2}$, I_{sink1} and I_{sink2}, each with a pulse-width of 50 ns (the choice of 50 ns is only for illustrative purposes). Each sub-current in Figure 11.23 is generated by the corresponding stimulator output stage: $I_{source1}$, $I_{source2}$ by current-source stages, and I_{sink1}, I_{sink2} by current-sink stages. Figure 11.24 shows the circuit schematic of the current-source stage [64] for conveying $I_{source1}$ to the stimulation load Z (representing the electrode-tissue impedance).

During the ON-intervals of $I_{source1}$, the blocking capacitor C_1 is charged and $I_{source1}$ is guided to the load via the diode D_1. During the 50 ns OFF-intervals of $I_{source1}$, the switch transistor M_3 is turned-ON, thereby enabling discharge of C_1 via the diode D_2. The voltage V_{dis1} at the gate of M_3 is either at the positive supply rail (V_{DD}) for ON, or at the negative supply rail (V_{SS}) for OFF. During the discharge phase, there is negligible current through Z because of the reversed bias of diode D_1. Using four such circuits (2 current-source and 2 current-sink stages) and summing their output currents in the stimulation load (Z), the resulting current through the load resembles I_{stim} of Figure 11.23(a). The difference between the current-source stage and the current-sink stage is the polarity of the diodes. This arrangement enables generation of balanced biphasic stimulus currents. Variants of this new type of output stage circuit are described in [65, 66].

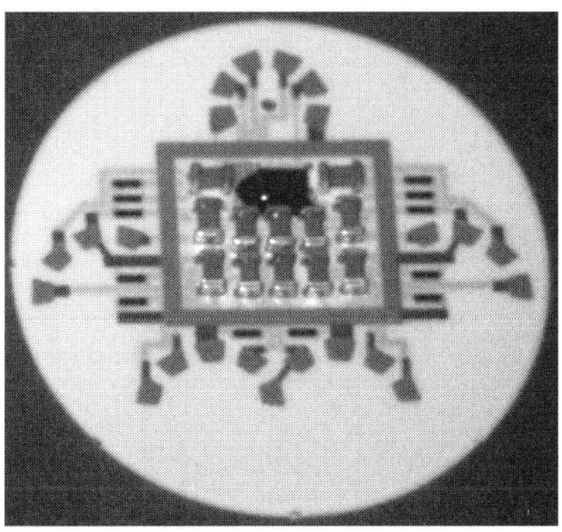

Figure 11.22 A subcutaneous nerve root stimulator made on a thick-film circuit [65]. The discrete off-chip capacitors dictate the implant volume. The integrated circuit is under the black "glob-top." Pads outside the seal rectangle are for cable connections.

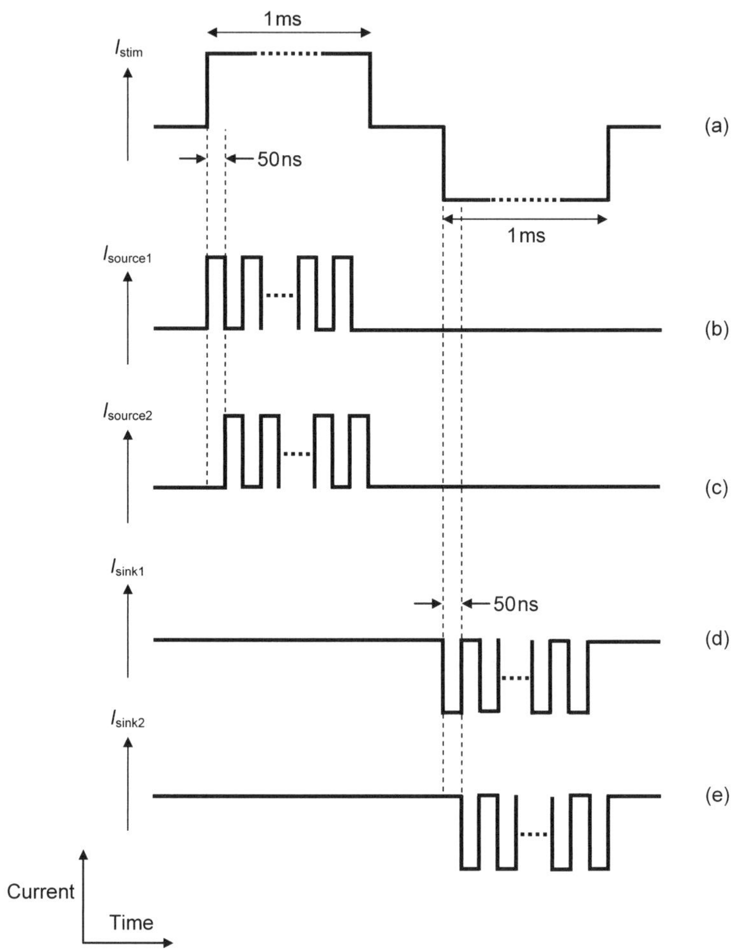

Figure 11.23 Generation of stimulus current I_{stim} from summation of 4 short current pulses [64].

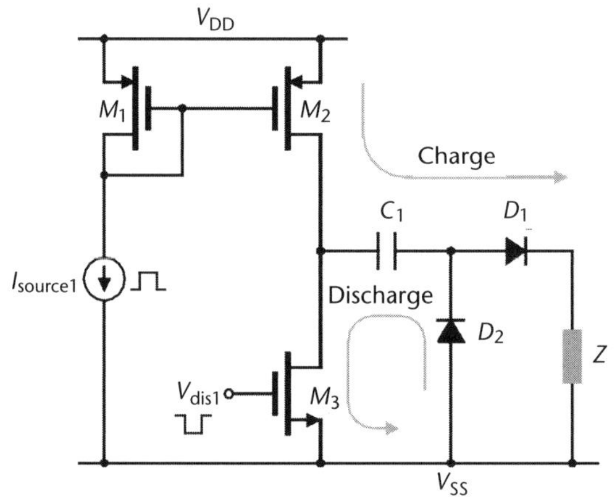

Figure 11.24 Circuit schematic of the current-source stage for conveying current $I_{source1}$ of Figure 23(b) to the stimulation load [64].

11.6.6 Stimulator Current Generator Circuits

Several current generator circuits for implantable neural stimulators have been reported in the literature. The full-scale output current varies from about 100 μA to 16 mA and the resolution from 3 to 8 bits, depending on the application. Desirable features for a current generator circuit for use in this application are: (i) large output voltage compliance, (ii) high output impedance, (iii) good linearity, (iv) low power consumption, and (v) small silicon area.

A current mirror is probably the easiest way to duplicate or scale the current-mode DAC output current, I_{DAC}, to the output current, I_{out}, through the load Z, as shown in Figure 11.25(a) [67–69].

However, both I_{DAC} and I_{out} branches consume power from the supplies. Although the power consumed by the I_{DAC} branch is only $1/n$ (usually, $n > 1$) of the power consumed by the I_{out} branch, it could be completely saved by moving the DAC in series with the load, keeping one branch only, as shown in Figure 11.25(b). By doing so, the DAC is functionally a current generator. Usually, an n-bit current-mode DAC is composed of n binary-weighted transistors [59, 70, 71]. Figure 11.26 shows the circuit schematic for a 4-bit nMOS current-mode DAC. The 4 digital input bits (d_0–d_3) decide whether the gates of the current sink transistors M_1–M_4 are connected to a common bias voltage, V_{bias}. If not, the individual transistor remains off by pulling its gate to 0 V (ground), contributing zero current to the total output current. If connected to V_{bias}, the current sink transistor generates a drain current of (ignoring second-order effects)

$$I_D = \mu C_{ox} \frac{W}{L}[(V_{bias} - V_T)V_{DS} - \frac{1}{2}V_{DS}^2] \tag{11.5a}$$

$$I_D = \frac{1}{2}\mu C_{ox} \frac{W}{L}(V_{bias} - V_T)^2 \tag{11.5b}$$

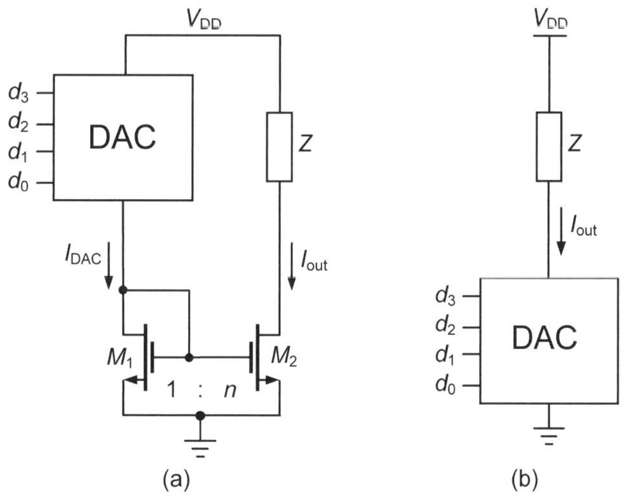

Figure 11.25 (a) Stimulation with a simple current mirror controlled by a current-mode DAC. (b) Stimulation with a current sink implemented by a current-mode DAC.

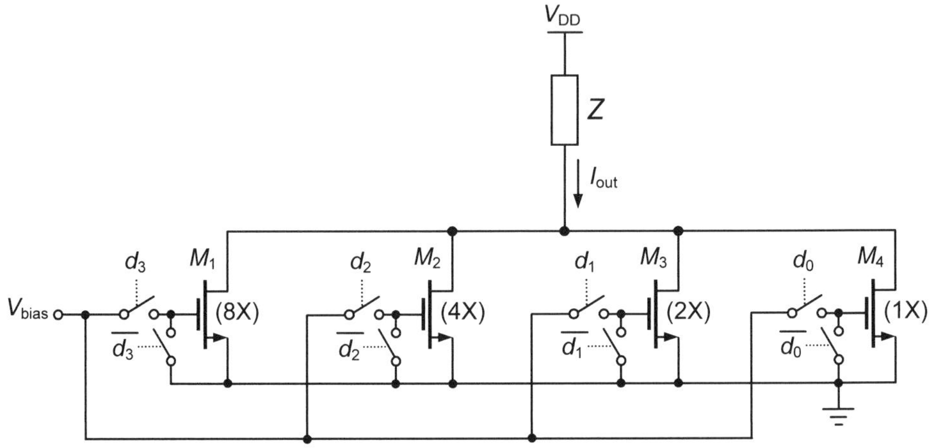

Figure 11.26 Stimulation with a current sink implemented by a current-mode DAC with binary-weighted transistors and fixed bias voltage. A 4-bit implementation is shown.

in the triode region Equation (11.5a) and saturation region Equation (11.5b), respectively; μ is the mobility, C_{ox} is the oxide capacitance per unit area, V_T is the threshold voltage, V_{DS} is the drain-source voltage, and W and L are the transistor width and length, respectively. In the circuit of Figure 11.26 the full-scale output current is 15 times the current supplied by the smallest transistor (M_4), i.e., the one controlled by the least significant bit d_0.

Figure 11.27(a) shows another implementation of the DAC that employs identical current sink transistors with "binary-weighted bias" [72]. Since transistors M_1–M_4 have the same dimensions and are subjected to the same drain-source voltage, the drain current will only be decided by the gate bias. If the multi-bias circuit in Figure 11.27(b) provides the gate biases in a binary-weighted manner, the drain currents of M_1–M_4 will also be binary-weighted.

In practice, the DAC current sink transistors are cascoded to increase the output impedance to maintain a constant output current, regardless of the voltage variation across the load. The cascode transistor is usually biased by a static voltage [59, 70–73] while it is also possible to increase the DAC output impedance by biasing the cascode transistor with active feedback [61].

In Figure 11.28, the high-gain amplifier locks the drain voltage of M_2 to be equal to the drain voltage of M_1 (i.e., the amplifier acts as a voltage follower). The same biasing conditions make the drain current of M_2, n times the current of M_1, the same as their aspect ratio difference. The output impedance of the active feedback current generator is given by

$$R_{out} = Ag_{m4}r_{o4}r_{o2} \tag{11.6}$$

where A is the amplifier gain, r_{o2} is the output resistance of M_2, and g_{m4} and r_{o4} are the transconductance and output resistance of M_4, respectively. The output impedance is $Ag_{m4}r_{o4}$ times larger than that of M_2 only.

It is also possible to achieve an adjustable current generator by using a voltage follower to bias a fixed resistor [74], as shown in 11.Figure 29. The input of the volt-

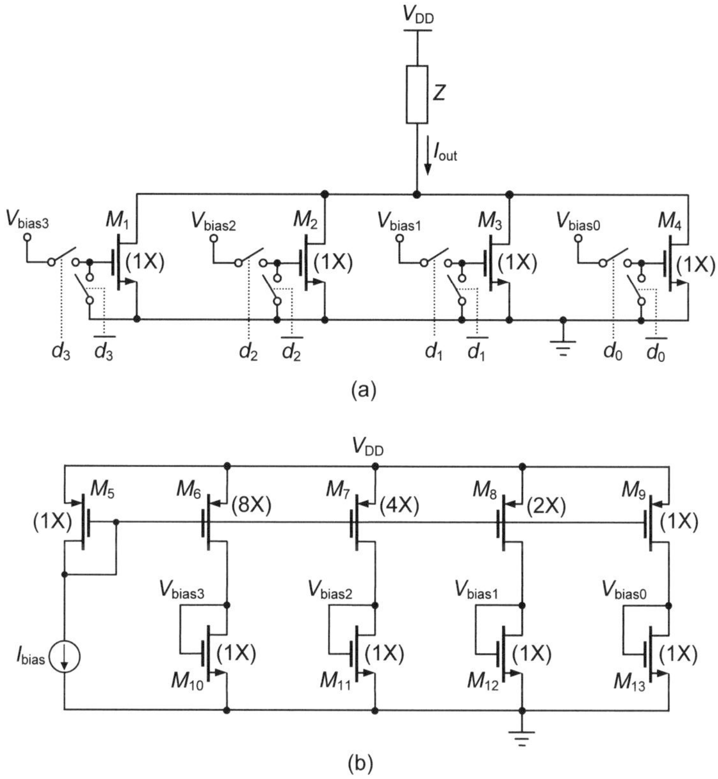

Figure 11.27 (a) Stimulation with a current sink implemented by a current-mode DAC with binary-weighted multi-bias [72]. A 4-bit implementation is shown. (b) Circuit schematic of the multi-bias voltage generator.

age follower, which is also the bias voltage across the resistor, is programmed by the DAC. The output current is given by

$$I_{out} = \frac{V_{DAC}}{R} \tag{11.7}$$

where V_{DAC} is the output voltage of the DAC and R is the fixed resistance. However, controlling I_{out} by changing V_{DAC} is not desirable because it changes the voltage compliance of the current generator circuit.

It is known from Equation (11.7) that the output current is also reciprocally proportional to the resistance. Thus, a voltage-controlled resistor with a constant bias will also make a current generator. The voltage-controlled resistor is usually implemented by a MOS transistor in the triode region, as shown in Figure 11.30 [63].

This configuration yields a current generator circuit with a large constant voltage compliance. When the bias voltage V_{ref} is small, in the range of several hundreds mV, M_1 operates in deep triode region and its drain current may be given by

$$I_{D1} = \mu_0 C_{ox} \frac{W_1}{L_1}(V_{DAC} - V_T)V_{ref} \tag{11.8}$$

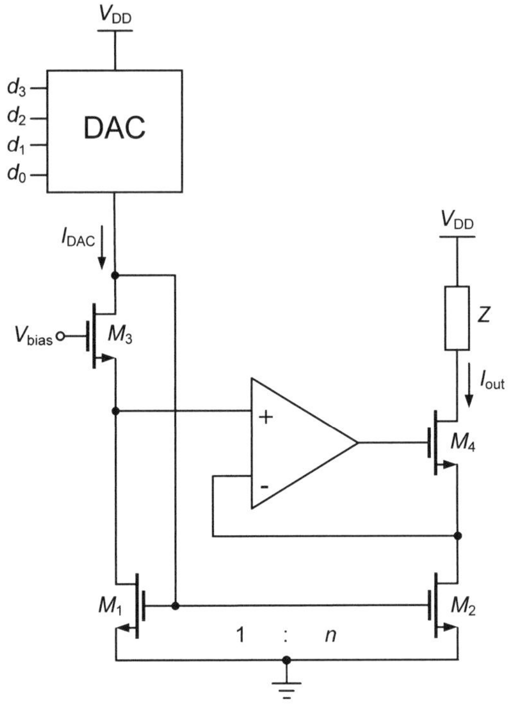

Figure 11.28 Stimulation with a current mirror employing active feedback to boost the output impedance. The input current is controlled by the current-mode DAC.

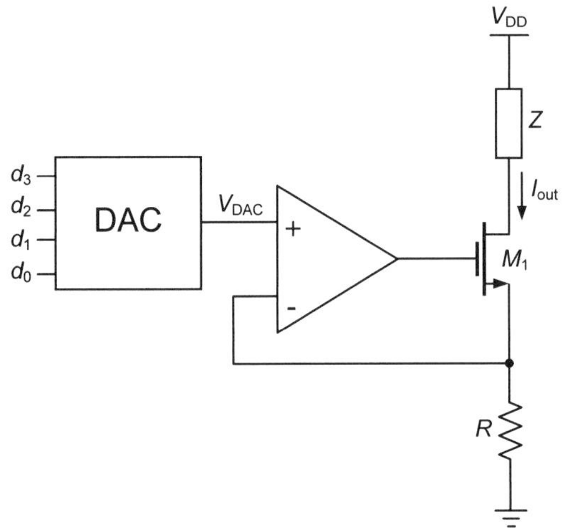

Figure 11.29 Stimulation with a voltage-to-current conversion circuit employing active feedback [74]. The output current is the ratio of the DAC output voltage over the fixed resistance.

which represents a linear resistor between the drain-source terminals equal to

$$R_{\text{DS1}} = \frac{1}{\mu C_{\text{ox}} \dfrac{W_1}{L_1} (V_{\text{DAC}} - V_T)} \tag{11.9}$$

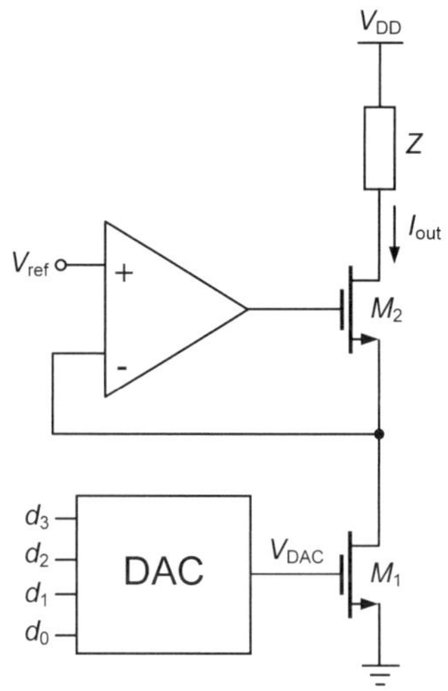

Figure 11.30 Stimulation with a current sink implemented by a voltage-controlled MOS resistor [63]. The active resistance is controlled by the voltage-mode DAC output.

However, at large gate-source voltages (i.e., for large V_{DAC}), mobility degradation due to the high vertical field cannot be neglected. To model this effect (in model level 3), the effective mobility is changed to

$$\mu_{eff} = \frac{\mu_0}{1+\theta(V_{DAC} - V_T)} \approx \mu_0[1-\theta(V_{DAC} - V_T)] \tag{11.10}$$

where μ_0 is the low-field mobility and θ is a fitting parameter; for the approximation in Equation (11.10) only the first two terms of the Taylor series expansion were retained. Because of the mobility degradation, the drain current will not be very linear to the overdrive voltage ($V_{DAC} - V_T$), especially for V_{DAC} values controlled by the most-significant bits of the DAC. This degrades the circuit's linearity, which may affect the charge balancing capability of the stimulator. To reduce nonlinearity, an extra current compensation circuit operating in the saturation region can be employed [63].

Table 11.1 compares the performance of various neural stimulator current generator circuits in terms of linearity, voltage compliance, output impedance, and silicon area.

Table 11.1 Comparison of Various Current Generator Circuits for Implantable Neural Stimulators

Current Generator	*Linearity*	*Output Impedance*	*Voltage Compliance*	*Silicon Area*
Binary-weighted transistors with single bias [59, 70, 71]	Low	Low	Medium	Medium
Identical transistors with binary-weighted bias [72]	Lowest	Medium	Small	Small
Active feedback [61]	High	High	Large	Medium
Voltage follower [74]	Medium	High	Large	Medium
Voltage-controlled resistor with analog DAC [63]	Medium	High	Large	Medium

11.7 Conclusion

This chapter has provided an introductory overview of recent advances in circuits and methods for implantable peripheral nerve recording and stimulation. The current research on neuroprosthetic implanted devices that interact with the nervous system is rapidly expanding. This provides an opportunity for collaborations among engineers, scientists, medical researchers, and practitioners to solve complex problems and to come up with technical innovations that can be applied to improve the health and quality of life of patients suffering from conditions such as spinal cord injury, incontinence, cochlear and retinal diseases, epilepsy, cerebral palsy, stroke, and multiple sclerosis, to name a few. As technology evolves, it is reasonable to expect that peripheral nerve neuroprostheses will advance more in the area of closed-loop "sense-and-stimulate."

References

[1] K.T. Ragnarsson, "Functional electrical stimulation after spinal cord injury: current use, therapeutic effects and future directions," *Spinal Cord*, September 2007.

[2] M. Sawan, H. Yamum, and J. Coulombe, "Wireless smart implants dedicated to multichannel monitoring and microstimulation," *IEEE Circuits Syst. Magazine*, vol. 5, no. 1, pp. 21–39, March 2005.

[3] M. Haugland, A. Lickel, J. Haase, and T. Sinkjaer, "Control of FES thump force using slip information obtained from the cutaneous electroneurogram in quadriplegic man," *IEEE Trans. Rehab. Eng.*, vol. 7, pp. 215–227, June 1999.

[4] L.A. Geddes and L.E. Baker, *Principles of Applied Biomedical Instrumentation.* John Wiley & Sons, 3rd edition, 1989.

[5] J.G. Webster, *Medical Instrumentation Application and Design.* Houghton Mifflin Company, 2nd edition, Boston, 1989.

[6] A.L. Hogkin and A.F. Huxley, "A quantitative description of membrane current and its application to conduction and excitation in nerve," *J. Physiol.*, vol. 117, no. 4, pp. 500–544, August 1952.

[7] I. Tasaki and G. Matsumoto, "On the cable theory of nerve conduction," *Bull. Math. Biol.*, vol. 64, no. 6, pp. 1069–1082, November 2002.

[8] M.S. Rahal, *Optimisation of Nerve Cuff Electrode Recordings for Functional Electrical Stimulation Applications.* Ph.D. thesis, Dept. Electronic & Electrical Eng., University College London, London, U.K., 2000.

[9] B.M. Bugbee, *An Implantable Stimulator for Selective Stimulation of Nerves.* Ph.D. thesis, Dept. Medical Physics & Bioeng., University College London, London, 2000.

[10] J. Malmivuo and R. Plonsey, *Bioelectromagnetism: Principles and Applications of Bioelectric and Biomagnetic Fields.* Oxford University Press, New York, 1995, ch. 22.

[11] W.L.C. Rutten, "Selective electrical interfaces with the nervous system," *Annu. Rev. Biomed. Eng.*, vol. 4, pp. 407–452, August 2002.

[12] K. P. Koch, "Neural prostheses and biomedical microsystems in neurological rehabilitation," *Acta Neurochir. Suppl.*, 97(Pt 1), pp. 427–434, 2007.

[13] J.J. Struijk, M. Thomsen, J.O. Larsen, and T. Sinkjaer, "Cuff electrodes for long-term recording of natural sensory information," *IEEE Eng. Med. Biol. Mag.*, vol. 18, pp. 91–98, May/June 1999.

[14] R.B. Stein, D. Charles, L. Davis, J. Jhamandas, A. Mannard, and T.R. Nichols, "Principles underlying new methods for chronic neural recording," *Can. J. Neurol. Sci.*, vol. 2, no. 3, pp. 235–244, 1975.

[15] G.G. Naples, J.T. Mortimer, A. Scheiner, and J.D. Sweeney, "A spiral nerve cuff electrode for peripheral nerve stimulation," *IEEE Trans. Biomed. Eng.*, vol. 35, no. 11, pp. 905–916, November 1988.

[16] K. Kallesoe, J.A. Hoffer, and K. Strange, *Implantable Cuff Having Improved Closure*. U.S. patent # 5,487,756, 1996.

[17] L.N.S. Andreasen and J.J. Struijk, "On the importance of configuration and closure of nerve cuff electrodes for recording," *Proc. EMBS'98*, vol. 6, Hong Kong, pp. 3004–3007, 1998.

[18] J.A. Hoffer, "Techniques to study spinal-cord, peripheral nerve, and muscle activity in freely moving animals," in *Neuromethods*, vol. 15: Neurophysiological Techniques: Application of Neural Systems, A.A. Boulton, G.B. Baker, and C.H. Vanderwolf, editors, Humana Press, pp. 65–145, 1990.

[19] J.J. Struijk, "The extracellular potential of a myelinated nerve fiber in an unbounded medium and in nerve cuff models," *Biophys. J.*, vol. 72, no. 6, pp. 2457–2469, June 1997.

[20] R.B. Stein, T.R. Nichols, J. Jhamanda, L. Davis, and D. Charles, "Stable long-term recordings from cat peripheral nerves," *Brain Res.*, vol. 128, no. 1, pp. 21–38, June 1977.

[21] I.F. Triantis, *An Adaptive Amplifier for Cuff Imbalance Correction and Interference Reduction in Nerve Signal Recording*. Ph.D. thesis, Dept. Electronic & Electrical Eng., University College London, London, U.K., 2005.

[22] Z.M. Nicolic, B.D. Popovic, B.R. Stein, and Z. Kenwell, "Instrumentation for ENG and EMG recordings in FES systems," *IEEE Trans. Biomed. Eng.*, vol. 41, no. 7, pp. 703–706, July 1994.

[23] J. Struijk and M. Thomsen, "Tripolar nerve cuff recording: stimulus artifact, EMG, and the recorded nerve signal," *Proc. 17th Int. Conf. IEEE-EMBS (EMBS'95)*, Montreal, Canada, vol. 2, pp. 1105–1106, 1995.

[24] M. Rahal, J. Taylor, and N. Donaldson, "The effect of nerve cuff geometry on interference reduction: a study by computer modelling," *IEEE Trans. Biomed. Eng.*, vol. 47, no. 1, pp. 136–138, January 2000.

[25] I.F. Triantis and A. Demosthenous, "The effect of interference source proximity on cuff imbalance," *IEEE Trans. Biomed. Eng.*, vol. 53, no. 2, pp. 354–357, February 2006.

[26] I. Pachnis, A. Demosthenous, and N. Donaldson, "Passive neutralization of myoelectric interference from neural recording tripoles," *IEEE Trans. Biomed. Eng.*, vol. 54, no. 6, pp. 1067–1074, June 2007.

[27] C. Pflaum, R. Riso, and G. Wiesspeiner, "An improved nerve cuff recording configuration for FES feedback control systems that utilise natural sensors," *Proc IFESS'95*, Vienna, Austria, pp. 407–410, 1995.

[28] A. Demosthenous and I.F. Triantis, "An adaptive ENG amplifier for tripolar cuff electrodes," *IEEE J. Solid-State Circuits*, vol. 40, no. 2, pp. 412–421, February 2005.

[29] E.A.M. Klumperink, S.L.J. Gierkink, A.P. van der Wel, and B. Nauta, "Reducing MOSFET 1/f noise and power consumption by switched biasing," *IEEE J. Solid-State Circuits*, vol. 35, no. 7, pp. 994–1001, July 2000.

[30] B. Dierickx and E. Simoen, "The decrease of 'random telegraph signal' noise in metal-oxide-semiconductors when cycled from inversion to accumulation," *J. Applied Physics*, vol. 71, no. 4, pp. 2028–2029, February 1992.

[31] C.C. Enz, E.A. Vittoz, and F. Krummenacher, "A CMOS chopper amplifier," *IEEE J. Solid-State Circuits*, vol. SC-22, no. 3, pp. 335–342, June 1987.

[32] A. Harb, Y. Hu, M. Sawan, A. Abdelkerim, and M.M. Elhilali, "Low-power CMOS interface for recording and processing very low amplitude signals," *Analog Int. Circuits Signal Proc.*, vol. 39, no. 1, pp. 39–54, April 2004.

[33] A. Uranga, X. Navarro, and N. Barniol, "Integrated CMOS amplifier for ENG signal recording," *IEEE Trans. Biomed. Eng.*, vol. 51, no. 12, pp. 2188–2194, December 2004.

[34] J. Neilsen and E. Bruun, "A CMOS low-noise instrumentation amplifier using chopper modulation," *Analog Int. Circuits Signal Proc.*, vol. 42, no. 1, pp. 65–76, January 2005.

[35] R. F. Yazicioglu, P. Merken, R. Puers, and C. Van Hoof, "A 60μW 60nV/√Hz readout front-end for portable biopotential acquisition systems," *IEEE J. Solid-State Circuits*, vol. 42, no. 5, pp. 1100–1110, May 2007.

[36] C.C. Enz and E.A. Vittoz, "Circuit techniques for reducing the effects of op-amp imperfections: autoeroing, correlated double sampling, and chopper stabilization," *Proc. IEEE*, vol. 84, no. 11, pp. 1584–1614, November 1996.

[37] R.R. Harrison and C. Charles, "A low-power low-noise CMOS amplifier for neural recording applications," *IEEE J. Solid-State Circuits*, vol. 38, no. 6, pp. 958–965, June 2003.

[38] B. Gosselin, A.E. Ayoub, and M. Sawan, "A low-power bioamplifier with a new active rejection scheme," *Proc. ISCAS'06*, Kos Island, Greece, pp. 2185–2189, 2006.

[39] R. Rieger, *Implantable Analogue Circuits for Improved Methods of Nerve Signal Recording*. Ph.D. thesis, Dept. Electronic & Electrical Eng., University College London, London, U.K., 2004.

[40] P. Langlois, J. Taylor, and A. Demosthenous, "Realization of a simple high-value grounded linear resistance in CMOS technology," *Proc. ESSCIRC'05*, Grenoble, France, pp. 383–386, 2005.

[41] R. Rieger, M. Schuettler, D. Pal, C. Clarke, P. Langlois, J. Taylor, and N. Donaldson, "Very low-noise ENG amplifier system using CMOS technology," *IEEE Neural Syst. Rehab. Eng.*, vol. 14, no. 4, pp. 427–437, December 2006.

[42] A.S. Sedra and K.C. Smith, *Mictroelectronic Circuits*. Oxford University Press, New York, 4th Edition, 2003.

[43] M. Degrauwe, E. Vittoz, and I. Verbauwhede, "A micropower CMOS-instrumentation amplifier," *IEEE J. Solid-State Circuits*, vol. SC-20, no. 3, pp. 805–807, June 1985.

[44] A.P. Brokaw and M.P. Timko, "An improved monolithic instrumentation amplifier," *IEEE J. Solid-State Circuits*, vol. SC-10, no. 6, pp. 417–423, December 1975.

[45] M.S.J. Steyaert and W.M.C. Sansen, "A micropower low-noise monolithic instrumentation amplifier for medical purposes," *IEEE J. Solid-State Circuits*, vol. SC-22, no. 6, pp. 1163–1168, December 1987.

[46] S.K. Kelly and J. Wyatt, "A power-efficient voltage-based neural tissue stimulator with energy recovery," *ISSCC'04 Dig. Tech. Papers*, San Francisco, CA, vol. 1, pp. 228–524, 2004.

[47] M. Ghovanloo, "Switched-capacitor based implantable low-power wireless microstimulating systems," *Proc. ISCAS'06*, Kos Island, Greece, pp. 2197–2200, 2006.

[48] R.K. Shepherd, J. Matsushima, R.E. Millard, and G.M. Clark, "Cochlear pathology following chronic electrical stimulation using non charge balanced stimuli," *Acta Otolaryngol*, vol. 111, vol. 5, pp. 848–860, 1991.

[49] T. Cameron, T.L. Liinamaa, G.E. Loeb, and F.J.R. Richmond, "Long-term biocompatibility of a miniature stimulator implanted in feline hind limb muscles," *IEEE Trans. Biomed. Eng.*, vol. 45, no. 8, pp. 1024–1035, Aug. 1998.

[50] P.R. Singh, *Micro-Stimulator Design for Retinal Prostheses*. M.Sc. thesis, North Carolina State University, USA, 2002.

[51] T. Klenzner, F. Knapp, F. Rohner, E. von Wallenberg, H. Mauch, P. Pedersen, A. Aschendorff, R. Laszig, and J. Lutterbach, "Influence of ionizing radiation on nucleus 24 cochlear implants," *Otol. & Neurotol.*, vol. 26, no. 4, pp. 661–667, July 2005.

[52] M.A. Khalil and C.L. Wey, "High-voltage stress test paradigms of analog CMOS ICs for gate-oxide reliability enhancement," *Proc. 19th IEEE VLSI Test Symp. (VTS'01)*, Marina Del Rey, CA, pp. 333–338, 2001.

[53] C.Q. Huang, R.K. Shepherd, P.M. Center, P.M. Seligman, and B. Tabor, "Electrical stimulation of the auditory nerve: direct current measurement in vivo," *IEEE Trans. Biomed. Eng.*, vol. 46, no. 4, pp. 461–469, April 1999.

[54] N. de N. Donaldson and P.E.K. Donaldson, "When are actively balanced biphasic ('Lilly') stimulating pulses necessary in a neurological prosthesis? II. pH changes; noxious products; electrode corrosion; discussion," *Med. Biol. Eng. Comput.*, vol. 24, no. 1, pp. 50–56, January 1986.

[55] D.L. Guyton and F.T. Hambrecht, "Capacitor electrode stimulates nerve or muscle without oxidation-reduction reactions," *Science*, vol. 181, no. 4094, pp. 74–76, July 1973.

[56] C. Donfack, M. Sawan, and Y. Savaria, "Implantable measurement technique dedicated to the monitoring of electrode-nerve contact in bladder stimulators," *Med. Biol. Eng. Comput.*, vol. 38, no. 4, pp. 465–468, July 2000.

[57] M. Schwarz and M. Maschmann, "Area saving stimulator cells for multielectrode arrays featuring adaptive waveform generation and monitoring," *Proc. 26th Annu. Int. Conf. IEEE Engineering in Medicine and Biology Society*, vol. 2, pp. 4314–4317, 2004.

[58] D. Hou, A. Asres, Z. Zhou, and Z. Zhu, "Stimulator for real time control of paralyzed muscles during functional electrical stimulation," *Proc. ICECS '96*, Rodos, Greece, vol. 2, pp. 1096–1099, 1996.

[59] M. Sivaprakasam, W. Liu, G. Wang, J.D. Weiland, and M.S. Humayun, "Architecture tradeoffs in high-density microstimulators for retinal prosthesis," *IEEE Trans. Circuits Syst. I: Reg. Papers*, vol. 52, no. 12, pp. 2629–2641, December 2005.

[60] X. Liu, A. Demosthenous, and N. Donaldson, "A Safe transmission strategy for power and data recovery in biomedical implanted devices," *Proc. ISCAS'07*, New Orleans, LA, pp. 2367–2370, 2007.

[61] M. Sivaprakasam, W. Liu, M.S. Humayun, and J.D. Weiland, "A variable range bi-phasic current stimulus driver circuitry for an implantable retinal prosthetic device," *IEEE J. Solid-State Circuits*, vol. 40, no. 3, pp. 763–771, March 2005.

[62] C.M. Zierhofer, I.J. Hochmair-Desoyer, and E.S. Hochmair, "Electronic design of a cochlear implant for multichannel high-rate pulsatile stimulation strategies," *IEEE Trans. Neural Syst. Rehabil. Eng*, vol. 3, no. 1, pp. 112–116, March 1995.

[63] M. Ghovanloo and K. Najafi, "A compact large voltage-compliance high output-impedance programmable current source for implantable microstimulators," *IEEE Trans. Biomed. Eng.*, vol. 52, no. 1, pp. 97–105, January 2005.

[64] X. Liu and A. Demosthenous, "Generation of balanced biphasic stimulus current with integrated blocking capacitor," *Proc. ECCTD'05*, Cork, Ireland, vol. 3, pp. 19–22, 2005.

[65] X. Liu, A. Demosthenous, and N. Donaldson, "A stimulator output stage with capacitor reduction and failure-checking techniques," *Proc. ISCAS'06*, Kos Island, Greece, pp. 641–644, 2006.

[66] X. Liu, A. Demosthenous, and N. Donaldson, "A fully integrated fail-safe stimulator output stage dedicated to FES stimulation," *Proc. ISCAS'07*, New Orleans, LA, pp. 2076–2079, 2007.

[67] J.D. Techer, S. Bernard, Y. Bertrand, G. Cathebras, and D. Guiraud, "New implantable stimulator for the FES of paralyzed muscles," *Proc. ESSCIRC'04*, Leuven, Belgium, pp. 455–458, 2004.

[68] B. Ziaie, M.D. Nardin, A.R. Coghlan, and K. Najafi, "A single-channel implantable microstimulator for functional neuromuscular stimulation," *IEEE Trans. Biomed. Eng.*, vol. 44, no. 10, pp. 909–920, October 1997.

[69] G. Gudnason, E. Bruun, and M. Haugland, "An implantable mixed analog/digital neural stimulator circuit," *Proc. ISCAS'99*, Orlando, Florida, vol. 5, pp. 375–378, 1999.

[70] W. Liu, K. Vichienchom, M. Clements, S.C. DeMarco, C. Hughes, E. McGucken, M.S. Humayun, E. De Juan, J.D. Weiland, and R. Greenberg, "A neuro-stimulus chip with

telemetry unit for retinal prosthetic device," *IEEE J. Solid-State Circuits*, vol. 35, no. 10, pp. 1487–1497, October 2000.

[71] K. Arabi and M.A. Sawan, "Electronic design of a multichannel programmable implant for neuromuscular electrical stimulation," *IEEE Trans. Neural Syst. Rehab. Eng.*, vol. 7, no. 2, pp. 204–214, June 1999.

[72] S.C. DeMarco, W. Liu, P.R. Singh, G. Lazzi, M.S. Humayun, and J.D. Weiland, "An arbitrary waveform stimulus circuit for visual prostheses using a low-area multibias DAC," *IEEE J. Solid-State Circuits*, vol. 38, no. 10, pp. 1679–1690, October 2003.

[73] K.E. Jones and R.A. Normann, "An advanced demultiplexing system for physiological stimulation," *IEEE Trans. Biomed. Eng.*, vol. 44, no. 12, pp. 1210–1220, December 1997.

[74] S. Boyer, M. Sawan, M. Abdel-Gawad, S. Robin, and M.M. Elhilali, "Implantable selective stimulator to improve bladder voiding: design and chronic experiments in dogs," *IEEE Trans. Neural Syst. Rehab. Eng.*, vol. 8, no. 4, pp. 464–470, December 2000.

CHAPTER 12

Neuromimetic Integrated Circuits

Timothée Levi, Noëlle Lewis, Sylvain Saighi, Jean Tomas, Yannick Bornat, and Sylvie Renaud

12.1 Introduction and Application Domain

This chapter presents the design of neuromimetic integrated circuits. These ICs are used in biomedical applications, and more particularly in the neurosciences. Computational neurosciences are a field of neurosciences dedicated to the modeling and exploration of neural networks. It relies commonly on software processing tools, but hardware-based solutions also exist to emulate neural networks. In Spiking Neural Networks (SNN), the information is encoded in the timing of the neurons' activity events (these events, named "spikes," correspond to electrical discharges that travel across the neuron membrane). In SNN, neuron models are chosen to describe the biophysics of spikes by computing the dynamics of the ionic currents flowing through the cell membrane. While software-based SNN can be configured for different types of models, hardware-based SNN are dedicated to a given type of models. The computational core of those systems consists of "neuromimetics ICs," i.e., integrated circuits specifically designed to reproduce the electrical activity of a nervous cell. In this chapter, we focus on the design of such circuits, which emulate parts of, or whole SNN. Most circuits present an analog core, in charge of the emulation of the electrical activity of the neurons. After a presentation of the possible models at the neuron and network levels, we list the possible architectures of ICs. The neuromimetic ICs can be dimensioned to run in biological absolute or average real time, they can also run an accelerated neural activity. Four versions of ASICs modeling conductance-based neurons and synapses are detailed; they represent different versions and architectures that depend on the applicative environment.

Hardware-based SNN are used in two types of experiments:

Experiments on hybrid living-artificial neural networks. In that case, they represent the artificial part, connected via artificial synapses to intra- or extra-cellular electrodes to a living neural network. This latter can consist of an in vitro or in vivo assembly of neurons. The living-artificial system is helpful for the exploration of the network as a whole, and for the characterization of its components. The artificial neurons can also be designedz to replace missing or altered cells.

In those experiments, real-time processing is mandatory to ensure a correct dialog between living and artificial neurons. Analog IC computation simplifies the communication between the circuits and the living neurons, as the electrodes measure an analog signal on the living cells and are also analog-controlled.

Experiments on artificial SNN. Such experiments exploit the hardware-based simulation tools in a way similar to the exploitation of software tools. The additional value of hardware is here the computation speed. Hardware computation is an efficient solution that can be used to implement the parallel computation stream, just by repeating circuitry on the ASIC. Analog circuitry computes non-linear functions by using the intrinsic voltage-current relationships of active components such as transistors.

Neuromimetic ICs present interesting features when designing artificial SNN. Such circuits are now frequently designed for multi-disciplinary projects, when a close-to-biology emulation of neural networks is necessary. However, this field is still in an emerging phase, and there is no doubt that it will benefit from the constant evolution of technology in microelectronics.

We present in a first section the neurons' possible models, corresponding to different levels of biological relevance. These models are implemented in hardware-based simulation platforms. We review the actual platforms based on analog neuromimetic ICs, and explain the possible design strategies of those ASICs, including IP-based synthesis solutions. Finally, we detail the implementation of a family of ASICs computing in biological real-time conductance-based models of small neural networks with dynamically adaptive synapses.

12.2 Neuron Models for Different Computation Levels of SNNs

12.2.1 Cell Level

In a biological neuron, ionic species with different concentrations of ions co-exist inside (soma) and outside the neuron membrane. The ionic currents flowing through the membrane are the support of the neuron electrical activity. Ionic currents are summed with the synaptic currents on the membrane capacitance to form the membrane potential (V_{mem}). A spiking neuron presents a V_{mem} composed of small pulses with a non-linear shape (*spikes*), which propagate along the axon and are transmitted to other neurons through synaptic nodes (see Figure 12.1). Models of spiking neurons reproduce the electrical activity of a neural element (soma, dendrite, axon, synapse) with a special attention to the dynamics of ionic or synaptic currents [Koch], [Gerstner].

Different families of models can be considered for the neuron models in SNN systems. Most models are point neuron models, in which a neuron is a single computational element, as opposed to compartmental models, which take into account the cells' morphology. Different levels of abstraction are also possible to describe point neuron models. One can focus on the properties of each ionic channel or prefer to choose a behavioral description. The user needs to select his model by finding an acceptable compromise between two contradictory criteria: faithfully reproduce the dynamics of V_{mem} and minimize the computational load on the simulation system.

12.2.1.1 Conductance-Based Models

In the most detailed family of models, known as conductance-based models, the neuron membrane is represented by a capacitor charged by the ionic and synaptic cur-

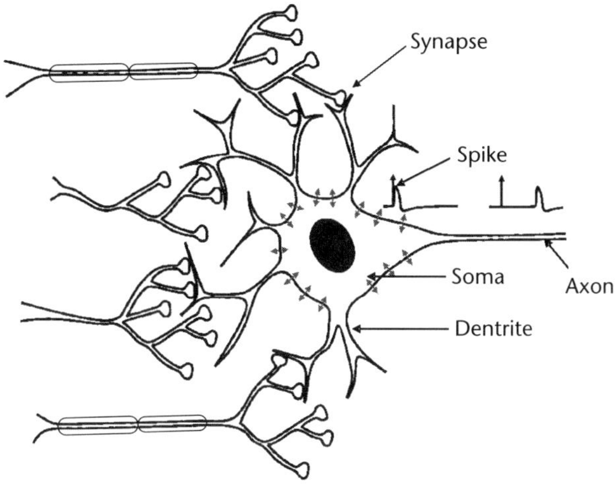

Figure 12.1 Anatomical description of a biological neuron.

rents [Gerstner], as described on Figure 12.2. All of these models find their origins in the Hodgkin & Huxley model (HH) [HH]. Each ionic channel (Sodium: Na, Potassium: K, leak, . . .) is represented by a time- and voltage-dependent conductance: this electrophysiological description makes these models particularly well-suited to an implementation involving analog electronics. The time-dependence traduces the kinetics of activation/inactivation process of the ionic channel. The hardware implementation uses intrinsic current-voltage dependence of transistors to implement those nonlinear relationships and specific circuitry for the kinetics (first-order differential equation).

Hodgkin-Huxley derived models have the same structure and include more or less the types of ion channels that enable the diversity of biological neurons to be suitably represented (see Figure 12.2).

Conductance-based models reduced to 2 dimensions are also very popular, as they can be entirely characterized using phase plane analysis. We can mention FitzHugh-Nagumo (FN) and Morris-Lecar models [FitzHugh], [Morris].

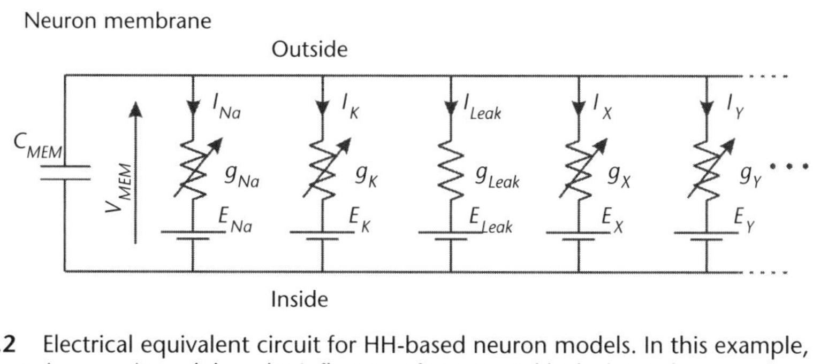

Figure 12.2 Electrical equivalent circuit for HH-based neuron models. In this example, additional conductances (x, y, . . .) modulate the influence of Na, K, and leak channels.

12.2.1.2 Threshold Type Models

Another class of models are the threshold-type models that reproduce, at a higher level of abstraction, the threshold effect in the initiation of an action potential. The shape of V_{mem} is not reproduced here, as ionic currents are no longer processed. These models are adjusted by fitting the firing time of the spikes and the threshold level. These phenomenological models are interesting in terms of computation cost, and are dedicated to the studies of neural coding and large network dynamics, as they are not precise at the neuron level. The Integrate-and-Fire model (IF) and Spike Response Model (SRM) belong to this family [Gerstner]. The Leaky Integrate-and-Fire model (LIF), which is able to compute the timing of spikes, is widely used for hardware SNN implementations (see Figure 12.3).

The LIF model computes V_{mem} on a capacitor, in parallel with a leaky resistor and an input current. When V_{mem} reaches a threshold voltage, the neuron fires and its dynamics are neutralized during an absolute refractory period [Gerstner]. From the hardware point of view, specific circuitry must implement the voltage comparison and the reset process. From the classical LIF, many extensions have been proposed [Gerstner], [Izhikevich], [Brette].

12.2.2 Network Level

The dynamics of a SNN and the formation of connectivity patterns are governed by synaptic plasticity [Koch]. In the structure of SNN, the synaptic weights w_{ij} (connection from neuron j to i) are the support of plasticity and can vary over the time, according to certain rules. A synapse can be reinforced (increase of w_{ij}), following a long-term potentiation (LTP) process, or can be weakened (decrease of w_{ij}), following a long-term depression (LTD) process. The procedure for adjusting the weights is the *learning rule*. The most classical and widely used learning rules are *Hebbian rules*, in the sense that synaptic changes are driven by correlated activity of pre- and post-synaptic neurons.

Among those learning rules, Spike-Timing Dependent Plasticity (STDP) algorithms [Gerstner] are often used in hardware-based SNN. Figure 12.4 illustrates the principle of standard STDP: when a post-synaptic spike arises after a pre-synaptic spike ($\delta t > 0$), the connection is reinforced ($\delta w > 0$), whereas in the opposite case it is weakened. When implemented on hardware, STDP leads to significant computational cost and requires a dynamic control of the synaptic connectivity [Badoual].

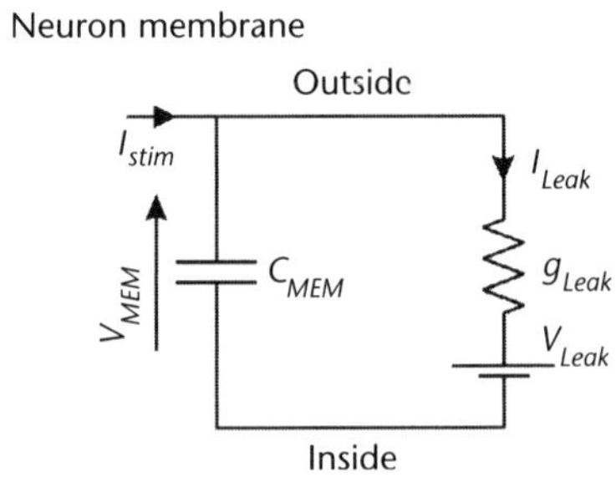

Figure 12.3 Electrical equivalent circuit of LIF neuron model.

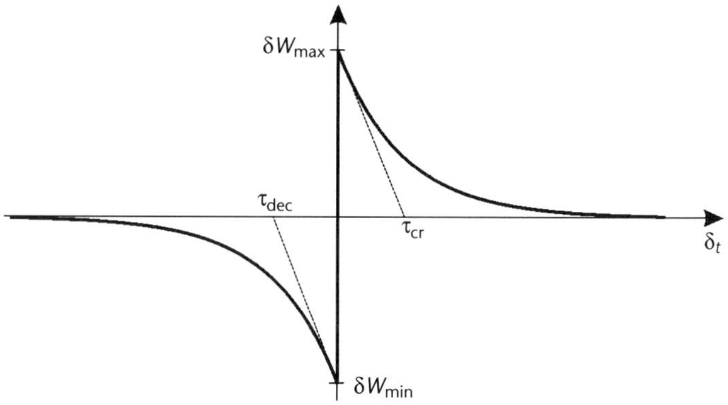

Figure 12.4 Variation of synaptic weight δW from neuron j (pre-synaptic) to i (post-synaptic), as a function of the time interval δt between t_i (post-synaptic spike) and t_j (pre-synaptic spike).

For large-scale networks, the connectivity between neurons becomes a critical issue and all-to-all adaptive connectivity may be impossible.

12.3 State of the Art of Hardware-Based SNN

As mentioned in the introduction, SNN can be implemented either onto software or hardware supports. Some dedicated software tools are well-known [Hines] and often used as a reference, but have the drawback of requiring prohibitively long computation times when it comes to simulating large or complex neural networks. Hardware-based SNN are developed around a neuromimetic IC and may contain additional software functionalities.

12.3.1 System Constraints and Computation Distribution

The whole system architecture is constrained by the application field and is closely related to the model choice. Applications can be purely artificial experiments—especially investigations on adaptation and plasticity phenomena on networks—or experiments on hybrid biological/artificial networks. The neuron models, which are very accurate and close to biology, require a high computation cost when they are digitally implemented. For this reason, many SNN solutions use analog cores at the lowest level of the network, thereby taking advantage of the natural parallel processing of neurons activities. Hence, one important issue is the optimal partition between analog and digital hardware, and between hardware and software processing.

12.3.2 Existing Solutions

During the last 15 years, few hardware-based SNN systems were developed: we list the most representative or more recently developed platforms, as well as pioneer platforms ([Mahowald], [Jung], [LeMasson]). Those systems make use of multi-compartmental [Hasler], point neuron conductance-based [Mahowald], [LeMasson], [Sorensen], [Binczak], [Renaud] or threshold-type models [Jung], [Liu], [Vogelstein],

[Glackin], [Indiveri], [Schemmel] of SNN, and simulate single neurons, small or large networks. Some platforms can be used for hybrid network experiments [Jung], [LeMasson], [Sorensen]. Figure 12.5 illustrates the level of neuron modeling and processing material used in these systems.

All presented SNN are partially or entirely implemented on hardware. Only one platform is a fully digital hardware system [Glackin], using FPGAs (Field Programmable Gate Array) for large-scale SNN topologies. Many processor cores are embedded in those FPGAs with a variable degree of parallelism in the distribution of computation.

All other solutions use analog hardware computation at the neuron level and even for plasticity. The simulated neural element can be either integrated on a single chip or distributed on multiple chips, due to integration constraints. The analog integrated circuits implement the models described previously (LIF, FN, HH). We labeled SHH the HH-inspired models in which some of the conductance functions are simplified or fitted, as opposed to the complete Hodgkin-Huxley description of non-linear and voltage- and time-dependent ionic conductances.

In the analog mode implementation, the signals are available as continuous variables, both in time and value. As a consequence, the simulation time scale can be precisely fixed (real-time or accelerated). In the case of real time (electrical time = biological time) and with biologically relevant neuron models, it is possible to construct mixed living-artificial networks, where the silicon neurons are interconnected with the biological cells to form "hybrid networks." Digital design presents a much lower fabrication cost, including a better time-to-market performance, and an easy re-configurability. But analog SNN can present two main advantages: a higher integration density, as one wire encodes one signal (instead of N wires to represent a N-bits digital signal) and a higher computational power.

For large-scale SNN, it may be interesting to accelerate the simulation of one or more orders of magnitude [Schemmel], in order to fasten simulation on large SNN.

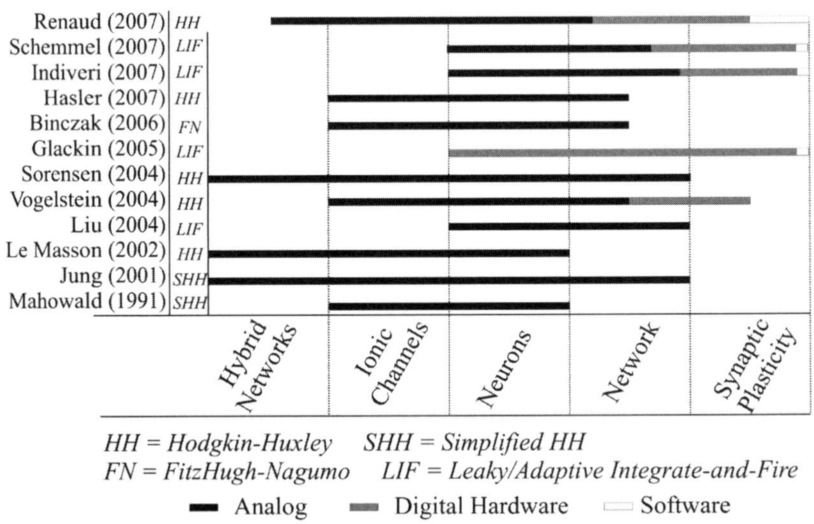

Figure 12.5 Neuron models and computation support in reviewed SNN systems.

For those applications, LIF neuron models are generally implemented as simple analog cells simulating a point neuron.

However, when the system reaches the network level or integrates plasticity rules, the digital hardware is the preferred support, for the connectivity computation and/or control. It becomes an efficient interface to the layer implanting the plasticity (hardware or software), through event-based protocols. More and more neuromimetic systems will present such mixed Analog/Digital architectures, as shown in Figure 12.5. The architecture of SNN platforms will finally be a compromise between the computational cost and the model complexity, which also constraints the achievable network size.

12.4 Criteria for Design Strategies of Neuromimetic ICs

This section presents the different design strategies for neuromimetic ICs. Different criteria have to be considered for defining the architecture and content of a neuromimetic IC. They are closely linked to the applicative field of the hardware neurons. We present here different design solutions: specific or generic mathematical operators, monosynapses or multisynapses, small or large networks, CMOS or BiCMOS technology. Then we describe an IP-based design method for a systematic evaluation of the solutions.

12.4.1 Specific or Generic Mathematical Operators

The Hodgkin-Huxley formalism has no analytic solution; thus, to calculate the membrane potential, numerical techniques are necessary. The analog circuits design requires more than six months time from scratch to test. Therefore, before starting the design of a new analog neuromimetic ASIC, we must define some criteria:

- The biological cell model (number of ionic channels, parameters of each ionic channel);
- The goal of the system development (parameters need to be tunable or could be fixed).

The number of applications for neuromimetic circuits grows exponentially: learning and plasticity study in neural networks, vision and audition prosthesis, epilepsy treatment, Parkinson treatment, etc. For that, the best solution is to design a library of the generic mathematical operators that are present in the Hodgkin-Huxley formalism. With the previous description (see the description of the cell level in Section 12.2.1), we can represent in Figure 12.6 the generic ionic current generator.

The repetition of mathematical operations within each ionic channel is an advantage for systematic developments of neuromimetic circuits if the circuitry allows each mathematical function to receive tunable parameters. The specifications of the mathematical functions must be set in collaboration with neuroscientists. This solution presents the best flexibility (design of a novel ASIC based on Hodgkin-Huxley formalism in a few weeks), but it is to the detriment of a more complex original design.

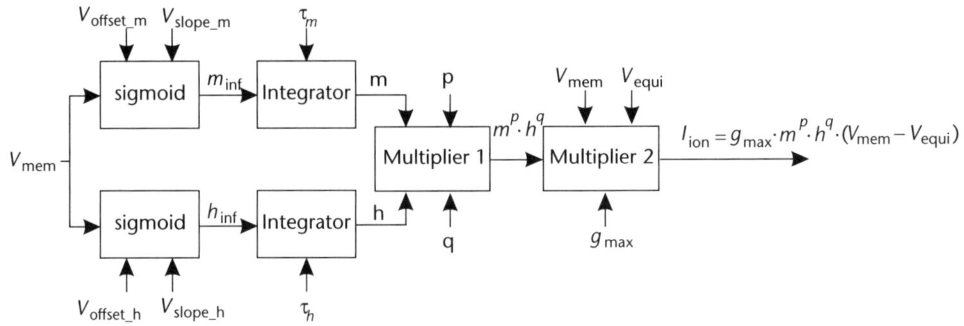

Figure 12.6 Generic ionic current generator for the Hodgkin-Huxley formalism.

12.4.2 Monosynapses or Multisynapses

Anyone who designs neuromimetic ICs for neural networks must pay particular attention to synapses: they are responsible for the dynamics in the information transmission within the network. A synapse model may only be relevant for a given category of SNN. We will not detail here all the models for synaptic transmission, but present the general principles and detail the most adapted to conductance-based neurons.

Synapse models are divided into 2 categories: monosynapses and multisynapses.

The *monosynapse model* is the most bio-realistic one. It consists in an ionic channel, which depends on both presynaptic and postsynaptic membrane potential. Presynaptic membrane voltage dependency may be very accurate (action potential shape and kinetics) to basic (action potential events). It can also include kinetics that reflects short-term plasticity effects (like saturation, delay modulation, etc.). However, such models need one hardware ionic channel for each incoming connection. Connectivity and size of the network depend of neuromimetic ICs' ability to receive large numbers of connections. This solution also requires a lot of silicon surface, which increases technical issues and production costs.

The *multisynapse model* is based on the statement that, in first approximation, all synaptic currents present an almost instantaneous positive step at the time of a presynaptic stimulation, and then decrease slowly following an exponential shape. Thanks to the exponential functions' properties, it is possible to express the current summation for synapses having the same decreasing kinetic into a single mathematical equation [Destexhe]. This cumulative current can therefore be implemented as a single function named multisynapse. Each function represents the sum of postsynaptic currents from a sub-ensemble of synapses of the same type (excitatory or inhibitory). With this model, IC designers only need to implement one multisynapse for each set of model parameters (V_{EQUI}, τ, etc.). The number of synaptic inputs (corresponding for the neuromimetic IC to a number of connections or a number of I/O pads) no longer limits the maximal size of the SNN. However, this solution has other consequences on the final network.

- Synaptic current response is standardized; then, it is less dependent on presynaptic spike characteristics.

- Presynaptic data from different neurons have to be multiplexed on the same input; it means that digital resources are required, with mixed circuits issues.
- A multisynapse loses all interest if we consider the origin of the incoming action potential. As a result, it is no more possible to compute short-term plasticity phenomenon. Therefore, computation of adaptation takes place in the network structures.

The simplest monosynapse uses the form:

$$G_{syn} = A_i \exp((t_i - t)/\tau)$$

where t_i and A_i are defined between events i and i+1.

But any function may be used like f(t) = t*exp(–t/tau). The only constraint is that, for each A, ta, B and tb, there is a C and tc so that: A f(t–ta) + B f(t–tb) = C f (t–tc). Thanks to this rule, it is only necessary to modify coefficients to take a new connection into account.

The choice of synaptic model depends on the size of the targeted neural network. For small networks, scientists need a very high accuracy to biology, and the designer should expect simulations focused on diversity. Monosynapses are interesting in the sense that they provide only one parameter for each connection and do not really need any architecture; a permanent wire is sufficient, weight is a parameter of the synapse, and a null weight codes no connection at all. On bigger networks, it is not interesting (or possible) to tune as many parameters per neuron anymore, the number of presynaptic neuron per synaptic type increases, and multisynapses become more interesting.

12.4.3 IC Flexibility vs. Network Specifications

We just saw that isolated artificial neurons have different interests depending on the size of the targeted network. For a small network simulation, users will focus on variability among neurons, and biological accuracy. For a bigger network, users will rather focus on plasticity or phenomenon at the network scale; in this case, a wide range of parameters for each neuron is not necessary. For extended networks, the user takes cell models from a limited number of standard types.

Designers have to strike a balance between full customizable models and predefined ones. On polyvalent circuits, parameters management takes a lot of development time. However, efforts on parameters also concern the system. An artificial neural network mixes two networks: a logical (simulated) network of neurons, and a physical network of ICs. To manage a high number of parameters, this physical network will require specific ICs and system complexity will be increased.

12.4.4 CMOS or BICMOS Technology

For the design of our ASICs, we can choose CMOS or BiCMOS technology. Most of our ASICs are made in BiCMOS technology. There is a main reason for that. Indeed, as we see in Figure 12.6, the ionic current is composed of a sigmoid function. The equation of this function is an exponential one. That is why a circuit using bipolar transistor (exponential equation) instead of CMOS transistor (quadratic equation) could easily create this function. Some experiments were made using a quadratic function in CMOS technology instead of the sigmoid function. Results are positive, but for the moment, no tests in silicium have been made.

To conclude, the BiCMOS technology is more appropriate for the design of our neuromimetic ASICs. However, there is one exception; the ASIC "Delphine" was made with the CMOS transistor under threshold. This ASIC will be presented later, and its advantages and its drawbacks will be mentioned.

12.4.5 IP-Based Design

The main objective of this part is to improve the design flow of these neuromimetic integrated circuits. The idea is to re-use the accumulated design knowledge that could be illustrated by the IP (Intellectual Property) concept. Then we organize these IPs to create a data base and we use it as a platform of automatic design.

12.4.5.1 Analog IP

This IP should give a precise characterization of already designed block; and it has to be described with adequate representations or models to enable the easy re-use of the block, along the complete design flow.

Table 12.1 shows the different descriptions (or *views*) that are embedded in our IP blocks. All these views have the same terminals and the same symbol.

For the *connectical*, *functional* and *behavioral* views, we use VerilogA language. These views are useful for multilevel simulations, especially in the verification phase of the design process. The *connectical* view is useful to test the supply voltage and the bias current of each block. The *functional* view describes the ideal equations of the function to be implemented. The *behavioral* one is more detailed; indeed there are refined equations that fit the schematic behavior.

One important point is to have a fluent and coherent design flow; that is why logical and mathematical links have been established between the different views.

The *datasheet* view is the most important view for the research of the corresponding IP. It contains information about the design and the re-use ability of the IP block. The technology, the supply voltage, the terminals and their validity domains, the links between the functional model and the behavioral model, the area of the layout and the cost of the design (which may be calculated with the technology and the area) are defined in this file.

Table 12.1 IP-AMS Hierarchical Description Levels

View name	*Description / Role*
Symbol	visualizes the function
Connectical	verifies connection between blocks (VerilogA)
Functional	models ideal electrical behavior (VerilogA)
Behavioral	models non-ideal electrical behavior, extracted from schematic (VerilogA)
Schematic	transistor-level schematic
Layout	
Datasheet	gives information about the circuit

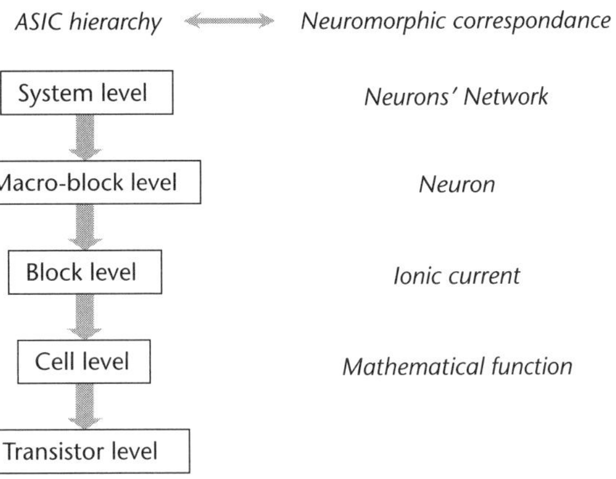

Figure 12.7 Description of the neuromimetic ASIC hierarchy.

The validity domain gives the range of input signals, where the circuit functionality is conserved. This information comes from systematic simulation of the primitive *cells* (*cell level*); then it is propagated to the *blocks* and *macro-blocks*. Figure 12.7 describes the hierarchy of a neuromimetic ASIC.

12.4.5.2 Creation and Exploration of the IP-Based Library

The data-base is implemented with MySQL formalism, using ten tables that describe the hierarchy of the system, the IP content, and validity domains. The objective of the data-base exploration is to find one ASIC solution according to the initial specifications. The chosen method is to perform a Top-Down exploration, from the *macro-block level* to the *cell level* (Figure 12.8) using the validity domain as a selection criterium. At the final step, a diagnostic is returned that quantifies the possibility to re-use IPs for a new ASIC project. In a case of re-use, IPs netlists are created for the designer.

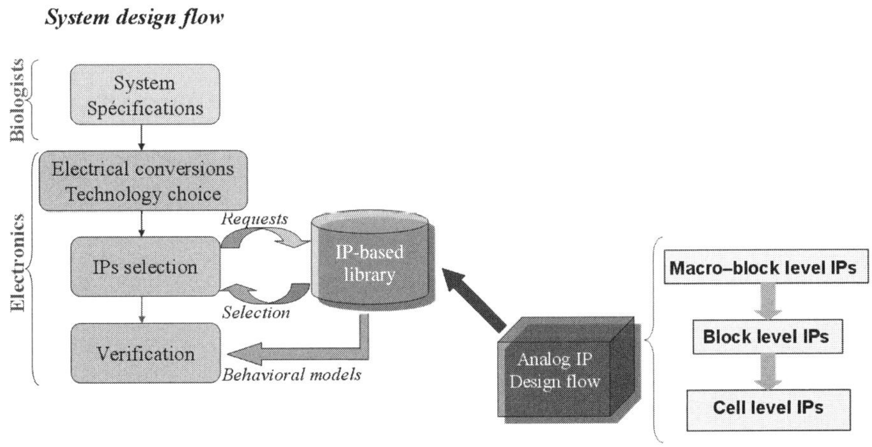

Figure 12.8 IP-based design flow.

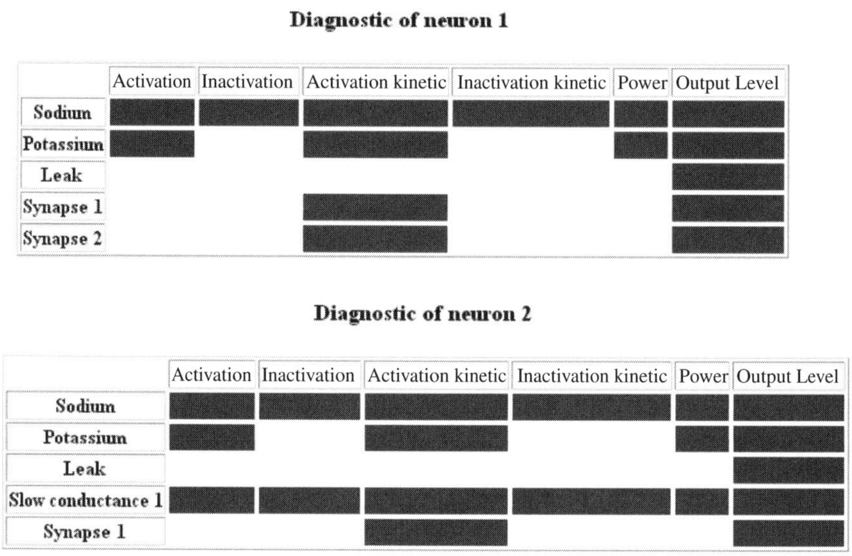

Figure 12.9 Diagnostics for one exploration.

12.4.5.3 Automated Design of a Neuromimetic ASIC

The data-base automatic exploration process has been tested for many plausible specification sets. We present here one of these examples: automatic design of one of our ASIC (Galway).

Neurosciences give us the biological specifications of the neurons' network. We convert them into electrical ones. Then there is an exploration of the IP-based library. Figure 12.9 gives the result of this exploration, and it shows that all the IPs have been found. The Bottom-Up phase verifies whether the proposed architecture really meets the specifications. The connectical, behavioral, and functional models are used to perform a multi-level simulation of the entire ASIC. To validate the whole circuit, only one block was described at the transistor level, while the others were described using behavioral description. As an example, a simulation for one neuron of type FS (Fast Spiking) with null synapses inputs lasts 2′17″ using *VerilogA* description and 149560 using transistor level description.

This IP-based library minimizes the design cost of our ASICs, as it shortens the development time and improves the design re-use. The library associates behavioral and schematic views of all blocks at all hierarchical levels and their ability to perform simulations of the whole chip in a reasonable CPU time.

12.5 Neuromimetic ICs: Example of a Series of ASICs

In this chapter, we describe four different ASICs. Each of them was dedicated with specific techniques and aims. But all of them share two main properties. The first one is that they respect a time scale of 1, i.e., the biological and the hardware models have identical timings. The second one is that the basic block of the ASICs is the ionic current generator. This block computes Equation (12.1) of the Hodgkin-Huxley formalism (see Sec. 12.2.1.1), in which I_{ION} is the current passing through the specific ionic channels, g_{max} is the maximal conductance value, m (opening/activation) and h (closing/inactivation) are the dynamic functions describing the permeability of membrane channels to this ion, V_{EQUI} the equilibrium potential and p, q integers.

$$I_{ION} = g_{\max} m^p h^q (V_{MEM} - V_{EQUI}) \tag{12.1}$$

In the block diagram of Figure 12.6 that describes the architecture chosen for the design of the ionic current generator, we can identify various electronic functions:

- sigmoid, integrator and power ones necessary to the computation of m^p and h^q
- multipliers necessary to the product of the different terms of Equation (12.1)

The four ASIC examples illustrate different combinations of technologies (CMOS 0.6 μm, BiCMOS 0.8 μm, BiCMOS 0.35 μm), routing techniques (full-custom, automatic P&R) and fixed of tunable parameters for the neuron model. All the front end (schematic, simulation) and back end (layout, verification) operations have been performed by the Cadence™ CAD software suite.

12.5.1 A Subthreshold CMOS ASIC with Fixed Model Parameters

This neuromimetic ASIC ("Delphine") was designed in current mode in a standard CMOS process, using MOS transistors in their weak-inversion region. Since the CMOS implementation consumes less power, more artificial neurons may be integrated on a single chip. Another important aspect of this design is that the on-chip voltage and current levels are identical to those encountered in biological neurons.

Parameters (g_{max}, V_{equi}, $V_{offsetm}$, V_{slopem}, τ_m, p, $V_{offseth}$, V_{slopeh}, τ_h, q) have to be set for each ionic current. They correspond to voltage values externally fixed on the chip pins. All the parameters and membrane voltages are in the –100 mV to +100 mV range and ionic currents are on the order of nanoamperes. As we use weakly inverted MOS transistors, we can exploit the translinear properties in order to implement complex operations like sigmoïdal functions or multiplications.

A prototype designed in a 0.6 μm CMOS process, routed in full-custom mode, was fabricated by austria*micro*system (AMS). Test points were inserted to provide access to intermediary variables. The circuit includes two ionic current generators (Na and K); one of them can also be used as a synaptic current generator. Monte-Carlo simulations were used to choose the transistor lengths. A compromise was made between minimizing the layout mismatch effects and chip size (thinking that we intend to integrate larger neural networks on a single chip). Cut-off frequency considerations are not of great importance since the neural activity operates at low frequencies. Most transistors have a 1.2 μm length and are of PMOS type, which ensures $V_{BS} = 0$ to avoid bulk-source effects on a P-type substrate. All current mirrors are of cascode type, to decrease the V_{DS} value of a single transistor, and limit the influence of the V_{DS} relative variations on the drain currents.

Figure 12.10 is a microphotograph of the circuit where the different modules are pointed out. The chip area with pads is 1.75 mm × 1.75 mm. We applied to the chip

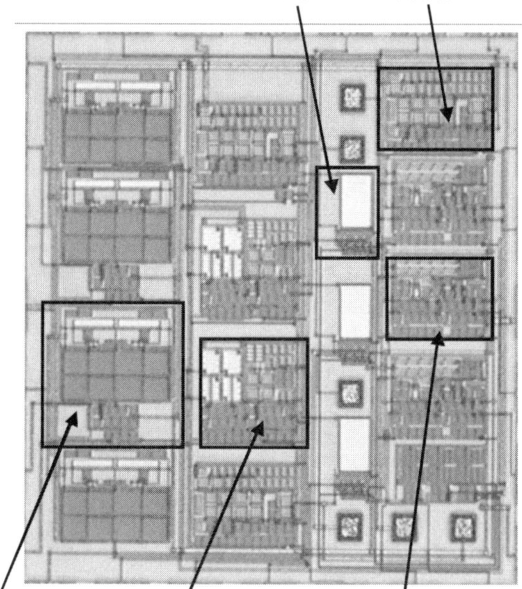

Figure 12.10 Microphotography of "Delphine" chip.

a voltage power supply of V_{cc} = 3.3 V. The measured power consumption for the whole chip is less than 60 μW, which respects the requested low power specification.

As indicated on Figure 12.11, we have built a simple spiking neuron with two ionic currents. The parameters have been set to model the sodium (Na) and potassium (K) channels. The Na current dynamics is described respectively with activation and inactivation processes, the K current with an activation process. This ASIC integrates one monosynapse for each neuron.

The chip output is the membrane potential V_{mem}; it spikes at 33 Hz (Figure 12.12). This is close, but not equivalent to the output predicted by the theoretical model. In a single period, three different phases typical in action potentials can be distinguished by: Na activation (phase 1) that depolarizes the neuron, Na inactivation and K activation (phase 2) that hyperpolarizes the neuron, and the leak current (phase 3) that slowly depolarizes the neuron back to phase 1.

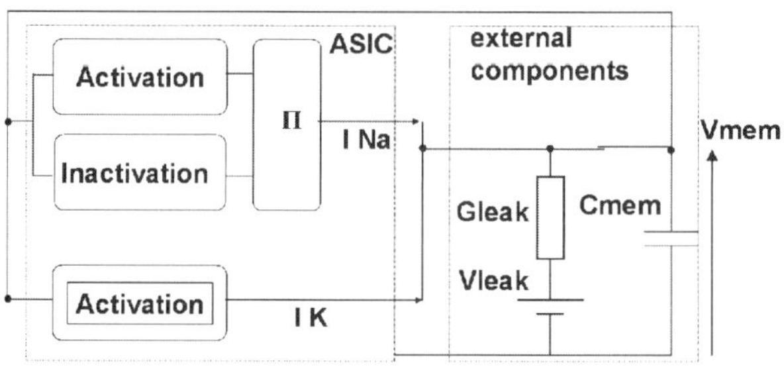

Figure 12.11 Spiking artificial neuron structure.

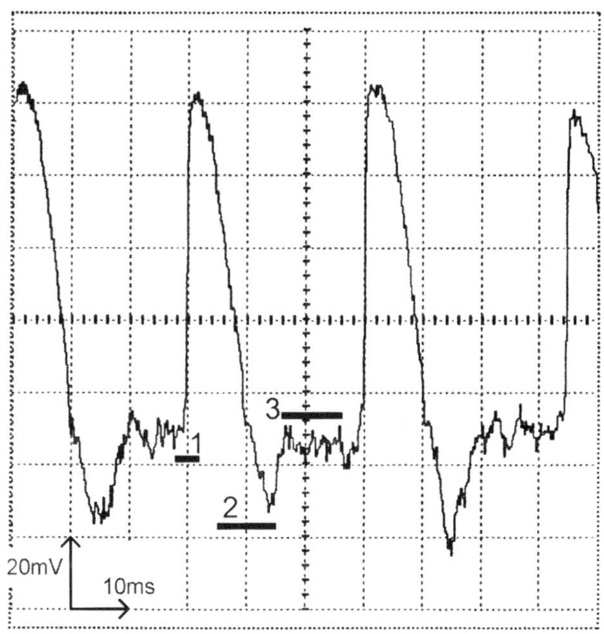

Figure 12.12 Measurement of V_{mem} membrane potential on the "Delphine" ASIC.

The use of CMOS transistors under threshold did not give results accurate enough to be exploited as a neural simulator. We found discrepancies between measurements and simulations, and the hardware neurons are too noise-sensitive for a proper use. The next ASICs, described in 12.5.2, were designed in BiCMOS technology.

12.5.2 A BICMOS ASIC with Fixed Model Parameters

The neuromimetic ASIC "Trieste" was also designed in current mode, but in a BiCMOS 0.8 μm process from AMS. To increase dynamic range and noise immunity, we decided to apply a $\times 10$ gain factor for electronic voltages and conductances. Still keeping a $\times 1$ factor for time, that choice implies $\times 100$ for currents and $\times 10$ for capacitance value. We limited the parameters choice to a few types of neurons, the most common among the neurons in the cortical area. Fixing the model parameters contributes to simplify the electronic implementation of each neural element and then to get a smaller area for the whole chip.

This chip is the computational analog core of a neural network simulator in which connectivity and plasticity are managed in digital mode. Each artificial neuron communicates in digital mode (2 digital inputs and 1 digital output) while all its internal variables (representing the membrane voltage and the ionic or synaptic currents) are analog and computed in continuous time. The structure of a neuron unit is given in Figure 12.13. The presynaptic signal "Trig" (synaptic control) is triggering the synaptic currents. The neuron spikes are detected and encoded on a 1-bit signal S ("neuron activity"). A computer collects and dispatches the digital signals according to programmable connectivity rules. In principle, this system is not limited in size; a large number of analog neurons can be integrated together in parallel.

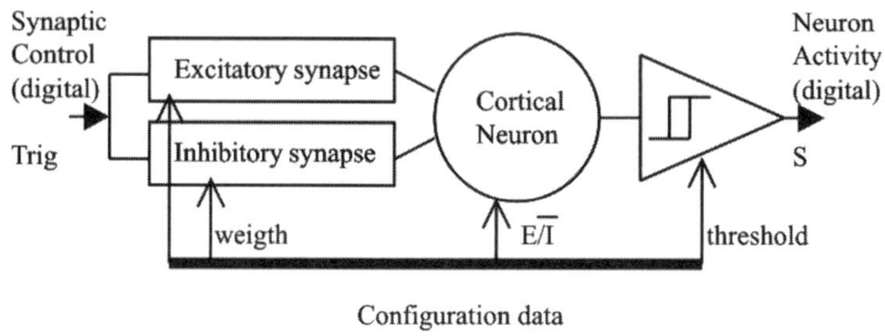

Figure 12.13 Neural element structure.

The simulation validation has been performed by comparison between results obtained from schematic and VerilogA description or computational neurosciences software, like "Neuron" [Hines]. The circuit includes different ionic current generators, each presenting two outputs: one connected to the membrane potential C_{mem} and the other connected to an external resistor for the single conductance characterization. Other extra pads have been added to access internal electrical information, like all the ionic currents generator parameters. Figure 12.14 is a microphotography of the chip (size 3.4 mm*3.4 mm). This circuit has been routed using Cell-Ensemble P&R software using a full custom library of elementary analog blocks. The power supply is 5 V with a middle point at 1.8 V corresponding to a biological value of 0 V. We have also integrated a 100 μA stable current source. Optimized analog layout procedures, such as common-centroïd, dummy devices, non minimum sizes and guard ring, have been used to implement critical structures.

To simulate the neuron activity, all the ionic current generators are connected to the membrane capacitance. Figure 12.15 presents the activity obtained for the inhibitory configuration and Figure 12.16 illustrates the oscillatory activity of an excitatory neuron that receives a stimulation current. In both cases, we obtain an activity very close to the theoretical one.

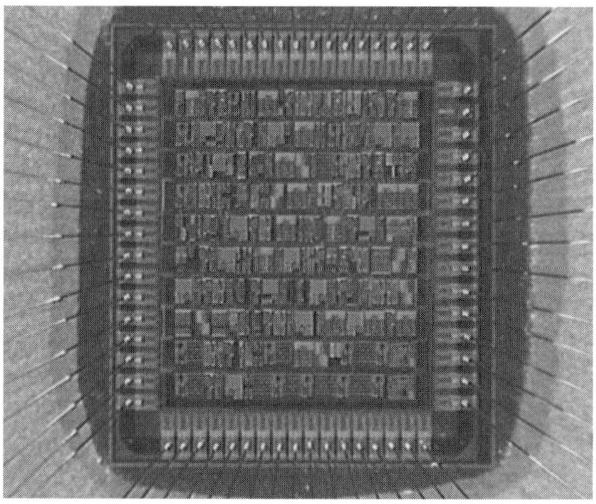

Figure 12.14 Microphotography of the "Trieste" ASIC.

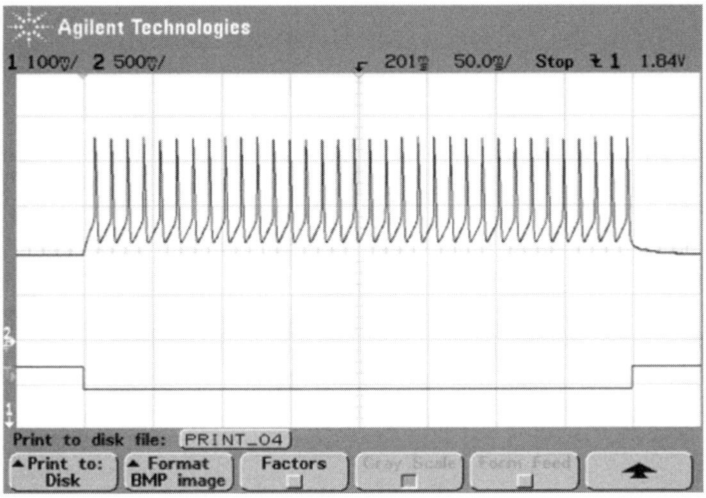

Figure 12.15 Fast spiking (inhibitory) neuron activity measured on "Trieste."

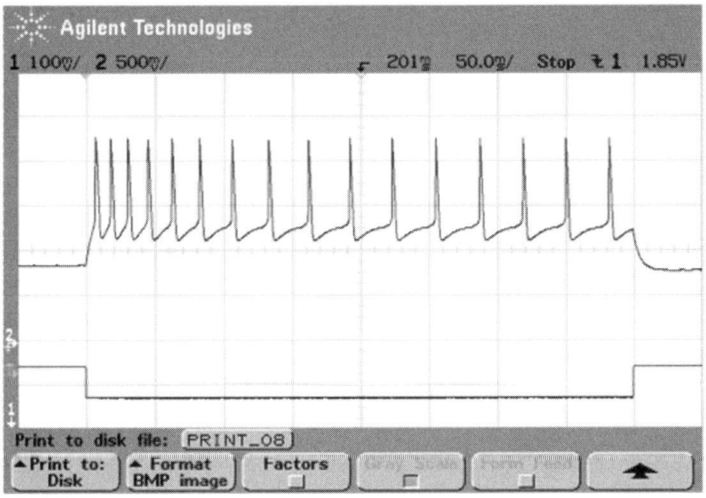

Figure 12.16 Regular spiking (excitatory) neuron activity measured on "Trieste."

12.5.3 A BICMOS ASIC with Tunable Model Parameters

The ASIC "Pamina" was designed around a library of mathematical functions for custom analog ICs. The functions can be assembled to form a set of ionic current generators. Digital functions are added to manage the core topology as well as analog memory cells to store the neuron model parameters.

Five ionic current generators are integrated in the IC analog core (Na, K, Ca, K(Ca) and Leak), 8 monosynapses for network applications, and one stimulation input (Figure 12.17).

All functions have two outputs: the first one can be connected to the external capacitor C_{mem} that represents the membrane capacitor; the second one is a display

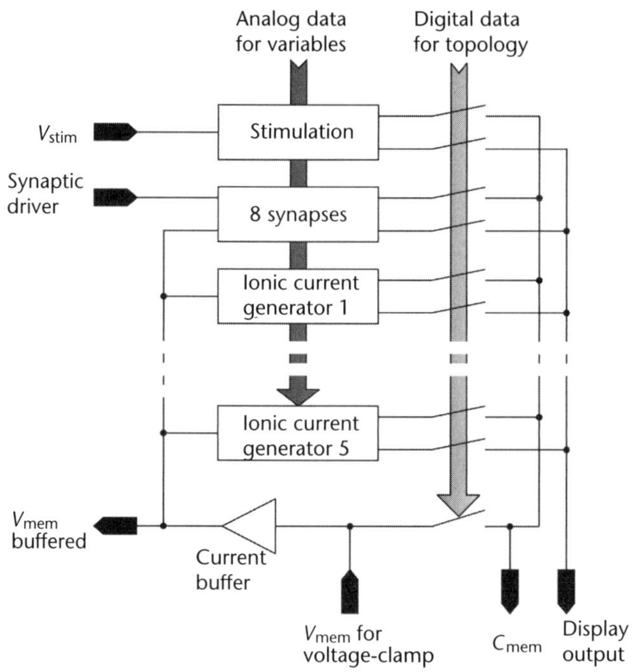

Figure 12.17 Analog core of the "Pamina" ASIC.

output used to observe each ionic or synaptic current. A current buffer authorizes through a third output the display of electrical membrane activity with a scope probe. The switch between the current buffer and the external capacitor could be closed for neuronal electrical activity simulation or could be opened for voltage-clamp experiments to identify individual channel parameters.

To minimize the chip area, only two analog computation cores were implanted in the "Pamina" chip. To build the hardware neuron, the user has to define, via the switches, which ionic or synaptic current generators are connected to the external capacitor C_{mem}; each switch in Figure 12.18 is controlled by a digital signal, stored in the topology memory (68 bits). DRAM analog memory cells store the 158 model parameters necessary for the two analog cores. The memory cells array is loaded by one external ADC, which sequentially refreshes the analog parameter values. This technique allows the dynamic modification of one or more parameters: one advantage of "Pamina" is the possibility of dynamical reprogramming of the neuron model while the simulation is still running.

The prototype ASIC was designed in full-custom mode with a BiCMOS SiGe 0.35 μm technology process from AMS (Figure 12.19). The ionic current generators have been designed in current mode, which means that the internal variables are physically represented by currents. Topology and analog memory cells can also be identified on the figure. The IC comprises 22000 elements, among which 71% are full-custom design (other than digital cells).

The library designed for this ASIC was re-used in the ASIC presented in 12.5.4. Functional measurements on "Pamina" are identical to those of Figure 12.22.

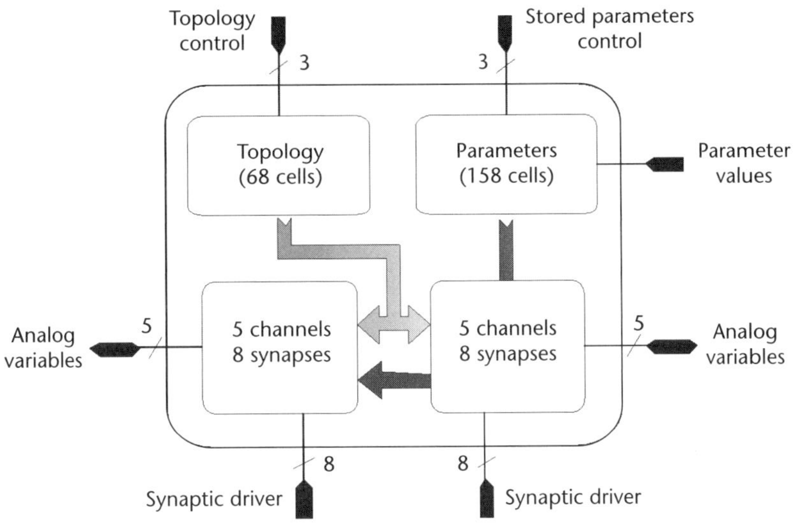

Figure 12.18 Architecture of the "Pamina" ASIC.

12.5.4 A BICMOS ASIC with Tunable Model Parameters and Multisynapses

The integrated circuit "Galway" was designed in a BiCMOS 0.35 μm process from AMS, using the functions library developed for "Pamina." Dedicated to the real-time simulation of adaptive neural networks, it integrates multisynapses inputs for each hardware neuron (see Sec. 12.4.2). The gain is ×10 for conductances, ×5 for voltages. The artificial neurons are configurable: the model parameters are not fixed, and can vary in a pre-defined range, representing standard neuron types or the cortex.

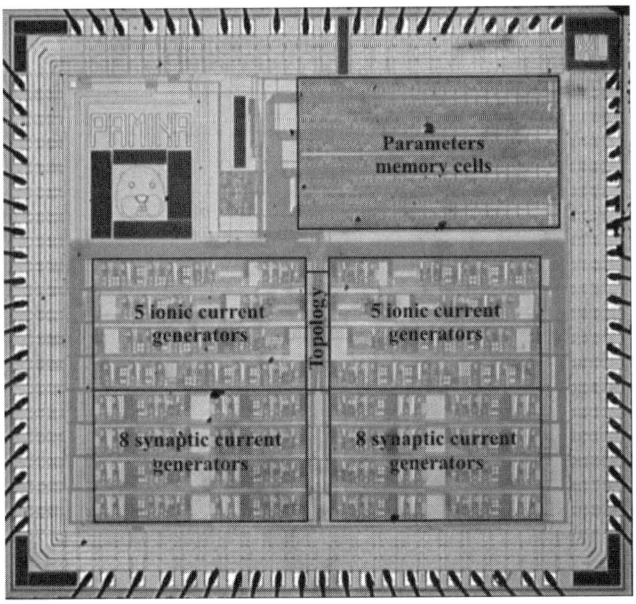

Figure 12.19 Microphotography of the chip "Pamina."

The ASIC provides a large variety of configurations. As in Sec. 12.5.3, subblocks in the ASIC compute ionic or synaptic current generators, with tunable parameters stored in on-chip analog memory cells.

Each "Galway" ASIC comprises (Figure 12.20):

- a ionic or synaptic current generators following a Hodgkin-Huxley type conductance-based model;
- spike-detection modules, to encode (1-bit) the neurons action potentials;
- multisynaptic input modules, that compute synaptic conductances with a digitally-controlled weight;
- an analog memory cells array, to store the conductances model parameters;
- a matrix of switches, to control the neurons topology (i.e., the arrangement of the conductance and synaptic modules that form the artificial neuron);
- digital functions to control data transfer from and to external devices.

"Galway" can compute in parallel up to five neural elements; each receives three multisynaptic currents—one for inhibitory input, one for excitatory input, and one for cortical background noise activity. The last ASIC "Pamina" contained eight synapses but with only three multisynapses; "Galway" can connect more neural elements. This difference improves the network possibilities.

To respect a biologically-realistic distribution of the neurons within a SNN, we have integrated (see the layout depicted in Figure 12.21):

- 1 Fast Spiking neuron (N1) constructed with 3 conductances I_{leak}, I_{Na}, I_K
- Regular Spiking neurons (N2,N3,N4) with 4 conductances I_{leak}, I_{Na}, I_K, I_{Ca}
- 1 Regular Spiking neuron (N5) with a fifth conductance identical to I_{Ca}.
- 1 extra conductance identical to I_{Ca}, that can be connected either to N4 or to N5
- the memory cell array storing the parameters of the neuron model card

The area of the chip is 10.5 mm^2, and it is composed of 47,000 devices.

Figure 12.22 illustrates one example of membrane voltages measured on N2, N3, and N5, with model parameters tuned as specified by biologists.

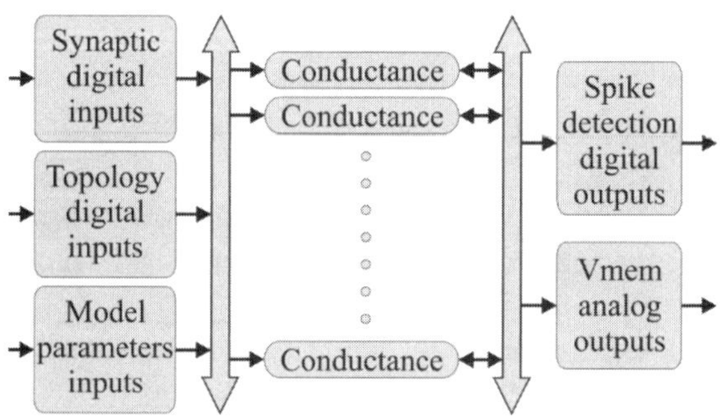

Figure 12.20 "Galway" chip architecture and data I/O.

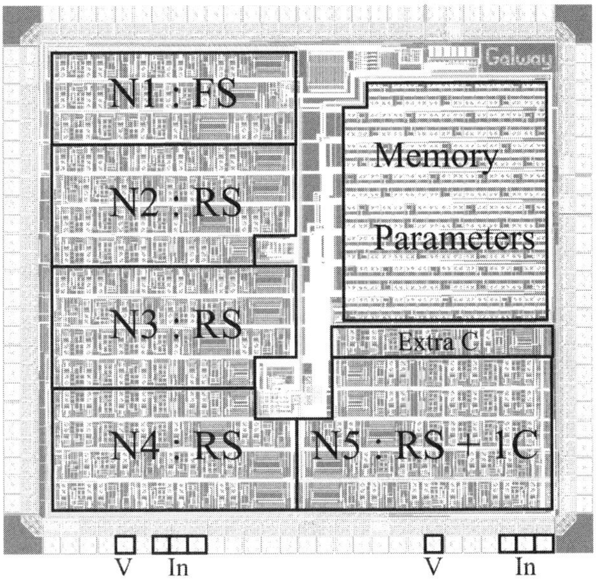

Figure 12.21 Layout of the "Galway" chip.

The "Galway" ASICs are integrated within a mixed software-hardware simulation system used to explore the computational paradigms of cortical neural networks (EU project *FACETS*, FET-IST-2004—15879). They are associated in the system with digital computation facilities (FPGA or software), in charge of the computation on biological real-time of the SNN learning rules. These rules change dynamically the synaptic weights depending on the relative activity of pre- and postsynaptic neurons. The whole set-up has been dimensioned to simulate up to 512 neurons (dispatched on ASICs) with all-to-all synaptic connections and learning rules. In such a configuration, the ASICs ensure the real-time computation of the SNN and give much better performance than classical software simulations. Furthermore, continuous and analog voltages and currents of neurons and synapses are available for a direct connection with living neurons, using extra- or intracellular microelectrodes.

We presented four examples of neuromimetic ASICs dedicated to the real-time simulation of conductance-based SNN. Each IC was designed to fit different criteria

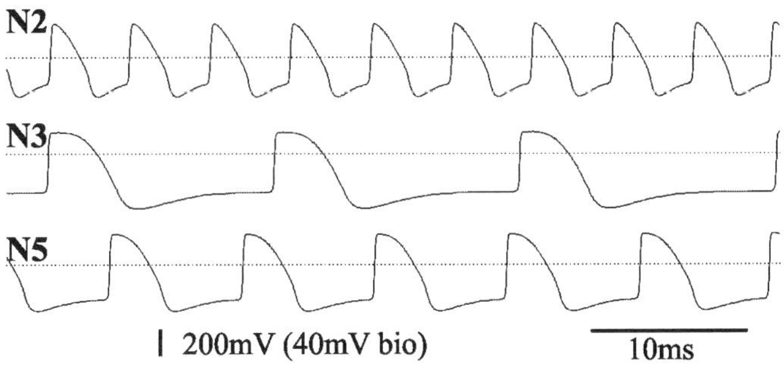

Figure 12.22 Spiking activity of neurons N2, N3, and N5 of "Galway."

Table 12.2 Synthesis of the Presented ASICs

ASICs	*Technology*	*Synapses*	*Mathematical operators*
Delphine	CMOS 0.6 μm	Monosynapse	Specific
Trieste	BiCMOS 0.8 μm	Multisynapses	Generic
Pamina	BiCMOS 0.35 μm	Monosynapse	Generic
Galway	BiCMOS 0.35 μm	Multisynapses	Generic

(technology, generic, or specific operators, etc.), specific to the foreseen applications (see Table 12.2).

This series of ASICs is characteristic of an evolutive design strategy. The design of the next ASICs' generation will be based on the IP-based platform (12.5).

12.6 Conclusion and Perspectives

We have seen the design context and considerations for neuromimetic ASICs. Such complex circuits do not compete with software simulators in terms of signal precision, but rather open a way for parallel computation of spiking neural networks. "Analog" neurons have intrinsic properties like noise and diversity, and perform non-repetitive simulations of SNN. This property is interesting in terms of biological relevance, although the hardware-based diversity may not reflect the reality of neural networks.

As an illustration of a SNN behavior, Figure 12.23 shows a simulation performed by neuromimetic ASICs interfaced with a computer. The processor computes the net-

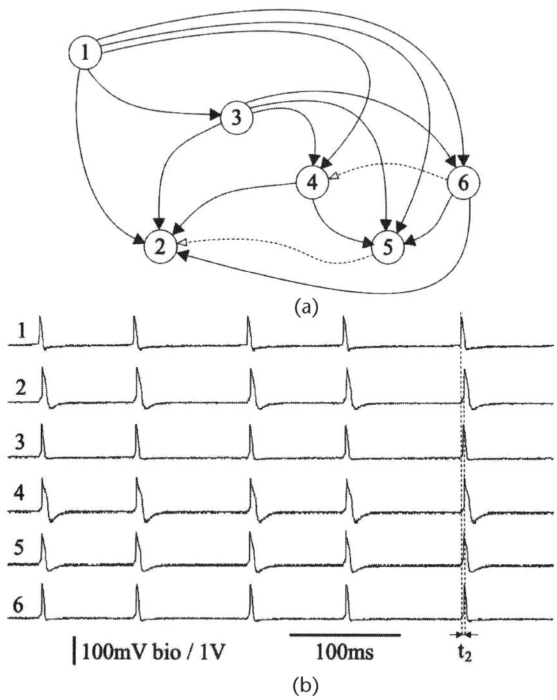

Figure 12.23 Example of hardware simulation with the associated network. (a) Network of six neuromimetic ASICs. (b) Activities of each neuron responding to a synaptic stimulation.

work level dynamics (synaptic adaptation) in real time. We obtain a synchronous activity in which neurons are sorted according to their ability to respond to a synaptic stimulation. This simulation involves six ASICs computing fixed parameter Hodgkin-Huxley neurons with multisynapses (see Sec. 12.4.2). The network's evolution obeys the rules of STDP.

Hardware simulation systems are frequently challenged by newborn powerful computing systems, but stay one step ahead thanks to the relative easiness they bring to parallel computing. They are still not equalled in equivalent computing power.

In parallel, understanding learning and adaptation phenomena in SNN is really an issue in neuroscience and in signal processing. Computing large SNN necessitates parallel operations on neurons and synapses, with a number of synaptic connections growing up exponentially with the network size. ASIC-based SNN have considerably evolved within the last 10 years, and the examples we have seen in this chapter have proved that they represent an alternative and bio-realistic approach to spiking neural networks.

References

[Badoual] M. Badoual, Q. Zou, A. Davison, M. Rudolph, T. Bal, Y. Frégnac, A. Destexhe, *Biophysical and phenomenological models of multiple spike interactions in spike-timing dependent plasticity*, International Journal of Neural Systems, no. 16, pp. 79–97, 2006.

[Binczak] S. Binczak, S. Jacquir, J.-M Bilbault, V.B. Kazantsev, V.I. Nekorkin, V.I. *Experimental study of electrical FitzHugh–Nagumo neurons with modified excitability*, Neural Networks, no. 19, pp. 684–693, 2006.

[Brette] R. Brette, W. Gerstner, *Adaptative exponential Integrate-and-Fire model as an effective description of neuronal activity*, Journal of Neurophysiology, no. 94, pp. 3637–3642, 2005.

[Destexhe] A. Destexhe, Z. Mainen, T. Sejnowski, *An efficient method for computing synaptic conductances based on a kinetic model of receptor binding*, Neur. Comp., no. 6, pp. 14–18, 1994.

[FitzHugh] R. FitzHugh, *Impulses and physiological states in models of nerve membrane*, Biophysic Journal, no. 1, pp. 445–466, 1961.

[Gerstner] W. Gerstner, W.M. Kistler, *Spiking Neuron Models: Single Neurons, Populations, Plasticity*, Cambridge University Press, 2002.

[Glackin] B. Glackin, T.M. McGinnity, L.P. Maguire, Q.X. Wu, A. Belatreche, *A novel approach for the implementation of large scale spiking neural networks on FPGA hardware*, Proceedings of IWANN 2005 Computational Intelligence and Bioinspired Systems, pp. 552–563, Barcelona, Spain, 2005.

[Hasler] P. Hasler, S. Kozoil, E. Farquhar, A. Basu, *Transistor Channel Dendrites implementing HMM classifiers*, Proceedings of IEEE International Symposium on Circuits and Systems, pp. 3359–3362, New Orleans, USA, 2007.

[HH] A.L. Hodgkin, A.F. Huxley, *A quantitative description of ion currents and its applications to conduction and excitation in nerve membranes*, Journal of Physiology (London), no. 117, pp. 500–544, 1952.

[Hines] M.L. Hines, N.T. Carneval, *The NEURON simulation environnement*, Neural Computation, no. 9, pp. 1179–1209, 1997.

[Indiveri] G. Indiveri, S. Fusi, *Spike-based learning in VLSI networks of integrate-and-fire neurons*, Proceedings of IEEE International Symposium on Circuits and Systems, pp. 3371–3374, New Orleans, USA, 2007.

[Izhikevich] E. Izhikevich, *Which model to use for cortical spiking neurons*, IEEE Transactions on Neural Networks, no. 15, pp. 1063–1070, 2004.

[Jung] R. Jung, E.J. Brauer, J.J. Abbas, *Real-time interaction between a neuromorphic electronic circuit and the spinal cord*, IEEE Transactions on Neural Systems and Rehabilitation Engineering, pp. 319–326, 2001.

[Koch] C. Koch, *Biophysics of Computation*, Oxford University Press, 1999.

[LeMasson] G. LeMasson, S. Renaud, D. Debay, T. Bal, *Feedback inhibition controls spike transfer in hybrid thalamic circuits*, Nature, no. 4178, pp. 854–858, 2002.

[Liu] S.-C. Liu, R. Douglas, *Temporal coding in a silicon network of integrate-and-fire neurons*, IEEE Transactions on Neural Networks, no. 15, pp. 1305–1314, 2004.

[Mahowald] M. Mahowald, R. Douglas, *A silicon neuron*. Nature, no. 354, pp. 515–518, 1991.

[Morris] C. Morris, H. Lecar, *Voltage oscillations in the barnacle giant muscle fiber,* Biophysic Journal, no. 35, pp. 193–213, 1981.

[Renaud] S. Renaud, J. Tomas, Y. Bornat, A. Daouzli, S. Saïghi, *Neuromimetic ICs with analog cores: an alternative for designing spiking neural network,* Proceedings of IEEE International Symposium on Circuits and Systems, pp. 3355–3358, New Orleans, USA, 2007.

[Schemmel] J. Schemmel, D. Brüderle, K. Meier, B. Ostendorf, *Modeling Synaptic Plasticity within Networks of Highly Accelerated I&F Neurons*, Proceedings of IEEE International Symposium on Circuits and Systems, pp. 3367–3370, New Orleans, USA, 2007.

[Sorensen] M. Sorensen, S. DeWeerth, G. Cymbalyuk, R.L. Calabrese, *Using a hybrid neural system to reveal regulation of neuronal network activity by an intrinsic current*, Journal of Neurosciences, no. 24, pp. 5427–5438, 2004.

[Vogelstein] R.J. Vogelstein, U. Malik, G. Cauwenberghs, *Silicon spike-based synaptic array and address-event transceiver*, Proceedings of ISCAS'04, pp. 385–388, 2004.

CHAPTER 13

Circuits for Amperometric Electrochemical Sensors

Mohammad M. Ahmadi and Graham A. Jullien

13.1 Introduction

Amperometric electrochemical sensors are widely used in many areas, including the food industry, environmental monitoring, and biotechnology. These sensors have both good sensitivity and good selectivity in detecting many chemical and biological species such as oxygen, glucose, toxic metals, etc. Basically, an amperometric electrochemical sensor responds to the chemical species of interest by generating an electrical current which is proportional to the concentration of that specie.

There is currently a growing interest in using amperometric electrochemical sensors in portable devices. Two examples are: (1) portable devices used to detect toxic metals in natural waters [1] and (2) implantable microsystems used to monitor the concentration of biological species, such as oxygen, glucose and cholesterol in the human blood [2]. These portable devices require highly integrated circuits with very low power consumptions.

The main goal of this chapter is to review the circuits required for interfacing with amperometric electrochemical sensors along with the challenges in the design of those circuits in advanced submicron CMOS technologies. The design of these circuits not only requires a good knowledge of circuit design, but also a relatively in-depth knowledge of electrochemistry. As a result, this chapter also provides some introductory material on electrochemistry and electrochemical sensors. In addition, it briefly reviews the methods and tools that are used to find the electrical-equivalent model of an electrochemical sensor.

13.2 Electrochemical Sensors

13.2.1 Electrochemistry and the Electrode Process

Electrochemistry is a branch of chemistry focused on the relation between electrical and chemical effects. In electrochemical systems, the processes and factors are studied that affect the transport of charge across the interface between chemical phases; for example, between an electronic conductor (an electrode) and an ionic conductor (an electrolyte) [3].

As an example, consider a silver electrode immersed in pure water (Figure 13.1). Some of the silver atoms dissolve in the solution (water) as positive ions (Ag^+), leaving their electrons in the electrode based on the following equation:

$$Ag \longrightarrow Ag^{+} + e^{-} \tag{13.1}$$

Very soon, the solution becomes so positive and the electrode so negative that the electric field created at the interface prevents more silver atoms from dissolving in the solution. The buildup of charge in the electrode and the solution causes an *interfacial potential difference*, which can affect the rate and direction of the reaction. Different electrodes have different interfacial potential differences. For example, when silver and copper electrodes are immersed in the water, more electrons build up in the copper than in the silver, thus copper is more negative in potential than silver.

Manipulation of the interfacial potential difference can be used as an external tool to control the reaction rate at an electrode surface. Moreover, since the dissolution of each of the atoms of the electrode in the solution involves the transfer of one (or more) electron(s) to the electrode, the reaction rate can be measured by monitoring the current flowing through the electrode [3].

Generally, by examining the voltage-current characteristic of an electrode/solution interface, and having some prior understanding about the system, a description about the reaction in the solution can be obtained. In fact, most of the importance of electrochemistry comes from the methods dealing with the interrelation between interfacial potential differences and the thermodynamics and kinetics of electrode reactions.

Two types of charge transfer reactions generally take place at an electrode solution interface: *oxidation* and *reduction*. In an oxidation reaction (similar to the silver electrode example), the chemical species pass electron(s) to the electrode, whereas, in a reduction reaction, the chemical species obtain electron(s) from the electrode. The resulting chemical reactions can respectively be represented by:

oxidation: $$R \longrightarrow O + ne^{-} \tag{13.2}$$

reduction $$O + ne^{-} \longrightarrow R \tag{13.3}$$

where O is the oxidized form of the species, R is the reduced form, and n is the number of transferred electrons in the reaction.

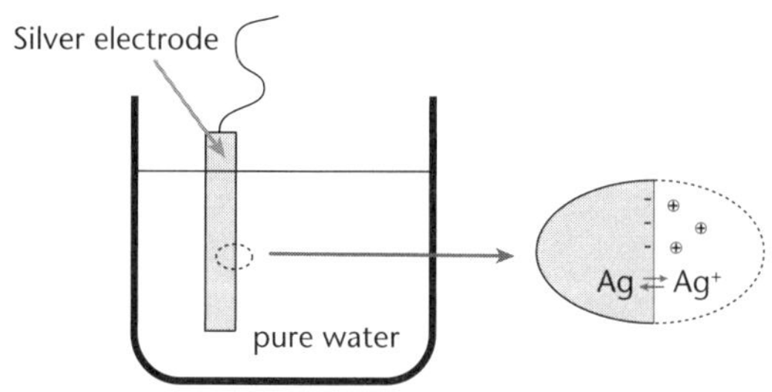

Figure 13.1 Oxidation of a silver electrode immersed in pure water.

It is worth mentioning that usually interfacial potential differences are limited to a few volts, but this potential difference is across a very short distance (in the range of nanometers) corresponding to a thin layer of solvent molecules and ions attached to the electrode surface. Consequently, a very large potential gradient exists on the electrode/solution interface. For example, a potential difference of only one volt across a thickness of one angstrom results in a potential gradient of 100 million volts per centimeter.

The interfacial potential difference, E, of an electrode can be calculated using the Nernst equation [3]:

$$E = E^o + \frac{RT}{nF}\ln\left(\frac{C_O}{C_R}\right) \tag{13.4}$$

where E^o is the standard potential of the electrode, R is the molar gas constant, T is the absolute temperature, n is the number of electrons transferred in the reaction, F is Faraday's constant, and C_O and C_R are the concentration of the oxidized and reduced forms of the species, respectively [3].

13.2.2 Electrochemical Cell

Measuring or controlling the interfacial potential difference between an electrode and a solution is impossible without immersing another electrode into that solution. Thus, an electrochemical cell, in its simplest form, consists of two electrodes separated by a solution (electrolyte) (Figure 13.2) [3].

The overall chemical reaction occurring in an electrochemical cell consists of two independent half-reactions describing the real chemical changes at each of the two electrodes. Each half-reaction responds to the interfacial potential difference at the corresponding electrode.

Usually the reaction in only one of the electrodes is of interest. This electrode is usually called the *sensing*, *indicator* or *working electrode* (WE). In order to focus on the reaction occurring at the working electrode, the other electrode should have a constant interfacial potential difference. This electrode is usually called the *reference electrode* (RE) [3].

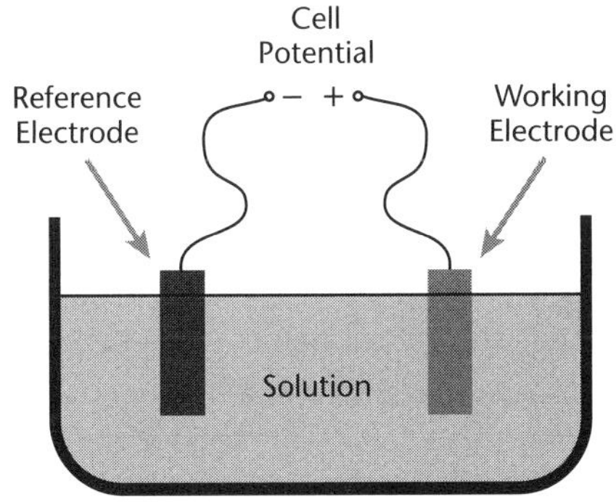

Figure 13.2 A simple electrochemical cell.

The internationally accepted primary reference electrode is the Normal Hydrogen Electrode (NHE), or sometimes called the Standard Hydrogen Electrode (SHE). The NHE consists of a platinum electrode immersed in a solution with constant hydrogen activity. The construction of the electrode is completed by bubbling pure hydrogen over the platinum electrode. The pressure of the gas should be 1 atmosphere (atm). The continuous stream of the hydrogen gas provides the solution with a constant hydrogen concentration [4].

Since it is somewhat difficult to use the NHE in experiments, potentials are often measured and reported with respect to reference electrodes other than the NHE. A more convenient reference electrode is the Reversible Hydrogen Electrode (RHE). The potential of an RHE depends on the pH of the solution. As an example, the potential of an RHE, when pH = 7, equals –0.413 V versus NHE at room temperature.

A more common reference electrode is the silver-silver chloride (Ag/AgCl) electrode, which has a potential of +0.197 V versus NHE at room temperature [3].

In an electrochemical experiment, it is very important to know the reference electrode to which the cell potential is referenced. Since the potentials of the standard Ag/AgCl electrode and the RHE (at pH = 7) are 0.197 V and –0.413 V versus NHE, respectively, the potential of the Ag/AgCl reference electrode versus RHE (at pH = 7) is 0.610 V. As an example, if the potential of an electrode is 0.6 V versus the Ag/AgCl reference electrode, it will be 0.797 V versus SHE and 1.210 V versus RHE (at pH = 7).

13.2.3 Electrochemical Sensors

Electrochemical sensors constitute the largest and oldest group of chemical sensors [5]. The principle of all electrochemical sensors consists of holding certain variables of an electrochemical cell constant while observing how the remaining variables (usually current, potential, or concentration) vary with changes in the controlled variables. Generally, electrochemical sensors are classified into three categories [5–6]:

- *Voltammetric* sensors, which are based on the measurement of the current-voltage relationship in an electrochemical cell. A potential is applied between the electrodes and the current flowing between them is measured. The measured current is related to the chemical species of interest. *Amperometric* sensors constitute a class in voltammetric sensors in which the potential of the electrochemical cell is kept constant while its current is measured. The current of the cell is related to the concentration of the electroactive species. It can be shown [3] that when the current of the electrochemical cell is limited by the transfer rate of electroactive molecules to the electrode surface (mass transfer-limited regime), the relationship between the current and the concentration of the electroactive species is linear. However, when the current is limited by the rate of the charge transfer at the electrode/solution interface (charge transfer-limited regime), the relationship is nonlinear. Thus, to have a linear proportionality between the current and the chemical specie of interest, the cell should be kept in the mass transfer-limited regime [3].
- *Potentiometric* sensors, in which the electrochemical cell is kept open circuit (cell current is zero) and cell potential is measured, which, according to

the Nernst equation, is proportional to the logarithm of the concentration of the chemical species of interest. Potentiometric sensors are very useful when the concentration of the chemical species of interest changes over several orders of magnitude (e.g., in the case of pH measurements). In other cases, in which the concentration changes over only one or two orders of magnitude (e.g., in the case of glucose concentration in physiological fluids), a sensor with a linear relationship between the output signal and the concentration is preferable (such as amperometric sensors) [7].

- *Conductometric* sensors, in which the conductance of the cell is measured by an alternating current bridge method. In this kind of sensor, the resistive component of the impedance of the solution is of interest. The sensing is carried out at one fixed frequency.

13.2.4 Three-Electrode Measurement System

In a voltammetry experiment, an external potential is applied to the electrochemical cell and the current that flows through the cell is measured. Precise control of the external applied potential is necessary in any voltammetry experiment, but this is not generally possible with a two-electrode system. The reason is that the solution part of the cell has some resistance, which generates a potential drop across the cell when current flows through the cell. Also, when current flows through the reference electrode, the electrode becomes slightly polarized, causing some changes in its interfacial potential difference. As a result, the interfacial potential difference of the working electrode cannot be precisely controlled with a two-electrode system. Moreover, material consumption in the reference electrode due to the current flow is another problem of two-electrode systems [4].

The above problems can be minimized by using a very large reference electrode and a very small working electrode. However, using a large reference electrode is not possible in many cases; e.g., when the goal is to miniaturize the electrochemical cell. A better approach to resolve the above issues is to use a three-electrode system, in which better potential control is achieved by introducing a new electrode into the electrochemical cell [4].

In a three-electrode system, as shown in Figure 13.3, the potential of the working electrode is controlled relative to the reference electrode, and the current is injected into the electrochemical cell by a third electrode called the *auxiliary* or

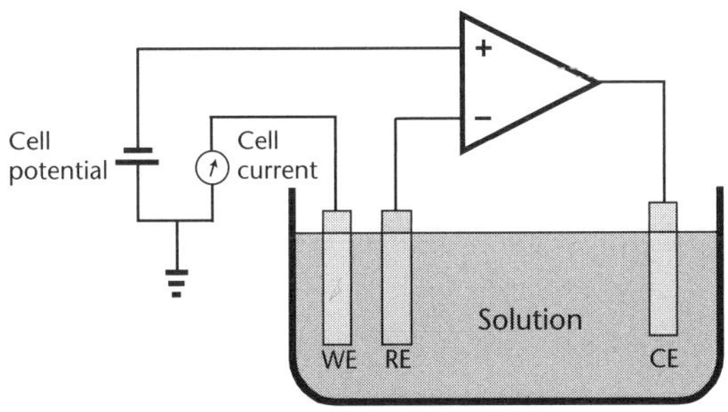

Figure 13.3 Three-electrode electrochemical measurement system.

counter electrode (CE) [3]. The current of the cell is measured at the working electrode. The current of the cell can also be measured at the counter electrode if no parasitic current path exists.

For realizing the three-electrode system, an electronic instrument, called a *potentiostat*, is required to control the potential difference between the working electrode and the reference electrode. The potentiostat implements this control using a negative feedback loop that injects the proper amount of current into the counter electrode to keep the potential difference between the working and reference electrodes at the desired potential [3, 4, 5].

13.3 Potentiostat

A potentiostat is an electronic instrument that controls the voltage difference between the working and reference electrodes of an electrochemical cell by sinking or sourcing a current from or into the electrochemical cell through the counter electrode. In almost all applications, the potentiostat measures the current flowing between the working and the counter electrodes [3].

As a result, a potentiostat has two tasks: (a) controlling the potential difference between the working and reference electrodes, (b) measuring the current flowing between the working and counter electrodes. Each of these tasks can be realized with a few different circuit configurations that are summarized in the following sections.

13.3.1 Potential Control Configurations

Controlling the cell potential can be realized in three configurations: *grounded working electrode*, *grounded reference electrode*, and *grounded counter electrode*. The first two configurations are electrically the same; thus, in fact there are only two different configurations [8].

The most popular configuration is the grounded working electrode. Figure 13.4 illustrates the basic implementation of this configuration. As shown, the working electrode is kept at the ground potential and an operational amplifier, called the *control amplifier*, controls the cell current, I_F, such that the cell potential, V_{CELL}, is kept at its desired preset potential, E_i.

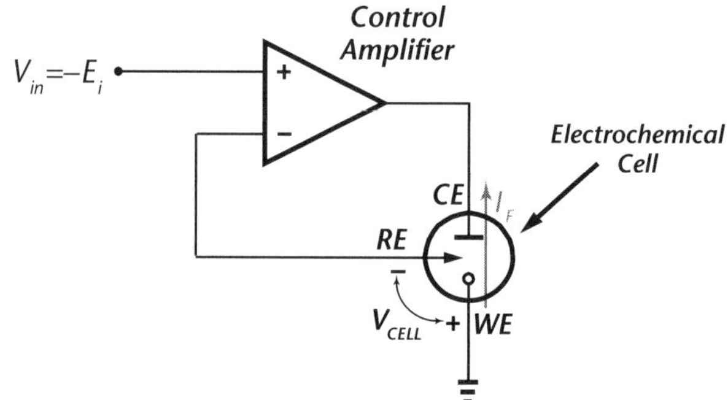

Figure 13.4 Potential control using the grounded working electrode configuration.

The principle of the operation is quite simple, but, like other opamp circuits, in actual realizations, the imperfections of the control amplifier limit the functionality of the potentiostat.

Since current flow in the reference electrode changes the potential of the reference electrode, the input bias current of the control amplifier should be extremely small (in the pA range or less) and the input resistance of the amplifier should be very large (a few GΩ or more) [9]. These specifications can be easily achieved if the circuit is implemented in a CMOS technology; however, in a bipolar technology, usually another operational amplifier, acting as a voltage buffer, is required to minimize current flow in the reference electrode (Figure 13.5).

The voltage gain and the input offset voltage of the control amplifier in Figure 13.4 define the accuracy of the potential control. The gain of the amplifier must be usually more than 10^4 and the input offset voltage less then 10 mV. Of course, depending on the target application, the limitations over the control amplifier parameters might be either tighter or more relaxed. The other important parameters of the control amplifier are its output voltage swing, input referred noise, and bandwidth.

Probably the most important parameter of the control amplifier is its stability. As shown in Figure 13.4, the electrochemical cell is the load and feedback network of the control amplifier. Since electrochemical cells are highly nonlinear and usually have frequency-dependent impedances, simulating the frequency and transient responses of the potential control loop is very complex and sometimes impossible. As a result, the design of a potentiostat should be such that it can provide stability over large ranges of operation, in order to handle a large diversity of electrochemical experiments. Even though commercial bench-top potentiostats consume considerable power to achieve the above capability, they can still become unstable and oscillate during an electrochemical experiment.

The grounded counter electrode configuration has recently been explored [8] as an alternative for the potential control. The basic realization of this configuration is shown in Figure 13.6. Clearly, this configuration is more complex than the grounded working electrode configuration and requires more components; thus it is more vulnerable to component mismatches. However, in some cases, it performs better than the grounded working electrode configuration [8].

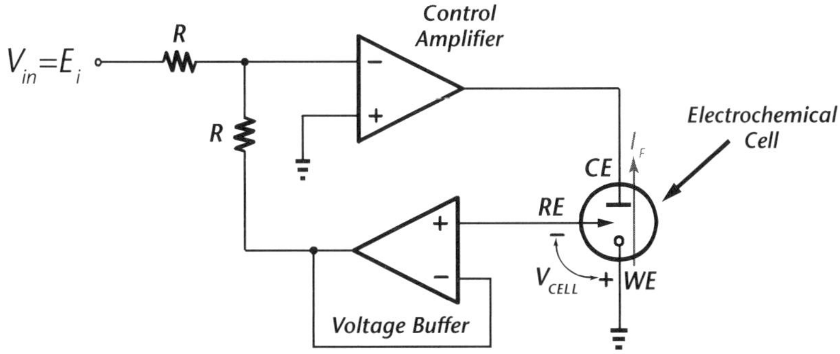

Figure 13.5 Using a voltage buffer to prevent current flow in the reference electrode.

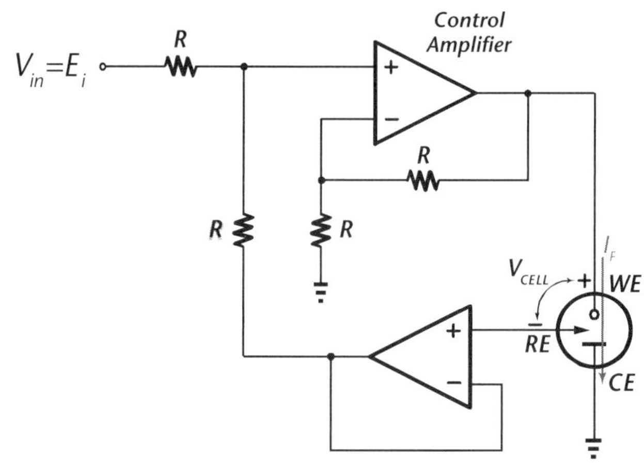

Figure 13.6 Potential control using the grounded counter electrode configuration.

The same considerations that were explained for the grounded working electrode configuration, regarding the imperfections of the operational amplifiers, are also valid for this configuration.

13.3.2 Current Measurement Approaches

A few different approaches exist for measuring the cell current, I_F. In this section, the current measurement approaches are explained for potentiostats using the grounded working electrode configuration; however, almost all of these approaches can be implemented for the potentiostats using the grounded counter electrode configuration.

Using a *transimpedance amplifier* is probably the most popular approach for current measurement. In this approach, as shown in Figure 13.7, a transimpedance amplifier forces a virtual ground at the working electrode and, at the same time, generates an output voltage linearly proportional to I_F.

This approach has a few advantages. First, it is relatively simple to realize. Second, very small currents can be measured by simply switching the current measurement resistor, R_M, to higher values (a dynamic range of 120 dB or more is achievable [9]). Third, both potential and current are measured with reference to ground.

The circuit has two main drawbacks. First, since the working electrode is not connected to a true ground, but instead to a virtual ground, it is vulnerable to noise and interference pick-up. This is mostly troublesome when measuring small currents for which large values for R_M are used. Second, the input resistance of the transimpedance amplifier behaves inductively. In other words, at low frequencies, it shows a very small impedance, but as the frequency increases, the impedance increases due to the roll-off in the gain of the transimpedance amplifier. Since the input impedance is in series with the electrochemical cell, which itself has very large capacitive components, the inductive behavior increases the possibility of instability and oscillation in the potential control loop. This drawback is also more troublesome when measuring small currents for which large values of R_M are required.

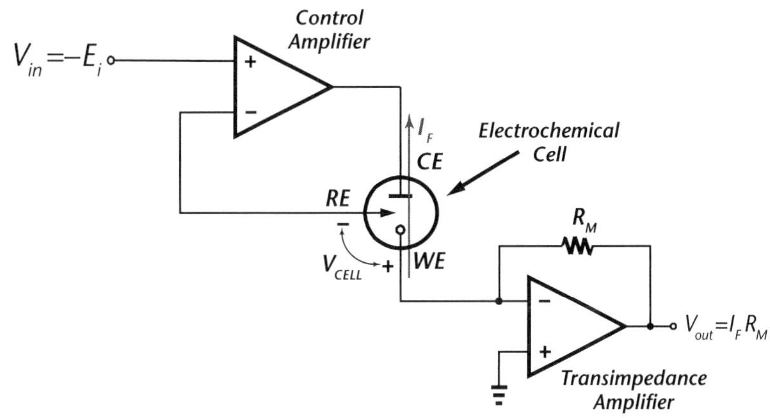

Figure 13.7 Current measurement using a transimpedance amplifier.

Since very large resistors are difficult to realize in integrated circuit form, the transimpedance amplifier is sometimes realized with switched capacitor circuits. A simple realization of this approach is shown in Figure 13.8 [10], in which, when the clock signal is low, I_F charges an integration capacitor, C_M to the following output voltage:

$$V_{out} = \frac{T}{2C_M} I_F \tag{13.5}$$

where T is the clock period. When the clock signal goes high, C_M is discharged, and this process repeats. The integration capacitor can be switched to a larger or smaller value depending on the intended measurement range.

In a more complicated realization, the sensor current can be injected directly into a current-input A/D converter [11], or into a current-input delta-sigma modulator [12]. In addition, the sensor current can be converted to variables other than voltage, such as frequency [2], or time [13].

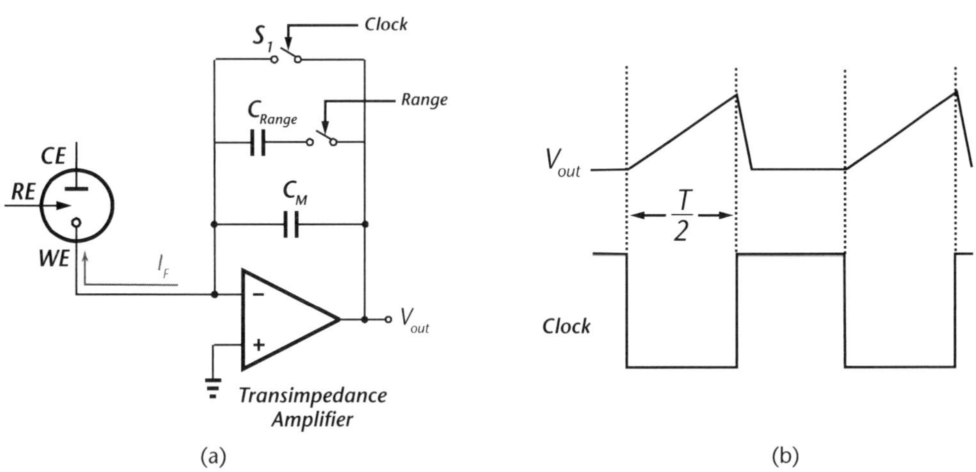

Figure 13.8 Realizing a transimpedance amplifier using a switch-capacitor circuit; (a) circuit, (b) timing.

An important consideration when using switch capacitor circuits for measuring the sensor current is that the capacitance of the input current source, i.e., the capacitance of the working electrode, is a few orders of magnitude larger than the integration capacitor, C_M. As a result, if the circuit is not properly designed, the errors due to charge injection during switching can be unacceptably high [14].

Another approach for the current measurement is to insert a resistor in the current path in the working electrode and measure the voltage developed across that resistor [9]. The voltage can also be amplified before measurement. Two realizations of this approach are shown in Figure 13.9. Clearly, the working electrode is no longer at the ground potential, but its potential changes depending on I_F. So, for proper potential control, its potential is measured and fed back to the control amplifier.

This approach is more complex than using a transimpedance amplifier and requires more active and passive components. As a result, it is noisier and more vulnerable to mismatch between the components. It also has the noise and interference pick-up issues at the working electrode. However, it has the important advantage that it is capable of measuring very small currents. Also, both current and voltage are measured with reference to ground.

Yet another approach for current measurement is to insert a resistor in the current path in the counter electrode and measure the voltage generated across that resistor [15]. Figure 13.10 illustrates this approach. As shown, an instrumentation amplifier measures the voltage generated across R_M. This approach needs more components than the previous two approaches, thus suffers more from mismatch in the components; however, it does have a few interesting advantages.

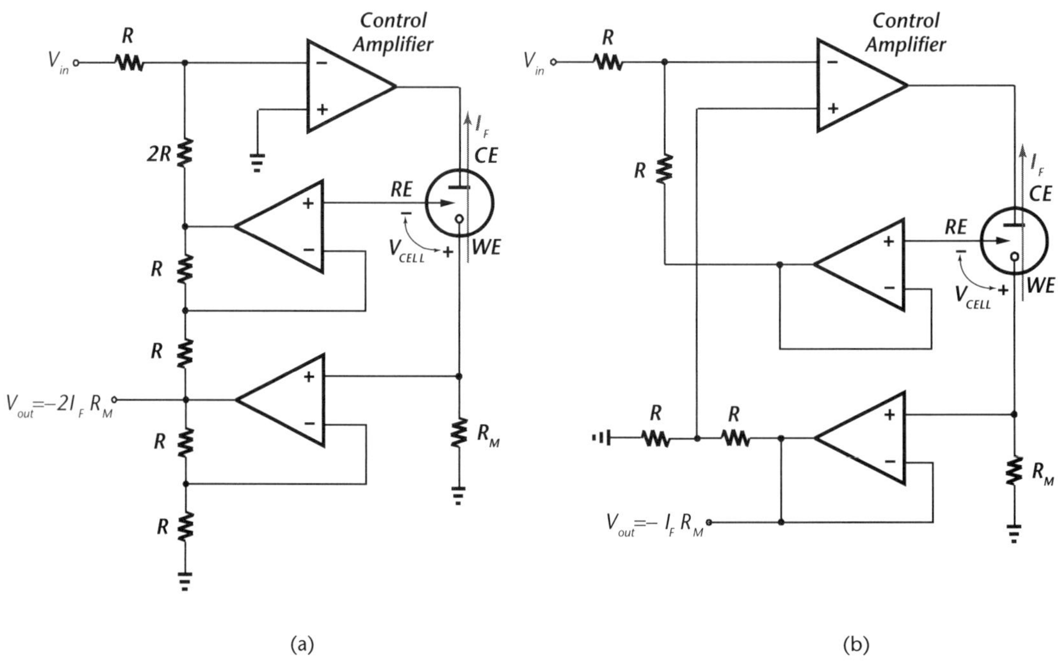

Figure 13.9 Parts (a) and (b) show two different circuits for current measurement by inserting a resistor in the working electrode.

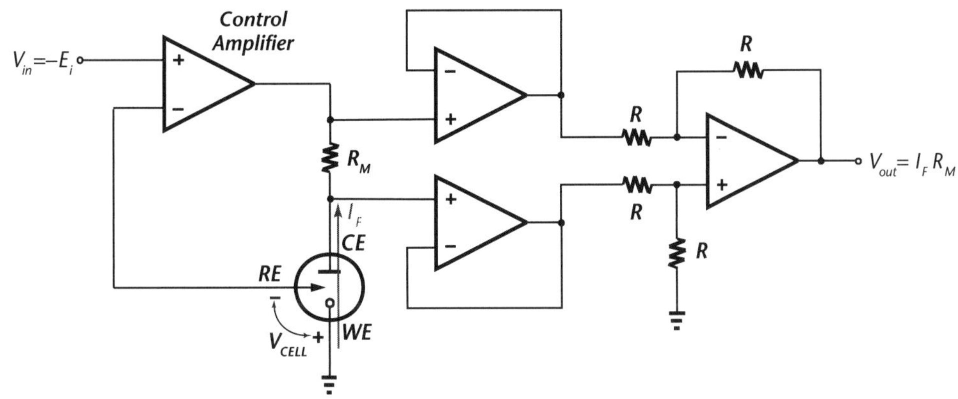

Figure 13.10 Current measurement by inserting a resistor in the counter electrode.

First, the working electrode is connected to a true ground, thus it is not vulnerable to noise and interference pick-up. Second, since there is no additional active component in the signal path, it has better stability than the previous approaches. Third, both measured voltage and current are referenced to ground.

13.4 Design Issues in Advanced CMOS Processes

Even though there are a number of reports on state-of-the-art potentiostats fabricated in CMOS technologies [2, 10–14], there is still a demand for devices with better functionality and with lower power consumption. As the feature size of CMOS processes decreases, the oxide and junction breakdown voltages decrease accordingly, necessitating the use of lower supply voltages for these processes [16–19]; this causes problems when the supply voltage falls below typical interfacial potential differences associated with many analytes. In fact, many analytes are not detectable with the conventional potentiostats working with supply voltages less than 1.8 V [19].

Another issue is the single-supply operation of the new technologies. This problem can be explained with two examples.

The two most widely used electrochemical glucose biosensors are oxygen electrode-based (O_2-based) and hydrogen peroxide electrode-based (H_2O_2-based) sensors. In O_2-based glucose sensors, the cell potential, V_{CELL}, should be about –0.6 V to –0.9 V (with reference to a standard Ag/AgCl reference electrode), and the output current of the sensor is the result of the reduction of oxygen at the surface of the working electrode. In other words, as shown in Figure 13.11(a), the reference electrode (in this case an Ag/AgCl electrode) is required to be maintained at a potential of about 0.6 V to 0.9 V above the potential of the working electrode, where the direction of the sensor current is from the counter electrode to the working electrode. Since the working electrode is at ground potential, maintaining the reference electrode at a potential above the working electrode is easily feasible as long as the cell potential is less than the supply voltage. However, for the transimpedance amplifier to work properly, the output voltage must move below the ground potential (because the direction of the sensor current is towards the working electrode), which is not possible in single-supply voltage circuits.

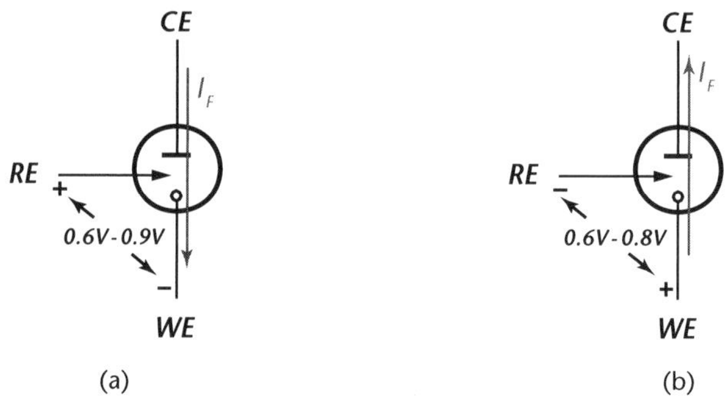

Figure 13.11 The current direction and the cell potential in (a) O_2-based and (b) H_2O_2-based electrochemical glucose biosensors.

For the H_2O_2-based glucose sensor, the situation is opposite but still presents single-supply voltage problems. In this case, the sensor current is the result of the oxidation of hydrogen peroxide at the surface of the working electrode, and so, as shown in Figure 13.11(b), the current flows from the working electrode to the counter electrode. But in this case, the cell potential, V_{CELL}, must be between 0.6 V and 0.8 V (assuming Ag/AgCl), meaning that the potential of the reference electrode must be kept between 0.6 V to 0.8 V below the potential of the working electrode, which again is not possible with a single positive supply because the working electrode is at the lowest potential in the circuit, which is the ground potential.

The issues of single-supply operation can be resolved to some extent by modifying the potentiostat circuit described earlier. For example, Figure 13.7 can be modified by shifting the potential of the virtual ground node to $V_{DD}/2$. The new circuit, shown in Figure 13.12, can be used for both of the O_2- and the H_2O_2-based glucose sensors if a supply voltage of at least 1.8 V is used. But still, the input drive voltage is limited to –0.9 V to +0.9 V which is not adequate for detecting many other analytes. As an example, the potential window for a platinum working electrode is about 3.0 V [19].

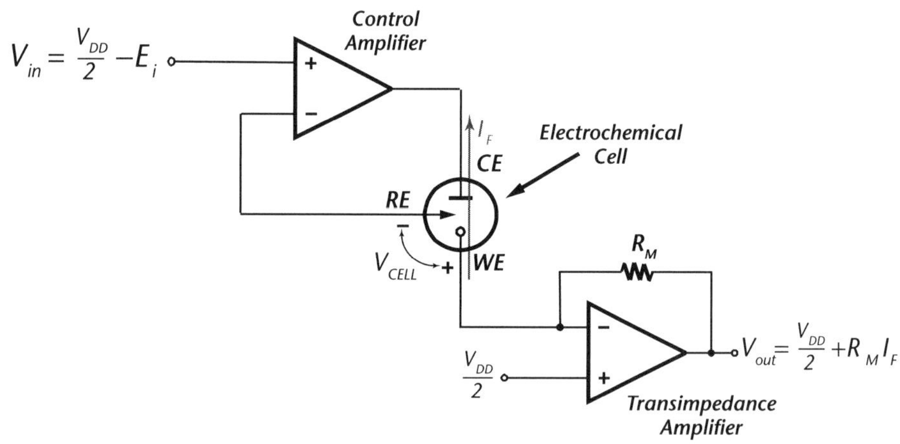

Figure 13.12 A conventional potentiostat working in a single-supply voltage chip.

To overcome the above issues, recently a fully differential potentiostat (Figure 13.13) was proposed [19]. This circuit has almost twice the voltage swing of the conventional potentiostat because neither the potential of the working electrode or reference electrode is fixed, instead both can change dynamically. Based on measurement results provided in [19], this circuit has more than 6 dB extra dynamic range compared to the conventional potentiostat structure (Figure 13.7). It also has a better common-mode rejection ratio. However, the circuit is clearly more complicated and has much larger power consumption. But, the main problems are that both input and output voltages are not referenced to ground, creating some difficulties in generating the input voltage and measuring the output voltage.

13.4.1 Generating the Input Drive Voltage

For a general-purpose potentiostat, the input drive voltage is usually set using a D/A converter. In other words, the user enters the input drive voltage digitally, and the D/A converter generates and applies the appropriate analog voltage to the input of the potentiostat.

However, for potentiostats dedicated for electrochemical sensors, the input drive voltage is usually a constant voltage. As an example, the cell voltage for an H_2O_2-based glucose sensor is usually fixed at 0.7 V, or for an O_2-based glucose sensor, it is usually fixed at –0.6 V.

Generating a reference voltage independent of temperature and process variations is accomplished using a bandgap circuit. In standard CMOS technologies, bandgap circuits are realized using native (parasitic) vertical PNP transistors (p^+/n-well/p-substrate). Conventional bandgap circuits generate a reference voltage of about 1.25 V or 2.5 V.

For electrochemical sensors, often input drive voltages of values other than 1.25 V or 2.5 V are required. In addition, it is sometimes required to generate a constant negative reference voltage (or in single-supply potentiostats, a constant bias voltage below V_{DD}). Here, two approaches for generating an arbitrary positive or negative constant voltage are described.

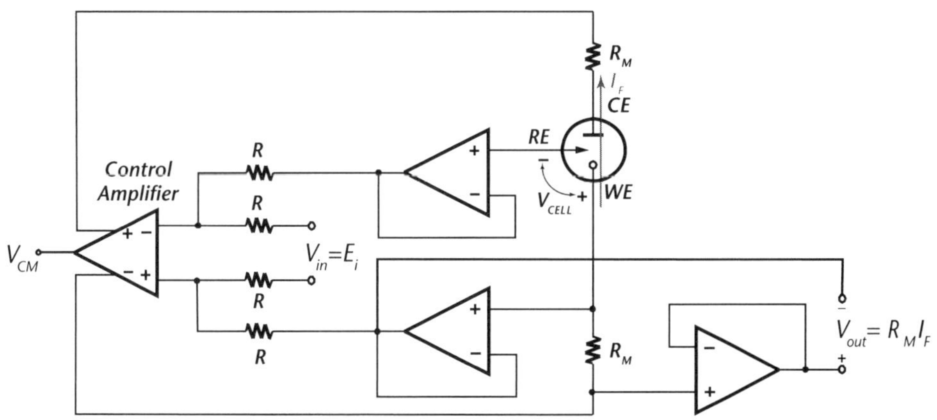

Figure 13.13 A fully differential potentiostat.

The first approach is achieved through the use of a conventional bandgap circuit. As illustrated in Figure 13.14, the bandgap voltage reference generated by the bandgap circuit is applied across a reference resistor, R_1, generating a reference current, I_{REF}. Then, I_{REF} is mirrored and injected into other resistors that are completely matched with R_1. As an example, in Figure 13.14, by changing the ratio of R_2/R_1, V_{BG2} can be set to the desired voltage reference. Similarly, by changing R_3/R_1, V_{BG3} can be set to an arbitrary voltage reference below V_{DD}. In addition to the ratio of the matched resistor, the ratio of the transistors in the current mirror can be used to achieve the desired voltage reference.

A better approach to generate arbitrarily-defined voltage references is to use a current-mode bandgap circuit.

Figure 13.15 illustrates a current-mode bandgap circuit [20].The operation of the circuit can be seen as follows. By assuming $V_X = V_Y$, and writing KCL at node V_Y, I_{REF} is calculated by:

$$I_{REF} = I_1 + I_2 = \frac{V_{EB1} - V_{EB2}}{R_1} + \frac{V_{EB1}}{R_3} = \frac{V_T \ln(mn)}{R_1} + \frac{V_{EB1}}{R_3} \tag{13.6}$$

where m is the area ratio of the bipolar transistors, Q_1 and Q_2, and n is the current ratio in those transistors. As a result of Equation (13.6), I_1 is a current with a positive temperature coefficient and I_2 with a negative temperature coefficient. Hence, by proper selection of the resistor ratio R_3/R_1, the temperature dependence of I_{REF} can be cancelled to the first order. As a result, I_{REF} is a current, which only depends on resistor variations, and V_{BG1} and V_{BG2} can respectively be calculated as follows:

$$V_{BG1} = R_4 I_{REF} = R_4 \left(\frac{V_T \ln(mn)}{R_1} + \frac{V_{EB1}}{R_3} \right) \tag{13.7}$$

$$V_{BG2} = V_{DD} - R_5 I_{REF} = V_{DD} - R_5 \left(\frac{V_T \ln(mn)}{R_1} + \frac{V_{EB1}}{R_3} \right) \tag{13.8}$$

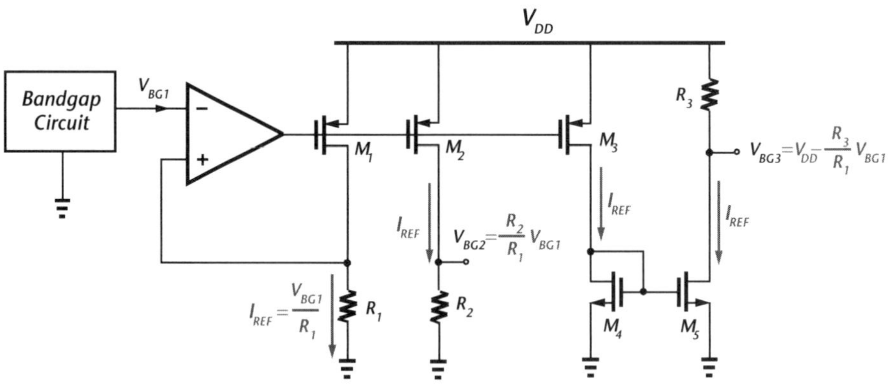

Figure 13.14 The normal approach for generating arbitrarily-defined bandgap references.

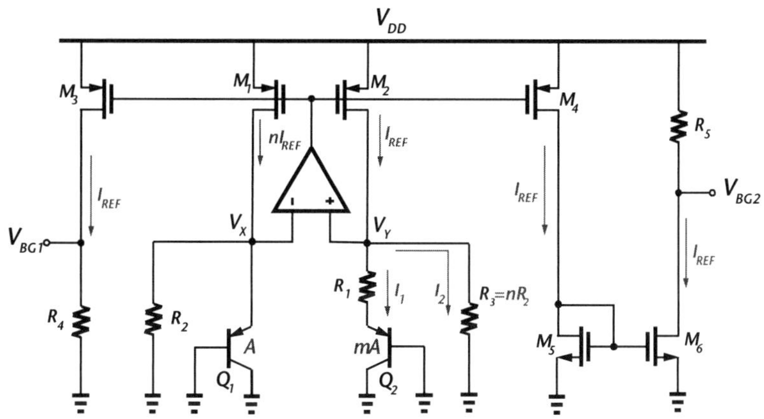

Figure 13.15 Using a current-mode bandgap circuit to generate arbitrarily-defined voltage references.

Therefore, if R_1 to R_5 are completely matched, V_{BG1} will be a positive reference voltage with a value that can be adjusted by changing R_4. Also, V_{BG2} is a reference voltage below V_{DD} with a value that can be adjusted by changing R_5.

The second circuit is advantageous in terms of power consumption and also the minimum required supply voltage for the proper operation of the circuit.

13.5 Electrical Equivalent Circuit Modeling

As explained earlier, the stability of a potentiostat is very important because if a potentiostat loses its stability, not only will it not provide correct measurements, but it also might damage the electrochemical sensor.

To properly design a potentiostat circuit, a comprehensive understanding of the electrical equivalent model of the electrochemical cell is necessary. This section aims to explain the physical model of an electrode/solution interface and develop a simple equivalent circuit for that interface. Secondly, the tools and approaches that are used in practice to find the equivalent circuits are explained.

13.5.1 Mathematical Circuit Modeling

For an ideal polarizable electrode, the impedance of the electrode consists of a capacitor, C_{dl}, so-called the double-layer capacitor, in series with the solution resistance, R_S (Figure 13.16(a)). Double-layer capacitance is very difficult to model as it is a nonlinear capacitance whose value depends on many parameters such as applied potential, temperature, ionic concentrations, types of ions, oxide layers, electrode roughness, impurity adsorption and so on [21]. However, C_{dl} can be approximated by

$$C_{dl} = K_{dl} A \tag{13.9}$$

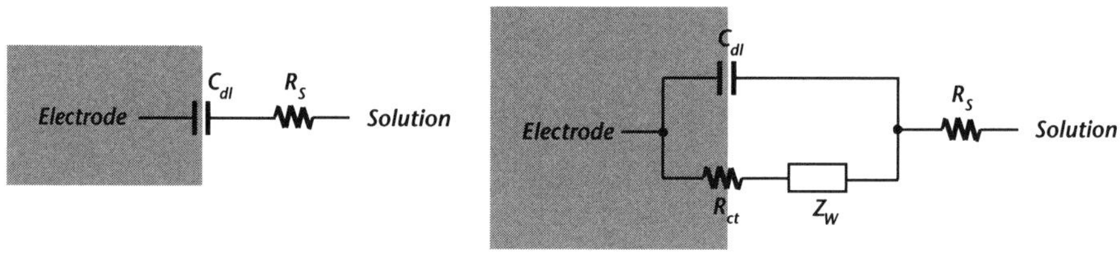

(a) (b)

Figure 13.16 (a) Equivalent circuit of an ideal polarizable electrode. (b) Randles' equivalent circuit.

where A denotes the area of the electrode, and K_{dl} is a constant typically in the range of 10–100 μF/cm^2 [22] (for some materials, such as iridium oxide, it can be orders of magnitude higher).

Solution resistance usually has a great effect on the impedance of an electrochemical cell. The resistance of an ionic solution depends on the ionic concentration, type of ions, temperature, and the geometry of the area in which current is carried [21, 22]. Assuming a uniform current is flowing though a bounded volume of the solution with an area of A and a length of l, the resistance can be calculated by

$$R_S = \rho \frac{l}{A} \tag{13.10}$$

where ρ is the solution resistivity [21]. Similar to the double-layer capacitance, solution resistance is also difficult to calculate because, in most electrochemical cells, there is not a uniform current distribution through a definite solution area, and it is very difficult to calculate the current flow path and the geometry of the solution in which current flows [21].

The circuit model of real electrodes is considerably more complicated. For example, double-layer capacitors do not behave like a linear capacitor, but they can be better modeled by a *constant phase element* (CPE). A constant phase element is considered to be a non-ideal capacitor whose impedance can be expressed by

$$Z_{CPE} = \frac{1}{C(j\omega)^{\alpha}} \tag{13.11}$$

For a capacitor, $\alpha = 1$, but for a constant phase element, α is less than one.

For a real electrode, when the electrode/solution potential is forced away from its open-circuit potential, an electric current flows through the electrode surface whose value is controlled by the kinetics of the reactions taking place at the electrode surface and by the rate of mass transfer of the reactants towards and away from the electrode surface [3].

Figure 13.16(b) shows Randles' equivalent circuit, which is a basic model and usually the starting point for modeling most electrode/solution interfaces. In the model, R_S and C_{dl} represent the solution resistance and the double-layer capacitance, respectively. R_{ct} is a resistance that represents charge transfer at the electrode surface and Z_W, called the *Warburg impedance*, is a general impedance representing the diffusion of species toward and away from the electrode. Unlike R_S, C_{dl} and R_{ct}, Z_W cannot be modeled with basic circuit elements, such as R, C and L, whose values are independent of frequency; instead, it is considered to be a general impedance [3].

To calculate the charge-transfer resistance, the following equation, which is the general relation between the potential and the faradaic current, is usually considered [21]:

$$i = i_0 \left[\frac{C_O}{C_O^*} e^{\alpha \frac{nF}{RT}\eta} - \frac{C_R}{C_R^*} e^{-(1-\alpha)\frac{nF}{RT}\eta} \right] \tag{13.12}$$

where η is the applied overpotential defined as $E - E_0$, where E and E_0 represent the applied and equilibrium (open circuit) potentials, respectively. i_o is the exchange current density, C_o is the concentration of oxidant at the electrode surface and C_o^* is concentration of oxidant in the bulk. C_R is the concentration of reductant at the electrode surface, and C_R^* denotes concentration of reductant in the bulk. α is the reaction order, and n is the number of electrons transferred. The overpotential, η, measures the degree of electrode polarization.

When the concentration in the solution bulk is the same as at the electrode surface, $C_o = C_o^*$ and $C_R = C_R^*$. Equation (13.12) is simplified to the so-called *Butler-Volmer equation* as:

$$i = i_0 \left[e^{\alpha \frac{nF}{RT}\eta} - e^{-(1-\alpha)\frac{nF}{RT}\eta} \right] \tag{13.13}$$

Stirring can minimize diffusion effects and keep the assumptions of $C_o = C_o^*$ and $C_R = C_R^*$ valid.

When the overpotential, η, is very small, the value of the charge transfer resistance can be simply calculated as [3]:

$$R_{ct} = \frac{RT}{nFi_0} \tag{13.14}$$

However, the amount of faradaic current is not just controlled by the kinetics of the reaction, but also by the diffusion of reactants towards and away from the electrode surface. The Warburg impedance, representing the diffusion, depends on the frequency of the excitation potential. It consists of a frequency-dependent resistance $R_W = \sigma/\omega^{0.5}$ in series with a pseudo-capacitance, $C_W = 1/(\sigma\omega^{0.5})$ [3]. Thus, the impedance of the Warburg impedance equals

$$Z_W = R_W + \frac{1}{C_W j\omega} = \frac{\sigma}{\omega^{0.5}} - j\frac{\sigma}{\omega^{0.5}} \tag{13.15}$$

where σ is the Warburg coefficient defined as [3]:

$$\sigma = \frac{RT}{n^2F^2A\sqrt{2}}\left(\frac{1}{C_O^*\sqrt{D_O}} + \frac{1}{C_R^*\sqrt{D_R}}\right) \tag{13.16}$$

where D_O is the diffusion coefficient of the oxidant, and D_R the diffusion coefficient of the reductant.

The above form of Warburg impedance is valid only if the diffusion layer has an infinite thickness; therefore it is called the *infinite Warburg Impedance*. Usually the assumption does not hold, thus, a more general form of the Warburg impedance can be used, namely the *finite Warburg Impedance* [21].

Randles' equivalent circuit is usually used for modeling very simple electrode processes. To consider more complex processes, such as those involving adsorption of electroreactants, multistep charge transfer and so on, many other more complicated equivalent circuits have been proposed [3].

13.5.2 Numerical Modeling

Unfortunately, closed-form mathematical circuit modeling of an electrochemical cell is usually difficult and sometimes impossible, due to all the factors mentioned previously. Thus, the impedance of an electrochemical cell is usually experimentally measured over a wide frequency range (usually from 1 mHz to 20 kHz [4]) and then, using a non-linear least squares fitting program, an equivalent circuit is fitted to the experimental data.

Measuring the impedance of an electrode over a frequency range is called *Electrochemical Impedance Spectroscopy* (EIS), which is a very powerful tool for the analysis of complex electrochemical systems and can provide a valuable and complete description of the electrode process [23].

Impedance measurement is possible in either the frequency domain, with a frequency response analyzer, or in the time domain using Fourier transformation with a spectrum analyzer [3].

Using a frequency response analyzer is more popular for modeling an electrode/solution interface. The principle of this approach is shown in Figure 13.17 [3]. The frequency response analyzer adds a very small AC signal, $e(t)$, with very small magnitude (5–10 mV peak-to-peak) to the DC potential applied to the cell, E_{dc}, and measures and saves the magnitude and the phase (or real and imaginary parts) of the AC current, $i(t)$, flowing though the cell [3].

This measurement is performed over the desired frequency range. Since the impedance of only one of the electrodes is usually of interest, a two-electrode system with a very large reference electrode or a three-electrode system has to be used.

The recorded data from the frequency response analyzer can be plotted either in a Nyquist plot or in a Bode plot. Electrochemists prefer the Nyquist representation, while engineers typically prefer a Bode plot [4].

In order to fit a circuit model to the impedance data, some prior knowledge of the electrochemical cell is necessary because two entirely different circuit networks can

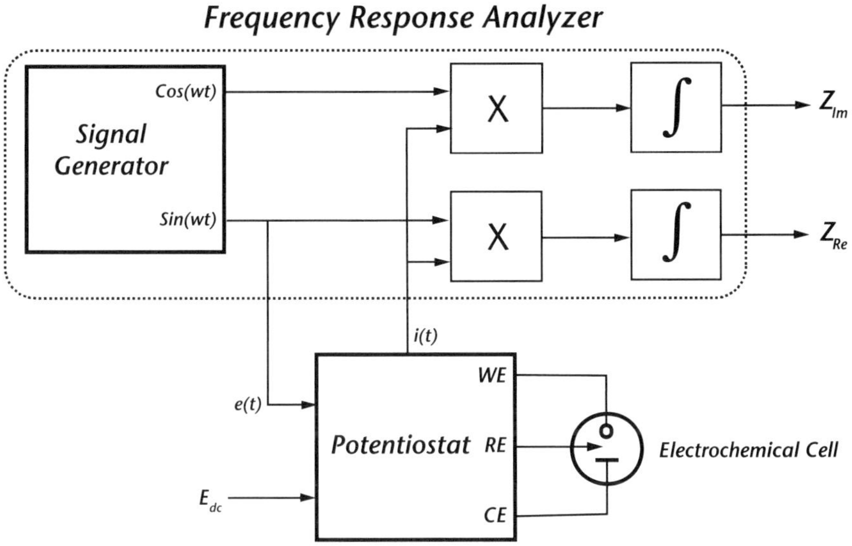

Figure 13.17 Block diagram of the system used for electrochemical impedance spectroscopy using a frequency response analyzer.

produce the same impedance spectrum. In fact, for a given phase and gain response, an infinite number of circuit networks exist [3].

It is worth mentioning that the equivalent circuit obtained from electrochemical impedance spectroscopy is valid only at the operating voltage point. In other words, it is a small-signal impedance and does not provide any information about the large-signal behavior of the electrochemical cell. The knowledge of the large-signal behavior of the electrochemical sensor is also important in the design of a potentiostat because, when the sensing process begins, the cell potential moves from its open-circuit potential to its desired cell potential. The large-signal behavior of the electrochemical cells are very non-linear and sometimes can show negative resistance characteristics; thus, sometimes the potentiostat might stick to a voltage point during start-up and begin to oscillate.

The knowledge of the large-signal behavior of an electrochemical cell can be obtained using a cyclic voltammetry experiment in which a large-signal triangular waveform is applied to the electrochemical cell and its output current is measured and plotted.

13.6 Conclusions

In this chapter, we started with a brief review of amperometric electrochemical sensors. Then, the three-electrode measurement system and potentiostat were introduced. Different approaches for the potential control and current measurement in potentiostat circuits were explained and the pros and cons of each approach were described. Next, the various challenges in the design of potentiostats in advanced submicron processes were presented. Finally, the methods and approaches for modeling electrochemical sensors were discussed.

Even though there has been considerable progress toward the full integration of potentiostats, there are still many issues that require further research. General-purpose potentiostats are required to interface with a large diversity of electrochemical sensors. The main design challenge here is the voltage head-room in low-voltage technologies. In addition, these circuits must have a high degree of stability. However, for portable applications that need low-power consumption, good stability together with low-power consumption cannot be easily achieved.

There is also a trend toward the microfabrication of electrochemical sensors and also other systems that use electrochemical principles such as neurochemical sensors, bimolecular detectors, and so on. This trend has meant that the area and consequently the output response of these sensors have been considerably reduced. Therefore, there will be a continuing requirement for the design of very low-noise and wide-range potentiostats with high accuracy and high resolution.

References

[1] S. M. Martin, F.H. Gebara, B.J. Larivee, and R.B. Brown, "A CMOS-Integrated microinstrument for trace detection of heavy metals," *IEEE J. Solid-State Circuits*, vol. 40; No. 12, pp. 2777–2786, 2005.

[2] M.M. Ahmadi and G. Jullien, "A low power CMOS potentiostat for bioimplantable applications," *Proceedings of the 5th International Workshop on System-on-Chip* (IWSOC'05), pp. 184–189, 2005.

[3] A.J. Bard and L.R. Faulkner, *Electrochemical Methods: Fundamentals and Applications*, Wiley, New York, 2001, 2nd Edition.

[4] M. Lambrechts and W. Sansen, *Biosensors: Microelectrochemical Devices*, IOP Publishing, 1992.

[5] A. Hierlemann, *Integrated Chemical Microsensor Systems in CMOS Technology*, Springer-Verlag, Berlin, 2005.

[6] B.R. Eggins, *Chemical Sensors and Biosensors*, Wiley, West Sussex, 2002.

[7] E. Wilkins and P. Atanosov, "Glucose Monitoring: state of the art and future possibilities," *Med. Eng. Phys.*, vol. 18, No. 4, pp. 273–288, 1996.

[8] L. Busoni, M. Carla, and L. Lanzi, "A comparison between potentiostatic circuits with grounded work or auxiliary electrode," *Review of Scientific Instruments*, vol. 73, No. 4, pp. 1921–1923, 2002.

[9] R. Doelling, "Potentiostats," *Bank Elektronik application note*, 2nd edition, March 2000.

[10] R. Kakerow, H. Kappert, E. Spiegel, and Y. Manoli, "Low-power single-chip CMOS potentiostat," *Proceedings of 8th International Conference on Solid-state sensors and actuators*, pp. 142–145, 1995.

[11] R. Reay, S. Kounaves, and G. Kovacs, "An integrated CMOS potentiostat for miniaturized electroanalytical instrumentation," *Proceedings of the IEEE International Solid-State Circuits Conference* (ISSCC), pp. 162–163, 1994.

[12] A. Gore, S. Chakrabartty, S. Pal, and E.C. Alocilja, "A multichannel femtoampere-sensitivity potentiostat array for biosensing applications," *IEEE Trans. on Circuits and Systems I: Regular Papers*, vol. 53, No. 11, pp. 2357–2363, 2006.

[13] H.S. Narula and J.G. Harris, "A time-based VLSI potentiostat for ion current measurements," *IEEE Sensors Journal*, vol. 6, No. 2, pp. 239–247, 2006.

[14] Richard Reay, "Microfabricated Electrochemical Analysis Systems," Ph.D. dissertation, Stanford University, 1995.

[15] R. Greef, "Instruments for use in electrode process research," *Journal of Physics E, Scientific Instruments*, vol. 11, pp. 1–12, 1979.

[16] R.F.B. Turner, D. Jed Harrison, and H.P. Baltes, "A CMOS potentiostat for amperometric chemical sensors," *IEEE J. Solid State Circuits*, vol. 22, No. 3, pp. 473–478, 1987.

[17] S.-J. Wei and H.C. Lin, "CMOS chopper amplifier for chemical sensors," *IEEE Trans. on Instrumentation and Measurement*, vol. 41, No. 1, pp. 77–80, 1992.

[18] A. Frey et al., "Design of an integrated potentiostat circuit for CMOS biosensor chips," *Proceedings of the IEEE International Symposium on Circuits and Systems* (ISCAS), Vol. 5, pp. 9–12, 2003.

[19] S. Martin, F. Gebara, T. Strong, and R. Brown, "A low-voltage, chemical sensor interface for systems-on-chip: the fully differential potentiostat," *Proceedings of the IEEE International Symposium on Circuits and Systems* (ISCAS), vol. 4, pp. 892–895, 2004.

[20] H. Banba et al., "A CMOS bandgap reference circuit with sub-1-V operation," *IEEE J. of Solid-State Circuits*, vol. 34, No. 5, pp. 670–674, 1999.

[21] "Electrochemical Impedance Spectroscopy Theory: A Primer," *Application Note*, Gamry Instrument.

[22] D.T. Sawyer, A. Sobkowiak, and J.L. Roberts Jr., *Electrochemistry for Chemists*, Wiley, New York, 1995 (2nd Ed.).

[23] S.-M. Park and J.-S. Yoo, "Electrochemical impedance spectroscopy for better electrochemical measurements," *Analytical Chemistry*, vol. 75, No. 21, pp. 455A–461A, 2003.

CHAPTER 14

ADC Circuits for Biomedical Applications

João Goes

14.1 Introduction

Most currently available sensors of biopotential signals operate in the analog mode, and the increased use of intensive digital signal processing has required analog-to-digital converters (ADCs) to interface with advanced digital processors and computers [1]. The advantages of digital signal processing include higher accuracy, repeatability, reliability, and immunity to noise. Additionally, there is an increasing demand for sensing biopotential signals using portable and wearable low-power devices that are efficiently integrated with wireless health-monitoring systems in order to allow patients to be permanently and remotely followed by doctors during long periods of time. It is unquestionable that monitoring the biopotentials of a person is a powerful diagnosing method. It is necessary to measure, record, and analyze several types of signals, depending on the area of concern. Currently, most of the equipment utilized to acquire these signals is very expensive and not easily transportable or wearable. On the other hand, the use of a standard CMOS technology, a mass production technology, provides affordable devices and the use of programmability will mean that one device can be re-configurable for different types of measurements. As a direct consequence, there is an increasing trend to produce cheap, battery-powered, light devices that may be used by a person collecting data for several days as well as from many different types of sensors.

The frequency content of different biopotential signals covers different portions of the spectrum, and signal bandwidths (*BW*) can range from near DC to about 10 kHz as illustrated in Figure 14.1 [1].

Some biopotentials have higher amplitudes than others, ranging from a few micro-Volts to several hundreds of mili-Volts. The A/D interface systems described in this chapter will be suitable for battery-powered (portable) medical equipment such as Electrooculogram (EOG), Electroencephalogram (EEG), Electrocardiogram (ECG), Electromyogram (EMG), and Axon Action Potential (AAP). On the other hand, these systems are supplied with several batteries of 1.5 V and dissipate a considerable amount of power. Both low-voltage operation and low-power dissipation are of great importance for portable applications. Low-voltage operation is demanded because it is desirable to use as few batteries as possible because of size and weight considerations. Low current consumption is necessary to ensure a reasonable battery lifetime.

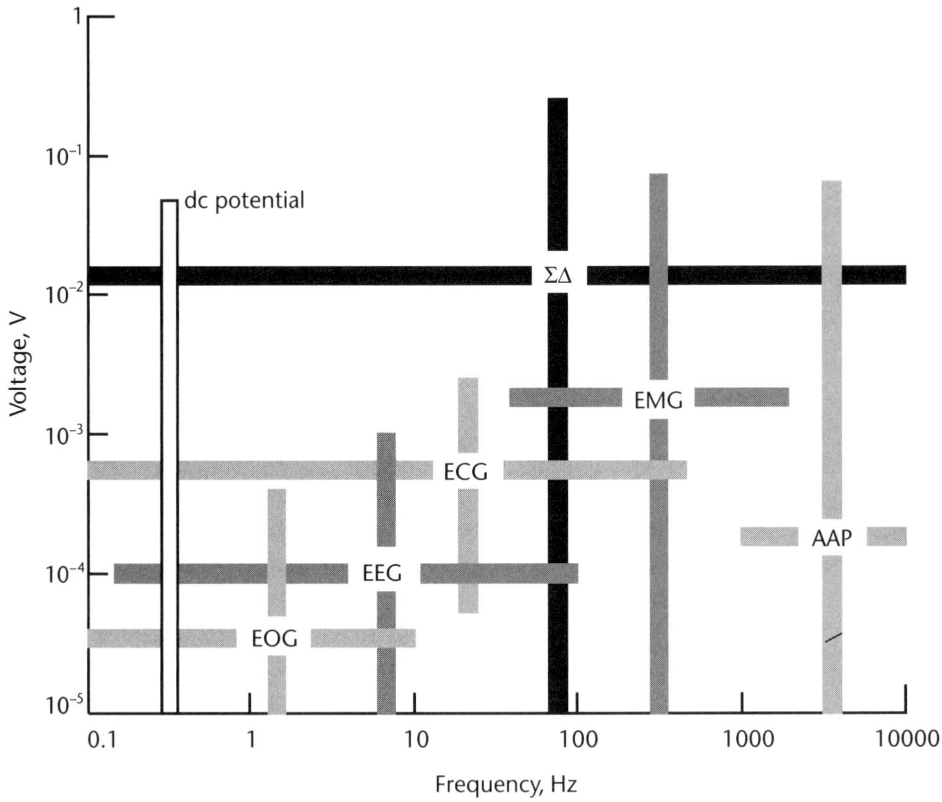

Figure 14.1 Voltages and frequency ranges of some common bio-potential signals (in gray color); dc potentials (in white color) include intracellular voltages as well as voltages measured from several points on the body; the black-color bars represent the required dynamic-range (DR) and bandwidth (BW) of the proposed ADC circuit (either Sigma-Delta or Nyquist-rate) [10].

Typical commercial data-acquisition systems such as the one illustrated in Figure 14.2 (a) have several performance limitations. They are normally based on ADCs with resolutions of around 10 to 12 bits, meaning that there is no dynamic range to deal simultaneously with a strong signal (such as the 50/60 Hz AC signal) and with the extremely small signals pretended to be measured/digitized. Moreover, as CMOS technologies continue to evolve towards smaller geometries, new design techniques need to be developed to simplify the design of such ADCs, while improving energy efficiency and reducing die area.

Many recent works have been published over the past years [2–9] based on A/D conversion architectures envisaging biomedical applications. Most of these architectures rely on sigma-delta structures [2–5, 7–9]. In [2, 3] an interesting switched-capacitor third-order ΣΔ modulator is described but with a limited DR of only 50 dB and a BW of 250 Hz, which makes it only suitable for low-speed applications, such as the acquisition of cardiac signals. In [4], a 0.6 V delta-sigma audio ADC (also suitable for multiple biomedical applications due to its 82 dB DR and 24 kHz BW) employs a 2-2 cascade structure and uses new switched-RC integrator circuits. This circuit has, however, the drawback of requiring a large silicon area. The ΣΔ modulator proposed in [5] follows a switched-current implementation that achieves quite

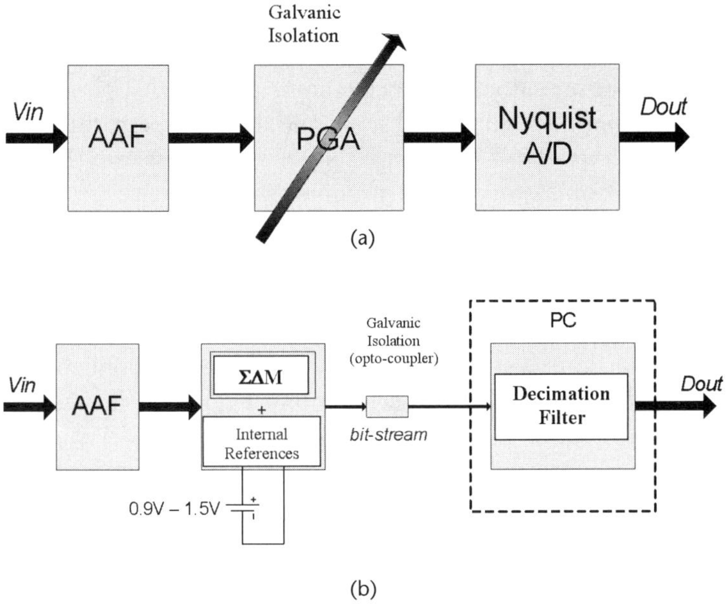

Figure 14.2 (a) Conventional biomedical acquisition systems; (b) proposed new architecture if a Sigma-Delta is used instead of a conventional Nyquist-rate ADC.

a small area. However, its DR is limited to about 60 dB (~10 bits), which is not enough to digitize some bio-potential signals. In [6], a completely different A/D architecture is proposed and it is based on a bio-inspired algorithm. Again, in this circuit, the effective resolution is limited to about 7.4 bits, although the power efficiency of this circuit is quite good. In [7], an hybrid incremental ΣΔ modulator is described but, due to its BW of the order of 1 MHz and its high power dissipation (~38 mW), it is only useful for digitizing bio-signals from arrays of many sensors. In [8], a very interesting reconfigurable ΣΔ modulator based on a MASH structure (with programmable BW and DR according to the specific application) is described and covers all referred applications. Likewise, the work proposed in [9] can be readily used in multiple biomedical applications. It relies on a continuous-time implementation of a third-order ΣΔ modulator using a new return-to-open DAC structure. This ADC is very power efficient and it needs only 0.5 V in the power supply for proper operation. However, as it is referred to later on in this chapter, the ΣΔ modulators reported in [4–5, 8–9] are quite power efficient but they are relatively poor in terms of power-and-area efficiency.

Two energy-and-area highly efficient single-amplifier architectures are selected and described in this chapter:

(1) A second-order ΣΔ modulator (ΣΔM) operating down to 0.9 V, which has the advantage of having a larger dynamic range (*DR*), followed by a decimation filter (DF) and by a programmable low-pass/band-pass digital filter (LP/BP). The ΣΔ architecture proposed here employs a single-phase scheme technique in order to improve the dynamic performance and, simultaneously, to reduce the circuit complexity, substrate noise, and area. The ΣΔM was fabricated in a 0.18 μm CMOS technology, occupies a die area of only 0.06 mm^2, dissipates 0.2 mW from a 0.9 V supply, and provides 80 dB SNDR and 83 dB DR over a 10 kHz BW.

(2) A Calibration-Free Low-Power and Low-Area 1.2 V 14-b resolution and 80 kHz BW (1.07 MHz clock frequency) two-stage algorithmic ADC. Due to the ultra-small area, the target performance is compatible with a power figure-of-merit better than 0.5 pJmm^2. The simulated static and dynamic performance is compatible with, at least, 12.2 bits (DNL, INL and ENOB) at Nyquist rate. The architecture consists of a cascade of 2 stages with minimum resolution per stage and the amplified residue is recycled during 7 clock cycles. Each stage comprises a low-resolution quantizer for local quantization and a 1.5-bit multiplying-digital-to-analog converter (MDAC) for residue computation and amplification. This MDAC is based in a mismatch insensitive multiply-by-two amplifier (MBTA) with an accurate gain of two, and it operates within a single clock cycle and uses only one amplifier. Note that, in the band of interest for a specific biomedical application, digital filtering can be applied due to the over-sampling factor which is at least 4, since for this Nyquist-rate ADC, the conversion-rate (Fs) is 154 kHz and the maximum band of interest is only, say, 20 kHz. If this type of filtering is used, the ENOB can be increased up to 13.7 bits since the SNR improves roughly by 12 dB.

14.2 A Second-Order ΣΔ Modulator (ΣΔM) with 80 dB SNDR and 83 dB DR Operating Down to 0.9 V

14.2.1 Introduction

The architecture proposed in [10] and shown in Figure 14.2 (b), employs a mixed clock-boosting/switched-opamp (CB/SO) second-order ΣΔ modulator, which has the advantage of having a larger dynamic range (DR), followed by a decimation filter (DF) and by a programmable low-pass/band-pass digital filter (LP/BP). The measured DR is about 83 dB ($ENOB$~14 bits) in a BW of 10 kHz and about 96 dB (ENOB~16 bits) only by re-programming the digital LP/BP filter to have a BW of 500 Hz (for ECG applications). The main advantages of this architecture are (1) it is flexible, since it is suitable for digitizing several bio-potential signals only by reconfiguring the LP/BP digital filter; (2) it is designed for low-voltage and low-power operation using a mixed CB/SO approach, i.e., suitable for portable equipment; and (3) the required Galvanic isolation can be performed in the digital domain, in the bit-stream of the modulator (using an opto-coupler), avoiding any type of analogue filtering.

14.2.2 Second-Order Sigma-Delta Architecture

Figure 14.3 shows the scaled modulator architecture that can operate with a positive power supply ranging from 1.5 V down to 0.9 V. As described in [11], a second-order non-cascaded topology is chosen due to the robustness against non-idealities. The optimized coefficients $gx1$, $gx2$, $gdac1$, $gdac2$ used are, respectively, 0.25, 0.5, 1/3 and 1/3. The differential reference voltage (V_{REF}) is nominally equal to 0.75 V (V_{REFp} = 0.875 V and V_{REFn} = 0.125 V). The over-sampling ratio (OSR) adopted is 256 and the nominal BW is 10 kHz ($F_{CLK} \approx 5.128$ MHz).

The modulator is scaled to meet the amplitude requirements resulting from the low supply voltage. In Figure 14.3, the filled-black areas of the voltage bars represent the permitted single-ended voltage levels at the different nodes. The integrator outputs

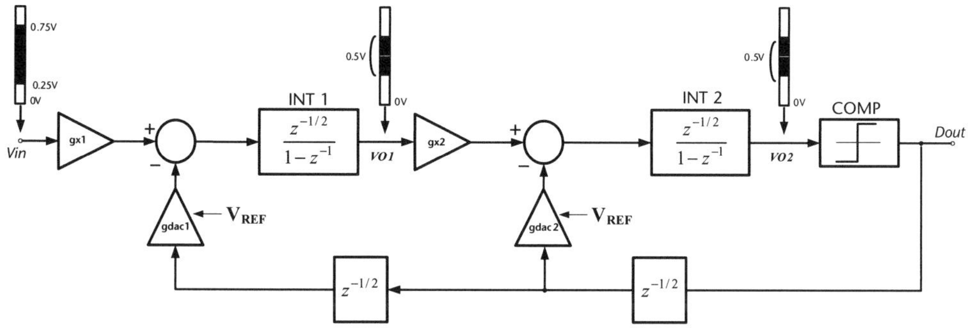

Figure 14.3 Scaled ΣΔ modulator topology. The filled black areas of the voltage bars represent the permitted single-ended voltage levels at the different nodes[11].

are designed for a peak-to-peak differential voltage range of 1 Vp-p. The modulator input is scaled so that the expected maximum SNDR is reached at an amplitude of 1 Vp-p. Digital half-delay D-type flip-flop (FF) stages are used in the modulator feedback path, to compensate for the effect of the SO half-delay integrators on the modulator transfer function.

There are several important techniques used in these ΣΔ modulators. The most important one is that the architecture proposed here employs the single-phase scheme described in [12], where all switches are driven by the same single clock-phase. Simulated results show that this new scheme is capable of improving the dynamic performance when compared with the conventional one. However, either at architecture or at circuit level, there are also other important differences when compared with [13–15]. At architecture level, all coefficients are optimized to avoid the need of using any input common-mode DC shifting capacitors, resulting in additional power and area savings. At circuit level, the integrators are realized using the SO technique, but two clock-bootstrapping (CBT) circuits are employed at the input switches overcoming the interface problem at the input and, on the other hand, strongly enhancing the linearity of the input sampling SC-network by keeping the gate-overdrive voltage practically constant. As it will be demonstrated by measured results, this enhancement of the linearity of the input sampling circuitry during the sampling operation together with the overall distortion reduction resulting from using the proposed single-phase scheme, has the result that the dynamic range of the modulator is pushed closer to the theoretical limit of an ideal second-order ΣΔ modulator.

14.2.3 Circuit Implementation

14.2.3.1 Mixed Clock-Boosted (CB) and Switched-Opamp (SO) Realization

The block diagram of the fully-differential ΣΔM circuit is shown in Figure 14.4.

Traditionally, four non-overlapping clocking phases are used to drive the SC network in the integrators (INTs). The first novelty in this circuit consists in using a single phase Φ_1 to drive all switches that are controlled by phases Φ_2, Φ_{2D} and Φ_{1D}. Likewise, switches driven by phases Φ_1, Φ_{1D} and Φ_{2D} are driven by a complementary phase Φ_1. Phases Φ_1 and Φ_1 are overlapping phases and, consequently, there is a certain fraction of time during which several switches conduct at the same time. This

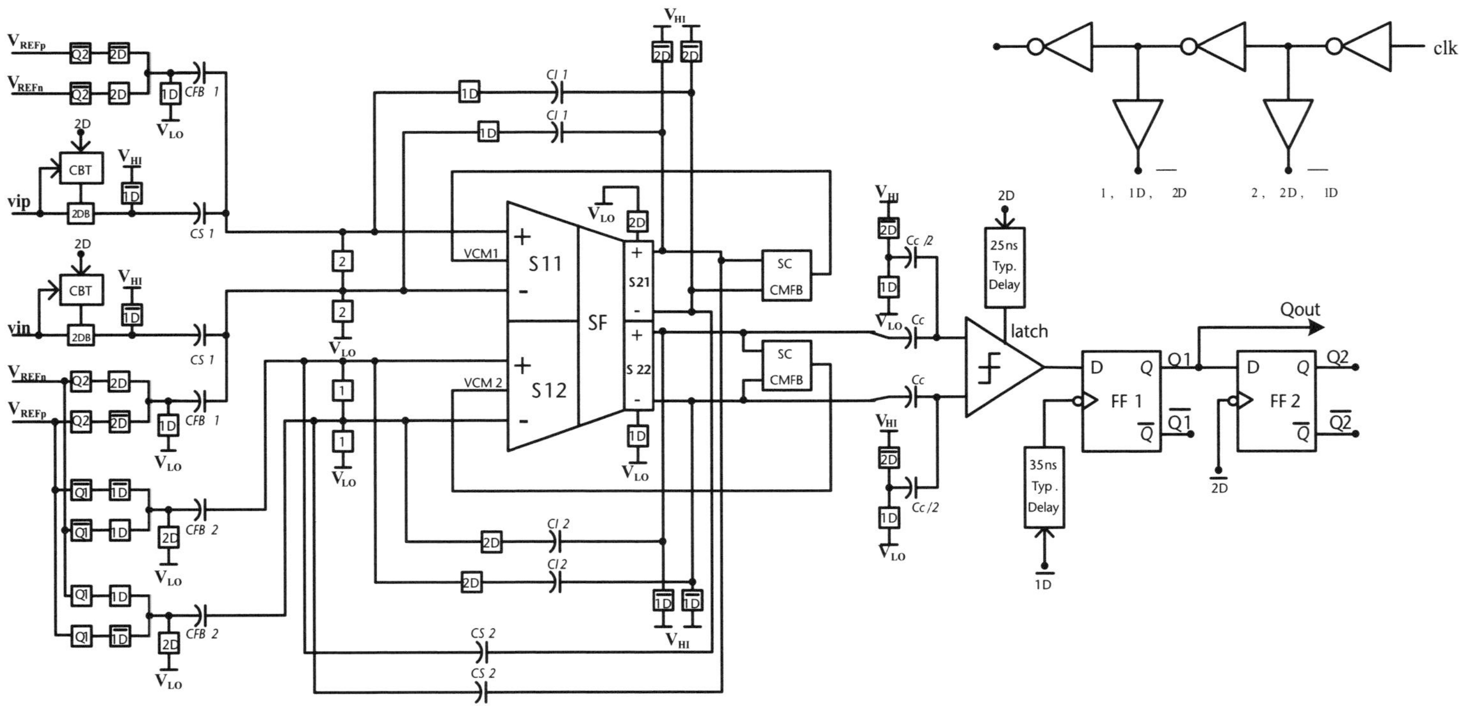

Figure 14.4 Second-order SO ΣΔ modulator architecture with amplifier sharing [11].

will produce a certain amount of charge that is lost when the charge is redistributed from the sampling and feedback capacitors into the integrating capacitors. However, as theoretically shown in [12], as long as the fall/rising time-delay, *td*, of the phases and the average equivalent conductance of the switches (g_{AVG}) during this overlapping time are both made small, the sampled signal degradation stemming from having various switches conducting simultaneously is negligible. With the evolution of CMOS technologies, the values of *td* and g_{AVG} are progressively being reduced. Hence, non-overlapping guard times might no longer be required in many SC circuits.

Moreover, in practical CBT circuits, there is always an inherent delay between the input clock phase and the generated boosted output phase that drives the sampling switches. Hence, this single-phase scheme offers another design simplification by eliminating the need to have delayed versions of the sampling phases necessary to avoid any signal-dependent charge injection. Furthermore, during the sampling operation of the SO circuits, the signal-dependent charge injection added by switching-off the output-stage of the amplifier (opamp) is very small, even if delayed phases are not employed. The reason is that the signal swing at the input of the output-stage of a 2-stage opamp is always very small, with the result that the amount of charge that must flow out of the channel region is practically signal-independent.

Since two half-delay integrators are used in a SO realization, the amplifier (opamp) can be shared by both integrators by employing a two-stage topology with a folded PMOS input stage followed by two common-source output stages operating in opposite phases, as suggested in [13], in order to realize the SO principle and, at the same time, saving a significant amount of power and area. The outputs of the integrators operate at a common-mode level of $V_{DD}/2$ (0.6 to 0.75 V) and the input common-mode level of the amplifiers is adjusted (by the capacitance values chosen) to about 50 to 250 mV (depending on the value of V_{DD}). As stated before, the modulator input is operated at a common-mode voltage of $V_{DD}/2$ and, therefore, two CBT circuits [16] are used in order to boost phase (2D) driving the input switches. One clock-boosting circuit *per* input switch in the signal path is required, in order to maintain reliability for lower-voltages technologies and, at the same time, overcomes the problem of the sampling switches at the inputs of this SO system.

For a peak SNDR better than 84 dB, values of 0.6 pF, 0.6 pF, 2.4 pF, 1.2 pF, 0.8 pF, and 0.4 pF are chosen (using a unique capacitor-array comprising only 0.2 pF unit capacitors), respectively, for sampling capacitors of the first and of the second integrators, *CS1*, *CS2*; for the integrating capacitors, *CI1*, *CI2*; and for the feedback coefficients, *CFB1* and *CFB2*. As already mentioned, using these values for *CFB1* and for *CFB2* and using the referred reference voltage, no input common-mode shifting capacitors are required.

14.2.3.2 Amplifier

The 2-stage opamp topology is presented in Figure 14.5. It comprises two input PMOS trifferential-stages (blocks A11, A12 comprising M_1, M_2 and M_c), folded into a common part (block AF comprising M_3 to M_5) and followed by two differential common-source output-stages (blocks A21, A22 comprising M_6 and M_7). CM input and output voltages of $V_{CMI} = V_{LO} = V_{SS}$ and $V_{CMO} = V_{HI}/2 = V_{DD}/2$, respectively, are used. Compensation is achieved by connecting capacitors C_{comp} to the sources of the

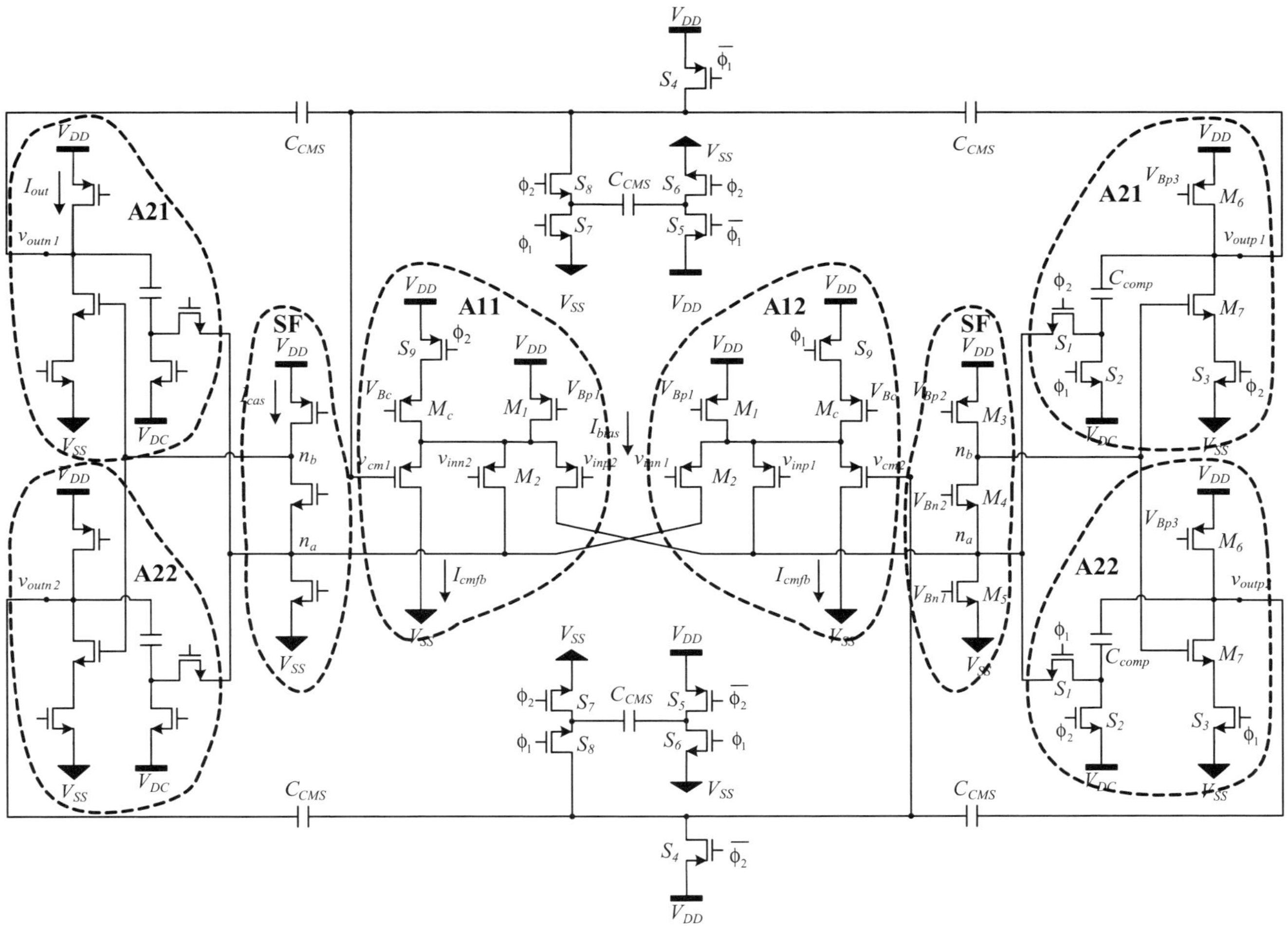

Figure 14.5 Two-stage cascade-compensated amplifier with CMFB circuitry [11].

NMOS cascode devices M_4 through switches S_1, when the corresponding output-stage is switched ON [17]. The output-stages are turned ON/OFF by turning ON/OFF switches S_3 and OFF/ON switches S_2. The opamp is designed to be efficiently shared by both INTs, thus resulting in significant power and area savings. Since two input stages, A11 and A12, are available, there is no need to use an input analog multiplexer as is done in [13], thus avoiding any memory parasitic effects that might degrade the performance of the INTs. Moreover, there is no extra burden in terms of circuitry and die area since when an input stage is being used by a given INT acting as a differential-pair (the 3rd input is switched OFF through S_9), the other input stage (in trifferential-mode) is also used to set the output CM to $V_{DD}/2$. This is done by adding the adjusting currents, I_{cmfb}, at the low-impedance nodes n_a [18]. Two auxiliary SC-networks comprising capacitors C_{CMS} and switches S_4 to S_8 are used to sense the CM at the outputs.

14.2.3.3 Comparator

The comparator is a simple regenerative resetable circuit [14, 15] as shown in Figure 14.6.

It consists of a PMOS differential-pair feeding into an NMOS type regenerative latch. In the reset phase (ϕ_{latch}), the outputs are reset to V_{SS} rather than to the meta-stable state in order to achieve low hysteresis. The operation of this comparator is as follows. When phase ϕ_{latch} is disabled, the switches driven by this phase turn OFF and the output nodes rise simultaneously to the meta-stable point, from which point on, the two outputs diverge. The low output is V_{SS} but the high output does not rise completely to V_{DD} because the full I_B continues to flow through the PMOS current source and the PMOS input transistor of the high-input side. When phase ϕ_{latch} is enabled, the output nodes are shorted to ground and a reset occurs.

As the output of the preceding integrator sampled to $V_{CMI} = V_{LO} \approx V_{SS}$ has a dc offset of about $V_{DD}/2$, a level shifting needs to be applied. Therefore, as illustrated in Figure 14.6, two dc shifting capacitors ($Cc/2$) are used in order to shift the input

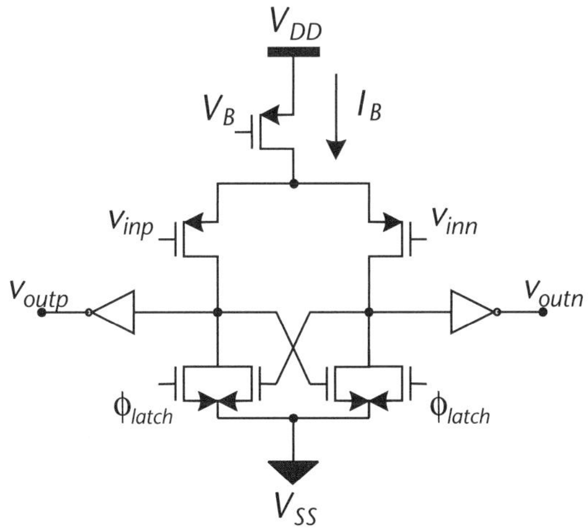

Figure 14.6 The regenerative comparator [10].

common-mode of the comparator to about V_{LO}. As the level shift at the comparator's inputs is performed synchronous to the modulator, two additional delayed clock phases are used to achieve a suitable timing margin [15]. Hence, two digital delay blocks are designed with typical delays of 25 ns and 35 ns.

14.2.4 Integrated Prototypes and Measured Results

The prototype IC was fabricated in a 0.18 μm CMOS process using MiM capacitors and the results were published in [11]. Only standard transistors with $V_{TN} \approx |V_{TP}| \approx 0.5$ V are employed and all transistors are biased in moderate inversion with V_{DSsat} = 50 to 150 mV. Figure 14.7 shows the chip microphotograph.

For comparison purposes, this IC includes, besides the described modulator, named ΣΔM-1, a second modulator, named ΣΔM-2, which is a replica of ΣΔM-1 that employs a conventional 4-phase clocking scheme to drive the SC switches. Modulator ΣΔM-1 occupies a die area of only 0.06 mm^2, while modulator ΣΔM-2 is 17% larger due to the phase generator block and the phase buses. Figure 14.8 shows the

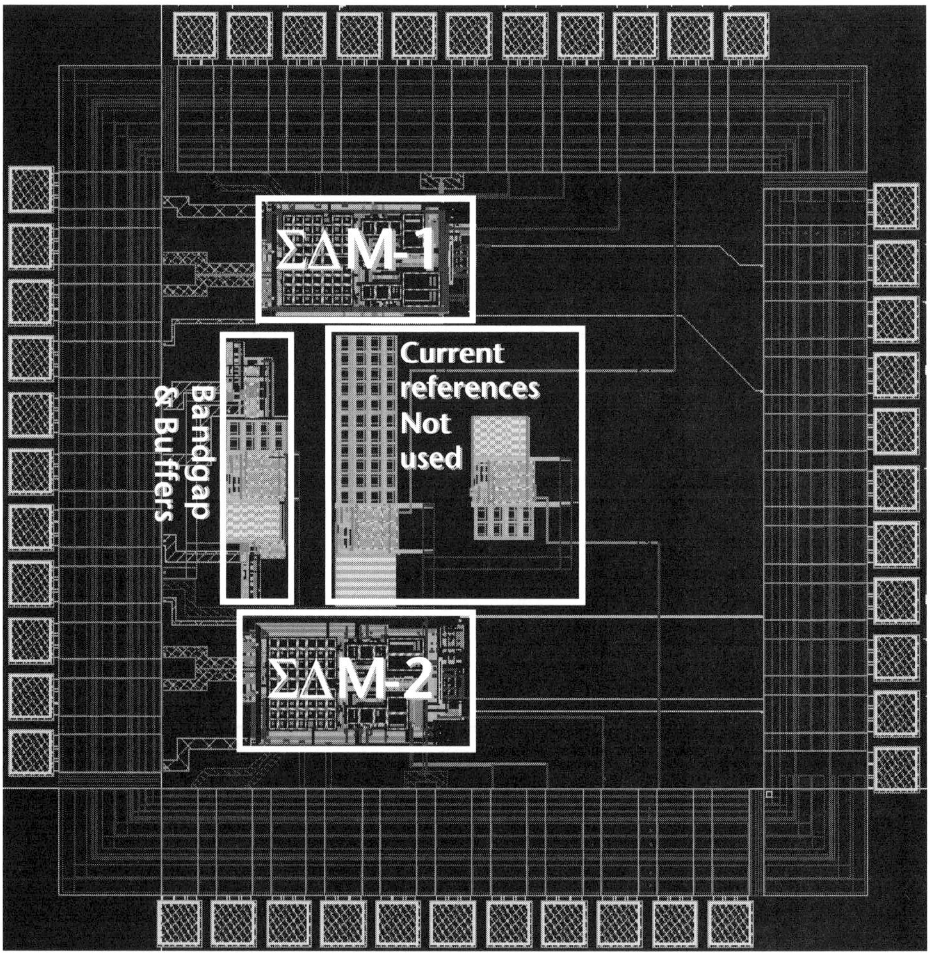

Fig 14.7 Chip layout [11].

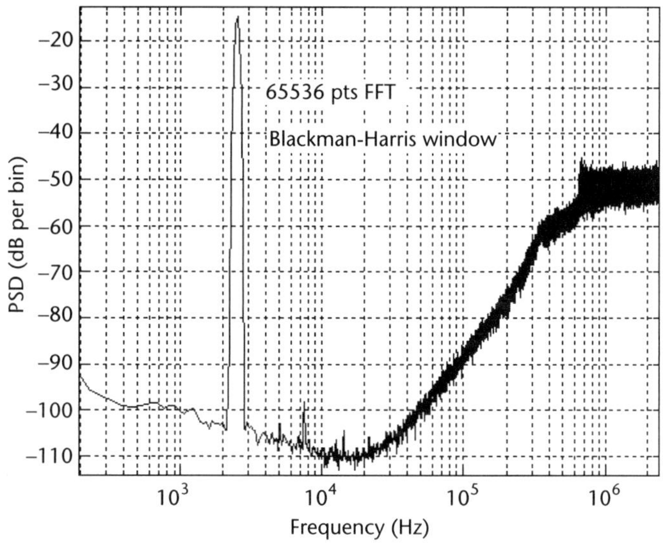

Fig 14.8 Measured 0.9 V ΣΔM-1 output spectrum with signal applied with an amplitude of –5.5 dBV [11].

measured FFT for ΣΔM-1 and Figure 14.9 displays the measured SNDR vs. signal amplitude for both modulators. These measurements are made for a 2.5 kHz signal frequency and 5 MHz clock frequency. At 0.9 V, ΣΔM-1 achieves 80 dB SNDR, 82 dB SNR, and 83 dB DR for a 10 kHz BW and dissipates only 0.2 mW from a 0.9 V supply. Both modulators have similar SNR and DR but ΣΔM-1 shows a 3.5 dB improvement in the SNDR due to the single-phase technique that improves the accuracy of the settling response. The key measurement results and a comparison between both modulators are summarized in Table 14.1.

The performance of this modulator is now compared with other state-of-the-art modulators. To compare performances, the common (figure-of-merit) $FOM = DR_{dB} + 10LOG(BW/P)$ equation is used. Table 14.2 summarizes this comparison and, as

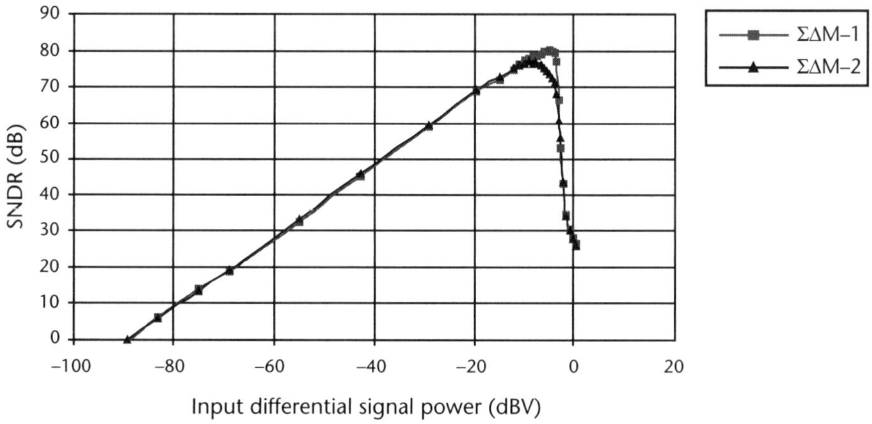

Figure 14.9 Measured SNDR vs. input signal level measured for ΔM-1 and for ΔM-2 and with VDD = 0.9V [11].

Table 14.1 Key Measured Results

	ΣΔ*M-1*		ΣΔ*M-2*
Technology		0.18 μm CMOS 1P-6M	
Supply Voltage		0.9 V	
Clock frequency, F_{CLK}		5 MHz	
OSR		256	
Signal BW		10 kHz	
Power Dissipation	0.2 mW		0.2 mW
Die area	0.06 mm^2		0.07 mm^2
Peak SNR		82 dB at −5.5 dBV input level	
Peak SNDR	80.1 dB at −5.5 dBV input level		76.7 dB at −9 dBV input level
DR		83 dB	

Table 14.2 Performance Comparison for 7 Different State-of-the-Art ΣΔ ADCs Suitable for Digitizing Different Biomedical Signals

Paper Ref. Author	*VDD (V)*	*Process (μm)*	*DR (dB)*	*BW (kHz)*	*Power (μW)*	*Area (mm^2)*	*FOM*	*FOM2 [15] (×10^{18})*
[4] Ahn	0.6	0.35	79	24	1000	2.880	153	0.06
[5] Cheng	0.8	0.18	60	5	180	0.050	134	0.45
[8] Hsu	1.8	0.18	98	1	360	0.320	162	0.56
[9] Pun	**0.5**	0.18	76	25	300	0.600	155	0.71
[11] Goes	0.9	0.18	83	10	200	0.060	160	**9.59**
[14] Peluso	0.9	0.5	77	16	40	0.850	**163**	2.71
[15] Sauerbrey	0.7	0.18	75	8	80	0.082	155	5.59

it can be observed, the ΣΔM described here and reported in [11] has the third best FOM from the power dissipation point of view. It can also be stated that all the modulators considered have very high FOM and operate at sub-1V supply (except [8]). Although the ΣΔM proposed in [14] has the best power efficiency and FOM, when die area is also taken into account and using a second and more complete figure-of-merit, $FOM2 = 10^{(DR[dB]-1.78)/20} \cdot BW/(P \cdot A)$, as suggested in [15], the modulator described here [11] has globally the best power-and-area efficiency.

14.3 A Calibration-Free Low-Power and Low-Area 1.2 V 14-b Resolution and 80 kHz BW Two-Stage Algorithmic ADC

14.3.1 Introduction

Two figures-of-merit (*FM*) for Nyquist-rate ADCs are usually employed and normally they are different from the ones used for sigma-delta modulators. The first one, FM_1, represents the used energy *per* conversion [19]:

$$FM_1 = \frac{P}{2^{ENOB} \cdot Min\{2 \cdot BW, Fs\}} \quad \text{(pJ)} \tag{14.1}$$

where Fs is the sampling rate, BW is the maximum bandwidth of the input signal, ENOB represents the effective-number-of-bits and P is the power dissipation.

A more complete figure-of-merit, FM_2, includes the area, A (in mm^2):

$$FM_2 = A \cdot FM_1 \quad (\text{pJmm}^2) \tag{14.2}$$

Sigma-Delta ($\Sigma\Delta$) architectures, either continuous-time (CT) [20] or switched-capacitor (SC) [21–23] can simultaneously achieve high BW, high resolution, and low power. Multi-bit SC implementations of $\Sigma\Delta$ modulators ($\Sigma\Delta$M) can reach FM_1 of the order of 0.5 pJ to 0.7 pJ [21-23] and FM_2 = 0.54 pJmm^2 is obtained in [21]; however, the decimation filter is not taken into account. In [20] a CT-$\Sigma\Delta$ realization includes the decimation filter, which dissipates an additional power of 50% and occupies an area of 30% of the $\Sigma\Delta$M. A high energy efficiency with FM_1 = 0.3 pJ is measured, but when area is also taken into account we end up with FM_2 = 2 pJmm^2. The state-of-the art is that CT-$\Sigma\Delta$ are, in general, 1.5 times more energy efficient than their SC counterparts, but less area efficient.

For signal BW above, a few MHz, self-calibrated pipeline ADCs have proved to be a better solution to minimize power and area. Although digital calibration does not require sophisticated analogue circuitry, it puts an extra burden on the digital part, and requires additional resolution in each stage, which results in increased area. A very energy efficient self-calibrated ADC can be found in [24], with FM_1 = 0.37 pJ, but the FM_2 is 1.18 pJmm^2, and the digital circuitry is not included. The ADC in [25] has FM_1 = 0.8 pJ and FM_2 = 0.8 pJmm^2 but, again, the digital self-calibration circuitry is implemented off-chip.

For ultra-low-area and low-signal bandwidth (BW), the best approach is to trade conversion-time for area. In this section, a two-stage algorithmic architecture is described in which a single amplifier is shared. Each stage uses a 1.5-bit mismatch-insensitive multiplying-DAC (1.5-bit MI-MDAC) for residue amplification. This 1.5-bit MI-MDAC is based in a multiply-by-two amplifier (MBTA) with an accurate gain of two and with parasitic compensation.

14.3.2 Architecture Description and Timing

The proposed A/D conversion architecture, depicted in Figure 14.10, consists of a cascade of two stages. Each stage comprises a 1.5-bit MI-MDAC and a 1.5-bit flash-quantizer (FQ).

During the first clock cycle, $MDAC_2$ acts as a sample-and-hold (S/H) with a closed-loop gain of 2 and samples the differential input signal. In the remaining 6 clock-cycles, the signal is successively recycled and amplified by 2 in an algorithmic manner. In each clock cycle, each 1.5-bit FQ provides 2 bits (4 bits total *per* clock cycle), and these bits are digitally synchronized and corrected, leading to a digital output with a net resolution of 14 bits. Since the two 1.5-bit MI-MDACs operate in opposite phases, they can share the same operational transconductance amplifier (OTA), allowing significant area and power savings. Moreover, since the failures in the comparators in the 1.5-bit FQs can be corrected digitally, the overall linearity of this A/D conversion architecture will be limited only by the gain accuracy of the 1.5-bit MI-MDACs (which should be accurately 2).

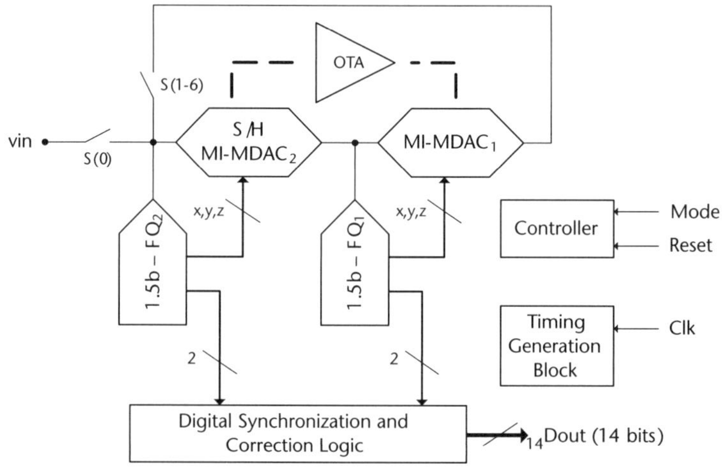

Figure 14.10 Proposed ADC architecture.

As stated before, to achieve simultaneously low power and low area, this architecture trades speed for low area. However, since two stages are used, this ADC has twice the speed efficiency of the conventional algorithmic architecture.

The output data latency and the timing of the different blocks are illustrated in Figure 14.11. The 1.5-bit FQs quantize the input signal at the middle of the sampling phase of the 1.5-bit MI-MDACs. This allows more time for the amplifier to settle with the required accuracy, since, during the beginning of the residue amplification, the x, y, z digital signals provided by the 1.5-bit FQ are already available.

The clock phases shown in Figure 14.11 are obtained using two D-type Flip-Flops (FFs), two standard non-overlapping clock-phase generators, and a few buffers, as depicted in Figure 14.12(a). One FF is used to divide the input clock (@2.15 MHz)

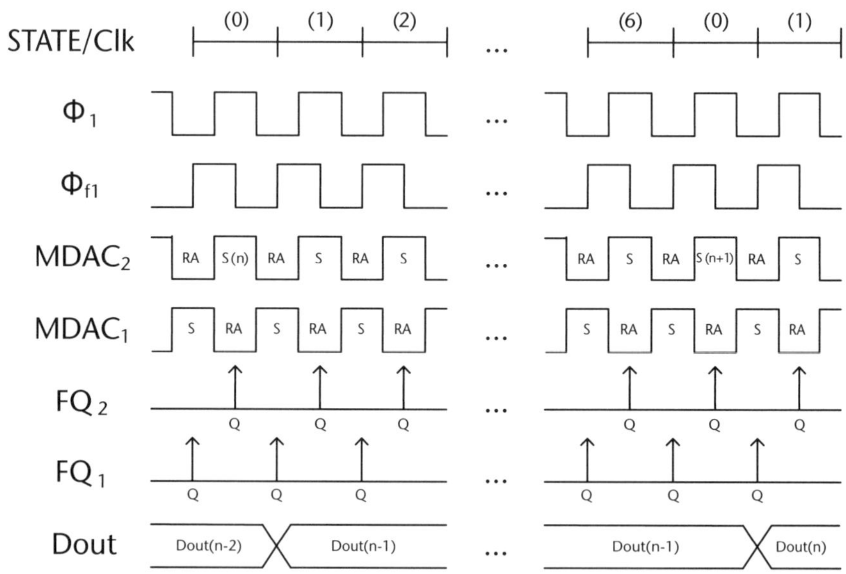

Figure 14.11 Timing of operation of the different blocks of the ADC.

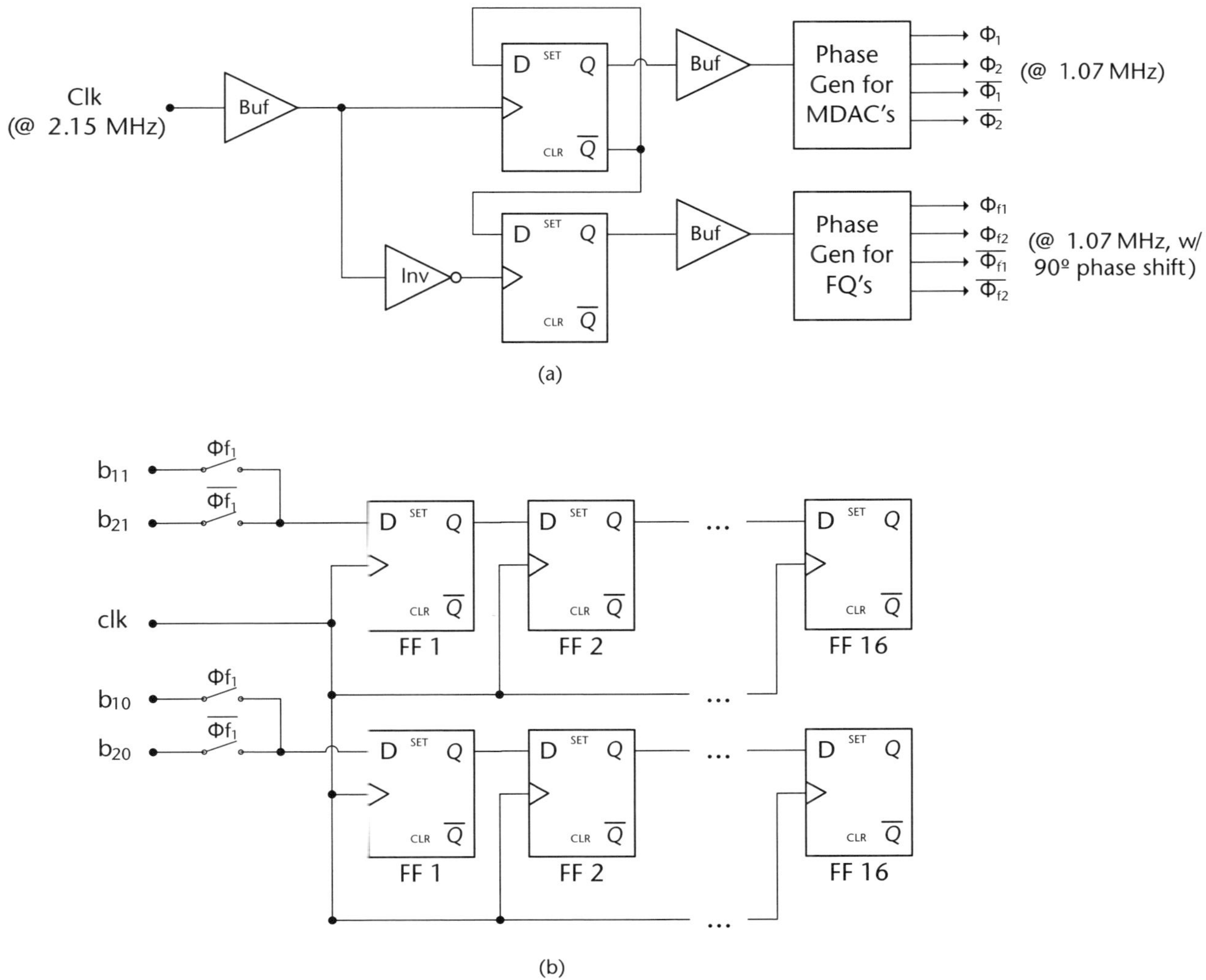

Figure 14.12 (a) Clock phase generation; (b) Synchronization logic.

by 2, and the other is used to obtain a 90° phase shift in the clock phases supplied to the 1.5-bit FQs. Shift registers (based also on simple D-type FFs) are used to synchronize the data supplied by the FQs; they have to switch their inputs between FQ_1 and FQ_2 at the appropriate time, and this is done using CMOS switches to multiplex the bits, as shown in Figure 14.12(b).

14.3.3 OTA and Comparators

The amplifier is shown in Figure 14.13. To achieve high gain, a differential regulated folded-cascode structure is used for the input-stage (two auxiliary fully-differential single-stage folded-cascoded amplifiers, *SatN* and *SatP*, are used to boost the gain). The common-source second-stage increases the gain and the output voltage swing (the supply voltage is only 1.2 V).

In each signal path, two compensation capacitors, C_a and C_b, provide hybrid cascaded-Miller compensation. Capacitors C_{sN} and C_{sP}, loading the auxiliary amplifiers, add an extra degree of freedom to control the frequency of the doublets (pole-zero pairs) caused by the gain-boosting loops. Optimization according to [26] leads to a settling time below 15 ns and an error smaller than 20 μV is obtained by simulation (the simulated dc gain is higher than 100 dB in the most important PVT corners). Due to noise constraints, the sum of C_a and C_b is 8 pF and the complete amplifier dissipates only 0.84 mW. Figure 14.14 shows the step response in a closed-loop with gain 2 of the OTA; the desired settling accuracy is within the available time slot. Two independent SC common-mode feedback circuits (CMFB) are used for the two stages.

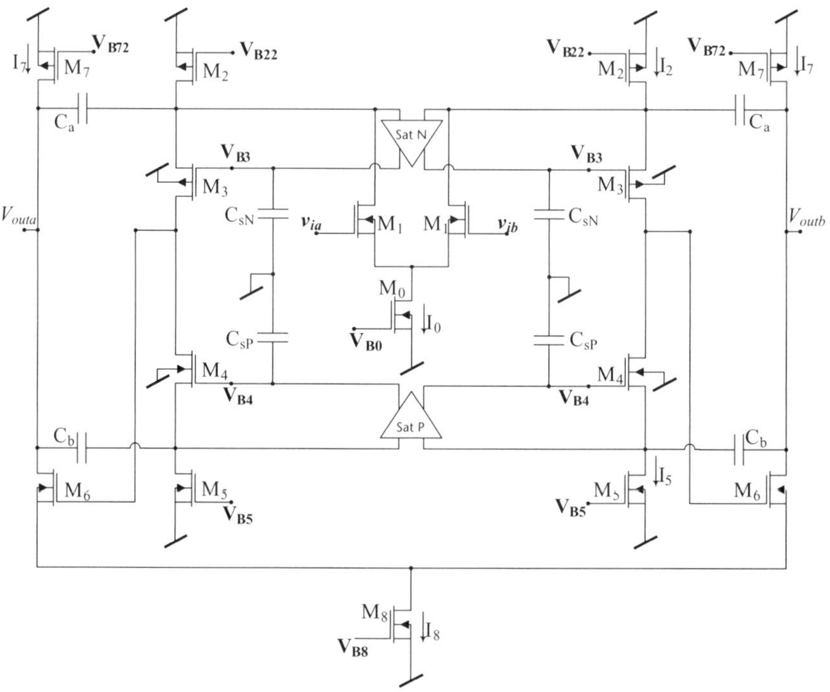

Figure 14.13 Schematic of the 2-stage fully-differential OTA shared by both 1.5-bit MI-MDACs (biasing and CMFB circuitry not shown).

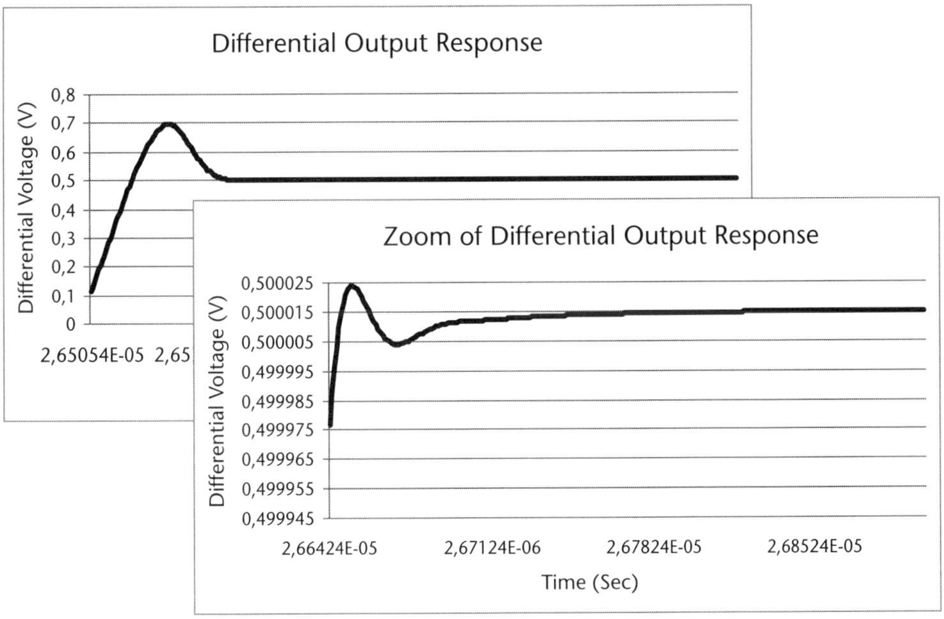

Figure 14.14 Simulated settling-response of the OTA.

Each 1.5-bit FQ consists of 2 comparators followed by a thermometer-to-binary digital encoder and by an x, y, z encoder. Each comparator comprises an input SC divider network to define the threshold level, followed by an ordinary dynamic preamplifier/positive-feedback latch. This comparator was optimized using exhaustive Monte-Carlo simulations in order to achieve low-offset, reduced kickback noise, high mean-time to failure, and low-power dissipation at the desired speed of operation.

14.3.4 The Mismatch-Insensitive Multiplying-DAC

High-resolution architectures of ADCs, such as pipeline and algorithmic, often employ MI-MDACs based on SC amplifiers with gain 2 (MBTA circuits). Since the linearity of high-resolution ADCs (e.g., above 10 bits) is usually limited by the accuracy of these gain blocks, it is mandatory to use self-calibration [27, 28] or, alternatively, to employ active [29, 30] or passive [31] capacitor error-averaging techniques. However, all these solutions either increase hardware complexity (e.g., digital self-calibration circuitry), or they trade speed for accuracy, by using more than one clock cycle to provide the accurate amplified value. We use instead a practical 1.5-bit MI-MDAC based on some modifications made to the mismatch-insensitive MBTA described in detail in [32].

Figure 14.15 shows the schematic in the two different clock phases of the new 1.5-bit MI-MDAC, based on the MBTA circuit in [32]. As depicted in Figure 14.15(a), during phase ϕ_1, capacitors C_{11}, C_{21}, C_{12} and C_{22} sample the differential input signal, v_{id}, into the bottom-plates. However, and this is the major difference of this circuit when compared with the MBTA circuit in [32], the top-plates of capacitors C_{11} and

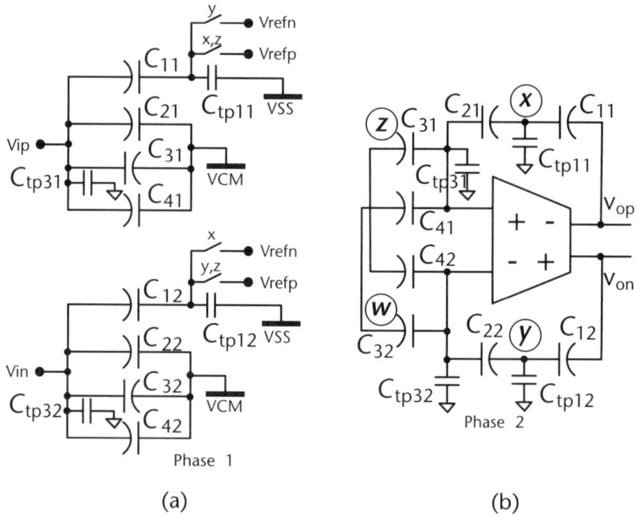

Figure 14.15 Two phases of the 1.5-bit MI-MDAC: (a) sampling-phase; (b) residue-amplification.

C_{12} are not connected to the common-mode voltage (VCM), but rather to V_{REFP} or to V_{REFN}, depending on the x, y and z outputs provided by the corresponding 1.5-bit FQ in this phase. During the amplification phase, ϕ_2, as illustrated in Figure 14.15(b), capacitors C_{11} and C_{21} in series are used as a feedback element in the positive path. Likewise, C_{12} and C_{22} are connected in series in the other signal path. Neglecting initially, for the sake of simplicity, the effects of parasitic capacitances (C_{tp11} and C_{tp12}), but allowing the main capacitances to be mismatched, the differential output voltage, v_{od}, at the end of the amplification phase, ϕ_2, is exactly $v_{od} = 2v_{id}$. However, the circuit comprising only the referred to four capacitors is highly sensitive to the top-plate parasitic capacitance (TPPC) of capacitors C_{11} and C_{12}, C_{tp11} and C_{tp12}, respectively.

As demonstrated in [32], to reach a completely stray-insensitive circuit, besides the main capacitors (C_{11}, C_{21}, C_{12}, and C_{22}), four auxiliary half-sized capacitors (C_{31}, C_{32}, C_{41}, and C_{42}) are used to compensate the TPPC of capacitors C_{11} and C_{12}. During the sampling-phase ϕ_1, capacitors C_{31} and C_{32} charge their TPPCs, respectively, C_{tp31} and C_{tp32} (expected to be half the values of C_{tp11} and C_{tp12}), to the differential input voltage (top-plate sampling). In the amplification phase, ϕ_2, the top-plates of C_{31} and C_{32} are connected to the inverting and non-inverting inputs of the OTA and, consequently, there is an opposite amount of charge that will cancel out the parasitic effects of C_{tp11} and C_{tp12}.

As shown in [32] (for z = "1"), if the parasitic capacitances are not considered, the differential output voltage is precisely $v_{od} = 2v_{id}$. With parasitics, we have

$$v_{od} \approx 2v_{id} \left[\begin{array}{l} 1+\dfrac{1}{8}\dfrac{\alpha(2\varepsilon_{P11}-2\varepsilon_{P31}-\varepsilon_{11}+\varepsilon_{21}+\alpha)}{1+\varepsilon_{11}+\varepsilon_{21}+\varepsilon_{11}\varepsilon_{21}} \\ +\dfrac{1}{8}\dfrac{\alpha(2\varepsilon_{P12}-2\varepsilon_{P32}-\varepsilon_{12}+\varepsilon_{22}+\alpha)}{1+\varepsilon_{12}+\varepsilon_{22}+\varepsilon_{12}\varepsilon_{22}} \end{array} \right] \tag{14.3}$$

where ε_{ij} are the random mismatches of the main and auxiliary capacitors, ε_{Pij} are the random mismatches of the top-plate parasitic capacitors, and α represents the average relative TPPC for the selected fabrication process.

In this equation, the first- and second-order terms are kept, but higher-order errors are neglected. This shows that the gain error becomes dependent on the products of the TPPC factor, α, and the mismatch errors of main and parasitic capacitances. Typical values in deep sub-micron CMOS technologies (e.g., 130 nm) with Metal-Insulator-Metal (MiM) capacitors are $\sigma(\varepsilon_{ij})$ = 0.2%, $\sigma(\varepsilon_{Pij})$ = 2%, and α = 0.25%. As shown in [32], the proposed circuit can, in theory, reduce the gain error from 0.1% down to 0.005%, when compared with the conventional circuit. This means a gain accuracy enhancement of 4 to 5 bits. Although auxiliary capacitors C_{31} and C_{32} sample the input voltage, they do not affect either the transfer function or the final gain accuracy. The reason is that capacitors C_{41} and C_{42} cancel out their charge and they are also connected in series during the amplification phase in order to cancel any mismatch effects.

14.3.5 Circuit Implementation and Simulation Results

An integrated prototype of the 1.2 V, 14-bit, 154 kS/s 2-stage algorithmic ADC was designed in a 130 nm 1P-8M CMOS technology with special MiM capacitor option. Figure 14.16 shows a plot of the layout. To achieve an input full-scale of 1 $V_{p\text{-}p}$ (differential) voltages $V_{REFP} = VCM = 0.8$ V, $V_{REFN} = 0.3$ V and $V_{CMO} = 0.55$ V are provided to the ADC. Dedicated switch-linearization control circuits (SLCs) are used to improve the conductivity of the most critical switches [33]. The active area of the complete ADC is about 0.36 mm^2. Figure 14.17 displays the FFT (256 bins) of the ADC output clocked at 1.075 MHz (after divided by 2) when a full-scale input of

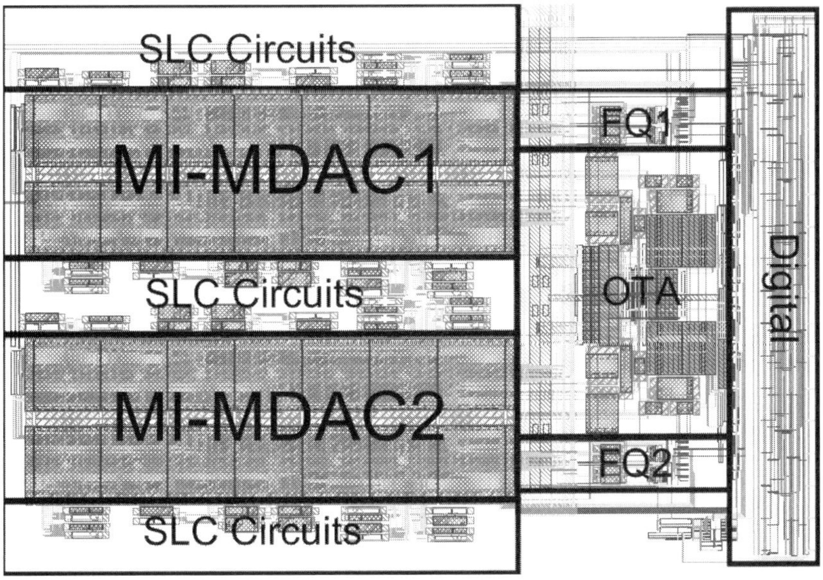

Figure 14.16 Plot of the layout of the 14-bit 1.54MS/s 2-stage ADC.

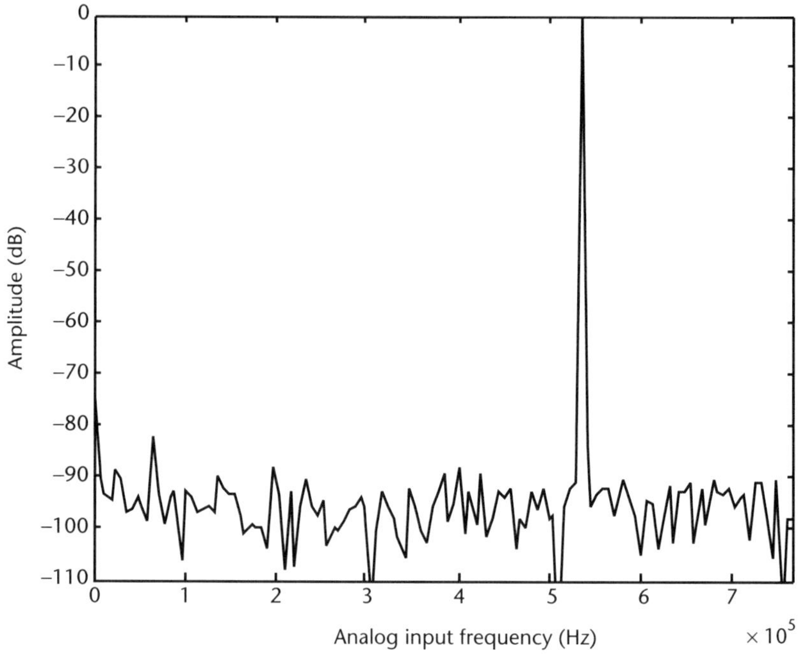

Figure 14.17 Simulated FFT spectrum with 256 bits for f_{clk} = 1.07 MHz (~80 kHz BW) and f_{in} = 53.4 kHz (coherent sampling).

53.4 kHz is applied. A peak SNR of 77 dB is obtained through analytical calculations when 4 pF unit capacitors are used to make $C_{11} = C_{21} = C_{12} = C_{22} = 8$ pF, $C_{31} = C_{32} = C_{41} = C_{42} = 4$ pF and $C_a = C_b = 4$ pF. Simulations show a THD of −79.4 dB, a SFDR of 82 dB, and a peak SNDR larger than 75 dB corresponding to an ENOB better than 12.2 bits. The circuit dissipates less than 1.0 mW with 1.2 V and at 153.6 kS/s corresponding to an area-and-energy efficiency better than 0.5 pJmm^2.

14.4 Conclusions

This chapter presented two possible energy-and-area highly efficient single-amplifier architectures of ADCs suitable for digitizing biomedical signals. First, a second-order ΣΔ modulator capable of operating down to 0.9 V was shown. This ΣΔM was designed and fabricated in a 0.18 μm CMOS technology [11], occupies a die area of only 0.06 mm^2, dissipates 0.2 mW from a 0.9 V supply, and provides 80 dB SNDR and 83 dB DR over a 10 kHz BW. Secondly, as a competitive alternative, a calibration-free low-power and low-area 1.2 V 14-b resolution and 80 kHz BW two-stage algorithmic ADC was also described. Due to the ultra-small-area, the target performance is compatible with a power figure-of-merit better than 0.5 pJmm^2. The simulated static and dynamic performance is compatible with, at least, 13.7 bits (DNL, INL, and ENOB) if an OSR of 4 is considered together with a BW of 20 kHz.

References

[1] "Medical Instrumentation—Application and Design," Edited by John G. Webster, ISBN 0-471-15368-0 John Wiley & Sons, 1998, pp. 258-259.

[2] A. Gerosa, A. Maniero and A. Neviani, "A fully integrated two-channel A/D interface for the acquisition of cardiac signals in implantable pacemakers," *IEEE Journal of Solid-State Circuits*, vol. 39, no. 7, pp. 1083–1093, July 2004.

[3] A. Gerosa and A. Neviani, "A 1.8-μW sigma-delta modulator for 8-bit digitization of cardiac signals in implantable pacemakers operating down to 1.8 V," *IEEE Transactions on Circuits and Systems—II: Express Briefs*, vol. 52, no. 2, pp. 71–76, Feb. 2005.

[4] Gil-Cho Ahn, et al., "A 0.6-V 82-dB delta-sigma audio ADC using switched-RC integrators," *IEEE Journal of Solid-State Circuits*, vol. 40, no. 12, pp. 2398–2407, Dec. 2005.

[5] C.-J. Cheng, S.-Y. Lee, and Y. Lo, "A low-voltage and area efficient adaptative SI SDADC for bio-acquisition microsystems," *Proc. IEEE Asian Solid-State Circuits Conference*, pp. 431–434, 2006.

[6] H.Y. Yang and R. Sarpeshhkar, "A bio-inspired ultra-energy-efficient analog-to-digital converter for biomedical applications," *IEEE Transactions on Circuits and Systems—I*, vol. 53, no. 11, pp. 2349–2356, Nov. 2006.

[7] A. Agah, K. Vleugels, P.B. Griffin, M. Ronaghi, J.D. Plummer, and B.A. Wooley, "A high-resolution low-power oversampling ADC with extended-range for bio-sensor arrays," *Proc. Symposium on VLSI Circuits*, pp. 244–245, June 2007.

[8] C.-M. Hsu, W.-S. Wang, and C. H. Luo, "The power-efficient biomedical acquisition system by variable-resolution sigma-delta modulator," *Proc. of the 29th Annual International Conference of the IEEE EMBS*, pp. 3152–3155, Aug. 2007.

[9] K.-P. Pun, S. Chatterjee, and P.R. Kinget, "A 0.5-V 74-dB SNDR 25-kHz continuous-time delta-sigma modulator with a return-to-open DAC," *IEEE Journal of Solid-State Circuits*, vol. 42, no. 3, pp. 496–507, March 2007.

[10] J. Goes, H. Pinto, R. Monteiro, N. Paulino, B. Vaz, and A.S. Garção, "Low power low-voltage CMOS A/D sigma-delta modulator for bio-potential signals driven by a single-phase scheme," special issue on "Biomedical Circuits and Systems: A New Wave of Technology," *IEEE Transactions on Circuits and Systems—I*, vol. 52, no. 12, pp. 2595–2604, Dec. 2005.

[11] J. Goes, B. Vaz, R. Monteiro, and N. Paulino, "A 0.9V SD modulator with 80dB SNDR and 83dB DR using a single-phase technique," *Proc. IEEE ISSCC'2006*, pp. 74–75, Feb. 2006.

[12] J. Goes, et al., "Switched-capacitor circuits using a single-phase scheme," *Proc. ISCAS*, pp. 3123–3126, Japan, 2005.

[13] V. Cheung, H. Luong, and W. Ki, "A 1-V 10.7-MHz switched-opamp bandpass ΣΔ modulator using double-sampling finite-gain-compensation techniques," *IEEE Journal of Solid-State Circuits*, vol. SC-37, no. 10, pp. 1215–1225, Oct. 2002.

[14] V. Peluso, P. Vancorenland, A.M. Marques, M.S.J. Steyaert, and W. Sansen, "A 900-mV low-power ΣΔ A/D converter with 77-dB dynamic range," *IEEE Journal of Solid-State Circuits*, vol. 33, no. 12, pp. 1887–1897, Dec. 1998.

[15] J. Sauerbrey, et al., "A 0.7-V MOSFET-only switched-opamp ΣΔ modulator in standard digital CMOS technology," *IEEE Journal of Solid-State Circuits*, vol. 37, no. 12, pp. 1662–1669, Dec. 2002.

[16] A. Abo and P. Gray, "A 1.5-V, 10-bit, 14.3-MS/s CMOS pipeline analog-to-digital converter," *IEEE Journal of Solid-State Circuits*, vol. 34, no. 5, pp. 599–606, May 1999.

[17] B.K. Ahuja, "an improved frequency compensation technique for CMOS operational amplifiers," *IEEE Journal of Solid-State Circuits*, vol. SC-18, no. 6, pp. 629–633, Dec. 1983.

[18] B. Vaz, J. Goes, and N. Paulino, "A 1.5-V 10-b 50 MS/s time-interleaved switched-opamp pipeline CMOS ADC with high energy efficiency," *Proc. 2004 Symposium on VLSI Circuits*, pp. 432–435, June 2004.

[19] F. Goodenough, "Analog technology of all varieties dominate ISSCC," *Electronic Design*, No. 19, pp. 96–111, 1996.

[20] G. Mitteregger, et al., "A 14 b 20 mW 640 MHz CMOS CT SD ADC with 20MHz signal bandwidth and 12b ENOB," *Proc. IEEE ISSCC*, pp. 62–63, 2006.

[21] S. Kwon and F. Maloberti, "A 14 mW multi-bit ΣΔ modulator with 82 dB SNR and 86 dB DR for ADSL2+," *Proc. IEEE ISSCC*, pp. 68–69, 2006.

[22] K.-S. Lee, S. Kwon, and F. Maloberti, "A 5.4 mW 2-channel time-interleaved multi-bit SD modulator with 80 dB SNR and 85 dB DR for ADSL," *Proc. IEEE ISSCC*, pp. 70–71, 2006.

[23] Y. Fujimoto, et al., "An 80/100 MS/s 76.3/70.1 dB SNDR ΣΔ ADC for digital TV receivers," *Proc. IEEE ISSCC*, pp. 76–77, 2006.

[24] J. Bjornsen, et al., "A 220mW 14b 40 MSPS gain calibrated pipelined ADC," *Proc. IEEE ESSCIRC*, pp. 165–168, 2005.

[25] P. Bogner, et al., "A 14b 100 MS/s digitally self-calibrated pipelined ADC in 0.13μm CMOS," *Proc. IEEE ISSCC'2006*, pp. 224–225, 2006.

[26] R. Tavares, et al., "Optimum sizing and compensation of two-stage CMOS amplifiers based on a time-domain approach," *ICECS'06*, Dec. 2006.

[27] A.N. Karanicolas, H.-S. Lee, and K.L. Bacrania, "A 15-b 1-Msample/s digitally self-calibrated pipeline ADC," *IEEE J. of Solid-State Circuits*, vol. 28, pp. 1207–1215, Dec. 1993.

[28] D. Fu, K. Dyer, S. Lewis, and P. Hurst, "Digital background calibration of a 10-b 40 Msample/s parallel pipelined ADC," *IEEE J. of Solid-State Circuits*, vol. 33, pp. 1904–1911, Dec. 1998.

[29] B.-S. Song, M.F. Tompsett, and K.R. Lakshmikumar, "A 12-bit 1-Msample/s capacitor error-averaging pipelined A/D converter," *IEEE J. of Solid-State Circuits*, vol. 23, pp. 1324–1333, Dec. 1988.

[30] H.-S. Chen, B.-S. Song, and K. Bacrania, "A 14-b 20-MS/s CMOS pipelined ADC," *IEEE J. of Solid-State Circuits*, pp. 997–1001, June 2001.

[31] Y. Chiu, "Inherently linear capacitor error-averaging techniques for pipelined A/D conversion," *IEEE Trans. on Circuits and Systems—II*, vol. 47, pp. 229–232, Mar. 2000.

[32] J. Goes, et al., "Switched-capacitor multiply-by-two amplifier insensitive to component mismatches," *IEEE Trans. on Circuits and Systems—II*, pp. 29–33, Jan. 2007.

[33] A. Galhardo, J. Goes, and N. Paulino, "Novel linearization technique for low-distortion high-swing CMOS switches with improved reliability," *IEEE Int. Symp. Circuits and Systems*, pp. 2001–2004, May 2006.

CHAPTER 15

CMOS Circuit Design for Label-Free Medical Diagnostics

Claudio Stagni, Sandro Carrara, Carlotta Guiducci, and Luca Benini

15.1 Introduction

In the last decade, micro-patterned arrays of DNA sites (known as DNA microarrays) have been massively employed in genetic expression analysis and polymorphisms studies. For instance, they led to important achievements in population genotyping [1] and research on cancer predisposition [2]. Their success and wide diffusion in gene-based studies have paved the way for their use in high-throughput personal tests for medical diagnostics.

DNA microarrays are fabricated on glass or quartz slides where different DNA probe molecules are immobilized in a two-dimensional array of small sites. Some of these devices, implemented with photolithographic techniques, can test a whole genome, with densities of a million sites per square centimeter [3]. They allow highly parallel and low-cost analysis. In fact, they host a large number of miniaturized detection sites on a single substrate where the DNA sample can be analyzed in very small volumes. Figure 15.1 depicts the working principle of such devices. Each site is specifically bio-functionalized by means of DNA molecules of known sequence immobilized on its surface (probes). Target molecules in the DNA sample bind only to probes with complementary sequences (hybridization): thus, their presence at specific sites reveals their composition.

Most of the existing microarrays require optically-active labels attached to the target DNA and instrumentation for fluorescence analysis. The DNA strands of the cell extract are usually labeled with fluorescent molecules during their processing and before the analysis with the microarray.

After the analysis of the DNA sample, the presence of detected molecules at matching sites of the array is measured by an optical scanner or a fluorescence microscope. Nevertheless, the high cost of the scanner poses critical limits to the use of these tools in point-of-care analysis. Some microarrays of more recent conception employ electrochemical labels (redox-active molecules or enzymes) that produce an electrical current through a conductive substrate in case of hybridization [4–6]. However, this approach meets, in the same way as the fluorescence technique, a more complicated processing of the sample due to the labeling step.

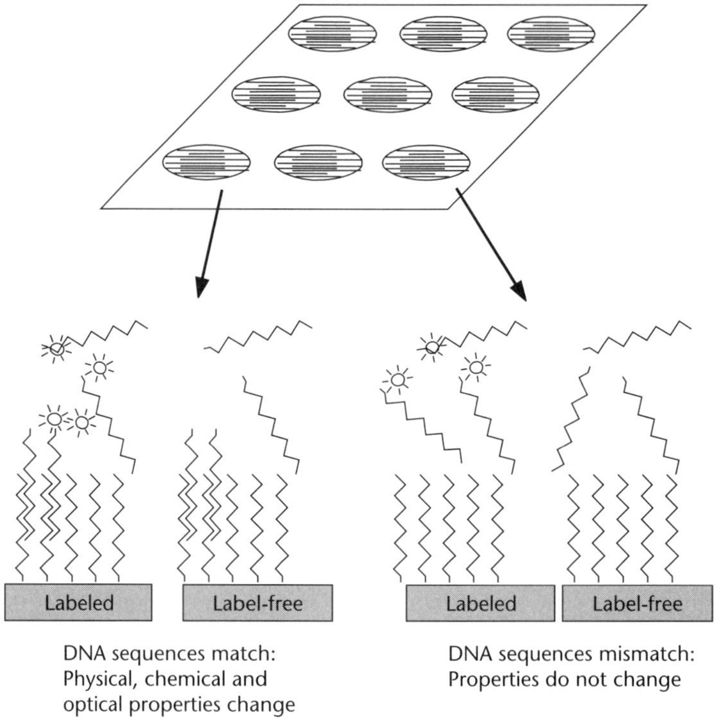

Figure 15.1 Schematic representation of DNA microarray principle.

Aiming to overcome these drawbacks, a large effort is devoted to the development of tools based on label-free techniques and suitable to be employed outside specialized laboratories. Several approaches based on mass sensing and mechanical oscillations have been proposed, which employ, in particular, piezoelectric devices [7, 8] and microfabricated cantilevers [9, 10]. Other techniques detect the changes of electrical properties of electrode/solution interfaces induced by DNA recognition. Within this category, a distinction can be made between devices where sites exploit passive electrodes [11] and sites which integrate semiconductor sensors [12–17]. These solutions are particularly advantageous, as they allow on-site sensing and direct-electrical readout whilst avoiding the labeling step of the DNA target molecules. Moreover, they are suitable for single-chip implementations that are characterized by portability and high parallelism and allow the integration of data processing functions.

This chapter aims at providing an overview of the working principles and system design issues for label-free DNA microarrays based on capacitive sensing. The chapter is organized as follows: Section 15.2 describes the electrical model of the electrode solution interface and Section 15.3 details how the DNA molecules are bound on gold. Section 15.4 illustrates the design and test of the electronic systems used to perform measurements and Section 15.5 presents results on DNA detection. A discussion on results, problems, and improvements is presented in Section 15.6. Finally, conclusions and perspectives are in Section 15.7.

15.2 Label-Free Molecular Detection with Electrochemical Capacitors

15.2.1 The Ideal-Capacitance Model

The approach presented in this chapter is based on interface capacitance measurements, whose conventional implementation consists of a three-electrode set-up for impedance spectroscopy [18, 19]. Much simpler two-electrode configurations, such as that used in this work, have also attracted significant interest. For example, a two-electrode set-up using a 2.4 mm^2 gold working electrode and an Ag/AgCl reference electrode has been employed successfully in capacitive detection of DNA at 20 Hz [20]. Moreover, it has already been shown that DNA hybridization can be detected by measuring interface capacitance by means of two gold electrodes (i.e., without the use of a reference terminal) [21]. Under suitable electrochemical conditions, bio-modified metal interfaces in saline solution exhibit a capacitive behavior, for instance, in the case of gold electrodes modified with short DNA strands immobilized by alkanethiol chain endings [18, 20], the capacitance values of electrode/solution interface have been estimated between 1 and 20 $\mu F/cm^2$ (these values depend strongly on the electrode characteristics and surface treatment).

A first-approximation model of the electrode/solution interface is the equivalent circuit depicted in Figure 15.2 (left) [22, 23], where R_S depends on the interface and solution characteristics; R_P is related to the insulating properties of the interface (for well-formed layers it can be considered infinite); C_P is mainly affected by the physical and chemical characteristics of the insulating bio-layer immobilized on the surface. In this model, the geometrical capacitance formed by the electrodes would be in parallel to C_P but, since it is several orders of magnitude smaller than the interface capacitance, its contribution is considered negligible in the first-approximation model.

This simple model provides an intuitive understanding of the basic sensing principle exploited here. Considering a capacitor formed by two neighboring electrodes of our chip, when a complementary DNA strand binds with the DNA probes on the

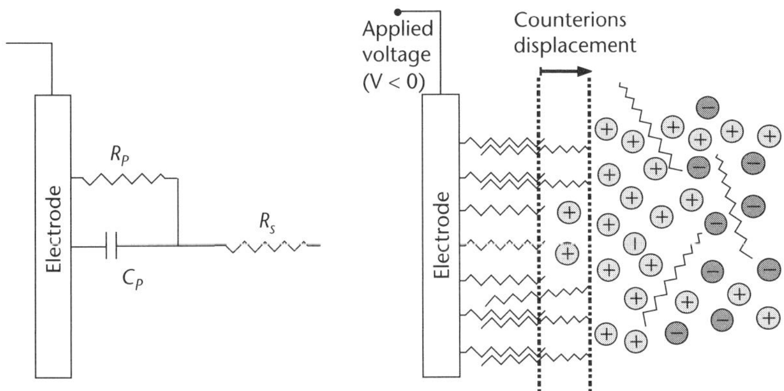

Figure 15.2 Left: Schematic representation of the lumped-element electrical model of the metal/solution interface of the capacitors used in this work. Right: Schematic illustration of the DNA hybridization process and the induced (further) displacement of counterions within the liquid solution. Elaborated from [26].

surface and the duplex is formed, the distance between the counterions of the solution and the polarized metal surface increases. This increases the distance between the two plates of the C_P capacitor [19–21] (Figure 15.2, right). Therefore, the capacitance decreases when hybridization occurs between complementary target DNA strands in the solution and the probe strands on the sensor surface. This change can be measured by a circuit integrated below the couple of electrodes.

15.2.2 The Constant Phase Element Model

In case of gold electrodes modified with alkanethiol chains layers [18] and even by layers of short DNA strands terminated with alkanethiol chains [24, 25] the ideal capacitive behavior is generally assumed. Under this assumption, the electrode/solution interface can be modeled by an equivalent circuit with a conventional capacitor that is the parameter to be measured.

However, a more precise characterization of the interface with DNA functionalized gold surface has demonstrated a nonideal behavior of Cp [26]. Recent work has shown that the frequency characterization of gold electrodes functionalized with DNA strands cannot be accurately described by a conventional capacitance model, and a different electrochemical model has been proposed to improve data interpretation in capacitive DNA sensors [27]. A more accurate model replaces the simple capacitor Cp with a Constant Phase Element (CPE) to describe the behavior of the ion layers at the gold/solution interface, (Figure 15.3).

This model is able to describe accurately the frequency-dependent capacitance behavior obtained from measurements on biochips. The model introduces two different fitting parameters, Cp and α (Eq. 15.1), and enhances the widely employed simple capacitive model significantly. These two parameters model the displacement and the movements of layering ions at the electrode/solution interface, as due to the different state configurations of the DNA molecules on the sensing electrodes of a biochip.

$$Z_{CPE} = \frac{1}{C_P(j\omega)^{\alpha}} = \frac{1}{\omega^{\alpha} C_P}\sqrt{1-\alpha^2} - j\frac{1}{\omega^{\alpha} C_P}\alpha \qquad (15.1)$$

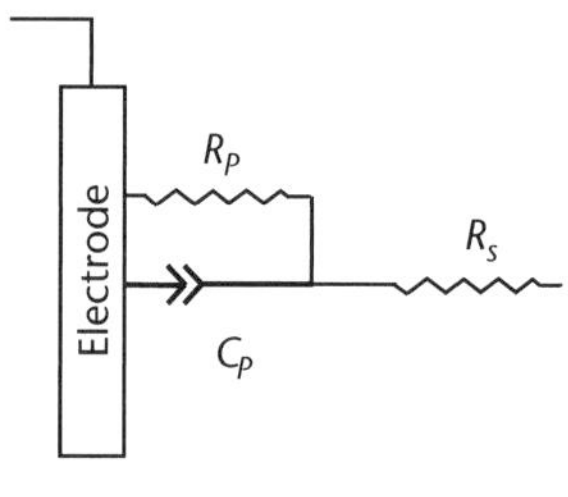

Figure 15.3 The correct model to be considered in the left of Figure 15.2.This model is based on a Constant Phase Element (CPE), which accounts not only for the capacitive but also to the conductive behavior of the DNA at the electrode/solution interface. Elaborated from [26].

Therefore, the model not only describes the insulating properties of the DNA layer, but also accounts for its conducting behavior. The changes of the reactance observed experimentally [27] are interpreted, as before, as the displacement of ions after hybridization, while the unchanged value of the resistance suggests that the formation of the DNA duplex does not modify the number of conductive pathways through the organic layer for the ions in the solution. This means that DNA hybridization affects mainly the reactance of the impedance in Equation (15.1). Therefore, the detection exploiting electronic systems like the CMOS-based circuit for label-free medical diagnostic can still be based on capacitance measurements, but without implicitly assuming a constant capacitance over a significant frequency range.

15.3 Electrodes Bio-Functionalization

The biochip electrodes have to be properly functionalized to enable capacitance detection. Moreover, the validation of the fabricated biochip may also be used to corroborate the proposed models for the interface behavior of the DNA layers. To do that, a particular kind of molecules (called probe molecules) are immobilized on the electrodes surface. They are selected to have biochemical affinity with the molecules to be detected (called target molecules). In the case of DNA, the probe and the target molecules are two single-stranded DNA molecules that are exactly complementary to each other. The nonspecific matching is usually checked by using a "nontarget" single-stranded DNA, which has a base sequence not complementary to that of the immobilized probe molecule.

In the following sub-section, we describe first a basic procedure that has been commonly used to immobilize DNA molecules on gold electrodes, then the required protocol to perform specific capturing of DNA targets, and, finally, we describe the step and the materials related to the detection of bound molecules on specific sites.

15.3.1 DNA Probe Immobilization

First, the gold electrodes on the biochip are cleaned by exposing the chip to oxygen plasma for 20 minutes at 200 W. Following this step, single-stranded DNA molecules modified with alkanethiol chains (a thiol reactive group and a spacer of 6 carboxylic groups) are immobilized on the gold electrodes by covalent S-Au bonds (a 3 μM DNA 1 μM Na_2HPO_4 solution is spread on the electrode surface for 18 hours). Two different probe molecules of the same length (25-mer) are attached to different electrodes on the same chip. To accomplish this, two separate droplets are deposited. After the incubation, the gold surfaces are extensively rinsed with ultrapure water to remove molecules that are not covalently bound to the gold electrodes. At this stage the electrode can be measured by wetting the surface with a suitable measurement solution.

15.3.2 DNA Target Hybridization

Target DNA solution (3 μM DNA 30-mer and TE 0, 3 M NaCl pH 7) is heated up to 80°C, spread on the electrodes, and cooled down to room temperature (for about

30 minutes). Finally, the surface is rinsed with the same saline solution (TE 0, 3 M NaCl pH 7) in order to remove the unbound DNA target.

15.3.3 DNA Detection

DNA detection is demonstrated by comparing measurements from electrode pairs subjected to the same reaction but with different DNA strands bound on the surface, complementary and noncomplementary to target molecules, respectively (the latter for negative control). All measurements are performed in the same saline solution used during the hybridization step (TE 0, 3 M NaCl pH 7). Since capacitances exhibit significant mismatches, a measurement after functionalization is performed and these values are used as a reference to be compared with the results obtained after (tentative) hybridization. In order to verify the biological steps previously described, an independent optical detection test based on fluorescence-labeled samples is performed [26]. It indicated a 80% hybridization efficiency on matching sites and less than 10% of nonspecific attachment on the other sites.

15.4 Chip Design for Capacitance Measurements

Recently, it has been shown that capacitance measurements can be done exploiting passive micro-fabricated electrodes [11]. Arrays made of passive electrodes are pad limited, as each electrode pair requires two pads for connecting to external measurement circuits. In such a context, this chapter presents the last achievements in CMOS circuit design for label-free diagnostic applications. Solutions with silicon chip featuring micrometric capacitors and on-chip logic for multiplexing on a limited number of I/O pins will be presented. The CMOS chips have been implemented with standard CMOS technology with the addition of gold deposition for capacitor electrodes.

15.4.1 Charge-Based Capacitance Measurements

In the first chip, capacitance measurements are performed by means of the Charge-Based Capacitance Measurement (CBCM) technique [28], which is suitable for low-complexity, small-area on-chip implementation. The chip includes the addressing circuitry, while the readout electronics has been realized externally by means of standard components in order to exploit the advantages of large experimental set-up flexibility (although it could eventually be easily integrated with the rest of the system). In Section 15.2, the two models of the sensing interface have been presented. In both cases, the detection of hybridization can be achieved by measuring the reactance part of the impedance and, therefore, the electrical detection in the CMOS circuit for label-free medical diagnostics may be based on capacitance measurements. Nevertheless, sensing of impedance variations requires a proper choice of the frequencies used for CBCM excitation waveforms. When measuring a capacitance with CBCM technique, an input square wave is applied to one electrode, while the current required to completely charge (or discharge) the capacitance is measured at the second electrode. The measured capacitance value equals the product of the average value of the output current, the applied voltage step, and the frequency of applied clock signal. With this technique, the measurement of the capacitive component of an impedance is independent of the resistive components provided that: (a) the charging and discharging current transients have the time to settle during the period of the square wave (i.e., all the charge stored in the reactive component is transferred); (b) the static current flowing through the R_P and R_S resistive path is negligible compared with the average output current (i.e., most of the charge transfer is due to the reactive component). Previous works on CBCM have demonstrated that both these requirements can be met in a practical experimental setting [21]. In the proposed CMOS circuit the transient discharging current has been driven to an external I/V converter (Figure 15.4) implemented off-chip by means of the operational amplifier OPA103AM and precision resistors.

The voltage signal at the op-amp output has been sampled by means of a National Instruments DAQ board (PCI-6032E [29]). Finally, the average value of the output voltage (V_{avg}) has been calculated by means of a trapezoidal integration and the average discharge current (I_{avg}) has been obtained as:

$$I_{avg} = V_{avg} / R_C \tag{15.2}$$

I_{avg} can be expressed as

$$I_{avg} = 2C\Delta Vf + I_{offset} \tag{15.3}$$

Here, ΔV, $((V+) - (V-))$, and f are controlled parameters, while C is the capacitance to be extracted from experimental data. For higher precision, the value of I_{avg} has been measured at nine different frequencies (from 60 Hz to 100 Hz and step of 5 Hz

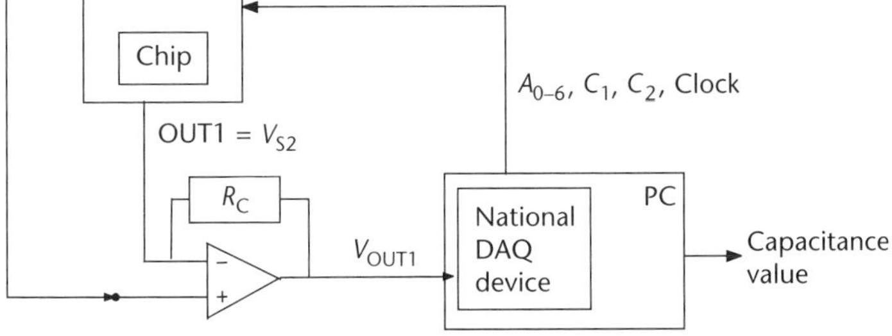

Figure 15.4 Schematic representation of measurement set-up. Elaborated from [26].

for each measurement) as the average of ten charging transients. Finally, C has been computed by least squares fitting on Equation 15.2 providing the slope m:

$$C = \frac{m}{2\Delta V} \tag{15.4}$$

A dedicated chip architecture has been designed in CMOS technology to implement this technique of capacitance measurement. Essentials of chip architecture and signal flow are shown in Figure 15.5(a).

Both analog and digital input signals are required. The former determine the voltage range used for the measurements, while the latter include a seven-bit address to select the sensing sites. An external clock has been used to provide the measurement frequency, which is the same as the external signal, as well as to synchronize the different blocks. Each sensing site features a block controlled by an external clock that generates a four square-wave signal with high timing precision. The on-chip address signals have been generated by means of two decoders. If one sensing site has been selected, the input signals coming from the pulse generator have been enabled and measurement has been performed. Only the output signal of the selected site has been connected to the shared output pad. At the output pad, the transient current has been

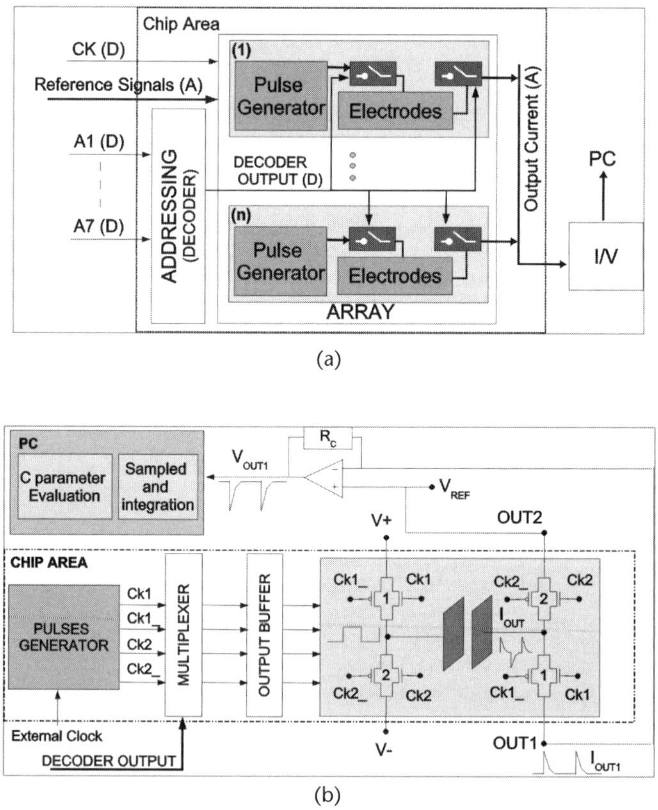

Figure 15.5 (a) The top illustration is a schematic representation of the system signal flow. (b) The bottom illustration represents the circuit under each pixel. Elaborated from [26].

converted by means of an external circuit into a voltage signal that has been sampled and processed by a PC in order to calculate the capacitance value. With respect to an on-chip implementation of the I/V conversion, this external solution allows larger flexibility in experimenting with different measurement parameters. The circuit implemented for each sensing site, illustrated in the dotted box in Figure 15.5(b), includes a pulse generator and four switches that selectively connect the electrodes of the sensing capacitances to one of three different reference voltages: V+, V–, and V_{REF}. A multiplexer has been inserted between the pulse generator and the switches and it allows the clock pulses to drive the electrodes of the sensing element only if it is selected. The switches have been implemented with both n- and p-channel transistors in order to exploit the full voltage range.

Exploiting its proximity with the switches, the (local) pulse generators provide very precise signals controlled by the external clock. A critical timing issue has to be considered in this regard, in that Ck1, Ck1– and Ck2, Ck2– must not close the switches at the same time in order to avoid shorting V+ and V–. For this reason, a suitable delay is inserted and non-overlapping clock signals are used in order to avoid that two transistors at the same time see a gate voltage larger than their threshold.

The delay used for this purpose is 1 ns and is obtained by means of the pulse generator block reported in Figure 15.6, also showing the output buffer following the multiplexer. The switches make it possible to connect the electrodes of the sensing capacitors either to V– and to V_{REF}, or to V+ and the voltage about V_{REF} at the negative input of the op-amp shown in Figure 15.5(b). When switching between these two bias conditions, a voltage step is applied at the sensing electrodes and a transient current is generated. With the circuits shown in Figure 15.5(b), the charging and discharging currents are driven to two different output pads, OUT 1 and OUT 2, thus allowing measurement of the average value using only one of them. The chip has been fabricated in a 60 n-well 0.5 μm CMOS process with two metal layers. The gold electrodes have been deposited after standard CMOS processing on silicon nitride (Si_3N_4) as described in [30]. Annealing steps have been introduced to guarantee good CMOS performance after gold deposition [30]. The area of the three sensing capacitors used in this work is 1 mm × 1 mm and the distance between them is 500 μm,

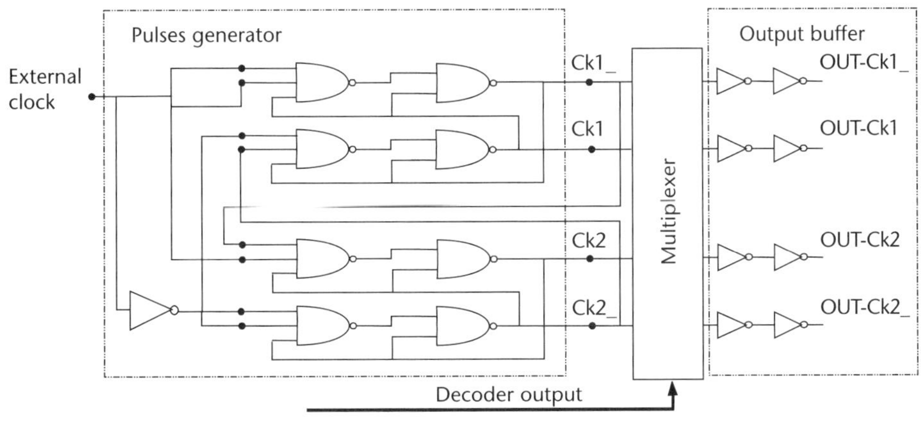

Figure 15.6 Schematic plot of the block used to generate clock signals that do not overlap. Elaborated from [26].

while that of the total chip, featuring 44 electrode couples of different size, is 6.5 mm × 4.6 mm. The parasitic capacitance between gold electrodes and substrate has been estimated to be 6 aF/μm^2, which is several orders of magnitude smaller than electrode/solution interface capacitance.

15.4.2 Frequency to Capacitance Measurements Technique

An alternative to the previously described technique to measure capacitances is a technique based on the conversion of the capacitance value to a frequency value [31], avoiding electrochemical labels [32]. In this case, the measurement technique used in the mixed-signal circuit is based on a very simple principle, as shown in Figure 15.7.

A periodic current excitation, I_{REF}, is provided to the electrodes. The electrodes react to the current pulses by changing their voltage difference in a transient waveform whose time constant is dominated by the capacitive component of the electrode-solution impedance. The inter-electrode potential is monitored by the crossings of two fixed reference values, $+V_{REF}$ and $-V_{REF}$.

In specific, the crossings of $+V_{REF}$ and $-V_{REF}$ produces a square waveform at the output of the comparator whose frequency is proportional to the rate of change of the voltage (as shown in Figure 15.7). If R_S is considered negligible, the crossing frequency obeys the following equation:

$$\frac{1}{f} = 2RC \ln \frac{1}{1 - \frac{V_{REF}}{I_{REF} R}} \tag{15.5}$$

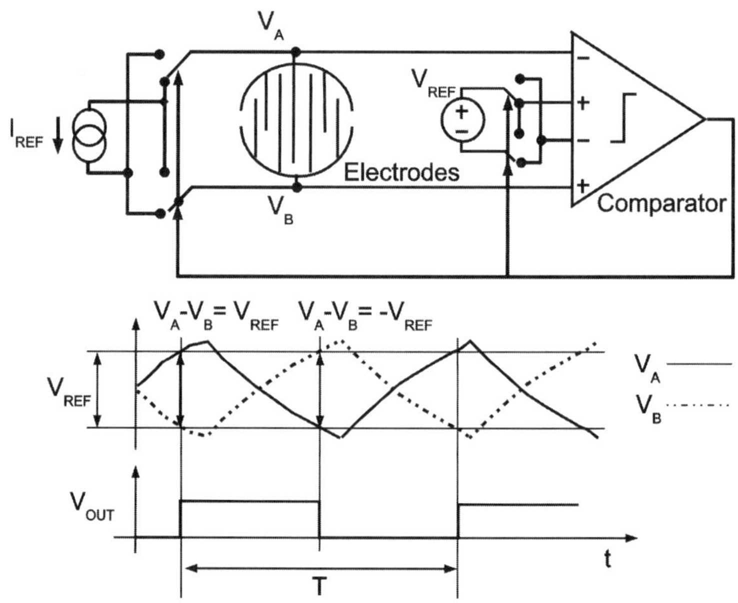

Figure 15.7 Measurement principle: interface capacitance determines the frequency of the electrodes charging and discharging transients. A comparator compares the inter-electrode potential with a reference voltage V_{REF} producing a digital signal at its output whose frequency is inversely proportional to capacitance. Elaborated from [31].

where R and C represent the contribution of the capacitance, C_P, and parallel resistance, R_P, of both electrode/solution interfaces. Moreover, if the frequency is not too low (i.e., I_{REF} is not too small) the first-order Taylor approximation of the logarithm returns the following equation:

$$\frac{1}{f} = \frac{2V_{REF}C}{I_{REF}} \tag{15.6}$$

The frequency is measured by means of a counter that is enabled to count the edges of the square waveform for a fixed time. The data stored in the counter can be read and the interface capacitance value of each electrode can be computed.

One major advantage of this technique is that the digital read-out of the frequency is almost trivial. In fact, an accurate estimate of the frequency value is obtained by counting the number of reference crossings in a given time interval. If the interval is long enough, very good frequency resolution can be obtained, assuming that the frequency is constant over the measurement interval. The circuit does not directly measure capacitance, but converts transient time into frequency of reference crossings. The chip architecture and signal flow developed to implement the frequency to capacitance measurements (FTCM) are summarized in Figure 15.8.

The chip interface requires both analog and digital I/O signals. Voltage references are analog DC signals, and they determine the voltage ranges used for measurements. Electrodes are selected using digital addressing lines A0–A6. Control logic includes reset and clock signal. The output is fully digital, as the chip performs internally the capacitance measurement and analog-to-digital conversion. Each sensing site features an analog part that converts the impedance value into frequency and outputs the data digitally.

Thus, 128 capacitance measurements and analog-to-digital conversions can be performed in parallel, and the results are then multiplexed on the shared output using

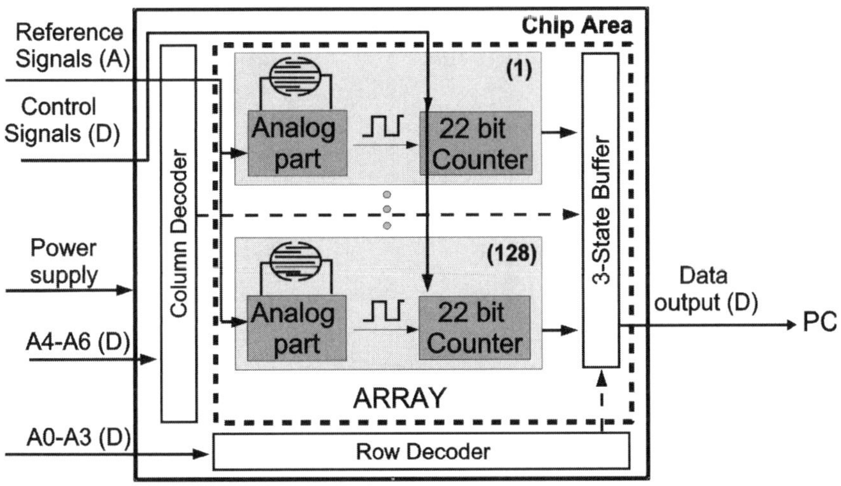

Figure 15.8 Schematic representation of the system and signal flow. A and D indicate analog and digital signals, respectively. Elaborated from [31].

the address signals that are generated on-chip by means of two decoders (Figure 15.8). At the output pad, the data are processed by a PC to calculate the capacitance value of the interface for each pixel. The mixed-signal circuit implemented for each sensing site is illustrated in Figure 15.9.

It includes an analog part (current source, comparator, and switches) and digital part (22-bit counter). The current pulses required for the circuit operation are provided by a current source based on a cascade stage followed by a pair of switches that alternatively connect the mirror to the electrodes in a current push or pull mode. The p-MOS source is part of an in-sensor site p-MOS current mirror biased by an n-MOS current source. The n-MOS current sources bias voltages are generated by an external circuit realized on a PCB. By adjusting the signal V_{MIRROR}, it is possible to change the reference current used for the measurements, thereby increasing the range of capacitance values that can be measured. In our case, V_{CASC} is set to 2 V to guarantee that n-MOS transistors work in the saturation region. If we neglect transistor mismatches and parasitic, I_{IN} is equal to I_{OUT} and to I_{REF}. The switches are implemented with parallel n- and p-channel transistors in order to have a full voltage range. Comparison of the electrode difference voltage with the reference difference voltage level is performed by a high-gain differential CMOS stage. The output of the gain stage is then buffered by a simple CMOS inverter, thereby becoming a digital signal. The number of oscillations within a given time is then counted by a digital 22-bit counter clock. After a user-settable time period, the counter is stopped, and the final count value can be transferred to the output via a shift register. The shift register is clocked from an external source resulting in a serial output of the counter's data bits at the chip's output. The counter/shift register circuit has already been described in [31]. A "reset" signal is activated before each measurement to set all the counters to zero. Then, a "count" signal is set at high value for a fixed time, called integration time, enabling the counter. Finally, a clock signal is used to read the data stored in the shift register of the counter. The described circuit guarantees that each pixel oscillates con-

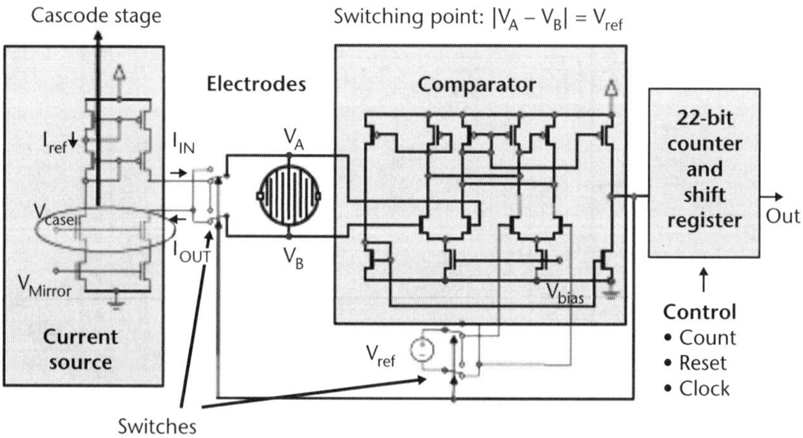

Figure 15.9 Schematic of the circuit associated with each sensing element. The current source is implemented by a current mirror circuit. The comparator features two differential input stages and a high-gain output stage. Finally, a 22-bit counter and shift register samples and stores measurement data. Elaborated from [31].

tinuously at a frequency determined by the interface capacitance. It is important to note that with this free-running oscillator concept the data from all sites are sampled simultaneously.

In this case, the chip is fabricated in a 60 n-well 0.5 μm CMOS process with three metal layers, the oxide thickness is 15 nm, and the supply voltage is 5 V. The gold electrodes are deposited after standard CMOS processing. After the gold deposition, an annealing step is introduced applying N_2/H_2 at 350°C for 30 minutes in order to guarantee sufficiently low values of the interface state density at the silicon/silicon dioxide interface [4]. The sensor sites consist of interdigitated electrodes with 1.2 μm line width and spacing; the diameter of the circular arrangement is 200 μm. The chip provides an 8×16 array of these sensors and the pitch is 250 μm. Total chip is 6.4 mm $\times$ 4.5 mm. The electrical interface includes analog as well as digital signals. Two different power supply and ground pads are also implemented on chip. A shield connected to ground is introduced to reduce noise between analog and digital circuits.

15.5 Biochip Application to DNA

The two CMOS chips previously described, based on CBCM and on FTCM method, respectively, were applied to detect target DNA molecules in label-free experiments. The typical experimental set-up is similar to that shown in Figure 15.4 (only the LabView™ program has been changed), where the developed chip is connected by ultra-sound bonding to a card enabling the I/O operations (Figure 15.10). A cell for fluidic handling has been placed on the top of the chip and inlet/outlet gates were used to inject the target samples as shown in Figure 15.10.

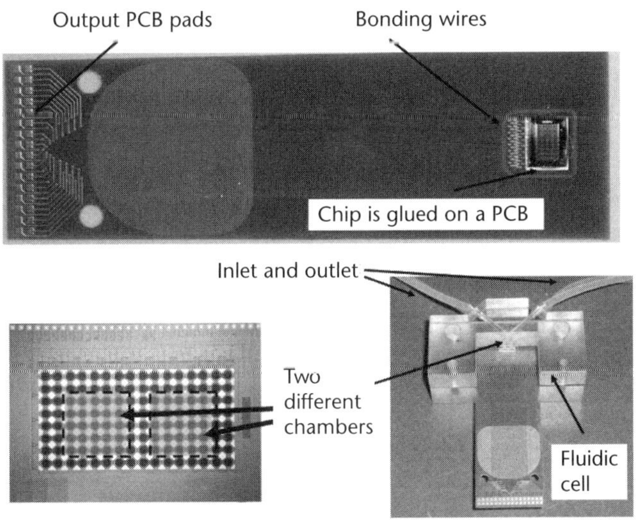

Figure 15.10 The final set-up for the testing of CMOS circuits. A fluidic cell with an inlet and an outlet for the injection of the target molecules is present in the set-up. The arrow on the left is indicating the chip sensing area. The pads in the photograph bottom are the I/O connections. Elaborated from [31].

As already discussed in subsection 15.3.3, DNA detection is achieved by comparing measurements on electrode couples subjected to the same reaction but with different DNA strands bound on the surface, complementary and noncomplementary to target molecules, respectively, (the latter for negative control).

All measurements are performed in the same saline solution of the hybridization step (TE 0, 3 M NaCl pH 7). Since capacitances exhibit significant mismatches, a measurement after functionalization is performed and these values are used as a reference to be compared with the results obtained after (tentative) hybridization. As reported in Figure 15.11(a), the absolute values of capacitance after DNA target/probe hybridization show an average decrease of about 48% with respect to the electrodes functionalized with the probe DNA molecules when the detection was done by means of the CBCM method [26]. On the other hand, the relative capacitance variations between clean electrodes and electrodes with DNA after DNA target/probe hybridization show a variation of about 65% with respect to the electrodes functionalized with the probe DNA molecules when the detection was done by means of the FTCM method, as reported in Figure 15.11(b) [31].

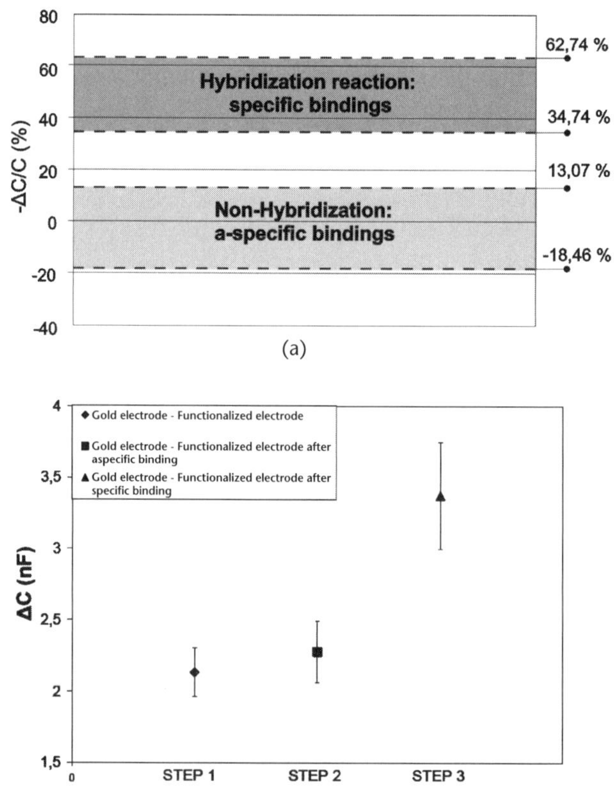

(b)

Figure 15.11 (a) Shows the capacitance variations due to specific and nonspecific bindings (upper and lower bands of measured capacitances, respectively). Positive values indicate capaictance decrease. Elaborated from [26]; (b) shows the average behavior of all the pixels, confirming that a nonspecific and specific binding are distinguishable. Elaborated from [31].

The two behaviors are not easily comparable because the first is related to the difference between the absolute capacitance values while the second is related to differences between the clean electrodes and the functionalized ones. However, the two experiments and set-up have shown the capability to clearly detect DNA hybridization reaction. Moreover, the two trends are showing a decrease in the average capacitance, confirming that both capacitance measurement methods are able to coherently detect the DNA hybridization at the electrode's interfaces.

Furthermore, the difference in the DNA detection discrimination between the two methodologies of capacitance determination (48% in one case, and 65% in the other) is not related to the difference in the two methods used for the capacitance detection. In fact, in the case of measurements done on test capacitances provided by solid-state capacitors, the output of the two CMOS circuits were similar and close to the nominal values. For example, the CBCM method returns a precision better than 1.4% in the range 100 nF to 1μF.

The complexity of these kinds of measurements can be easily understood by observing Figure 15.12, which shows the data measurement in the case of the FTCM method. Two phenomena can be highlighted: (1) a decreasing trend during measurement and (2) a transient when the measurement re-starts. Possible reasons related to issues concerning the biomodified electrode/solution interfaces are discussed in detail in the next section.

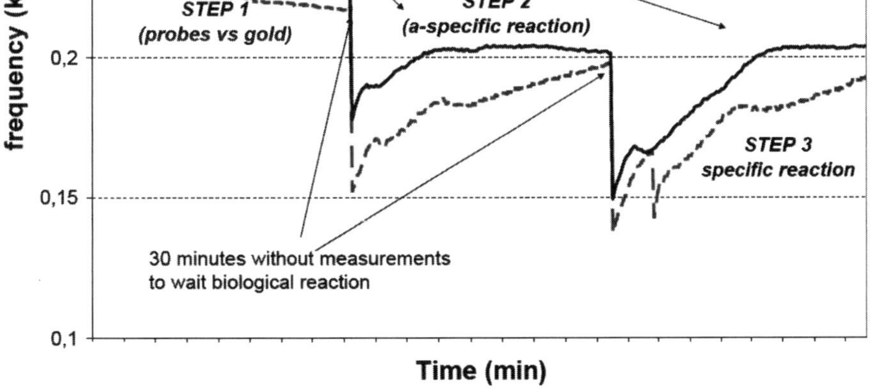

Figure 15.12 Frequency changes of the average of reference electrodes (continuous line), and the average of functionalized electrodes (dashed line) show a larger gap after the DNA hybridization step, considering the stable value reached at the end of the transient. Elaborated from [31].

15.6 Discussion on Results: Analysis and Future Perspectives

In this paragraph we will show that the difference in the DNA detection results observed with the two capacitance measurement techniques are related to the different behavior of the DNA layer at the interface with the solution in the two types of experiments shown previously. In fact, it was also shown that capacitance of the DNA layers changes with frequency [27], thus, the comparison of data acquired within different frequency ranges can be misleading. Moreover, it was also shown by using impedance spectroscopy that the ability to distinguish the single- and double-stranded DNA may reverse when the trend in frequency of the phase is considered [33]. In subsection 15.6.1, the electrical analysis in frequency and problems related to electrical measurement will be discussed, while in subsection 15.6.2 improvements to measurement and DNA detection from a biochemical point of view will be presented.

15.6.1 Frequency Analysis of Electrical Measurements

A clearer view of the surface biophysics can be obtained by performing capacitance measurements of the gold biomodified interfaces at different frequencies. The frequency range to be considered is a crucial issue. In fact, if the capacitance changes with frequency, the method to estimate the capacitance implemented in CMOS may result in a wrong estimation of the capacitance values.

In what follows, we report simulations obtained implementing the CBCM method to estimate the capacitance in a situation in which the DNA behavior at the electrode's interface is strongly dependent on the frequency. Figure 15.13(a) shows this situation for three different electrodes (clean electrodes, DNA probes, DNA target).

In particular, Figure 15.13(a) shows simulations based on the model of the CPE element (cfr. paragraph 15.2.2) and plots three trends in the range 1 to 1000 Hz. Figure 15.13(b) simulates the average current acquisitions based on Equation (15.3), but using the capacitance value coming from the trend reported in Figure 15.13(a). Figure 15.13(b) also reports the linear fitting to determine the parameter "m" of Equation (15.4), which is used to determine the value of the estimated capacitance (here the capacitance is estimated following the CBCM method). The CPE leads to a 30–40% decrease and a 100% increase in the capacitance parameter C of Equation (15.1) as due to different DNA layers on the electrodes and the consequent equivalent capacitance is in the range of variation tested as shown in Table 15.1.

However, Table 15.1 reports the effective capacitance values in the considered frequency range for the average current acquisition and the mean capacitance estimated by using the CBCM method. The table shows a large discrepancy between the estimated average capacitance and the capacitances varying into the considered frequency range, as shown in Figure 15.13(a). This means that the estimated capacitance value is inaccurate, even if Figure 15.13(b) shows a frequency trend for the average current close to that expected from a linear regression.

Therefore, attention should be paid when considering capacitance estimation in DNA detection because the DNA surface shows strong capacitance vs. frequency variations. Similar problems may be found when employing the FTCM method.

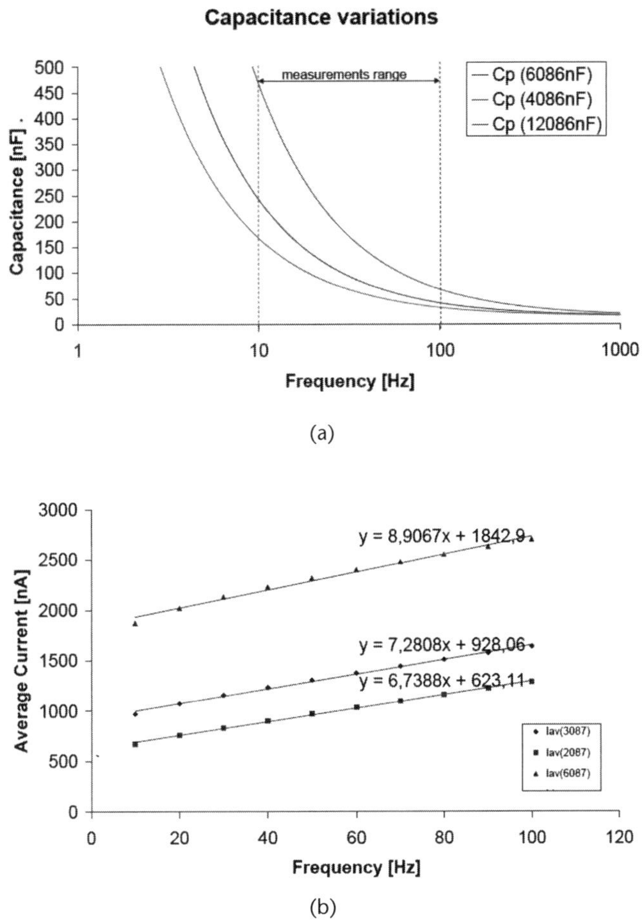

Figure 15.13 (a) Simulation of capacitance variation on frequency. (b) Simulation of the average current variations as calculated from the capacitance trend shown in (a).

15.6.2 Discussion on Biochemical Issues

In this section, we describe how we can improve the biochip interface behavior by changing the functionalization of the electrode surface to approach an ideal capacitance behavior (see paragraph 15.2.1). Our aim is to obtain functionalized surfaces with capacitance behavior that does not strongly depend on frequency, in order to stabilize and improve the DNA detection capability and reliability. Fortunately, there

Table 15.1 Three Different Ranges of Capacitance

C range [nF]	*Measured with CBCM [nF]*
41–242	18
32–167	17
68–468	22

From Figure 15.13(a) extracted from 10 to 100 Hz and the average values estimated with CBCM in the same frequency range coming from data in Figure 15.13(b).

is a possibility to obtain a capacitance close to the ideal one. In fact, it is possible to close the charge exchange pathways to the electrode's surface by using a tightly packed and stable sub-layer. To create such a sub-layer, it is possible to use thiols having a long alkyl chain that tend to produce highly packed films, and a glycol segment [34]. Moreover, this kind of thiols has a high capability to resist nonspecific adsorption, thereby improving the specificity of the sensing surface for biosensor applications [35]. Two different alkanethiol molecules are used just after silanization to form an insulating *Self-Assembly Monolayer* (SAM) on the electrode surface. Both molecules are composed by a mercapto-group, for the immobilization of the molecule on gold; an alkylic part of 11 carbons, for the ordered self-assembly of the molecules, and a glycol part $(OCH_2CH_2)n$, functionalized with a OH or COOH group. The glycol part improves electrode stability significantly, because after equilibration, these functional groups form an ordered layer that prevents solution ions from reaching the electrode. Thus, parasitic electron transfer between solution and electrode surface is almost completely avoided. The formation of SAM produces a slight decrease in capacitance value due to the increased gap between solution ions and metal interface, while the glycol chain leads to measurements that are 10 times more stable with respect to the ones obtained with simple alkanethiol molecules. Preliminary results show an almost ideal capacitive behavior. In Figure 15.14, the capacitance vs. frequency acquired on a self-assembly glycol-thiols monolayer is plotted. This relationship is close to a constant in the frequency domain.

15.7 Conclusions and Perspectives

The possibility to fabricate biochips based on CMOS technology creates the opportunity to push DNA detection technology out of research laboratories, toward point-of-care. CMOS electronics may be employed to develop DNA and Protein Chip to be used in personalized therapy. In this chapter we presented two CMOS architectures implementing a fully-electrical, label-free detection method. Two different architectures based on different principles used to estimate the capacitance of the molecules at the electrode/solution interface have been presented and both are highly reliable.

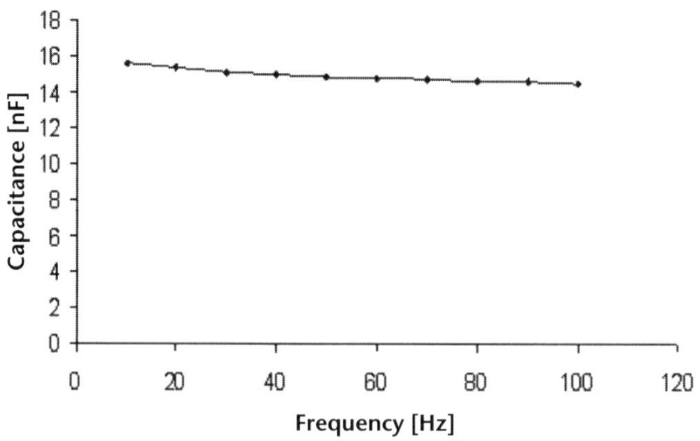

Figure 15.14 The frequency trend of the capacitance measured by the CBCM method on a gold electrode functionalized with three-glycol thiols.

The possibility to apply these architectures to DNA detection was demonstrated. However, application to point-of-care diagnostic requires high stability and repeatability of the electrical measurements, which becomes very problematic if probe layers do not show ideal capacitor behavior, as reported in Section 15.2. Therefore, the procedure used for functionalization is a crucial step for biochip applications. Big improvements in stability are achievable by exploiting advanced biofunctionalization techniques such as the ones reported in Section 15.6. Looking into the future, it is important to note that the same transduction techniques used for DNA sensing could be applied for protein detection. In fact, even protein electrode functionalization can be performed on glycol layers [35] and the capacitance detection principle can also be applied and investigated to this case. Hence, this technology may have an important role for the development of simple and low-cost biochips for point-of-care diagnostics, for both genomic and proteomic. In the case of market products, a cost of 0.5$ per chip for a CMOS-based DNA biochip is achievable. This opens the possibility to enter the market with low-cost, handy, point-of-care technologies in medical diagnostics.

References

[1] S. Mouterau, R. Narwa, C. Matheron, N. Vongmany, E. Simon, and M. Goossens, "An improved electronic microarray-based diagnostic assay for identification of MEFV mutations," *Human Mutation*, vol. 23, no. 6, pp. 621–628, 2004.

[2] P.K. Riggs, J.M. Angel, E.L. Abel, and J. DiGiovanni, "Differential gene expression in epidermis of mice sensitive and resistant to phorbol ester skin tumor promotion," *Molecular Carcinogenesis*, vol. 44, no. 2, pp. 122–136, 2005.

[3] G.C. Kennedy, H. Matsuzaki, S. Dong, W.-m. Liu, J. Huang, G. Liu, X. Su, M. Cao, W. Chen, J. Zhang, W. Liu, G. Yang, X. Di, T. Ryder, Z. He, U. Surti, M. S.Phillips, M.T. Boyce-Jacino, S.P. Fodor, and K.W. Jones, "Large-scale genotyping of complex DNA," *Nature Biotechnology*, vol. 1, no. 10, pp. 1233–1237, 2003.

[4] Motorola Life Sciences Inc.—www.motorola.com.

[5] C. Yu, Y. Wan, H. Yowanto, J. Li, C. Tao, M.D. James, C.L. Tan, G.F. Blackburn, and T.J. Meade, "Electronic detection of single-base mismatches with ferrocene-modified probes," *J. Am. Chem. Soc.*, vol. 123, no. 45, pp. 11:155–11:161, 2001.

[6] M. Schienle, C. Paulus, A. Frey, F. Hoffmann, B. Holzapfl, P. Schindelr-Bauer, and R. Thewes, "A fully electronic DNA sensor with 128 positions and in-pixel A/D conversion," *IEEE Journal of Solid-State Circuits*, vol. 39, no. 12, pp. 2438–2444, 2004.

[7] R. Gabl, E. Green, M. Schreiter, H.D. Feucht, H. Zeininger, R. Primig, and D. Pitzer, "Novel integrated FBAR sensors: a universal platform for bio- and gas detection," *Proc. IEEE Sensors*, vol. 2, pp. 1184–1188, 2003.

[8] R. Brederlow, S. Zauner, A. L. Scholtz, K. Aufinger, W. Simburger, C. Paulus, A. Martin, M. Fritz, H.-J. Timme, H. Heiss, S. Marksteiner, L. Elbrecht, R. Aigner, and R. Thewes, "Biochemical sensors based on bulk acoustic wave resonators," *IEDM Tech. Digest*, pp. 992–994, 2003.

[9] Y. Li, C. Vancura, C. Hagleitner, J. Lichtenberg, O. Brand, and H. Baltes, "Very high Q-factor in water achieved by monolithic, resonant cantilever sensor with fully integrated feedback," *Proc. IEEE Sensors*, vol. 2, pp. 809–813, 2003.

[10] K.-U. Kirstein, Y. Li, M. Zimmermann, C. Vancura, T. Volden, W.H. Song, and J. Lichtenberg, "Cantilever-based biosensors in CMOS technology," *Proc. DATE05*, vol. 2, pp. 210–214, 2005.

[11] C. Guiducci, C. Stagni, A. Fischetti, U. Mastromatteo, L. Benini, and B. Riccò, "Microfabricated two-terminal capacitors for label-free DNA sensing/recognition," *IEEE Sensors*, vol. 6, no. 5, pp. 1084–1093, 2006.

[12] H. Berney, J. West, E. Haefele, J. Alderman, W. Lane, and J. Collins, "A DNA diagnostic biosensor: development, characterisation and performance," *Sensors and Actuators B*, vol. 68, pp. 100–108, 2000.

[13] F. Uslu, S. Ingebrandt, S. Bcker-Meffert, D. Mayer, M. Krause, M. Odenthal, and A. Offenhusser, "Label-free fully electronic nucleic acid detection system based on a field-effect transistor device," *Biosensors and Bioelectronics*, vol. 19, no. 12, pp. 1723–1731, 2004.

[14] J. Fritz, E.B. Cooper, S. Gaudet, P.K. Sorger, and S.R. Manalis, "Electronic detection of DNA by its intrinsic molecular charge," *Proceedings of the National Academy of Science*, vol. 99, no. 8, pp. 14142–14146, 2000.

[15] F. Pouthas, C. Gentil, D. Côte, and U. Bockelmann, "DNA detection on transistor arrays following mutation-specific enzymatic amplification," *Applied Physics Letters*, vol. 84, pp. 1594–1596, 2004.

[16] E. Souteyrand, J. Cloarec, J. Martin, C. Wilson, I. Lawrence, S. Mikkelsen, and M. Lawrence, "Direct detection of the hybridization of synthetic homo-oligomer DNA sequences by field effect," *J. Phys. Chem. B*, vol. 101, pp. 2980–2985, 1997.

[17] F. Perkins, S.J. Fertig, K.A. Brownt, D. McCarthy, L. Tender, and M. Peckerar, "An active microelectronic transducer for enabling label-free miniaturized chemical sensors," in *Technical Digest. International Electron Devices Meeting (IEDM'00)*, San Francisco, USA, Dec. 2000.

[18] R.P. Janek, W.R. Fawcett, and A. Ulman, "Impedance spectroscopy of self-assembled monolayers on Au(111): Evidence for complex double-layer structure in aqueous NaClO4 at the potential of zero charge," *J. Phys. Chem. B*, vol. 101, pp. 8550–8558, 1997.

[19] C. Berggren, P. Stalhandske, J. Brundell, and G. Johansson, "A feasibility study of a capacitive biosensor for direct detection of DNA hybridization," *Electroanalysis*, vol. 3, no. 11, pp. 74–84, 1999.

[20] M. Riepl, V.M. Mirsky, I. Novotny, V. Tvarozek, V. Rehacek, and O.S. Wolfbeis, "Optimization of capacitive affinity sensors: drift suppression and signal amplification," *Analytica Chimica Acta*, vol. 392, no. 1, pp. 77–84, 1999.

[21] C. Guiducci, C. Stagni, G. Zuccheri, A. Bogliolo, L. Benini, B. Samorì, and B. Riccò, "DNA detection by integrable electronics," *Biosensors and Bioelectronics*, vol. 19, no. 8, pp. 781–787, 2004.

[22] J.R. Macdonald, *Impedance Spectroscopy*. New York: John Wiley and Sons, 1987.

[23] J. Israelachvili, *Intermolecular and Surface Forces*. London: Academic Press, 1992.

[24] C. Berggren, P. Stalhandske, J. Brundell, and G. Johansson, "A feasibility study of a capacitive biosensor for direct detection of DNA hybridization," *Electroanalysis*, vol. 11, no. 3, pp. 156–160, 1999.

[25] C. Guiducci, C. Stagni, G. Zuccheri, A. Bogliolo, L. Benini, B. Samorí, and B. Riccó, "DNA detection by integrable electronics," *Biosensors and Bioelectronics*, vol. 19, no. 8, pp. 781–787, 2004.

[26] C. Stagni, C. Guiducci, L. Benini, B. Riccò, S. Carrara, B. Samorì, C. Paulus, M. Schienle, and R. Thewes: "A fully-electronic label-free DNA sensor chip," *IEEE Sensor Journal*, vol. 7, no. 4, pp. 577–585, 2007.

[27] S. Carrara, F.K. Gürkaynak, C. Guiducci, C. Stagni, L. Benini, Y. Leblebici, B. Samorì, and G. De Micheli, "Interface layering phenomena in capacitance detection of DNA with biochips," *Sensors & Transducers Journal*, vol. 76, pp. 969–977, 2007.

[28] A. Bogliolo, L. Vendrame, L. Bortesi, and E. Barachetti, "Charge-based on-chip measurement technique for the selective extraction of crosscoupling capacitances," in *Proceedings of IEEE Signal Propagation on Interconnects*, Castelvecchio Pascoli, Pisa (Italy), 2002.

[29] National Instruments—www.ni.com.

[30] F. Hoffmann, A. Frey, B. Holzapfl, M. Schienle, C. Paulus, P. Schindelr-Bauer, D. Kuhlmeier, J. Krause, E. Hintsche, E. Nebling, J. Albers, W. Gumbrecht, K. Plehnert, G. Eckstein, and R. Thewes, "Fully electronic DNA detection on a CMOS chip: device and process issues," in *IEDM Tech. Dig.*, pp. 488–491, 2002.

[31] C. Stagni, C. Guiducci, L. Benini, B. Ricco, S. Carrara, B. Samorì, C. Paulus, M. Schienle, M. Augustyniak, and R. Thewes, "CMOS DNA sensor array with integrated A/D conversion based on label-free capacitance measurement," *IEEE Journal of Solid-State Circuits*, vol. 41, no. 12, pp. 2956–2964, 2006.

[32] M. Schienle, C. Paulus, A. Frey, F. Hoffmann, B. Holzapfl, P. Schindler-Bauer, and R. Thewes, "A fully electronic DNA sensor with 128 positions and in-pixel A/D conversion," *IEEE Journal of Solid-State Circuits*, vol. 39, no. 12, pp. 2438–2444, 2004.

[33] K.-S. Ma, H. Zhou, J. Zoval, and M. Madou, "DNA hybridization detection by label free versus impedance amplifying label with impedance spectroscopy," *Sensors and Actuators B*, vol. 114, pp. 58–64, 2006.

[34] S. Carrara, V.K. Bhalla, C. Stagni, and B. Samorì, "Three-glycol alkyl thiols surfaces for application in sensors and biosensors array based on capacitance detection," submitted for publication.

[35] J. Lahiri, L. Isaacs, J. Tien, and G. Whitesides, "A strategy for the generation of surfaces presenting ligands for studies of binding based on an active ester as a common reactive intermediate: a surface plasmon resonance study," *Analytical Chemistry*, vol. 71, pp. 777–790, 1999.

CHAPTER 16

Silicon-Based Microfluidic Systems for Nucleic Acid Analysis

Levent Yobas

16.1 From Tubes to Chips

The idea of replacing *vacuum tubes* with an *integrated circuit* (IC) about half a century ago has sparked a new era of opportunities under the field of Microelectronics. Inspired by the success of miniaturization in electronics, researchers have now set the goal to extend the trend over the life sciences by replacing simple *test tubes* with *microfluidic chips*. If proved successful, such technology has the potential to decentralize bioanalytical processes that are mainly limited to the clinical laboratory settings. The current practice requires piling together clinical samples before processing them all at once through liquid-handling robots. These robots are the analogue of bulky mainframe computers that once occupied research laboratories before personal computers entered into daily life by becoming smaller, cheaper, and more powerful.

Similarly, a key motivation behind these research efforts is to develop a portable miniaturized system such that complicated and skill-laden bioanalytical processes can take place on a tiny chip or cartridge that can be used by a relatively unskilled person outside the laboratory. Such a device is also broadly referred to as "Lab-on-a-Chip (LOC)" or "Micro Total Analysis System (μ-TAS)." Further benefits that come with the miniaturization include reduced sample and reagent consumption, faster bioanalysis, higher efficiency and accuracy. Of the bioanalytical assays, molecular tests that screen for the presence of a specific target sequence of nucleic acids are known as nucleic acid probe assays and offer much higher sensitivity and specificity.

The vision of a point-of-care device based on the detection of a target nucleic acid is conceptually shown in Figure 16.1 [1]. The device accepts the raw sample from the body as an input and automatically produces the test result as an output without any intervention. The device utilizes LOC or μ-TAS to execute three essential tasks in consecutive steps: (1) extraction and purification of nucleic acid from a given raw sample, (2) amplification, and (3) detection of an existing target sequence. Amplification of nucleic acids involves a biochemical reaction that can synthesize many copies of the target sequence to detectable levels. Ideally, it is desired to perform all these three tasks on a "self-contained" and "fully-enclosed" disposable cartridge where the required reagents and the reactions' waste are stored in isolated compartments. "Self-contained" means that the cartridge needs only the raw sample to be supplied

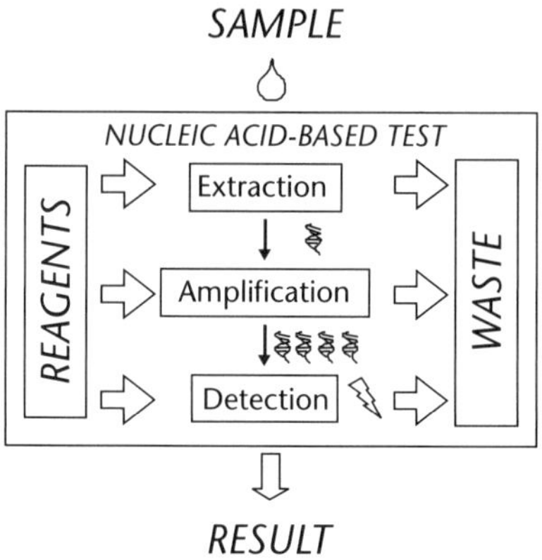

Figure 16.1 Concept diagram of a *self-contained* and *fully-enclosed* point-of-care device (sample-in-result-out system) for a portable nucleic acid probe assay [1].

by the user, whereas "fully-enclosed" implies that the cartridge, once supplied with the raw sample, forms a truly enclosed system that does not expose any of its contents to outside. Both features are critical for its safe use in the field with samples and reagents potentially hazardous to health and the environment.

The purpose of this chapter is to give a brief account of each of these three essential tasks (extraction, amplification, and detection of nucleic acids) by highlighting some of the landmark developments in the field. It should be noted that, although the field initially emerged from the silicon-based technology (semiconductor processing) more than a decade ago, it has quickly ventured into other materials such as glass, poly(dimethylsiloxane) (PDMS), and other polymers by adopting non-silicon fabrication methods such as soft lithography, hot embossing, and injection moulding. This transformation has been mainly driven by the following needs: (1) a transparent substrate that is more suitable for optical detection of nucleic acids in the visible range; (2) an insulating substrate that can withstand high voltage pulses applied during the electrophoretic separation of nucleic acids; and (3) a lower manufacturing cost per unit device. However, the silicon-based technology has a great potential to deliver a point-of-care device for nucleic acid analysis that is fully integrated, high-performance, rapid, automated, reliable and most of all manufacturable. Optical detection of nucleic acids, although it has been well established, is mainly indirect and requires the extra step of labeling. Moreover, most optical detection schemes are against the spirit of integration and have to rely on off-chip external modules including lenses, photodiodes, or photomultiplier tubes. In contrast, electronic detection of nucleic acids is rather direct, as no labeling is needed and may lead to a portable miniaturized system.

16.2 Nucleic Acid Extraction

Nucleic acids, in the form of either DNA or RNA, are well protected inside living organisms such as cells, bacteria, and viruses, being enveloped by a membrane of lipid or protein coating. For detection of a specific sequence of DNA or RNA, nucleic acids have to be extracted out first and purified from macromolecules such as proteins, nucleases, and hemoglobin that may hinder their amplification. This is routinely performed in forensic laboratories for suspect identification via DNA fingerprinting, in clinical laboratories for diagnosis of genetic mutations and infectious diseases, and in the food and agriculture industry for developing disease-resistant produce and inspecting livestock. Particularly in forensic cases, the scarcity of typical samples found at a crime scene as potential evidence might greatly benefit from a microextraction device that requires only minute quantities of raw samples and reagents. In addition, a point-of-care device that screens suspects for the presence of viral infection should be able to extract and detect viral nucleic acids from bodily samples. Viruses are simple organisms carrying a small amount of genetic material in the form of either DNA or RNA but not both. For instance, the corona virus that causes atypical pneumonia, also known as Severe Acute Respiratory Syndrome (SARS), contains only a single-strand RNA. For many of the above applications, time-to-result is a pressing factor.

Extraction of nucleic acids from a given raw sample, also known as the sample preparation, is the very first stage of a fully integrated system. Yield and selectivity of this process can determine the performance requirement of the subsequent amplification and detection steps. Despite the importance of this initial stage, the topic of on-chip sample preparation previously received little attention from the research community in comparison with the subsequent stages of nucleic acid amplification and detection [2]. This could be attributed to the complexity of the problem, which poses technical hurdles like diversity of raw biological samples to deal with (e.g., tissue, blood, saliva, urine, etc.) and/or scarcity of the target sequence of nucleic acids present in these samples (e.g., those from rare cells or few virus particles).

A major challenge in the chip-based nucleic acid extraction is to attain a certain degree of purity so that nucleic acids can be amplified and detected. Unless the extraction is sufficiently free of impurities that may inhibit the subsequent stage, nucleic acids cannot be amplified to detectable levels. Integrity of the extracted nucleic acids is also important to be able to preserve and amplify the target sequence. If nucleic acids get exposed to excessive shear during the extraction process, the target sequence may break into fragments and hence cannot be multiplied (amplified) later. Another challenge lies with the extraction of RNA because RNA, unlike DNA, is known to be unstable due to its backbone being susceptible to degradation.

Design of a microfluidic system for extraction and purification of nucleic acids has to be specific to the biochemical protocol of choice. Protocol for nucleic acid extraction may vary depending on the type of nucleic acids and the nature of raw samples being targeted. For instance, extracting genomic DNA from human blood involves isolation of white blood cells (WBC) from red blood cells (RBC). Genomic DNA resides in the nucleus of WBC, whereas RBC lacks a nucleus (hence contains no DNA) and carries a high level of hemoglobin, which is known to inhibit the subsequent stage of nucleic acid amplification. Depending on the approach, this task can be daunting, as the relative population of RBC to that of WBC is overwhelming (typical counts of WBC $< 25,000$ and of RBC $>10^6$ in a given 1 mL of blood).

Separation of target cells or virus particles from a given sample is conventionally performed in clinical laboratories by subjecting the sample to (ultra)-centrifuge or chemicals that can selectively break open (lyse) unwanted cells. The former is not amenable to miniaturization, but the latter, the process of selective chemical lysis, can be implemented on chip. The cells or virus particles can also be separated on chip according to their physical properties using techniques such as filtration [3, 4], dielectrophoresis [5], and acoustophoresis [6]. Some of these methods can be time consuming (e.g., filtration), whereas others can be highly sensitive to buffer composition (e.g., dielectrophoresis). If none of the physical properties can be utilized as a distinguishing factor, a further method involves tagging the target cells with antibody-conjugated magnetic beads and then trapping them in an externally-applied magnetic field [7].

Once the particles of interest (cell, virus, bacteria, etc.) are isolated, they must be broken open (lysed) to release their nucleic acids (DNA or RNA). There are several ways of lysing cells on chip: mechanical, electrical, chemical, enzymatic, osmotic, and thermal in nature. Mechanical lysis, (i.e., the physical disruption of the cell membrane), can be easily implemented by pressurizing cells through sharp microstructures or micro nozzles [8, 9]. A highly efficient mechanical lysis method utilizes high-frequency ultrasound waves and creates small bubbles expanding and imploding violently [10]. The electrical and thermal methods are easy to miniaturize but may not be that efficient for lysing all cell types [4, 11]. The chemical lysis method is rather efficient but may require relatively large amounts of organic solvents such as chaotropic agents to be injected into the chip [12]. These reagents have to be subsequently removed, as they can inhibit the nucleic acid amplification.

With the disruption of cells, the real challenge becomes the purification of nucleic acids from a complex matrix of cellular debris including proteins and membrane fragments. Fortunately, this can be accomplished by adopting selective and reversible binding of nucleic acids to a glass or silica surface [13]. It is well-known that nucleic acids bind to a silica-based surface in the presence of chaotropic salts such as 6 M of guanidine hydrochloride (GuHCl). Chatropic salts solubilize proteins, dissolve cell membrane, and denature DNA. They also dehydrate nucleic acids and enhance the intermolecular attractions that bind them to the glass surface. This property is the basis of modern-day kits for the extraction and purification of DNA and RNA. A typical protocol requires several wash steps whereby the glass or silica surface is sequentially exposed to (1) a sample having been lysed and mixed with a binding buffer containing chaotropic agents to promote selective binding of nucleic acids, (2) a wash buffer containing ethanol to precipitate nucleic acids on the surface while removing salt and the cellular impurities, and (3) an elution buffer containing no salt or a low concentration of salt to recover nucleic acids from the surface.

The commercial kits typically utilize a column of silica-gel membrane or filter whereby each wash step is performed by passing the corresponding solution through the column via centrifugal spinning [14]. Since the kits require repetitive steps of pipetting and spinning, they are manually involved and prone to human error. They also suffer from low extraction efficiency if the starting copy number of nucleic acids is extremely low. Nevertheless, a similar extraction protocol can be automated in microfluidics by implementing a flow-through concept wherein each solution is sequentially injected through a silica-based microfluidic device. A clear advantage of the silicon-based technology is that it readily offers a silica-based surface for nucleic acid binding. Such a surface can be prepared on silicon substrates by techniques such as thermal oxidation or chemical vapor deposition.

Christel et al. utilized this advantage and showed that the oxidized silicon microstructures can be used to concentrate nucleic acids [15]. Using deep reactive ion etching (DRIE), the authors crafted a forest of pillars in a silicon substrate (Figure 16.2) to increase its surface area and hence nucleic acid binding capacity.

The experiments on the oxidized silicon pillars showed that the pillars can capture and concentrate fragments of short DNA (500 bp) and medium size DNA (48 kbp) dissolved in binding buffer (GuHCl). The results revealed a binding capacity 40 ng/cm^2 for input solutions in the range 0.1 to 1 mg/mL. For dilute samples containing bacteriophage lambda DNA, the authors reported an extraction efficiency of 50% and a concentration factor of $\times$ 10. Cady et al. further investigated the capability of the pillar structures for purifying DNA from intact cells [16]. The authors used either bacteriophage lambda DNA or bacterial chromosal DNA from Esherichia coli (*E. coli*) cells directly lysed in binding agent guanidinium isothiocyanate (GuSCN). They demonstrated a binding capacity 82 ng/cm^2 and managed to recover ~10% of the bound DNA in the first 50 μl of elution buffer. The authors further reported that the silicon pillars can remove ~87% of the protein from a lysate of *E.coli* cells and that the DNA recovered from the pillars can be efficiently amplified.

These earlier reports used simple microstructures and proved the feasibility of purifying and concentrating nucleic acids on the silicon-based platforms. Subsequently, Yobas and colleagues reported on more advanced designs that integrated all the functional components necessary for an automated sample preparation on a single silicon-glass chip [1, 17–20]. They demonstrated two particular designs, each about the size of a 2-cm-by-2-cm die and specific to preparation of either genomic DNA or viral RNA from whole blood (Figure 16.3).

Both designs offer multiple inlets for injecting whole blood and reagents (e.g., buffers for chemical lysis, binding, wash, and elution steps) as well as multiple outlets for collecting waste and purified nucleic acids. The designs share a common set of components such as spiral-shaped chaotic mixer, a filter structure made by close arrangement of silicon pillars, and binder. The designs also differ in their arrangement of components and in the specific function of their filters. For example, the filter in the genomic DNA chip is designed to trap WBC while passing RBC, whereas the filter in the viral RNA chip separates plasma along with virus particles (typically < 1 μm) from the remaining blood. The latter adopts a flow-through concept to handle a relatively large volume of blood (400 μl) since there are usually few virus

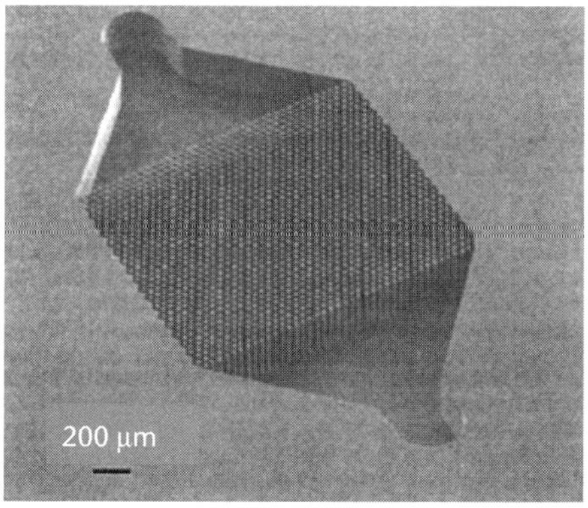

Figure 16.2 Scanning electron microscopy image showing forest of silicon pillars (each 18 μm diameter and 34 μm apart) developed for capturing and concentrating nucleic acids [15].

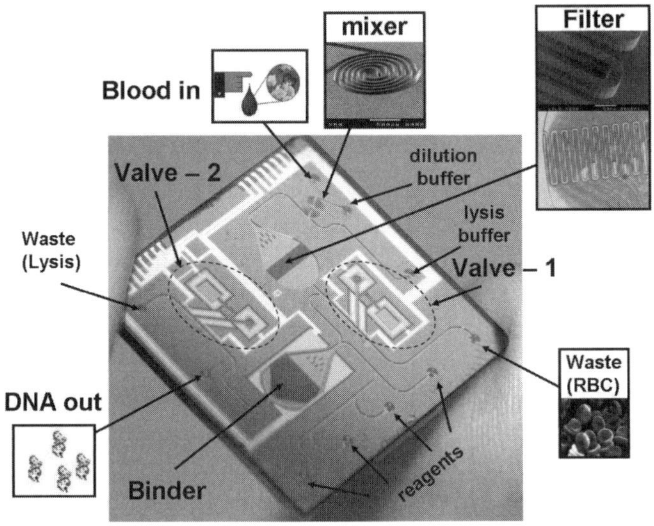

(a)

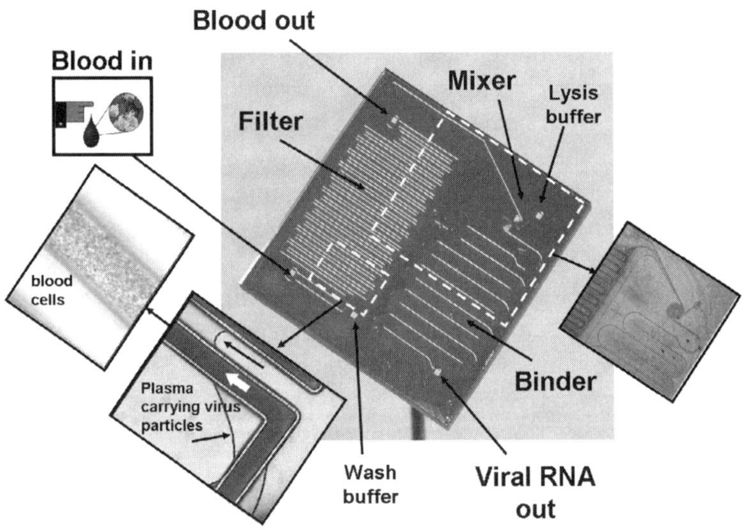

(b)

Figure 16.3 Protocol-specific microfluidic designs integrated in silicon-based chips for extraction and purification of (a) genomic DNA and (b) viral RNA from whole blood [1, 17–20].

particles in a given blood sample at the onset of a disease [21]. The genomic DNA chip further integrates thermally-actuated paraffin-based valves for one-time use only. Either chip illustrates the protocol-specific nature of microfluidic designs for sample preparation and the capability of silicon-based integration.

Other investigators also studied the chip-based extraction of nucleic acids from relatively crude biological samples but their approach involved creating microchannels in glass substrates and filling them with silica beads or a hybrid matrix composed of silica beads and sol-gel [22–25]. These structures, although they provided a solid phase that can selectively and reversibly adsorb nucleic acids under favorable chemistries, suffered from a problem of aging and shrinkage that resulted in voids.

These voids not only decreased the total surface area for nucleic acid binding but also degraded the mechanical integrity of the solid phase.

16.3 Nucleic Acid Amplification

Among the nucleic acid amplification methods, polymerase chain reaction (PCR) stands out because of its simplicity. PCR is an *in vitro* technique in molecular biology for enzymatically replicating the target DNA sequence flanked by a pair of specific DNA primers. For RNA, a reverse transcriptase (RT) step is required to build complementary DNA (cDNA), which then can be amplified through PCR. The PCR technique amplifies (multiplies) a target sequence exponentially to a level that can be easily detected. The technique consists of periodic cycles of three reaction steps each conducted at a specific temperature. These three steps are, namely, denaturation (~94°C), primer annealing (~50°C), and primer extension (~72°C). The temperature profile in each step is critical and any thermal inaccuracy or non-uniformity could lead to failure of the enzymatic reaction.

PCR is conventionally carried out in a thermal cycler, a machine that heats up and cools down individual reaction tubes to the precise temperature point of each step. It typically takes several hours to complete a PCR reaction due to slow heat transfer through the plastic tubes. Northrup et al. demonstrated that PCR performed in a silicon-based microfabricated reactor (micro-PCR) with an integrated heater takes minutes rather than hours [26]. This enhancement is mainly due to the reduced thermal mass of the overall reactor. Earlier versions of Northrup's reactor involved a single heater design with a glass top, whereas later designs incorporated two-heater chambers. Based on the miniaturized reactors, Northrup and colleagues introduced a portable thermal cycling instrument that can amplify and optically detect the presence of target DNA (Figure 16.4) [27]. The instrument was capable of completing a 35-cycle reaction in 10 min with the typical heating and cooling rates 30°C/s and 4°C/s, respectively. Following Northrup's landmark demonstration, numerous

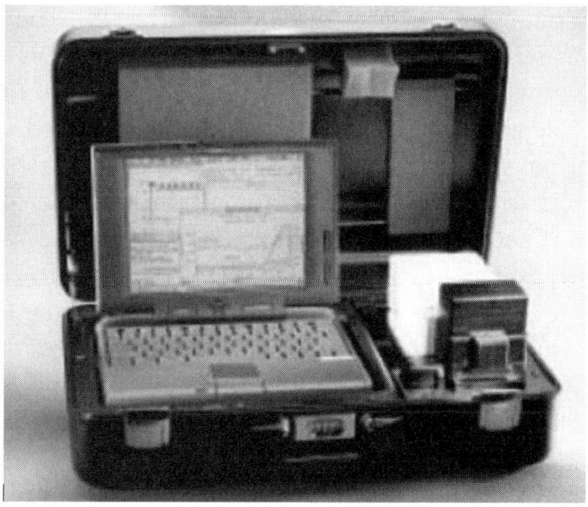

Figure 16.4 Photograph of a portable thermal cycling instrument that can amplify and detect DNA in real-time using the silicon-based micro-PCR devices [27].

research projects have been undertaken worldwide to improve the micro-PCR. These developments have been discussed in recent reviews [28, 29].

The superior thermal conductivity of silicon (150 W/mK) is attractive for rapid thermal cycling, but one has to implement a proper thermal isolation around the reactor to maintain a uniform temperature profile during each temperature cycle. Accordingly, Zou et al. demonstrated a micromachined thermal reactor in silicon where the silicon substrate remains unheated during thermal cycling of the reaction chamber because of its thermal isolation design (Figure 16.5(a)) [30].

This design led to further development of a miniaturized multichamber thermal cycler that is independently controllable with multiplex thermal protocols (Figure 16.5(b)) [31]. A single unit of the design involves a reaction microchamber created on a thin silicon membrane that is tethered with a pair of silicon beams from opposing sides while being physically and thermally isolated elsewhere. The silicon beams provide excellent heat transfer during cooling, whereas the physical isolation around the microchamber reduces the thermal mass that needs to be ramped up during heating. The device maintains a uniform temperature profile (±0.3°C) by means of a unique side-heating scheme (joint-heating) that strategically locates thin-film resistors near the silicon beams. This is unlike other reactors, which usually heat up a whole microchamber. Typical characteristics of the reactor with a 10 μl microchamber have been reported as: 15–100°C/s ramping rate, 10–70°C/s cooling rate, ±0.3°C temperature nonuniformity, ±0.2°C temperature inaccuracy, 2 W heating power, and 8 V operating voltage.

It should be noted that bare silicon inhibits PCR and has to be covered with a layer of silicon oxide or silicon oxynitride. Northrup and colleagues reported that PCR fidelity increases with surface silanization of silicon, silicon dioxide, and silicon nitride and improves occasionally with bovine serum albumin added directly to the reaction [27]. Moreover, they reported a significant enhancement of reaction fidelity with various polymer liners, the best being polypropylene, the material commercial PCR tubes are made of. The liner approach has also been adopted by other researchers since it offers the added advantage of reusing the silicon heater after replacing the liner. For instance, Zou et al. introduced a hybrid device for a relatively high throughput micro-PCR (maximum 16) [32]. The device, shown in Figure 16.5(c), consists of two parts: a disposable polyethylene terephthalate (PET) sheet hot-embossed with 4-by-4 passive microchambers (400 μm deep and 5 mm square) and a reusable array of silicon heating blocks mounted on a printed circuit board (PCB). After pipetting the samples, the microchambers are sealed with polypropylene tape to prevent evaporation. The bottom of the PET microchambers is kept relatively thin (100 μm), as the thermal conductivity of PET (0.2 W/mK) is fairly poor, being at least three orders of magnitude less than that of silicon. Consequently, a 30-cycle reaction on a 20 μl sample takes no more than 8 min at full speed.

By applying the same strategy, Neuzil and colleagues demonstrated a micro-PCR device (Figure 16.6) where reactions can occur in individual droplets placed on an inexpensive microscope glass cover slip, as the disposable item [33]. The aqueous droplets are encapsulated in oil, forming a virtual reaction chamber on the surface that is treated to be both hydrophobic and oleophobic. The cover slip is simply placed on a re-usable silicon chip that is directly soldered to a PCB. The chip applies

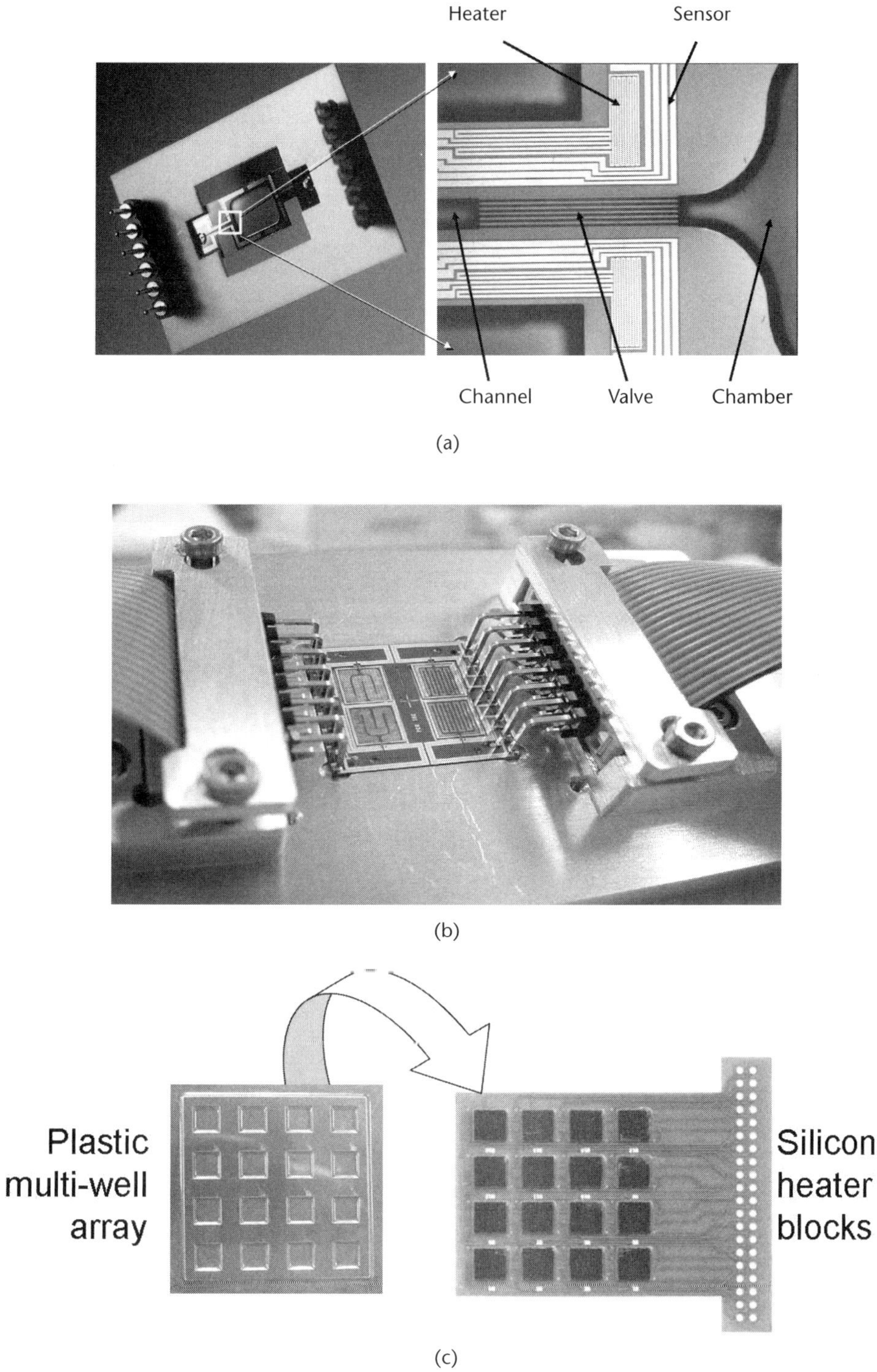

Figure 16.5 Photographs showing various silicon-based micro-PCR devices [1]: (a) a thermally-isolated single-chamber device (with a close-up picture showing its side-arm) [30], (b) a multichamber (2-by-2) device with four independently controllable thermal protocols [31], and (c) a multichamber (4-by-4) device using a plastic-based liner (left) directly placed on silicon heating blocks (right) [32].

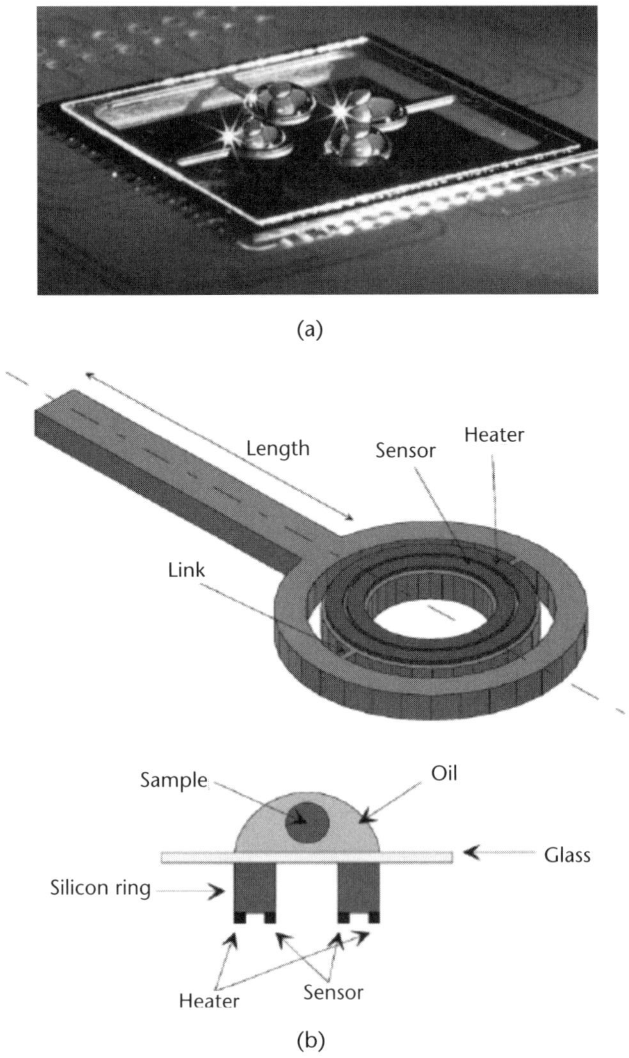

Figure 16.6 (a) Photograph of a micro-PCR device whereby the reactions take place in aqueous droplets encapsulated in oil placed on a square microscope glass cover slip. The cover slip is in direct contact with a silicon heater soldered to a printed circuit board (PCB). (b) Schematics of an individual silicon heater [33].

localized contact heating by means of thin-film resistors integrated on the tip of a cantilever that is sculpted out of a single crystal silicon using deep reactive ion etching. Thermal isolation at the tip of the cantilever is established by two concentric silicon rings with the inner ring supporting both the heater as well as the sensor. Thermal response of the device has been further improved by replacing the inner ring with a solid disk and scaling the overall size by a factor of ½. Thus, a relatively fast thermal time constant 0.27 s has been achieved with heating and cooling rates up to 175°C/s and –125°C/s. Successful amplification has been reported from 0.1 μL droplets encapsulated in 1.1 μL mineral oil at the conclusion of a 40-cycle PCR completed in less than six minutes.

Many of the research efforts have been geared toward a cost-effective chip that can efficiently cycle the temperature of a reaction chamber (physical or virtual).

Meanwhile, Manz and colleagues introduced the concept of a continuous flow-through PCR based on the idea of time-space conversion (Figure 16.7) [34].

That is, instead of cycling the temperature of a fixed location that retains the reaction fluid, the reaction fluid is flowed through the chip, repeatedly passing through individual temperature zones that are maintained constant over time. This approach offers the following advantages: (1) the thermal inertia of the system is reduced to that of the reaction fluid only; (2) the reaction speed can be changed by changing the flow rate of the reaction fluid; (3) the reaction volume is not pre-defined by the chip design and can vary over a range. The approach, however, is not without disadvantages that may adversely affect the PCR performance: (1) the formation of gas bubbles in the reaction fluid flowing through the chip; (2) a progressive sample dispersion due to hyperbolic flow profile of the reaction fluid under pressure-driven flow; (3) increased surface adsorption of molecules with the increased surface-to-volume ratio; (4) the difficulty of regulating the flow between the temperature zones and the requirement of an external precision pump; and (5) a fixed number of reaction cycles per given fluidic design. Some of these disadvantages can be overcome by adopting a ferrofluid-driven circular PCR in which the temperature zones are defined around a fluidic loop [35]. The number of reaction cycles can be varied by deciding how many times the reaction fluid shall go around the loop.

A further innovative concept reminiscent of the continuous flow-through PCR came from Burns and colleagues [36]. This concept harnesses Rayleigh-Benard convection, the steady buoyancy-driven circulatory flow naturally occurring in a confined fluid between surfaces maintained at two fixed temperature points. This convection shuttles the reaction fluid through the temperature zones associated with each stage

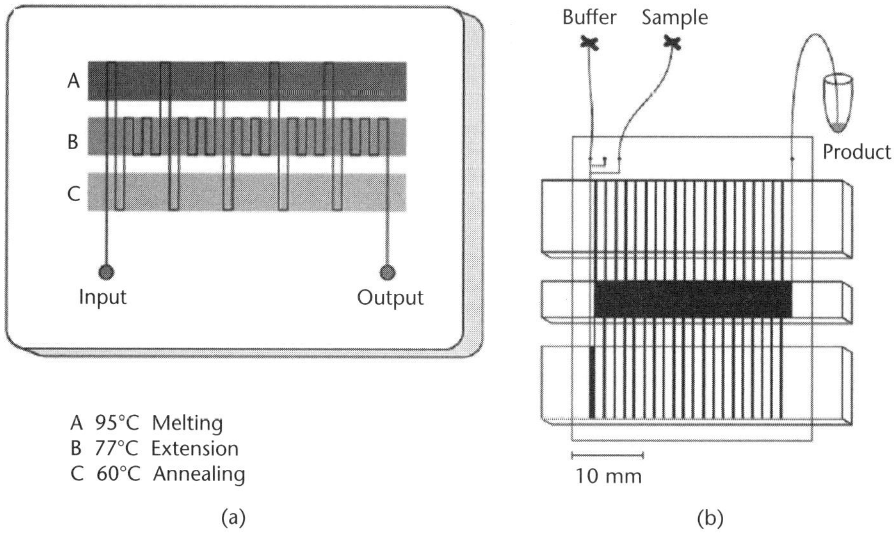

Figure 16.7 Schematics of a continuous flow-through micro-PCR device: (a) the chip layout with a single channel passing through three temperature zones defines the thermal cycling process and (b) the experimental setup in which the whole chip is placed on thermostated copper blocks to establish three well-defined temperature zones at 95°, 77°, and 60°. The sample along with a constant buffer flow is passed through the channel etched into the chip incorporating 20 identical cycles [34].

of the reaction. The reaction is primarily controlled by the geometry of the confinement and requires no external pump, thereby greatly simplifying the external control hardware. Ugaz and colleagues recently used this concept in a flow-loop reactor made of fluoropolymer tube in contact with two thermoelectric heaters [37]. They demonstrated multiplex amplification of five different human respiratory infections associated with targets in 50 minutes with a 16-μL flow loop. They also constructed a pocket-sized battery-operated convective-flow PCR by further simplifying the heater arrangement. Either concept of continuous flow-through PCR or convective-flow PCR is suitable for realizing in silicon-based platforms.

PCR, since its Nobel-prize winning development by Mullis in the early 1980s and its miniaturization by Northrup in the early 1990s, continues to be a fruitful area of research open to scientific and engineering innovations. For instance, digital PCR, introduced in the late '90s by Kalinina et al. [38] and further developed by Vogelstein and colleagues [39], partitions the reaction fluid into many individual compartments such that each compartment may contain no more than a single copy of a nucleic acid molecule prior to thermal cycling. Since the efficiency of PCR may vary depending on a given reaction, this approach allows a more accurate measure of the absolute number of starting copies (quantity). This is done by simply counting the number of reaction chambers that present detectable levels of end-product. Digital PCR has been recently adopted in microfluidic platforms and may benefit the point-of-care diagnostic devices [40].

16.4 Nucleic Acid Detection

Numerous techniques have been investigated for on-chip detection of nucleic acids including electrical [41–46, 48–50, 55, 56], optical [57–65], and electrochemical methods [66, 67]. Some of these methods are more amenable to on-chip miniaturization and integration than others. Among those, electrical methods are label-free and leverage from CMOS electronics and signal processing. In many of the detection techniques, selectivity is achieved through hybridization whereby a target sequence of nucleic acid (target probe) binds to its complementary pair (capture probe) immobilized on a solid support. Prior to hybridization, optical and other label-dependent methods required target probes to be attached with reporter molecules such as fluorescent dyes so that they could emit signals upon excitation. Hence their hybridization could be detected. Although such labels can increase the detection sensitivity greatly, their use is undesired since they are costly and necessitate an extra step of sample preparation.

Nucleic acids carry a negative electrical charge per base at their sugar-phosphate backbone. This intrinsic molecular charge can act as a native label that can be detected electronically using a field-effect device. Field-effect transistors (FETs) have been previously demonstrated for detecting DNA hybridization under constant drain current mode or capacitive mode [41, 42]. To configure the device structure of FET as a field-effect sensor, gate dielectric must be exposed to electrolyte that contains charged molecules such as nucleic acids. A voltage bias can be applied to the electrolyte by means of a reference electrode. Binding of charged molecules on the dielectric surface varies the surface potential and modifies the charge distribution (space charge region) in the silicon underneath. The surface potential can then be measured as a conductivity or capacitance change in the transistor.

Manalis and colleagues demonstrated field-effect sensors that can detect and distinguish label-free 12-mer oligonucleotides at nanomolar concentrations with a single base mismatch within minutes [43]. The authors created 50 × 50 μm^2 sensing regions at the terminus of two silicon cantilevers 500 μm long, 75 μm wide, and 3 μm thick (Figure 16.8).

The surface potential sensitivity of these sensors was enhanced by employing a low doping level (~10^{15} atoms per cm^3) and an extremely thin insulator thickness (~2 nm layer of chemically grown oxide). A low-ionic strength solution was utilized to maximize the sensitivity in the field-effect detection. Rapid hybridization at this

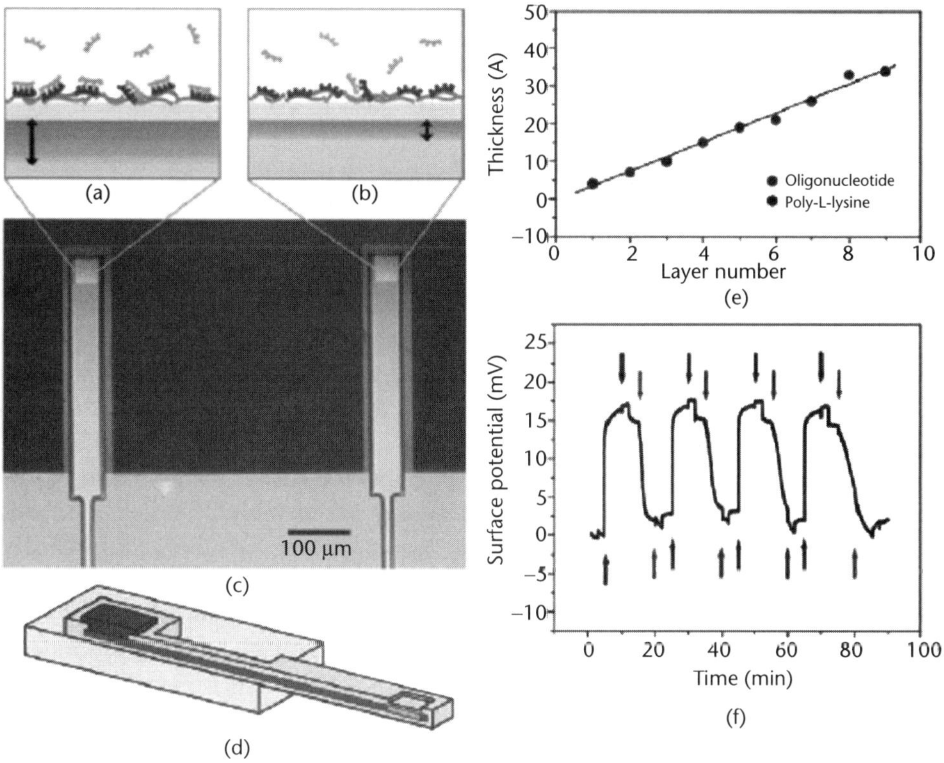

Figure 16.8 (a) and (b) Schematic description of the field-effect sensing concept that utilizes a layer of poly-L-lysine to electrostatically immobilize capture probes on the sensor. Binding of negatively charged target probes complementary to capture probes at the sensor surface extends the depletion region (arrow) in the silicon portion of the sensor compared with (b) where no binding occurs to non-complementary capture probes. (c) Photomicrograph of the device with sensor regions formed at the terminus of two cantilevers and (d) a schematic description of the cross-sectional profile of each cantilever with a layer of highly doped silicon electrically connecting the sensor region at the cantilever terminal to a metal contact on the substrate. (e) and (f) PLL-DNA multilayer growth as monitored (e) by ellipsometry measurements on silicon substrates prepared identically to the field-effect sensor surfaces and (f) by surface potential measurements on the field-effect sensor. Arrows indicate injections of PLL and DNA, each twice and followed by an injection of buffer. While ellipsometry measurements indicate a linear increase in thickness, the sensor surface potential alternates according to the charge of the adsorbed layer (positive for PLL and negative for DNA). The same concentrations of PLL and DNA were used for either measurement [43].

low-ionic strength was facilitated by depositing a positively charged layer of poly-L-lysine (PLL), a cationic polypeptide, on the sensing area. This positive layer helped to compensate electrostatic repulsion between the negatively-charged complementary DNA strands (target and capture probes) and accelerated their hybridization. By functionalizing either sensing area of the dual cantilever configuration with a distinct capture probe, a parallel differential detection was performed and the background signal was corrected by subtraction.

Detection of PCR products through hybridization requires an extra step of sample preparation to denature double-stranded DNA into single-stranded pairs. This usually involves product heating followed by rapid cooling to prevent renaturation of the pairs or in vitro transcription of double-stranded products to generate single-stranded RNA. Manalis and colleagues further demonstrated a technique whereby the field-effect sensing can be directly applied to detect PCR products without the hybridization [44]. The authors created a field-effect sensor inside a microfluidic channel that acts as a variable capacitor whose impedance is sensitive to the charge density of the surface-bound molecules (Figure 16.9).

Instead of using capture probes immobilized on the surface as in hybridization, they utilized a thin layer of PLL deposited on the charge-sensitive region of the sensor to electrostatically attach double-stranded DNA on the surface. The sensor can quantitatively and reproducibly differentiate duplex DNA in the PCR relevant range 1–80 ng/μL. Moreover, the sensor can be recovered for a new measurement without degrading its sensitivity by depositing a fresh layer of PLL directly on the surface-bound nucleic acids. This layer-by-layer assembly allows sequential analysis of PCR products on the same sensor at various reaction cycles. The authors also integrated this detection technique into a micro-PCR, achieving thermocycling rates up to 50°C/s [45].

One-dimensional field-effect devices in the form of silicon nanowires (SiNWs) exhibit an increased sensitivity to charge-based molecular detection due to their extremely high surface-to-volume ratio. Binding of charged molecules on the nanowire surface can affect the entire conduction pathway because it is structurally formed through the bulk of the nanowire, unlike those electronically defined beneath the surface of conventional FETs. Sensitivity of SiNWs can be reproducibly tuned by tailoring their dopant concentration and/or their critical dimension (width or diameter). By reducing the width of SiNWs from 200 nm to 50 nm, sensitivity to surface potential variations can be increased by an estimated factor of 20 [46]. Further sensitivity increase may not be practical due to 1/f noise increasing inversely with the nanowire cross-sectional area [47]. SiNWs can be fabricated by process techniques using either a "bottom-up" or "top-down" approach. The former builds SiNWs by starting from the atomic level and applying fundamental steps of nucleation and growth. The latter sculpts them out from bulk materials by applying semiconductor manufacturing techniques. Disadvantages of the bottom-up approach include the lack of controlled growth of uniform nanowires and their challenging "pick and place" assembly into a high density functional array with reliable ohmic contacts.

Hahm and Lieber reported the use of p-type SiNWs for real-time label-free detection of DNA at concentrations down to tens of femtomolar range [48]. They used a bottom-up approach, vapor–solid–liquid (VLS) technique, whereby SiNWs can be synthesized by chemical vapor deposition (CVD) using gold nanoclusters as catalysts

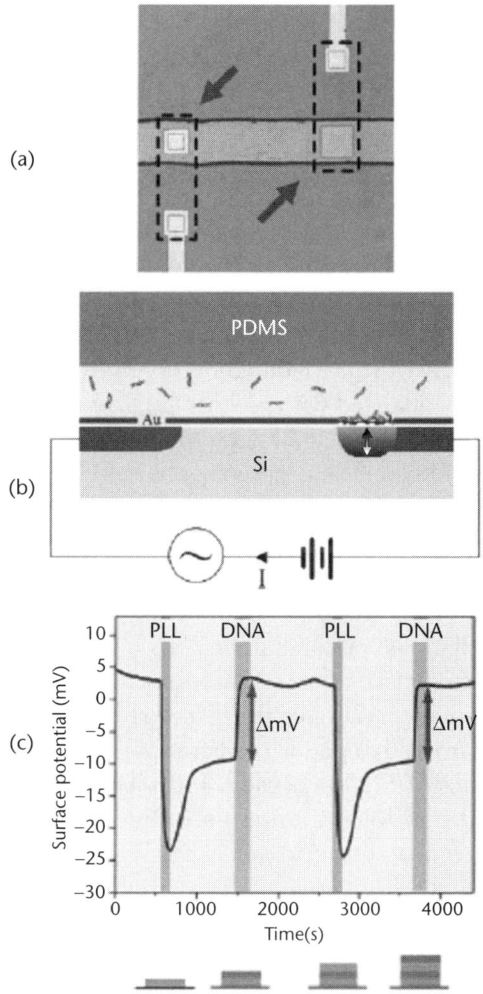

Figure 16.9 (a) Photomicrograph of a PDMS-defined microfluidic channel enclosing a gold signal electrode (arrow, left) and a p-type field-effect sensor (arrow, right) separated by 400 μm. Both are connected to their respective electrical leads away from the channel through highly-doped buried conductive traces (dotted lines). (b) The device schematic describing the measurement concept: Binding of DNA on the surface changes the device capacitance by altering the distribution of positive mobile charge carriers in silicon and modulating the depletion depth (arrow). This capacitance change is determined by measuring the current through the solution and across the DC voltage-biased variable capacitor, which is modulated by the surface potential, in response to an AC voltage applied to the gold electrode through the buried conductive trace in silicon (dark gray). An implanted ground plane (not shown) is fixed at a potential to minimize parasitic effects from the bulk silicon. A layer of silicon nitride and silicon dioxide passivate the inactive areas. (c) Electronic detection of DNA-PLL multilayer growth by flowing the device with alternating cycles of PLL for 3 min followed by 10-min rinse buffer and then DNA for 5 min followed by 15-min wash. The lower diagram indicates the expected monotonic increase in film thickness due to alternating exposures to PLL and DNA [44].

and silane (SiH_4) as a vapor-phase reactant. In their study, SiNWs were grown with an average diameter of 20 nm, and then suspended in ethanol before being deposited on oxidized silicon substrates. Electrical contacts to SiNWs terminals were defined through electron-beam lithography. SiNWs were functionalized with peptide nucleic acids (PNA) as the capturing probes since the PNA probes are known to bind to target complementary DNA with much greater affinity and stability than the DNA probes. The PNA probes were biotinylated and then linked to avidin proteins immobilized on the oxide surface. These probes were designed to recognize a specific mutation site in a transmembrane receptor gene responsible for the fatal genetic disease cystic fibrosis.

Williams and colleagues demonstrated DNA detection on SiNWs 50 nm wide, 60 nm high, and 20 μm long fabricated through a top-down approach whereby silicon-on-insulator (SOI) wafers were subjected to a combination of electron-beam lithography (for nanowires), optical lithography (for electrical leads) and reactive ion etching (RIE) [49]. A thin layer of thermal oxide (3 nm) was grown on SiNWs to decrease the density of surface dangling bonds and increase the stability of sensors. SiNWs were functionalized with 12-mer capture probes (DNA) covalently linked to a self-assembled monolayer (SAM) on the oxide surface. To minimize the screening effect of counter ions on the negatively-charged DNA molecules, target DNA molecules were introduced in high–purity water. A lower detection limit of 25 pM was reported at a signal-to-noise ratio > 6. By switching the capture probes from DNA to PNA, the detection limit was further lowered down to 10 pM but still remained three orders of magnitude larger than the value reported for the synthesized SiNWs with a relatively small cross-sectional area [46].

The choice of surface functionalization chemistry to convert SiNWs into molecular sensors plays a crucial role in their performance. Heath and colleagues investigated this role by studying how the nature of the inorganic/organic interface affects the characteristics of SiNWs sensors [50]. They used a high-density array of 400 SiNWs, each ~2 mm long, 20 nm wide and at 35 nm pitch (Figure 16.10) fabricated through a top-down approach, namely superlattice nanowire pattern transfer (SNAP).

This approach transfers nanowire patterns onto silicon by utilizing a physical template made of selectively etched GaAs/$Al_xGa_{(1-x)}$As superlattice synthesized via molecular beam epitaxy (MBE) [51]. The method can be further combined with spin-on glass doping and low-energy high-frequency fluorine-chemistry-based RIE to minimize process-induced defects [52]. Two surface functionalization chemistries were compared for DNA detection on the SiNWs: an amine-terminated alkyl monolayer directly grown on a hydrogen-terminated silicon surface and an amine-terminated siloxane monolayer on the native oxide surface of silicon. The former showed significantly enhanced sensitivity with an accompanying improvement of two orders of magnitude in the dynamic range of sensing. The limit of detection (LOD) increased from 1 nM to 10 pM, while the real-time, label-free detection of DNA 16 mers was realized in physiologically relevant (0.165 M) electrolyte solution. This enhancement was probably due to the possibility that the capture probes (DNA) electrostatically adsorbed onto the amine-terminated surface have brought hybridization events closer to SiNWs and hence managed to disengage Debye screening as an inhibiting factor for the field-effect detection.

Highly ordered SiNWs sensors can be manufactured through CMOS-compatible alternative methods such as self-limiting dry oxidation and orientation-dependent wet etching. It is well-known that dry oxidation of silicon structures with extremely small radii is a self-limiting process due to stress-induced retardation [53]. This process is capable of transforming silicon in structures patterned via traditional meth-

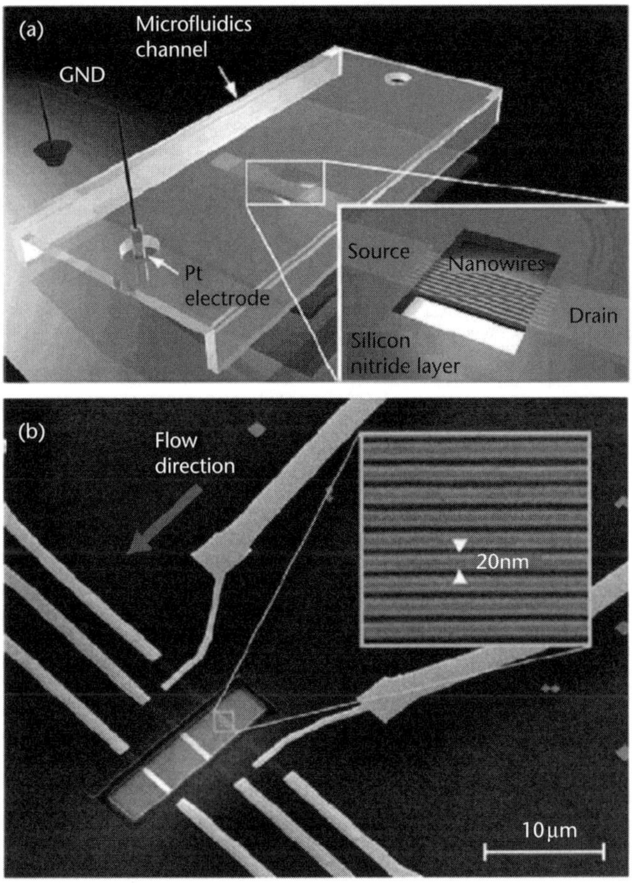

Figure 16.10 SiNWs fabricated through SNAP process. (a) Concept diagram of SiNWs integrated in a microfluidic channel via PDMS encapsulation and (b) a scanning electron microscopy image showing a section of SiNWs arranged in three independent segments. Each segment contains about 10 SiNWs and six such sections are included in a fully integrated device. The wafer is covered with Si_3N_4 except for the exposed active regions containing SiNWs 20 nm wide [50].

ods (e.g. optical lithography and RIE) into SiNWs down to 5 nm diameter and up to 1 mm length (Figure 16.11) [54].

Gao and colleagues demonstrated that such SiNWs once functionalized with PNA capture probes can detect DNA hybridization as low as 10 fM and satisfactorily discriminate against single base-pair mismatches [55]. Alternatively, SiNWs can be produced by utilizing the fact that Si (111) planes etch about hundred times slower than all other crystallographic planes in an anisotropic wet etch such as tetramethylammonium hydroxide (TMAH). Reed and colleagues used this fact and introduced SiNWs with a trapezoidal cross-sectional profile and an exposed surface mainly dominated by Si (111) planes, the preferred surface for selective functionalization [56]. Such SiNWs possess high-quality electrical characteristics since their fabrication avoids RIE that unacceptably degrades device performance. These SiNWs, although they have yet to be tested for the detection of nucleic acids, have been demonstrated for label-free detection of specific antibodies below 100 fM and real-time monitoring of cellular immune response.

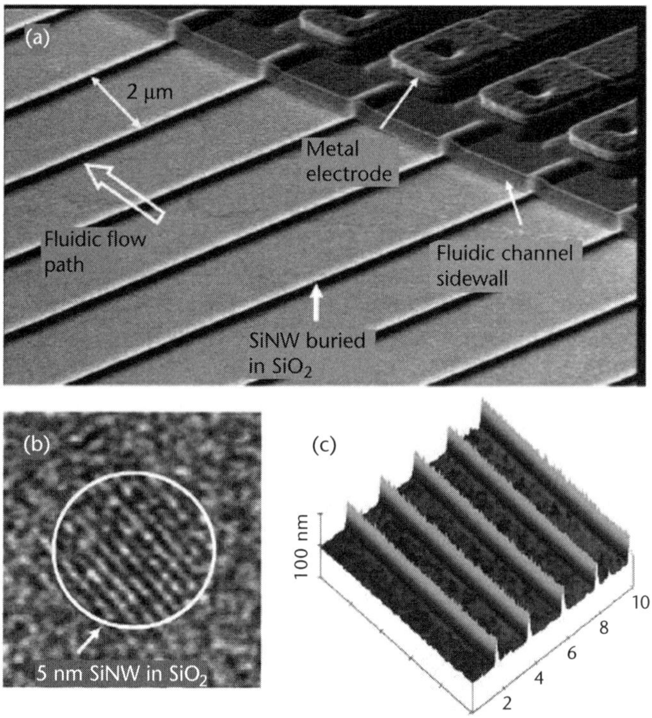

Figure 16.11 SiNWs fabricated through self-limiting dry oxidation of silicon fin structures. (a) Scanning electron microscopy image showing an array of SiNWs where each nanowire has its own electrical contacts and can be independently addressed, (b) transmission electron microscopy image showing a cross section of a single nanowire about 5 nm diameter, and (c) atomic force microscopy image of the SiNWs [55].

16.5 Discussion

For a system level integration of all three modules (nucleic acid extraction, amplification, and detection), several challenges remain to be addressed. Of those, microfluidic integration that deals with fluidic valving and control is extremely important and has to be planned accordingly. Liquids transferred to a downstream module must match the requirement of that module with accurate volume, concentration, and purity in order to ensure successful amplification and detection. Moreover, the flow has to be carefully timed to minimize cross-contamination between various reagents. For instance, chaotropic salts and ethanol employed by the extraction module are known to inhibit the PCR reaction and have to be removed before the thermal cycling can begin. During the thermal cycling, expansion and evaporation of the liquid must be prevented. Furthermore, fluidic control (e.g., liquid pumping and valving) has to be addressed without resorting to external bulky hardware or sophisticated miniaturized components that may complicate the fabrication process, compromise the system reliability, and increase its cost. For instance, electrochemical or thermo-pneumatic pumps and thermally-actuated paraffin-based microvalves can be efficiently utilized in such an integrated system [68, 69].

A further challenge may arise from the process integration point of view when fabricating all three modules on a monolithic silicon substrate. Realizing the extraction and amplification modules on the same substrate may not be too problematic since both share nearly identical fabrication steps such as deep reactive ion etching to form microfluidic structures and thermal-isolation slits, and metallization to define thin-film heaters and sensors. For instance, the DNA extraction chip shown in Figure 16.3(a) integrates heaters/sensors and thermal isolation slits around the binder as well as around the thermally-actuated valves. In this particular case, the binder temperature is controlled to increase the yield of nucleic acids because binding and elution kinetics of nucleic acids depend on temperature. However, same hardware architecture also applies to micro-PCR. Integration of a silicon field-effect sensor into micro-PCR has also been realized for label-free detection of PCR products [45]. These parallel developments indicate the feasibility of integrating all three modules into a monolithic silicon chip.

Once such a chip for nucleic acid analysis is attained by overcoming the challenges relevant to microfluidic and process integrations, it should be packaged in a self-contained fully-enclosed cartridge for field use by a relatively unskilled person. A truly self-contained system should be able to accommodate storage of reagents and reaction waste without exposing them to the environment. Some of these reagents, however, require special storage conditions such as refrigeration to prevent them from being degraded or becoming ineffective. One alternative method to avoid refrigeration is to store the reagents in a specially formulated dry state after a lyophilization (freeze-dry) process [70]. This process may prolong their shelf-life at room temperature to several months. Lyophilized reagents are also not sensitive to climatic conditions and can be wetted with the sample itself before use [2].

16.6 Conclusion

The silicon-based microfluidic systems provide an ideal platform for the miniaturization and automation of the essential tasks involved in a typical nucleic acid probe assay. For the extraction and purification of nucleic acids from a raw sample, these systems readily offer a silica-based surface that can selectively bind to nucleic acids under favorable conditions. Surface chemistry for silica is relatively well understood and can be utilized to further enhance surface affinity for nucleic acids. Silicon also offers high thermal conductivity and thermally-isolated microreactors in silicon enable rapid thermal cycling for efficient PCR amplification of nucleic acids. Further, silicon, being an electronic material, can be configured as a field-effect sensor for detecting nucleic acids through their intrinsic molecular charge without the requirement of extrinsic labels. Particularly, one-dimensional SiNWs show extreme sensitivity and realize label-free detection of nucleic acids down to the femtomolar range. Highly-ordered and electrically-addressable SiNWs can be fabricated through CMOS-based (top-down) processes and they can be functionalized with an array of distinct capture probes for multiplexed and label-free detection of various target probes simultaneously. Practical integration and packaging of all these components in a "self-contained" "fully-enclosed" point-of-care device will be rewarding but requires overcoming major challenges relevant to process and microfluidic integration.

Acknowledgments

The author gratefully acknowledges financial support from the Agency for Science, Technology, and Research (A*STAR), Singapore. The author thanks members of Biosensor Focused Interest Group (BFIG) and staff of the Silicon Process Technologies at the Institute of Microelectronics (IME), Singapore.

References

[1] L. Yobas, H. Ji, W. Hui, Y. Chen, T-M. Lim, C-K. Heng, and D-L. Kwong, "Nucleic acid extraction, amplification, and detection on Si-based microfluidic platforms," *IEEE Journal of Solid-State Circuits* (2007), 42(8), 1803–1813, 8 Aug. 2007.

[2] Y. Huang, E.L. Mather, J.L. Bell, and M. Madou, "MEMS-based sample preparation for molecular diagnostics," *Anal. Bioanal. Chem.*, 372, 49–65, 2002.

[3] H.M. Ji, V. Samper, Y. Chen, C.K. Heng, T.M. Lim, and L. Yobas, "Silicon-based microfilters for whole blood cell separation," *Biomedical Microdevices*, 10, 251–257, 2008.

[4] P. Wilding, L.J. Kricka, J. Cheng, G. Hvichia, M.A. Shoffner, and P. Fortina, "Integrated cell isolation and polymerase chain reaction analysis using silicon microfilter chambers," *Analytical Biochemistry*, 257, 2, 95–100, 1998.

[5] J. Voldman, R.A. Braff, M. Toner, M.L. Gray, and M.A. Schmidt, "Holding forces of single-particle dielectrophoretic traps," *Biophys. J.*, 80(1), 531–541 (2001).

[6] A. Nilsson, F. Petersson, H. Jonsson, and T. Laurell, "Acoustic control of suspended particles in micro fluidic chips," *Lab Chip*, 4(2), 131–135 (2004).

[7] M.A.M. Gijs, "Magnetic bead handling on-chip: new opportunities for analytical applications," *Microfluidics and Nanofluidics*, 1(1): 22–40, 2004.

[8] D. Di Carlo, K.H. Jeong, and L.P. Lee, "Reagentless mechanical cell lysis by nanoscale barbs in microchannels for sample preparation," *Lab Chip*, 3(4), 287–291, 2003.

[9] L. Yobas, R.K. Sharma, R. Nagarajan, V.D. Samper, and P.S.R. Naidu, "Precise profile control of 3D lateral junction traps by 2D mask layout and isotropic etching," *J. Micromech. Microeng.*, 15(2), 386–393, 2005.

[10] M.T. Taylor, P. Belgrader, B.J. Furman, F. Pourahmadi, G.T.A. Kovacs, and M.A. Northrup, "Lysing bacterial spores by sonication through a flexible interface in a microfluidic system," *Anal. Chem.*, 73(3), 492–496, 2001.

[11] H. Lu, M.A. Schmidt, and K.F. Jensen, "A microfluidic electroporation device for cell lysis," *Lab Chip*, 5(1), 23–29, 2005.

[12] H.J. Tian, A.F.R. Huhmer, and J.P. Landers, "Evaluation of silica resins for direct and efficient extraction of DNA from complex biological matrices in a miniaturized format," *Analytical Biochemistry*, 283(2): 175–191, Aug. 1, 2000.

[13] B. Vogelstein and D. Gillespie "Preparative and analytical purification of DNA from agarose," *Natl. Acad. Sci., USA*, 76, 2, 615–619 (February 1979).

[14] QIAamp® DNA Mini and Blood Mini Handbook, http://www1.qiagen.com/literature.

[15] L.A. Christel, K. Peterson, W. McWilliam, and M.A. Northrup, "Rapid, automated nucleic acid probe assays using silicon microstructures for nucleic acid concentration," *J. Biochemical Engineering—Trans. ASME*, 121(1): 22–27 Feb. 1999.

[16] N.C. Cady, S. Stelick, and C.A. Batt, "Nucleic acid purification using microfabricated silicon structures," *Biosensors and Bioelectronics*, 19(1), 59–66, 2003.

[17] W.C. Hui, L. Yobas, V.D. Samper, C.K. Heng, S. Liw, H.M. Ji, Y. Chen, L. Cong, J. Li, and T.M. Lim, "Microfluidic systems for extracting nucleic acids for DNA and RNA analysis," *Sensors and Actuators, A-Physical*, 133(2): 335–339, 2007.

[18] H.M. Ji, V. Samper, Y. Chen, W.C. Hui, H.J. Lye, F.B. Mustafa, A.C. Lee, L. Cong, C.K. Heng, and T.M. Lim, "DNA purification silicon chip," *Sensors and Actuators A-Physical*, 139(1–2): 139–144, 2007.

[19] L. Yobas, W. Hui, H.M. Ji, Y. Chen, S.S.I. Liw, J. Li, C.S. Chong, X. Ling, C.K. Heng, H.J. Lye, S.R. Bte, K. Lee, S. Swarup, S.M. Wong, and T.M. Lim, "Microfluidic chips for viral RNA extraction and detection," *IEEE Sensors* 2005, 49–52.

[20] L. Yobas, H.M. Ji, W.C. Hui, Y. Chen, T.M. Lim, C.K. Heng, and D.L. Kwong, "Nucleic acid extraction, amplification, and detection on Si-based microfluidic platforms," *Proceedings of the IEEE 2006 Custom Integrated Circuits Conference*, 465–472, 2006.

[21] L. Yobas, E.L. Gui, H.M. Ji, J. Li, Y. Chen, W.C. Hui, S.R.B.M. Rafe, S. Swarup, S.M. Wong, T.M. Lim, and C.K. Heng, "A flow-through shear-type microfilter chip for separating plasma and virus particles from whole blood," *Micro Total Analysis Systems*, 2004, 2(297), 7–9, 2005.

[22] H.J. Tian, A.F.R. Huhmer, and J.P. Landers, "Evaluation of silica resins for direct and efficient extraction of DNA from complex biological matrices in a miniaturized format," *Analytical Biochemistry*, 283(2): 175–191, Aug. 1, 2000.

[23] K.A. Wolfe, M.C. Breadmore, J.P. Ferrance, M.E. Power, J.F. Conroy, P.M. Norris, and J.P. Landers, "Towards a microchip-based solid-phase extraction method for isolation of nucleic acids," *Electrophoresis*, 23(5): 727–733, March 2002.

[24] M.C. Breadmore, K.A. Wolfe, I.G. Arcibal, W.K. Leung, D. Dichson, B.C. Giordano, M.E. Power, J.P. Ferrance, S. Feldman, P.M. Norris, and J.P. Landers, "Microchip-based purification of DNA from biological samples," *Anal. Chem.*, 75(2003): 1880.

[25] Q. Wu, J.M. Bienvenue, B.J. Hassan, Y.C. Kwok, B.C. Giordano, P.M. Norris, J.P. Landers, and J.P. Ferrance, "Microchip-based macroporous silica sol-gel monolith for efficient isolation of DNA from clinical samples," *Anal. Chem.*, 78(2006): 5704–5710.

[26] M.A. Northrup, M.T. Ching, R.M. White, and R.T. Watson, "DNA amplification with a microfabricated reaction chamber," Transducers'93, *Seventh International Conference on Solid State Sensors and Actuators*, 1993, p. 924.

[27] M.A. Northrup, B. Benett, D. Hadley, P. Landre, S. Lehew, J. Richards, and P. Stratton, "A miniature analytical instrument for nucleic acids based on micromachined silicon reaction chambers," *Anal. Chem.*, 70, 918–922, 1998.

[28] C. Zhang, and D. Xing, "Miniaturized PCR chips for nucleic acid amplification and analysis: latest advances and future trends," *Nucleic Acids Research*, 1–15, 2007.

[29] C.S. Zhang, J.L. Xu, W.L. Ma, and W.L. Zheng, "PCR microfluidic devices for DNA amplification," *Biotechnology Advances*, 24(3): 243–284, 2006

[30] Q.B. Zou, U. Sridhar, Y. Chen, J. Singh, E. Seluanayagam, T.M. Lim, Y. Tie, I. Rodriguez, and M.L. Lesaicherre, "A micromachined integrable thermal reactor," *IEEE IEDM* 01-371 2001.

[31] Q.B. Zou, U. Sridhar, Y. Chen, and J. Singh, "Miniaturized independently controllable multichamber," *IEEE Sensors Journal,* 3(6): 774–780, Dec. 2003.

[32] Q.B. Zou, Y.B. Miao, Y. Chen, U. Sridhar, C.S. Chong, T.C. Chai, Y. Tie, C.H.L. Teh, T.M. Lim, and C.K. Heng, "Micro-assembled multi-chamber thermal-cycler for low-cost reaction chip thermal multiplexing," *Sensors and Actuators A*, 102(1–2):114–121 Dec. 1, 2002.

[33] P. Neuzil, J. Pipper, and T.M. Hsieh, "Disposable real-time microPCR device: lab-on-a-chip at a low cost," *Molecular Biosystems*, 2(6–7), 292–298, 2006; P. Neuzil, C. Zhang, J. Pipper, S. Oh, and L. Zhuo, "Ultra fast miniaturized real-time PCR: 40 cycles in less than six minutes," *Nucleic Acids Research*, 34(11), e77, 2006.

[34] M.U. Kopp, A.J. de Mello, and A. Manz, "Chemical amplification: continuous-flow PCR on a chip," *Science*, 280, 1046, 1998.

[35] Y. Sun, Y.C. Kwok, and N.T. Nguyen, "A circular ferrofluid driven microchip for rapid polymerase chain reaction," *Lab Chip*, 7(8): 1012–1017, 2007.

[36] M. Krishnan, V.M. Ugaz, and M.A. Burns, "PCR in a Rayleigh-Benard convection cell," *Science*, 298(5594): 793, 2002.

[37] N. Agarwal, Y.A. Hassan, and V.M. Ugaz, "A pocket-sized convective PCR thermocycler," *Angew. Chem. Int. Ed.*, 46(23): 4316–4319, 2007.

[38] O. Kalinina, I. Lebedeva, J. Brown, and J. Silver, "Nanoliter scale PCR with TaqMan detection," *Nucleic Acids Research*, 25(10): 1999–2004, 1997.

[39] B. Vogelstein, and K.E. Kinzler, "Digital PCR," *Proc. Natl. Acad. Sci. USA*, 96, 9236–9241, 1999.

[40] E.A. Ottesen, J.W. Hong, S.R. Quake, and J.R. Leadbetter, "Microfluidic digital PCR enables multigene analysis of individual environmental bacteria," *Science*, 314, 1464, 2006.

[41] E. Souteyrand, J.P. Cloarec, J.R. Martin, C. Wilson, I. Lawrence, S. Mikkelsen, and M.F. Lawrence, "Direct detection of the hybridization of synthetic homo-oligomer DNA sequences by field effect," *J. Phys. Chem. B*, 101, 2980–2985, 1997.

[42] H. Berney, J. West, E. Haefele, J. Alderman, W. Lane, and J.K. Collins, "A DNA diagnostic biosensor: development, characterization and performance," *Sensors and Actuators B Chem.*, 68, 100–108, 2000.

[43] J. Fritz, E.B. Cooper, S. Gaudet, P.K. Sorger, and S.R. Manalis, "Electronic detection of DNA by its intrinsic molecular charge," *PNAS*, 99(22): 14142–14146, Oct. 29, 2002.

[44] C.S.J. Hou, N. Milovic, M. Godin, P.R. Russo, R. Chakrabarti, and S.R. Manalis, "Label-free microelectronic PCR quantification," *Anal. Chem.*, 78(8): 2526–2531, April 15, 2006.

[45] C.S.J. Hou, M. Godin, K. Payer, R. Chakrabarti, and S.R. Manalis, "Integrated microelectronic device for label-free nucleic acid amplification and detection," *Lab on a Chip*, 7, 347–354, 2007.

[46] Z. Li, B. Rajendran, T.I. Kamins, X. Li, Y. Chen, and R.S. Williams, "Silicon nanowires for sequence-specific DNA sensing: device fabrication and simulation," *Appl. Phys. A: Mater. Sci. Process.*, 2005, 80, 1257.

[47] S. Reza, G. Bosman, A.S. Islam, T.I. Kamins, S. Sharma, and R.S. Williams, "Noise in silicon nanowires," *IEEE Trans. Nanotechnol.*, 2006, 5, 523.

[48] J. Hahm and C.M. Lieber, "Direct ultrasensitive electrical detection of DNA and DNA sequence variations using nanowire nanosensors," *Nano Letters*, 4(1): 51–54, 2004.

[49] Z. Li, Y. Chen, X. Li, T.I. Kamins, K. Nauka, and R.S. Williams, "Sequence-specific label-free DNA sensors based on silicon nanowires," *Nano Letters*, 4(2): 245–247, 2004.

[50] Y.L. Bunimovich, Y.S. Shin, W.-S. Yeo, M. Amori, G. Kwong, and J.R. Heath, "Quantitative real-time measurements of DNA hybridization with alkylated nonoxidized silicon nanowires in electrolyte solution," *J. Am. Chem. Soc.*, 128, 16323–16331, 2006.

[51] N.A. Melosh, A. Boukai, F. Diana, B. Gerardot, A. Badolato, P.M. Petroff, and J.R. Heath, "Ultrahigh-density nanowire lattices and circuits," *Science*, 300, 112, 2003.

[52] R.A. Beckman, E. Johnston-Halperin, N.A. Melosh, Y. Luo, J.E. Green, and J.R. Heath, "Fabrication of conducting Si nanowire arrays," *J. of Applied Physics*, 96(10): 5921, 2004.

[53] H.I. Liu, N.I. Maluf, R.F.W. Pease, D.K. Biegelsen, N.M. Johnson, and F.A. Ponce, "Oxidation of sub-50 nm Si columns for light emission study," *J. Vac. Sci. Technol. B*, 10(6): 2846, 1992.

[54] N. Singh, A. Agarwal, L.K. Bera, T.Y. Liow, R. Yang, S.C. Rustagi, C.H. Tung, R. Kumar, G.Q. Luo, N. Balasubramanian, and D.L. Kwong, "High-performance fully depleted silicon-nanowire (diameter <= 5 nm) gate-all-around CMOS devices," *IEEE Electron Device Lett.*, 27, 383–385, 2006.

[55] G. Zhiqiang, A. Agarwal, A.D. Trigg, N. Singh, C. Fang, C.-H. Tung, Y. Fan, K.D. Buddharaju, and J. Kong, "Silicon nanowire arrays for label-free detection of DNA," *Anal. Chem.*, 79(9): 3291–3297, 2007.

[56] E. Stern, J.F. Klemic, D.A. Routenberg, P.N. Wyrembak, D.B. Turner-Evans, A.D. Hamilton, D.A. LaVan, T.M. Fahmy, and M.A. Reed, "Label-free immunodetection with CMOS-compatible semiconducting nanowires," *Nature*, 445, 519–522, 2007.

[57] M.A. Burns, B.N. Johnson, S.N. Brahmasandra, K. Handique, J.R. Webster, M. Krishnan, T.S. Sammarco, P.M. Man, D. Jones, D. Heldsinger, C.H. Mastrangelo, and D.T. Burke, "An integrated nanoliter DNA analysis device," *Science*, 282(5388): 484–487, Oct. 16, 1998.

[58] R. Pal, M. Yang, R. Lin, B.N. Johnson, N. Srivastava, S.Z. Razzacki, K.J. Chomistek, D.C. Heldsinger, R.M. Haque, V.M. Ugaz, P.K. Thwar, Z. Chen, K. Alfano, M.B. Yim, M. Krishnan, A.O. Fuller, D.T. Burke, and M.A. Burns, "An integrated microfluidic device for Influenza and other genetic analyses," *Lab on a Chip*, 5(10): 1024–1032, 2005.

[59] A.T. Woolley, D. Hadley, P. Landre, A.J. deMello, R.A. Mathies, and M.A. Northrup, "Functional integration of PCR amplification and capillary electrophoresis in a microfabricated DNA analysis device," *Anal. Chem.*, 1996, 68, 4081–4086.

[60] C.N. Liu, N.M. Toriello, and R.A. Mathies, "Multichannel PCR-CE microdevice for genetic analysis," *Anal. Chem.*, 2006, 78, 5474–5479.

[61] E.T. Lagally, I. Medintz, and R.A. Mathies, "Single-molecule DNA amplification and analysis in an integrated microfluidic device," *Anal. Chem.*, 2001, 73, 565–570.

[62] C.A. Emrich, H. Tian, I.L. Medintz, and R.A. Mathies, "Microfabricated 384-lane capillary array electrophoresis bioanalyzer for ultrahigh-throughput genetic analysis," *Anal. Chem.*, 2002, 74, 5076–5083.

[63] B.M. Paegel, C.A. Emrich, G.J. Weyemayer, J.R. Scherer, and R.A. Mathies, "High-throughput DNA sequencing with a microfabricated 96-lane capillary array electrophoresis bioprocessor," *PNAS*, 99(2): 574–579, Jan. 22, 2002.

[64] Y.N. Shi, P.C. Simpson, J.R. Scherer, D. Wexler, C. Skibola, M.T. Smith, and R.A. Mathies, "Radial capillary array electrophoresis microplate and scanner for high-performance nucleic acid analysis," *Anal. Chem.*, 71(23): 5354–5361, Dec. 1, 1999.

[65] J. Reichert, A. Csaki, J.M. Kohler, and W. Fritzsche, "Chip-based optical detection of DNA hybridization by means of nanobead labeling," *Anal. Chem.*, 72(24): 6025–6029, Dec. 15, 2000.

[66] A.T. Woolley, K.Q. Lao, A.N. Glazer, and R.A. Mathies, "Capillary electrophoresis chips with integrated electrochemical detection," *Anal. Chem.*, 70(4): 684–688, Feb. 15, 1998.

[67] C.J. Yu, Y.J. Wan, H. Yowanto, J. Li, C.L. Tao, M.D. James, C.L. Tan, G.F. Blackburn, and T.J. Meade, "Electronic detection of single-base mismatches in DNA with ferrocene-modified probes," *Journal of the American Chemical Society*, 123(45): 11155–11161, Nov. 14, 2001.

[68] R.H. Liu, J. Yang, R. Lenigk, J. Bonanno, and P. Grodzinski, "Self-contained, fully integrated biochip for sample preparation, polymerase chain reaction, amplification and DNA microarray detection," *Anal. Chem.*, 76(2004): 1824.

[69] M.A. Burns, B.N. Johnson, S.N. Brahmasandra, K. Handique, J.R. Webster, M. Krishnan, T.S. Sammarco, P.M. Man, D. Jones, D. Heldsinger, C.H. Mastrangelo, and D.T. Burke, "An integrated nanoliter DNA analysis device," *Science*, 282(5388): 484–487, Oct. 16, 1998.

[70] V. Siegmund, O. Adjei, P. Racz, C. Berberich, E. Klutse, F. Van Vloten, T. Kruppa, B. Fleischer, and G. Bretzel, "Dry-reagent-based PCR as a novel tool for laboratory confirmation of clinically diagnosed *Mycobacterium Ulcerans*–associated disease in areas in the tropics where *M. Ulcerans* is endemic," *J. of Clinical Microbiology*, 43, 1, 271–276, Jan. 2005.

CHAPTER 17

Architectural Optimizations for Digital Microfluidic Biochips

Bharat Joshi, Arindam Mukherjee, Siddhartha Datta, and Arun Ravindran

17.1 Introduction

Microfluidics-based biochips constitute an emerging category of mixed-technology micro systems [13]. Recent advances in microfluidics technology have led to the design and implementation of miniaturized devices for various biochemical applications. These micro systems, referred to interchangeably in the literature as microfluidics-based biochips, lab-on-a-chip, and bioMEMS [15,16], promise to revolutionize biosensing, clinical diagnostics, and drug discovery, and have created tremendous opportunities and interesting challenges in the areas of enzymatic analysis, DNA analysis, proteomic analysis involving proteins and peptides, immunoassays, implantable drug delivery devices, and environmental toxicity monitoring [28]. Biochips based on microfluidics automate highly repetitive laboratory tasks by replacing cumbersome equipment with miniaturized and integrated systems, and they enable the handling of micro and nanoliter volumes of fluids. Thus, compared to traditional methods, these biochips allow ultra-sensitive detection at significantly lower cost and higher throughput.

The first generation of microfluidic biochips contained permanently etched structures and operated on the principle of continuous fluid flow [33]. Liquid flow was achieved through external pressure sources, integrated mechanical micropumps, or electrokinetic mechanisms such as electro-osmosis. Recently, a novel microfluidics technology, known as *digital microfluidics* has been developed to manipulate liquids as discrete microliter/nanoliter droplets. Compared to continuous-flow systems, digital microfluidics offers the advantage of dynamic reconfigurability and architectural scalability.

The level of system integration and the complexity of digital microfluidics-based biochips are expected to increase in the near future due to the growing need for multiple and concurrent bioassays on a chip [16]. However, shrinking processes, new materials, and the underlying multiple energy domains will make these biochips more susceptible to manufacturing defects. Moreover, some manufacturing defects are expected to be latent, and they may manifest themselves during field operation of the biochips. In addition, harsh operational environments may introduce physical defects such as particle contamination during field operation. Consequently, robust off-line and on-line test techniques are required to ensure system dependability as biochips are deployed for safety-critical applications such as field diagnostics tools to monitor infectious disease, decode genes, and biosensors to detect biochemical toxins and other pathogens.

The microfluidic biochip is based on the manipulation of micro-liter/nano-liter droplets using the principle of electrowetting-on-dielectric (EWOD). Electrowetting refers to the modulation of the interfacial tension between a conductive fluid and a solid electrode coated with a dielectric layer by applying an electric field between them. An imbalance of interfacial tension is created if an electric field is applied to only one side of the droplet; this tension gradient forces the droplet to move.

There are two types of EWOD-based digital microfluidic biochips. One is considered to be a one-plane system (shown in Figure 17.1 (a)) and the other a two-plane system (shown in Figure 17.1 (b)). The two-plane system has the advantages of faster droplet transportation and less evaporation of droplets. Nowadays, the two-plane system is considered useful for all operations. It consists of two parallel glass plates. The bottom plate contains a patterned array of individually controllable electrodes, and the top plate is coated with a continuous ground electrode. The control electrodes in the bottom plate are formed by a 200 nm-thick layer of chrome, which is further coated with a layer of Parylene C (800 nm) as a dielectric insulator. This microfluidic array uses a 1.0 mm electrode pitch size. A 50 nm-thick film of Teflon AF 1600 is added as the hydrophobic thin film to the top and bottom plates to decrease the wettability of the surface and to add capacitance between the droplet and the control electrode. A layer of optically transparent indium tin oxide (ITO) in the top glass plate is used as the continuous ground electrode. The 600 μm gap between the top and bottom plates is set using a glass spacer. The droplet containing biochemical samples and the filler medium, such as the silicone oil, are sandwiched between the plates; the droplets travel inside the filler medium.

In order to move a droplet, a control voltage is applied to an electrode adjacent to the droplet (shown in Figure 17.1(a)) and at the same time the electrode just under the droplet (shown in Figure 17.1(b)) is deactivated. Thus, the charge in the droplet/insulator interface that is accumulated over the activated electrode results in an interfacial tension gradient, which consequently causes the droplet transport. By varying the electrical potential along a linear array of electrodes, micro-liter/nano-liter

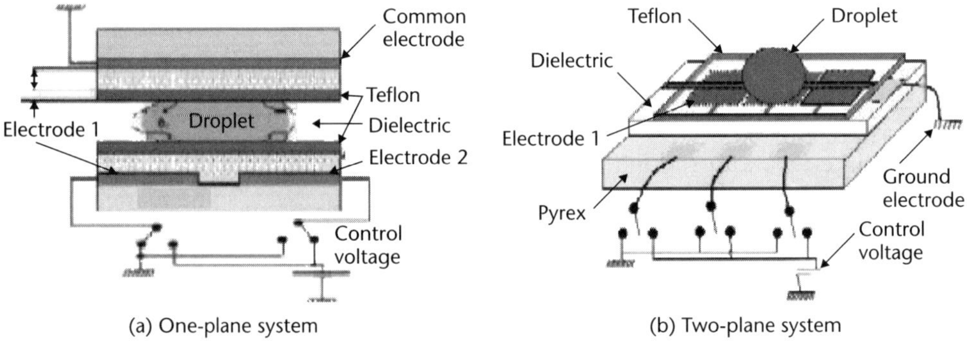

Figure 17.1 The two types of digital microfluidic biochips.

volume droplets can be transported along this line of electrodes. This method of transportation of the droplets is often referred to as "Direct Reference." The velocity of the droplet can be controlled by adjusting the control voltage (0 ~ 90 V), and droplets have been observed to move with velocities up to 20 cm/s. Furthermore, based on this principle, droplets can be transported freely to any location on a two-dimensional array without the need for micro pumps and micro valves that are required in continuous-flow systems.

Using a two-dimensional microfluidic array, many common operations for different bioassays can be performed, such as sample movement (*transport*), temporary sample preservation (*store*), and the mixing of different samples (*mix*). For instance, the *store* operation is performed by applying an insulating voltage around the droplet. The *mix* operation is used to route two droplets to the same location and then turn them about some pivot points. Note that these operations can be performed anywhere on the array, whereas in continuous-flow systems they must operate in a specific micro mixer or micro chamber. This property is referred to as the reconfigurability of a digital biochip. The configurations of the array, (i.e., the droplet transport routes and their rendezvous points, are programmed into a microcontroller that controls the voltages of electrodes in the array). The experimental set-up of the biochip is shown in Figure 17.2.

Concepts from VLSI design can be efficiently utilized to assign functionalities to the cells and schedule the bioassays. Typically, a microfluidic module library is provided to the designer after experimental characterization. This module library, analogous to the standard/custom cell library used in cell-based VLSI design, includes different microfluidic functional modules such as mixers and storage units. Each module is characterized by its function (mixing, storing, detection, etc.) and parameters such as width, length, and operation duration. During the biochip design, the microfluidic assay operations are mapped to the grid to the available microfluidic modules, and then use architectural-level synthesis techniques to determine a schedule of sets of bioassays subject to constraints imposed by the corresponding assay protocols [24]. The locations of the modules on the microfluidic array are then determined by efficient placement algorithms. These configurations of the microfluidic array are loaded into a microcontroller that controls the voltages of electrodes in the array. Therefore, these modules can be dynamically formed by activating the

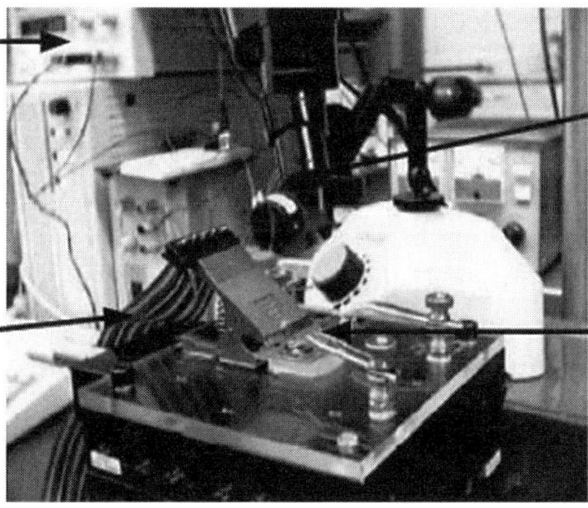

Figure 17.2 Experimental setup (Courtesy Duke University [22]).

corresponding control electrodes during run-time. In this sense, they can also be viewed as virtual devices. Henceforth a EWOD-based digital microfluidic biochip will be simply referred to as a biochip.

The focus of this chapter is to explore techniques to schedule biochips efficiently for fast analysis, to test and reconfigure biochips for quality assurance and yield enhancement at the time of manufacture, and to increase the reliability and extend the lifetime of the biochip during field operation.

The organization of the chapter is as follows. In Section 17.2, new challenges created by the advances in relevant technologies are discussed. While testing and reconfiguration strategies are described in Section 17.3, scheduling and resource allocation methodologies are discussed in Section 17.4. In Section 17.5, testing, reconfiguration, and scheduling and resource allocation methodologies are integrated to form off-line and on-line (concurrent) testing methodologies. Off-line testing strategies are applied to the biochips only during the time intervals when no bioassays are being analyzed. Concurrent testing implies that while the biochip is being tested for faults it is also being used by the bioassays. Future trends and applications of biochips are identified in Section 17.6.

17.2 Challenges

The level of system integration and the complexity of digital microfluidics-based biochips are expected to increase in the near future due to the growing need for multiple and concurrent bioassays on a chip and advances in technologies. Packaging a biochip to control a large number of active electrodes, and efficiently implementing complex bioassays on the biochip are two of the most significant challenges. For example, a 100×100 array of cells in a biochip would require 10,000 pins to control each active electrode individually in the direct-referencing scheme. This number is more than 10-fold higher than the existing integrated circuit packaging technologies that have pins per package on the order of a few hundreds. Since the dimension of such a biochip is expected to be around 5 cm $\times$ 5 cm, precision manufacturing of contacts, packaging, and designing the circuit board that controls the active electrodes with multiple metal layers for routing 10,000 control-pin-to-active-electrode wires are required. Thus, in the future a scheme would be needed in which a group of electrodes could be controlled by a common voltage, thereby reducing the number of control pins. Such a method is typically known as cross referencing [35].

With emerging applications that demand more complex bioassays to be concurrently executed on a biochip, and with the use of biochips in often critical and real-time applications, there is a need to deliver an advanced level of computer-aided design support to the biochip designer. Moreover, an optimized design can potentially reduce the number of independently controlled electrodes required. Current design practices for mapping applications onto biochips are ad-hoc and inefficient. An automated design flow is required for optimal realizations of application-specific biochip designs. The authors of [24, 25] made a significant effort in this direction by optimizing the placement of mixers on a biochip, for a given bioassay schedule and a fixed architecture.

Moreover, the International Technology Roadmap for Semiconductors has identified the integration of electrochemical and electrobiological techniques as one of the design challenges that will be faced beyond 2009 when feature sizes are expected to shrink below 50 nm [27]. Shrinking feature sizes and new materials and processes will make these biochips more susceptible to manufacturing defects. Moreover, some manufacturing defects are expected to be latent, and may manifest during field operation of the biochips. In addition, harsh operational environments may introduce physical defects such as particle contamination during field operation. Some of these faults are caused by dielectric breakdowns, shorts between adjacent electrodes, degradation of the insulator, and opens in the metal connection between the electrode and the control source [23]. Consequently, effective test techniques are required to ensure system dependability as biochips are deployed for safety-critical applications such as field diagnostics tools to monitor infectious disease and decode genes, as well as biosensors to detect biochemical toxins and other pathogens.

17.3 Testing and Reconfiguration Strategies

Several test strategies for digital microfluidic systems have been proposed in the literature [17, 18, 23-26]. Physical defaults in such systems were analyzed and faults were classified as being either catastrophic or parametric when drawn from the analogy of analog and mixed signal devices. In all these strategies, faults are detected by electrically controlling and tracking the motion of test droplets. Prior work on the testing of digital microfluidics-based biochips is based on simplistic assumptions regarding the impact of certain defects on droplet flow. For example, a common defect seen in fabricated microfluidic arrays is a short circuit between two adjacent electrodes [23–25]. It was assumed in [26] that this defect causes a droplet to get stuck at one of the two electrodes, irrespective of the orientation of liquid flow. Based on this assumption, Hamiltonian paths are used to detect catastrophic faults in microfluidic arrays [22, 30]. A Hamiltonian path is a path in an undirected graph that visits each vertex exactly once. One of the problems with this approach is that although finding Hamiltonian paths in grid structures is well-known, checking the existence of a Hamiltonian path in a graph is NP-complete [9]. Thus, it would be expensive to determine such paths in the microfluidic array after it is reconfigured based on results of the fault diagnosis.

The strategy proposed in [4] is an improvement over the previous method. One source/sink was used and the droplets were sequentially transferred across their predetermined paths and retrieved at the sink. If a droplet does not reach the sink, then that particular path is considered faulty and the droplet is assumed to be stuck at an electrode before the faulty electrode in its path. A method was developed to retrieve this droplet using a procedure similar to binary search method and the location of the faulty electrode or edge was determined. The paths were divided into the outer path, inner horizontal paths, and inner vertical paths. All these paths were traversed sequentially, which took a considerable amount of time. Analysis and simulations of this algorithm indicated that the complexity of the algorithm is quite high. It can be seen that since each edge has to be tested, the lower bound on the testing problem is $\Omega(mn)$ where m and n are the number of rows and columns in the grid. It can be seen that if multiple sources/sinks are available, then the testing time for a realistic biochip can be reduced by partitioning the chip in such a way that all the partitions are tested simultaneously. In this case an ideal speedup of N is possible where N is the number of partitions. In Section 17.3.1 a strategy based on the portioning technique is described in detail.

17.3.1 Testing Technique Based on Partitioning the Grid for Multiple Sources and Sinks

This method is based on the assumption that several sources through which test droplets can be administered, and sinks through which droplets can be retrieved are available. One particular partitioning that is very effective involves dividing the grid into two halves and then each half is further divided into sub-grids equaling the number of sources/sinks available (Figure 17.3).

All the sub-grids can be tested in parallel with the other grids. Each source/sink dispenses test droplets to two sub-grids. Thus the number of sub-grids is equal to twice the number of sources/sinks available. The method of the division of the total grid size into the sub-grids is based on Equations 17.1, 17.2 and 17.3. It is assumed that the grid size is (N, M) and sub-grid size is $\{n, m\}$. As shown in Figure 17.3 the size of the sub-grids decreases as the number of sources/sinks increases.

The total number of sub-grids (IG) is given by:

$$IG = 2 \times num\_sources \tag{17.1}$$

For $\{2 \times (M \bmod num\_sources)\}$ sub-grids:

$$(n,m) = \left(\frac{N}{2}, \left\lfloor \frac{M}{num\_sources} \right\rfloor + 1\right) \tag{17.2}$$

For remaining $\{IG - [2 \times (M \bmod num\_sources)]\}$ sub-grids:

$$(n,m) = \left(\frac{N}{2}, \left\lfloor \frac{M}{num\_sources} \right\rfloor\right) \tag{17.3}$$

Each sub-grid is tested using a testing procedure described in [4]. The algorithm is listed below for the sake of completeness.

*Algorithm MFDL * Microfluidic array fault detection and location algorithm **

Step 1

1. ***While*** *not(done)*
2. *Dispense a test droplet from the source into the outer loop (initially boundary nodes and edges) in the clockwise direction.*

   If the droplet is retrieved at the sink after \E\ units of time then
3. *outer loop is fault-free*

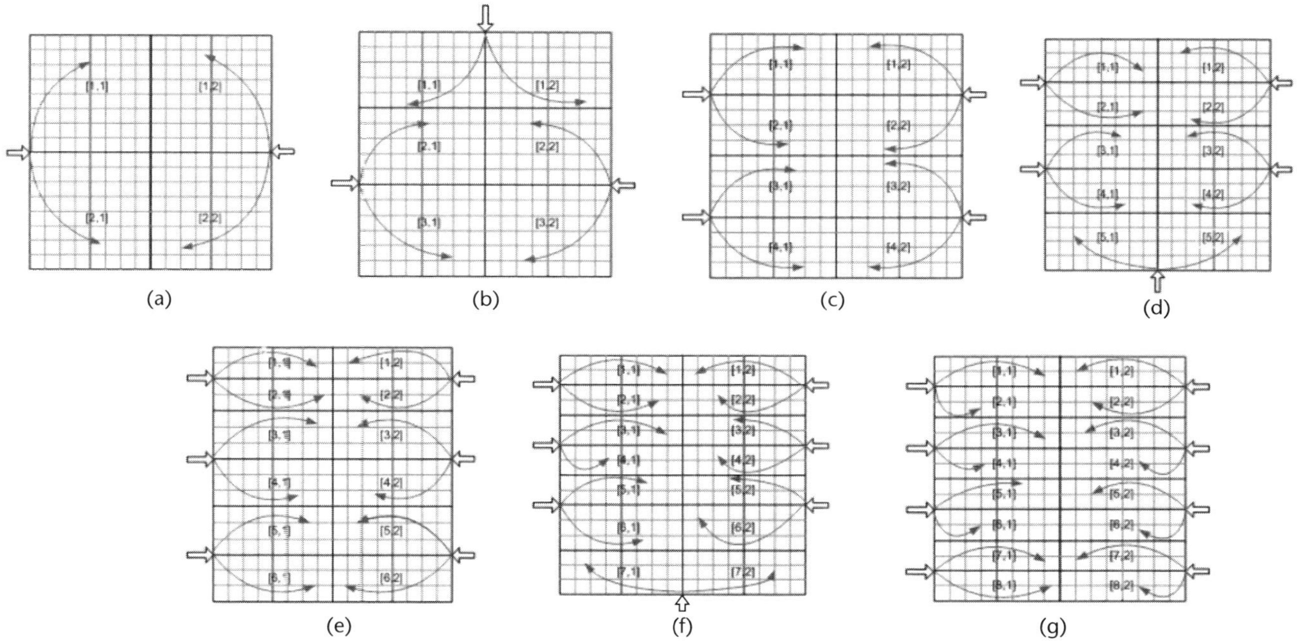

Figure 17.3 Partitioning of a grid based on different number of source/sinks.

4. * \E\ is the number of edges in the loop. It is assumed that a droplet takes one unit of time to traverse an edge *\
5. **Else**
6. edge = 0, node = 0
7. FaultLocation (loop, source, sink, edge, node)
8. ReconfigureOuter (edge, node)
9. **Endif**
10. **If** (outer Loop is fault-free) OR (microfluidic array useless)
* An example of a microfluidic array becoming useless - a critical resource is disconnected from the rest of the system *\
11. done = true
12. **EndIf**
13. **EndWhile**

End Step 1

Step 2

1. Dispense a test droplet from the source to each of the horizontal loops whose three sides are a path from the Outer Loop (Figure 17.2(a)) starting from the smallest loop at an interval of 3 time units in the clockwise direction
2. Mark each loop *i* from whom the droplet was not retrieved in (\E$_i$\ + d_i) units of time where \E$_i$\ is the number of edges in the loop *i* and d_i is the delay in the droplet dispensing * Faults are detected in horizontal loops *\
3. **For** each marked loop
edge = 0, node = 0
FaultLocation (loop, source, sink, edge, node)
4. **EndFor** * All the faulty nodes and all the faulty horizontal edges have been identified *\
5. **For** each node identified faulty
6. ReconfigureInner (node)
7. **EndFor**
8. Dispense a test droplet from the source to each of the vertical loops whose three sides are a path from the Outer Loop (Figure 17.2(b)) starting from the smallest loop at an interval of 3 time units in the clockwise direction
9. Mark each loop *i* from whom the droplet was not retrieved in (\E$_i$\ + d_i) units of time where \E$_i$\ is the number of edges in the loop *i* and d_i is the delay in the droplet dispensing * Faults are detected in vertical loops *\
10. **For** each marked loop
FaultLocation (loop, source, sink, edge, node)
11. **EndFor** * All the faulty vertical edges have been identified *\

End Step 2

Retrieve (node_and_edge, path, firstNode, lastNode, done)

1. **If** (node-edge) then
2. Apply voltages to electrodes sequentially starting from the counterclockwise neighbor of the lastNode

```
Else
    Apply voltages to electrodes sequentially starting from the clockwise
      second neighbor of the lastNode
EndIf
If droplet is retrieved then
    done = true
Else
    done = false
EndIf
End Retrieve
```

```
FaultLocation (loop, source, sink, faultyEdge, faultyNode)
located = false
retrieved = false
nodeEdge = true
path = first half of the loop starting from source
lastNode = sink
size = 0
While not (located)
    Retrieve (nodeEdge, path, source, lastNode, retrieved)
    If not (retrieved)
        path = path U p1, where p1 is the first half of the remaining loop
        lastNode = last node in the path
        size = number of nodes in p1
    Else
        Dispense test droplet in the path by applying voltages to the electrodes
          in the clockwise direction starting from the source
        path = first half of the path
        If (size == 1)
            Retrieve (nodeEdge, path, source, lastNode, retrieved)
            located = true
            FaultSet = {node in p1, clockwise edge of the node in p1}
        EndIf
    EndIf
EndWhile
Dispense test droplet from the sink in the counter-clockwise direction till
  the candidate faulty node
lastNode = second clockwise neighbor of the candidate faulty node
nodeEdge = false
Retrieve (nodeEdge, path, source, lastNode, retrieved)
If (retrieved)
    faultEdge = edge between the candidate faulty node and the clockwise
      neighbor
Else
```

30. faultyNode = candidate faulty node
31. ***EndIf***
End FaultLocation

ReconfigureOuter (edge, node)
1. ***If*** *node is faulty then*
2. Delete faulty node and the edges incident on that node
*3. Reconfigure the loop * if n_{i1} is faulty then reconfigure*
$n_{i-1,1} \rightarrow n_{i-1,2} \rightarrow n_{i,2} \rightarrow n_{i+1,2} \rightarrow n_{i+1,1}$. *Similarly for others **
4. ***EndIf***
5. ***If*** *edge is faulty then*
6. Delete faulty edge
7. Reconfigure loop to bypass the faulty edge
8. ***EndIf***
End ReconfigureOuter

ReconfigureInner (node)
1. Delete faulty node and the edges incident on it
2. Reconfigure loop to form an inner vertical loop using the nearest neighbors
End ReconfigureOuter

Detailed analysis of the MFDL algorithm is presented in [4]. It can be observed that the droplet paths of any sub-grid are disjointed from others and the edges connecting the adjacent sub-grids are not tested. To accommodate the testing of these edges, the droplet paths are modified to enable the test droplets to traverse a subset of the outer edges of its adjacent sub-grids. This results in the adjacent sub-grids test droplets' paths to overlap. Referring to Figure 17.4, the outer and inner horizontal paths of each test droplet of sub-grid {1, 1} is changed to traverse through the left most column of {1, 2} and the uppermost row of {2, 1}. Similarly, the test droplets

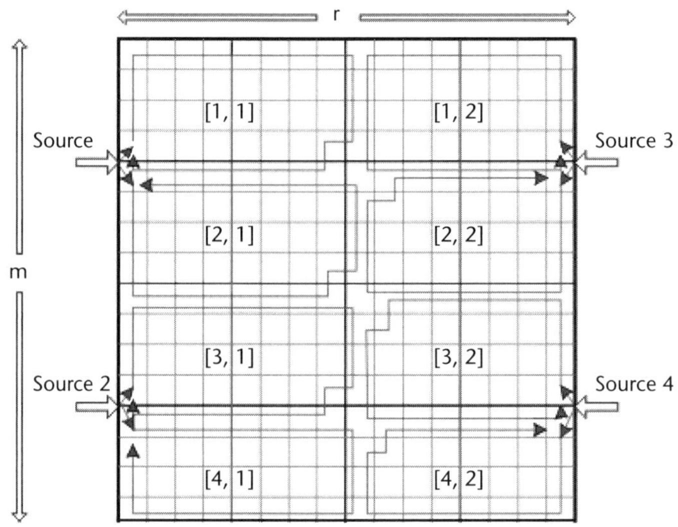

Figure 17.4 Example illustrating the paths of test droplets through their respective internal grids.

programmed to traverse the inner vertical paths of {1, 1} are modified to traverse through the uppermost row of {2, 1}. Thus the path length of these test droplets increases by the number of extra electrodes to be traversed. In this way, every sub-grid's dispensed test droplets' paths are modified. The modification in the paths is not the same for all sub-grids. It depends on the orientation of the sub-grid on the total grid space. In Figure 17.4, {4, 2} would have no changes made in its test droplets' paths. This is because {4, 2} does not have any sub-grid located below or to its right.

Furthermore, as described in [22, 24], a typical electrode in a digital microfluidic-based biochip has the capacity of holding no more than two droplets. Accumulation of more than two droplets will flood the electrode, leading to corruption of the entire chip [24]. Thus, an effective and efficient scheduling scheme is needed to avoid flooding while all the sub-grids are being tested. Figure 17.4 shows how the outer paths of each internal grid are modified to allow only two test droplets to pass through each electrode. The paths of {1, 1} of a (16, 16) grid with four sources/sinks are demonstrated in Figure 17.4. Based on this, a schedule is designed in which the sub-grids are tested in different phases. Sub-grids placed diagonally to one another are tested simultaneously. For example, (Figure 17.5), sub-grids {1, 1}, {2, 2}, {3, 1} and {4, 2} are tested simultaneously in phase 1. Once these are tested, the remaining sub-grids, (i.e., {1, 2}, {2, 1}, {3, 2} and {4, 1}), are tested during phase 2. By this method, there

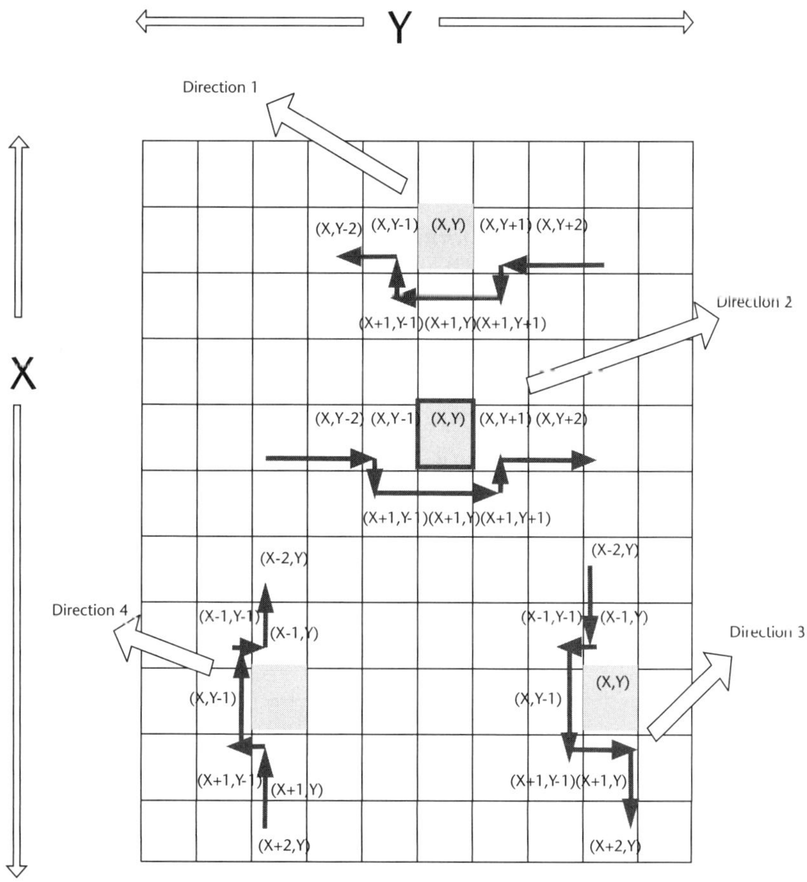

Figure 17.5 Reconfiguration of droplet paths.

is significant reduction of any two internal grids' droplets traversing through the overlapping rows and columns. The only overlap that still occurs is between internal grids {1, 2} and {2, 1}, {2, 2} and {3, 1} and {3, 2} and {4, 1}. The overlap is of one electrode and the scheduler controls it.

17.3.1.1 Partitioning Algorithm for Generating Sub-Grids

The partitioning algorithm is presented below.

Partition_test *( )*

1. *Check for the number of sources/sinks (num_sources) specified by the user*
2. *Total grid size is (N, M)*
3. *Number of internal grids is twice the number of sources/sinks available for dispensing test droplets*
4. *Each source/sink is assigned to 2 internal grids*
5. *{2 × (M mod num_sources)} internal grids will be of size: N/2 electrodes by (M/ (num_sources)) + 1 electrodes*
6. *Remaining internal grids will be of size: N/2 electrodes by (M/ (num_sources)) electrodes*
7. *For every [n, m] sized internal grid, there will be one outer path, m–2 inner horizontal paths and n–2 inner vertical paths to be tested*
8. *Extra rows and columns to be tested by each internal grid are considered*
9. *Routes of each test droplet through each internal grid are calculated*
10. *The scheduler calculates the number of time steps taken by each test droplet to reach back to the source and stores it*
11. *Assignment of the internal grids is now done serially*
    [1, 1] is internal grid 1, [1, 2] is 2, [2, 1] is 3 and so on
12. *If the internal grid_number mod4 = {0,1}, then go to step 13 else go to step 14*
13. *First shift of the testing method begins. Go to step 15*
14. *Second shift of the testing method begins*
15. *All these internal grids are tested simultaneously using the method described in [4]*
16. *If a fault is detected, location procedure is performed according to method in [4]*
17. *After location of the fault, the test droplet reconfigures its path around the fault using* ***Reconfigure****(node, edge) (subset of MFDL) from [4] to test the remaining part of its path*
18. *Location of multiple faults is complete*

It can be easily shown that the complexity of the algorithm is $O(max(m^3, n^3))$.

17.3.2 Reconfiguration Techniques for Fault Isolation

In this section, reconfiguration techniques for both bioassay droplets traversal paths and mixer locations are considered. The primary purpose of reconfiguration is to isolate the faults that were identified during the fault diagnosis phase.

17.3.2.1 Reconfiguration of Bioassay Droplets Traversal Routes

Various techniques [31] have been proposed for replacing modules affected by faulty areas by unused fault-free areas on the chip.

The algorithm discussed in this article does not trace unused areas to accommodate entire modules affected by faulty regions. The modules can remain as is and the paths of the droplets can be reconfigured around the detected faulty regions. The reconfiguration process begins as soon as a fault is detected in a droplet's path. The first step is to determine the direction of the droplet's path, (i.e., if the droplet was moving towards the right, left, top, or bottom) (Figure 17.5). The algorithm assigns numeric values to each of these directions. Once the direction of the droplet's path is known, the algorithm creates two paths to maneuver the droplet around the fault. One of the paths is considered to be the default path. This path is usually considered unless it cannot be implemented within the grid limits or any of these electrodes in the reconfigured path are detected faulty. The default paths for droplets moving in every direction are shown in Figure 17.8. For example, if a droplet's path is $(x-2, y) \rightarrow (x-1, y) \rightarrow (x, y) \rightarrow (x+1, y) \rightarrow (x+2, y)$ and the fault is detected at (x, y). The droplet is calculated to have been downwards, (i.e., the direction assigned is 3). The two possible paths around the fault are:

1. $(x-2, y) \rightarrow (x-1, y) \rightarrow (x-1, y-1) \rightarrow (x, y-1) - (x+1, y-1) \rightarrow (x+1, y) \rightarrow (x+2, y)$
2. $(x-2, y) \rightarrow (x-1, y) \rightarrow (x-1, y+1) \rightarrow (x, y+1) \rightarrow (x+1, y+1) \rightarrow (x+1, y) \rightarrow (x+2, y)$

This algorithm is recursive in nature because if any of the electrodes in the second path is also found faulty, then the droplet's path will be reconfigured around that faulty electrode and routes itself back to its original path.

Algorithm Reconfigure (fault locations, droplet path description)

1. *Fault is detected at (x, y)*
2. *If the droplet's path passes through (x, y) then go to step 3 else get out of the loop*
3. *If the droplet is moving from electrode $(x, y+1) \rightarrow (x, y)$, the direction = 1*
4. *If the droplet is moving from electrode $(x, y-1) \rightarrow (x, y)$, the direction = 2*
5. *If the droplet is moving from electrode $(x-1, y) \rightarrow (x, y)$, the direction = 3*
6. *If the droplet is moving from electrode $(x+1, y) \rightarrow (x, y)$, the direction = 4*
   */**

   *Depending on the direction value the droplet re-routes its path around the fault in the shortest possible way */*
7. *If direction = 1, the droplet reconfigures its route to $(x, y+1) \rightarrow (x+1, y+1) \rightarrow (x+1, y) \rightarrow (x+1, y-1) \rightarrow (x, y-1)$. If any of these electrodes are detected faulty or if these electrodes are at the edge of the grid or outside the grid then the reconfigured path is $(x, y+1) \rightarrow (x-1, y+1) \rightarrow (x-1, y) \rightarrow (x-1, y-1) \rightarrow (x, y-1)$*
8. *If direction = 2, the droplet reconfigures its route to $(x, y-1) \rightarrow (x+1, y-1) \rightarrow (x+1, y) \rightarrow (x+1, y+1) \rightarrow (x, y+1)$. If any of these electrodes*

are detected faulty or if these electrodes are at the edge of the grid or outside the grid then the reconfigured path is (x, y – 1) → (x – 1, y – 1) → (x – 1, y) → (x – 1, y + 1) → (x, y + 1)

9. *If direction = 3, the droplet reconfigures its route to (x – 1, y) → (x – 1, y – 1) → (x, y – 1) – (x + 1, y – 1) → (x + 1, y). If any of these electrodes are detected faulty or if these electrodes are at the edge of the grid or outside the grid then the reconfigured path is (x – 1, y) → (x – 1, y + 1) → (x, y + 1) → (x + 1, y + 1) → (x + 1, y)*
10. *If direction = 4, the droplet reconfigures its route to (x + 1, y) → (x + 1, y – 1) → (x, y – 1) → (x – 1, y – 1) → (x – 1, y). If any of these electrodes are detected faulty or if these electrodes are at the edge of the grid or outside the grid then the reconfigured path is (x + 1, y) → (x + 1, y + 1) → (x, y + 1) → (x – 1, y + 1) → (x – 1, y)*
11. *If the final reconfigured path also contains faulty electrodes, then go to step 1*
12. *else*
13. *Follow the reconfigured path and route around the faulty electrodes.*

17.3.2.2 Reconfiguration Techniques for Mixer Locations

A group of electrodes in which certain specific assay droplets move continuously over some period of time to form another compound is defined as a mixing operation. This group of electrodes is known as the mixer location. If the location of a mixer or reservoir is found faulty, then a diverse reconfiguration algorithm is implemented. Now if any electrode of this group is detected faulty, there are two options of reconfiguration. One would be that the mixer location remains the same and the reconfiguration algorithm is applied. The second option would be to shift the entire mixer to bypass the faulty electrode. Observations indicate that the latter method results in less latency and complexity.

The mixer is shifted in any four directions by one electrode spacing, (i.e., top, bottom, left, or right to avoid the faulty electrode). The default direction is shifting the mixer location one electrode to the right. After shifting the mixer location to the right, if the new mixer location gain has a detected faulty electrode, then the mixer is moved back to its original position and then shifted to the left. This procedure continues until all the possible directions are checked. If none of the new positions located are fault free, then the mixer will be shifted right by two electrodes' spacing. This algorithm is recursive in nature and continues until a fault-free area is located for accommodating the mixer or storage operation.

Algorithm for reconfiguration of the mixers' locations:

Reconfigure_mixer_loc *(mixer location, fault locations)*

1. *Assign the electrodes to mixer location. Assign original position to be (x, y) → (x, y + 1) → (x + 1, y + 1) → (x + 2, y + 1) → (x + 2, y) → (x + 1, y) → (x, y)*
2. *Initialize variable count = 1*

3. *count = count + 1*
4. *Check if any of these electrodes are detected faulty. If detected faulty, then go to step 5 else go to step 21*
5. *Shift the entire mixer location to the right (→) by one electrode spacing*
6. *Check if any of these electrodes are detected faulty or exceeds grids boundaries. If detected faulty, then go to step 7 else go to step 21*
7. *Shift the entire mixer location back to original position*
8. *Shift the entire mixer location to the left (←) by one electrode spacing*
9. *Check if any of these electrodes are detected faulty or exceeds grids boundaries. If detected faulty, then go to step 10 else go to step 21*
10. *Shift the entire mixer location back to original position*
11. *Shift the entire mixer location to the top (↑) by one electrode spacing*
12. *Check if any of these electrodes are detected faulty or exceeds grids boundaries. If detected faulty, then go to step 13 else go to step 21*
13. *Shift the entire mixer location back to original position*
14. *Shift the entire mixer location to the bottom (↓) by one electrode spacing*
15. *Check if any of these electrodes are detected faulty or exceeds grids boundaries. If detected faulty, then go to step 16 else go to step 21*
16. *If count = 2 then shift original position of mixer to the right by one electrode spacing, i.e., to:* $(x, y + 1) \rightarrow (x, y + 2) \rightarrow (x + 1, y + 2) \rightarrow (x + 2, y + 2) \rightarrow (x + 2, y + 1) \rightarrow (x + 1, y + 1) \rightarrow (x, y + 1)$ *and go to step 3*
17. *If count = 3 then shift original position of mixer to the left by one electrode spacing, i.e., to:* $(x, y - 1) \rightarrow (x, y) \rightarrow (x + 1, y) \rightarrow (x + 2, y) \rightarrow (x + 2, y - 1) \rightarrow (x + 1, y - 1) \rightarrow (x, y - 1)$ *and go to step 3*
18. *If count = 4 then shift original position of mixer to the top by one electrode spacing, i.e., to:* $(x - 1, y) \rightarrow (x - 1, y + 1) \rightarrow (x, y + 1) \rightarrow (x + 1, y + 1) \rightarrow (x + 1, y) \rightarrow (x, y) \rightarrow (x - 1, y)$ *and go to step 3*
19. *If count = 5 then shift original position of mixer to the bottom by one electrode spacing, i.e., to:* $(x + 1, y) \rightarrow (x + 1, y + 1) \rightarrow (x + 2, y + 1) \rightarrow (x + 3, y + 1) \rightarrow (x + 3, y) \rightarrow (x + 2, y) \rightarrow (x + 1, y)$ *and go to step 3*
20. *If still no fault free location is assigned for the mixer operation then go to step 16 and count = 2*
21. *This is the final location of the mixer*

17.4 Scheduling and Resource Allocation for Pin-Constrained Biochips

As mentioned in Section 17.2, emerging applications that require more complex bioassays to be concurrently executed on a biochip and the use of biochips in critical and real-time applications have created an urgent need for an advanced computer-aided design toolset that will enable designers to develop optimal biochips that will potentially reduce the number of independently controlled electrodes required.

Physical design automation for integrated circuits, particularly module placement, is a fairly matured area. Heuristics such as the Timber Wolf placement method [15], based on simulated annealing, are extensively used for custom cell placements [23]. The placement problem is often formulated as a 2-D rectangle packing predicament

[23]. Fault tolerance, reliability, and module placement are critical design factors for most digital microfluidic biochips. Previous techniques [31] for module placement utilize the dynamic reconfigurability characteristic of these 2-dimensional arrays. Programming the module placement on biochips is very similar to that used for Dynamically Reconfigured Field Programmable Gate Arrays (DRFPGAs). The difference between DRFPGAs and Digital Microfluidic-based biochips is that the DRFPGAs are limited by the well-defined roles of interconnect and logic blocks. Interconnect cannot be used for storing information, and logic blocks cannot be used for routing, whereas digital microfluidics-based biochips simplify programmability. The cells in the microfluidic array are multifunctional because they can be used for storage and functional operations, as well as transportation of droplets. Dynamic reconfiguration of the microfluidic-based biochips convert the problem into a 3-D packaging one. Each microfluidic module is modeled by a 3-D box [31], the base of which denotes the rectangular area of the module and the height of which denotes the time-span of its operation. Microfluidic biochip placement can now be viewed as the problem of packing these boxes to minimize the total base area while avoiding overlaps. Along with the placement problem, various other issues are also addressed, for example, the base of these 3-D boxes have to be placed on the grid in such a way that minimum time is spent in traversing to these locations by droplets from their sources and returning to the sinks on completion of these functional operations. Analyses are done extensively for all the paths that can be traversed by the droplets to reach the module location. The module placement and selection of the path for each droplet problem for electronic design is known to be NP-complete [9]. There are always $|x_1 - x_2| + |y_1 - y_2| + 1$ number of shortest distant paths between any source (x_1, y_1) and destination (x_2, y_2). Consequently, heuristics are needed to solve these problems in a computationally efficient manner. Simulated annealing is a well-studied combinatorial optimization method, and it has been extensively used for traditional module placement problems [8, 10–12]. An advantage of simulated annealing is that it explores the configuration space of the optimization problem while allowing hill-climbing [14] moves, that is, the acceptance of new configurations that increase the cost. In this chapter, a simulated annealing-based algorithm is presented to solve the problems for digital microfluidics-based biochips for both direct and cross-referencing schemes. There are several constraints imposed by both the direct and cross-referencing schemes that have to be carefully considered in any scheduling and resource allocation strategy.

17.4.1 EWOD Droplet Constraints

The relative constraints between droplets due to the fluidic principles of EWOD, which are applicable to both direct-referencing and cross-referencing schemes, are discussed. Consider that at time instant T_k, droplet D_l is located at cell (i_1, j_1), and droplet D_m is located at cell (i_2, j_2). Here "i" denotes the row that is numbered starting from the top and incrementing downward, while "j" denotes the column that is numbered starting from the left and incrementing toward the right.

Constraint 1: An electrode gap of at least two has to be maintained when droplets are moving along the same direction in a column or row to prevent either of the droplets from splitting and merging with each other. This condition is shown in Figure 17.6(a), where the droplets D_l and D_m are in the same column ($j_1 = j_2$), and are separated by only one row. In this case, if D_l is moved simultaneously with D_m toward cells $(i_1 - 1, j_1)$ and $(i_2 - 1, j_2)$, respectively, D_l might move to $(i_1 + 1, j_1)$ because the active electrode at $(i_1 + 1, j_1)$ will have to be made high for attracting D_m, and hence D_l might merge with D_m as shown in the figure. It is also possible that D_l might get split between $(i_1 - 1, j_1)$ and $(i_1 + 1, j_1)$.

Constraint 2: When droplets are placed diagonally to each other in neighboring cells, the movement of droplets toward each other or in the same direction is not possible. This condition is indicated in Figure 17.6(b).

Constraint 3: When droplets are placed next to each other in neighboring cells, movement of droplets is possible in all directions except toward each other. This constraint is shown in Figure 17.6(c).

17.4.2 Additional Constraints Due to Cross Referencing

Basic assumptions: Droplet d_l is located at electrode (i_1, j_1), connected to pins $P(r_a)$ and $P(c_b)$ at time instant T_k. Droplet d_m is located at electrode (i_2, j_2) connected to pins $P(r_c)$ and $P(c_d)$ at time instant T_k. "i" indicates the row number starting from the top and incrementing downward.

"j" indicates the column number starting from the left and incrementing toward the right.

Constraint 4:

If $[P(c_d) = P(c_b) + 1 \wedge P(r_a) \neq P(r_c)]$ and d_l is scheduled to move to electrode $[(i_1 \pm 1, j_1) \vee (i_1, j_1 - 1)]$ at time instant T_{k+1} and d_m is scheduled to move to electrode $(i_2, j_2 - 1)$ at time instant T_{k+1},

OR

If $[P(c_d) = P(c_b) - 1 \wedge P(r_a) \neq P(r_c)]$ and d_l is scheduled to move to electrode $[(i_1 \pm 1, j_1) \vee (i_1, j_1 + 1)]$ at time instant T_{k+1} and d_m is scheduled to move to electrode $(i_2, j_2 + 1)$ at time instant T_{k+1},

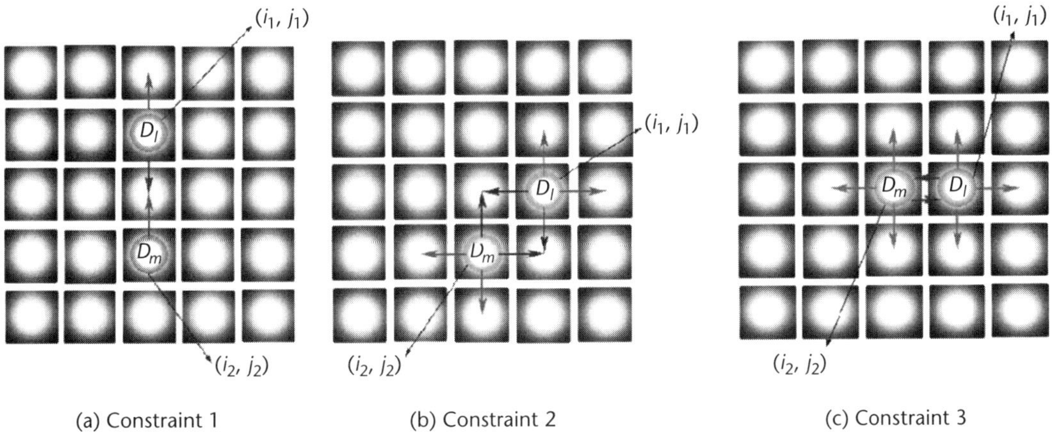

Figure 17.6 EWOD-related droplet constraints.

then depending on the potentials applied to the pins, one of the droplets undergoes a split condition or enters a state of metastability.

Constraint 5:
If $[P(r_c) = P(r_a) + 1 \wedge P(c_d) \neq P(c_b)]$ and d_l is scheduled to move to electrode $[(i_1, j_1 \pm 1) \vee (i_1 - 1, j_1)]$ at time instant T_{k+1} and d_m is scheduled to move to electrode $(i_2 - 1, j_2)$ at time instant T_{k+1},

OR
If $[P(r_c) = P(r_a) - 1 \wedge P(c_d) \neq P(c_b)]$ and d_l is scheduled to move to electrode $[(i_1, j_1 \pm 1) \vee (i_1 + 1, j_1 + 1,)]$ at time instant T_{k+1} and d_m is scheduled to move to electrode $(i_1 + 1, j_1)$ at time instant T_{k+1}, then depending upon the potentials applied to the pins, one of the droplets undergoes a split condition or enters a state of metastability.

Constraint 6:
If $[P(r_c) = P(r_a) \wedge P(c_d) \neq P(c_b) \wedge i_1 = i_2]$ and d_l is scheduled to move to electrode $(i_1 + 1, j_1)$ at time instant T_{k+1} and d_m is scheduled to move to electrode $(i_2 - 1, j_2)$ at time instant T_{k+1},

OR
If $[P(r_c) = P(r_a) \wedge P(c_d) \neq P(c_b) \wedge i_1 = i_2]$ and d_l is scheduled to move to electrode $(i_1 - 1, j_1)$ at time instant T_{k+1} and d_m is scheduled to move to electrode $(i_2 + 1, j_2)$ at time instant T_{k+1}, then depending upon the potentials applied to the pins, one of the droplets undergoes a split condition or enters a state of metastability.

Constraint 7:
If $[P(c_b) = P(c_d) \wedge P(r_c) \neq P(r_a) \wedge j_1 = j_2]$ and d_l is scheduled to move to electrode $(i_1, j_1 + 1)$ at time instant T_{k+1} and d_m is scheduled to move to electrode $(i_2, j_2 - 1)$ at time instant T_{k+1},

OR
If $[P(c_b) = P(c_d) \wedge P(r_c) \neq P(r_a) \wedge j_1 = j_2]$ and d_l is scheduled to move to electrode $(i_1, j_1 - 1)$ at time instant T_{k+1} and d_m is scheduled to move to electrode $(i_2, j_2 + 1)$ at time instant T_{k+1}, then depending on the potentials applied to the pins, one of the droplets undergoes a split condition or enters a state of metastability.

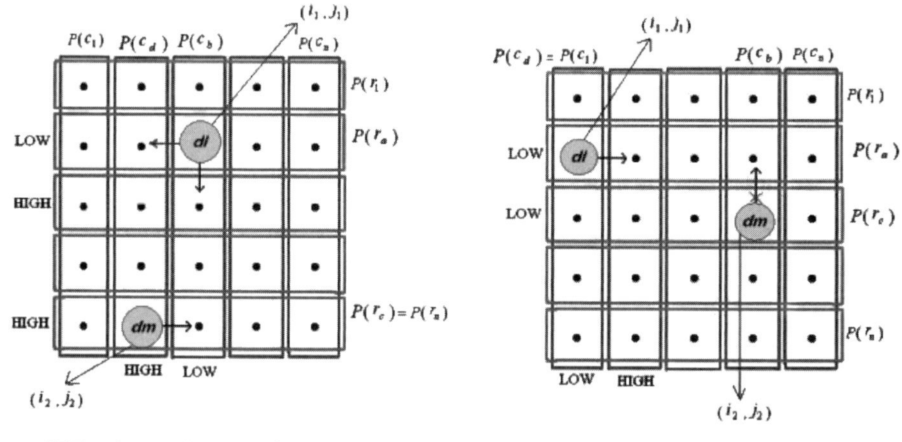

Figure 17.7 Constraints 4 and 5.

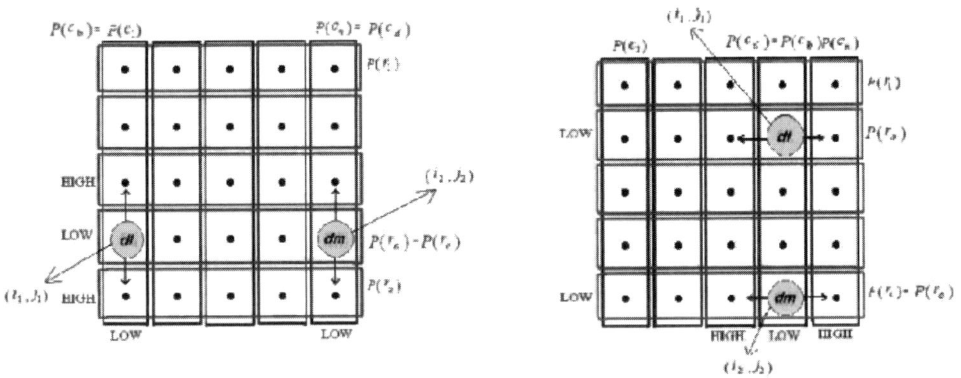

Figure 17.8 Constraints 6 and 7.

17.4.3 Optimization

Given a biochip with a fixed two-dimensional array of cells, along with a fixed number and specified locations of detection cells and droplet dispensing/collection reservoirs, the optimization goal is to reduce the total latency of executing a set of bioassays on the biochip. The set of bioassays is expressed as a directed dependence graph G, with vertices representing the four basic operations: droplet mixing, droplet optical detection, droplet dispensing from reservoirs, and droplet collection at reservoirs (Figure 17.9). An edge exists between two vertices if the output of the parent vertex is an input to the child vertex. There are delay values associated with each vertex, and these delays depend on the types of input droplets. Delays of all droplet dispensing and collection operations are zero. Delays associated with the edges represent droplet routing delays, including the stalls necessary to satisfy EWOD droplet constraints (constraints 1–3 for direct referencing and constraints 1–7 for cross referencing).

The optimization is based on two significant concepts, namely the macro and micro steps. A macro step is defined as a collection of operations that operate simultaneously without depending on any other operation results. A micro step is the actual time taken for any bioassay droplet to traverse between an electrode and its adjacent electrode. The value of every micro step is 62.5 milliseconds [22]. Variables in the optimization include the assignment of operations corresponding to different vertices in G to different macro steps during scheduling; binding the relevant vertices to physical architectural components like mixers, detectors and reservoirs; placing these architectural components on the biochip; and selecting bus layouts for droplet routing on the biochip. A macro step in the schedule includes the droplet routing delays, along with the delays associated with different operations. Since a cell on the biochip can be configured to mix, move, or store droplets, the positions and numbers of architectural components like mixers and buses are also variables in each schedule macro step. Hence, the architecture for executing the bioassays on the biochip is a variable in each schedule macro step.

Figure 17.9 represents a typical bioassay-directed dependency graph (G). Different numbered vertices correspond to different operations such as droplet dispensing/collection, mixing and detection. M is a variable assigned to mixers and V variables

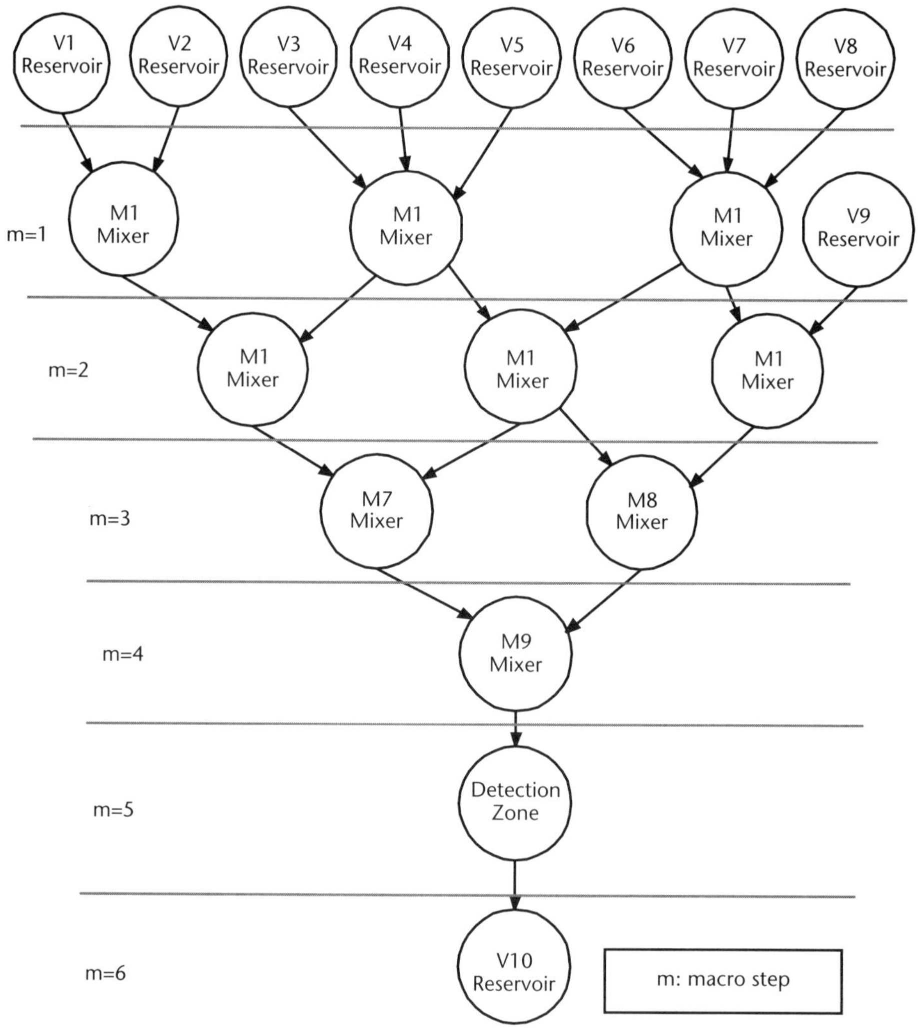

Figure 17.9 Bioassay dependence graph.

are assigned to reservoirs (sources/sinks required for dispensing the bioassay droplets). There are nine droplet dispensing, and one droplet collection reservoir(s) in the figure. The dotted lines demarcate the different macro steps in the example schedule. Depending on the size of the total grid space and mixers, the maximum number of mixers that can be paced at any macro step is calculated by $\left\lfloor \frac{(n-2)(m-2)}{(mixer\_length+2)(mixer\_breadth+2)} \right\rfloor - 1$ for a grid size (n, m). In this example, we have considered a (20, 20) grid size and the mixers are of size (2, 3). So a maximum of 15 mixers can be placed at each macro step "m". For this example, only one detection zone is considered.

The optimization procedure takes place in the following sequence.

1. **Resource Allocation:** The sources or reservoirs are placed on the grid space prior to the optimization. The sources are placed at the edges of the grid. The objective is to minimize latency. So the input bioassay droplets should be dispensed by reservoirs or sources physically located close to one another. For example, four sources located at electrodes S1:<1, 1>, S2:<5, 1>, S3:<1, 15>, and S4:<1, 20> are to be mapped to four input droplets D1, D2, D3 and D4. Further, D1 and D2 mix and D3 and D4 mix. The optimizer minimizing the latency maps D1 and D2 to S1 and S2 and D3 and D4 to S3 and S4. Any other mapping would result in an increase in the delay. Thus, this step is included in the optimization.
2. **Mixer Locations:** Considering the example shown in Figure 17.4, the locations of mixers M1, M2, and M3 are determined using the Geometric Centroid Theorem. The location of every mixer is calculated by averaging the X and Y co-ordinates of its sources. If reservoirs V1 and V2 are located at (x_1, y_1) and (x_2, y_2), then the mixer's first electrode is located at $x\_mixer_1 = \frac{x_1 + x_2}{2}$ and $y\_mixer_1 = \frac{y_1 + y_2}{2}$. The considered mixer size is (2, 3), so the location of the mixer 1 is: (x_mixer_1, y_mixer_1), $(x\_mixer_1 + 1, y\_mixer_1)$, $(x\_mixer_1, y\_mixer_1 + 1)$, $(x\_mixer_1 + 1, y\_mixer_1 + 1)$, $(x\_mixer_1, y\_mixer_1 + 2)$, $(x\_mixer_1 + 1, y\_mixer_1 + 2)$. Similarly, the locations of mixers M2 – M6 are calculated. This method remains permanent irrespective of the mixer sizes. The location of mixers present in macro step $m > 1$ are calculated by considering the first electrode location of input mixers as sources. For example, the location of the first electrode of mixer 6 is: $x\_mixer_6 = \frac{x\_mixer_3 + x_9}{2}$ and $y\_mixer_6 = \frac{y\_mixer_3 + y_9}{2}$. Note that this may not always be the final location of the mixer because of overlap with (1) fixed detection cells or (2) mixers already present at that location. There is always a two-electrode difference between any two mixer locations (so that a droplet can traverse through the mixers in operation). The algorithm is listed below.

1. *Assign the electrodes to mixer location. Assign original position to be (x, y) → (x, y + 1) → (x + 1, y + 1) → (x + 2, y + 1) → (x + 2, y) → (x + 1, y) → (x, y)*
2. *Initialize variable count=1*
3. *count = count+1;*
4. *Check if any of these electrodes are assigned to another mixer. If detected, then go to step 5 else go to step 21*
5. *Shift the entire mixer location to the right (→) by one electrode spacing*
6. *Check if any of these electrodes are assigned to another mixer or exceeds grid's boundaries. If detected, then go to step 7 else go to step 21*
7. *Shift the entire mixer location back to original position*

8. *Shift the entire mixer location to the left (←) by one electrode spacing*
9. *Check if any of these electrodes are assigned to another mixer or exceeds grid's boundaries. If detected, then go to step 10 else go to step 21*
10. *Shift the entire mixer location back to original position*
11. *Shift the entire mixer location to the top (↑) by one electrode spacing*
12. *Check if any of these electrodes are assigned to another mixer or exceeds grid's boundaries. If detected, then go to step 13 else go to step 21*
13. *Shift the entire mixer location back to original position*
14. *Shift the entire mixer location to the bottom (↓) by one electrode spacing.*
15. *Check if any of these electrodes are assigned to another mixer or exceeds grid's boundaries. If detected, then go to step 16 else go to step 21*
16. *If count = 2 then shift original position of mixer to the right by one electrode spacing, i.e., to:* $(x, y + 1) \rightarrow (x, y + 2) \rightarrow (x + 1, y + 2) \rightarrow (x + 2, y + 2) \rightarrow (x + 2, y + 1) \rightarrow (x + 1, y + 1) \rightarrow (x, y + 1)$ *and go to step 3*
17. *If count = 3 then shift original position of mixer to the left by one electrode spacing, i.e., to:* $(x, y - 1) \rightarrow (x, y) \rightarrow (x + 1, y) \rightarrow (x + 2, y) \rightarrow (x + 2, y - 1) \rightarrow (x + 1, y - 1) \rightarrow (x, y - 1)$ *and go to step 3*
18. *If count = 4 then shift original position of mixer to the top by one electrode spacing, i.e., to:* $(x - 1, y) \rightarrow (x - 1, y + 1) \rightarrow (x, y + 1) \rightarrow (x + 1, y + 1) \rightarrow (x + 1, y) \rightarrow (x, y) \rightarrow (x - 1, y)$ *and go to step 3*
19. *If count = 5 then shift original position of mixer to the bottom by one electrode spacing, i.e., to:* $(x + 1, y) \rightarrow (x + 1, y + 1) \rightarrow (x + 2, y + 1) \rightarrow (x + 3, y + 1) \rightarrow (x + 3, y) \rightarrow (x + 2, y) \rightarrow (x + 1, y)$ *and go to step 3*
20. *If still overlap exists at location assigned for the mixer operation then go to step 16 and count = 2;*
21. *This is the final location of the mixer*

3. **Calculation of Critical Paths:** Subsequent to the selection of mixer locations, critical paths (Δ_m) in every macro step are calculated. The critical path is defined as the shortest path between any source and destination of a droplet. The ASAP (As Soon As Possible) scheduling algorithm is implemented to calculate each Δ_m. The initial step is the calculation of the minimum distance to be traversed by the droplet from its source to destination. From Figure 17.4, consider the droplet traversing from reservoir V1 to mixer M1 location. Thus the minimum path length is calculated by: $path\_len = |x\_mixer_1 - x_{V1}| + |y\_mixer_1 - y_{V1}| + 1$. There are $|x_1 - x_2| + |y_1 - y_2| + 1$paths of the minimum path length joining the source to destination. The optimization algorithm considers three paths, as shown in Figure 17.10. The optimizer was programmed to simplify the complexities of optimization and scheduling. Observations indicate that path1 and path2 result in minimum clashing with other droplets, once the scheduling process begins.
4. **Scheduler:** The next step is to actually traverse the droplets over the grid, avoiding any clashes between droplets or violating any EWOD droplet constraints. The scheduler monitors all the droplets of every macro step. If there occurs, at any time step, a constraint violation or droplet clash, it stalls one of the droplets till its movement stops violating any of the constraints.

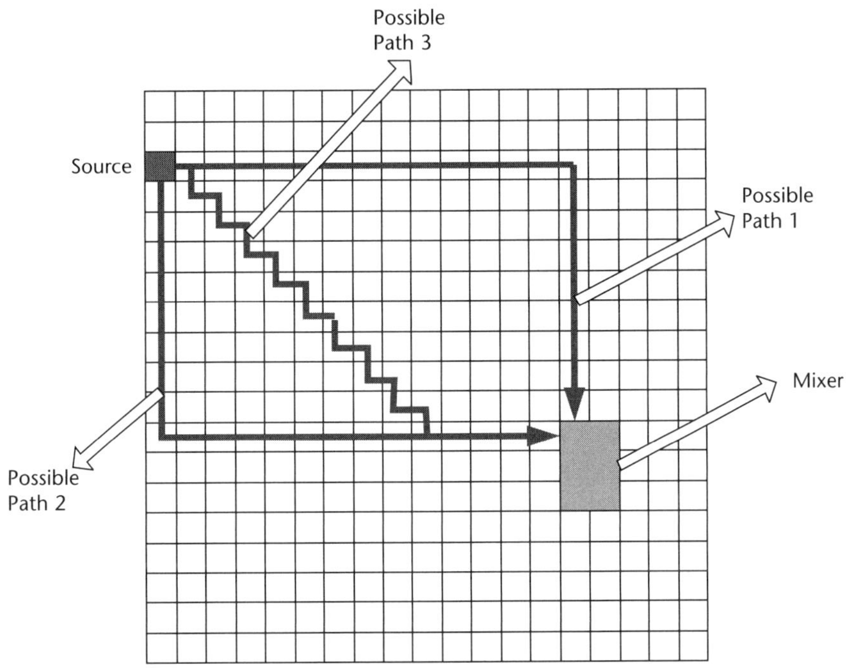

Figure 17.10 Multiple shortest paths created between source and destination.

The scheduler sets priorities to every edge of the current macro step after every elapsing micro step of the dependency graph G (droplet traversal) used to stall droplets when required. The priorities are set according to the distance left to be traversed by every droplet. The scheduler does priority-based scheduling [21] to assign priorities to each droplet. The droplet having the maximum distance to traverse gets the highest priority and so on. The number of time steps a droplet is stalled depends on which EWOD constraint is violated stated in Table 17.1.

5. **Simulated Annealing:** The scheduling of the dependence graph *G* uses a simulated annealing (SA)-based algorithm [14] to minimize a cost function that is the total latency of executing the bioassays on the biochip, and equals the summation of the critical path delays of all the macro steps and mixing operations. SA is a very well known optimization technique that falls in the category of hill-climbing heuristics. This method accepts temporarily

Table 17.1 Stalling Due to EWOD Constraints

Constraint Number	*Number of Time Steps the Droplet Is Stalled for if Violated*
1	2
2	2
3	2
4	3
5	3
6	3
7	3

inferior solutions with the hope of overcoming locally optimal solutions and obtains globally optimum ones. We start with a random assignment of weights to vertices in G; these weights determine the priority of scheduling vertices to macro steps. Solutions are obtained by the function *get_possible_schedule*. This function randomly selects one of the three paths created initially. In this manner, all the reservoir locations, mixer locations, and the critical paths are calculated. The complexity of this algorithm increases if the number of mixer operations during a macro step exceeds the limit. In that case the extra mixing operations are reallocated into the next macro step. The mixer products of the current macro step continue to move to their next destinations in the next macro step but have to avoid the electrodes where droplets are mixing. This is an added criterion to select the critical path for any droplet. The scheduler creates a virtual path length for each droplet. The virtual path lengths initially are equal to the actual path length of every droplet, but as droplets get stalled, their virtual path lengths are updated and the stalled time steps (added latency) are added to their values. These virtual path lengths are used by the scheduler to compute the latency value taken to execute an assay. The total latency is the summation of the latency issued by individual droplets and mixing operations of various macro steps. This latency value returned by ***get_possible_schedule*** is the cost function of the schedule. A parameter used in the SA algorithm, temperature, starts off initially at a high value and gradually cools down during the heuristic. A scheduling solution is accepted if either the cost function of the new schedule is better than the previous best, or if a randomly generated number is smaller than a threshold selected by the increase in cost function and the current temperature. Note that the higher the temperature, the higher the tendency of the algorithm to accept inferior solutions and overcome local minima. Of course, each solution point has to be feasible and satisfy all constraints. The best scheduling solution is always saved if the latency of the schedule is the minimum over all schedules that have been tried out. The number of iterations of the inner loop is increased, and the temperature is decreased inside the outer loop as the algorithm continues executing. The complete algorithm is presented below.

```
Simulated_Anneal (G)
begin
Iteration = I0;                        /* initial number of iterations*/
SA_Counter = 1000;                     /* SA run time*/
T = T0;                         /* initial temperature*/
initialize vertex weights (G);
CFNbest = get_possible_schedule (G);
loop SA_Counter times
loop Iteration times
perturb_weights (G);
CFNnew = get_possible_schedule (G);
if (CFNnew < CFNbest or random ( ) < exp((CFN_best – CFN_new)/kT) ) then
```

```
if (CFNnew < CFNbest) then
update_best_schedule (G);
CFNbest = CFNnew;
        end if;
end if;
end loop;                         /* inner loop ends*/
T = α* T ; Iteration = β* Iteration ; /* α < 1,β > 1*/
end loop;                         /* Simulated Annealing is out of time*/
end Simulated_Anneal;
get_possible_schedule (G)
begin
macro step m = 1;
if(m = 1)
{input (grid size, number of bio-assays, location of source);
for (i = 0, i < = number of bio-assays, i + + )
input (bio-assay[i]);
}
for (i = 1; i < = number of bio-assays; i + +)
{
num_inp++;
}
for (i = 1; i < = num_inp; i + +)
{
for (j = 1; j < = all_source locations; j + +)
{
if ([j] is repeated)
assign same location of previous input to i;
else
{
k = Min_path_length(source_loc[j](x,y), source_loc[j+1](x,y));
s = min (k);
source_loc[j](x,y) = i;
source_loc[j + 1](x,y) = i;
}
macro step m = 2;
while (unscheduled operation in G)
{
ASAP_Schedule unscheduled operations in macro step m choosing the
  highest weighted ones first; /* subject to availability of mixers in m*/
Allocate_Resources (m, G);    /*Bind operations to mixers and detectors*/
Analyze_next_macro step(m + 1, G, nearby);
Place_Mixers (m, G, nearby);/*Place mixer at/near the centroid of the
  locations of the droplets to be mixed—location of a droplet is considered at
  the start of the macro step m */
```

```
Route_Droplets_to_Inputs (m, G);
/*Route droplets from their locations at the start of m to the inputs of mixers/detectors/sink reservoirs*/
for (i = 1; i < = all inputs for present macro step; i + +)
{
Δm = Get_Critical_Path (current macro step input[i], G); /*using shortest distance algorithm, the shortest paths are calculated*/
}
Analyze_present _macrostep(all inputs of current macro step, mixer locations, G); /*to determine which path to select for each droplet to minimize constraint violations*/
Route_Droplets_from_Outputs (m, G);
/*Route droplets from outputs of mixers/detectors/source reservoirs towards their probable use locations in step m + 1*/
/*these movements are restricted to droplets that complete mixing/detection in less than Δm time */
increment m by 1;
}
return Latency = Σ_m Δm;
end get_possible_schedule;
Analyze_next_macrostep(m + 1, G, nearby)
{
For (all mixing operations of step m + 1)
{
If (mixing operation depends upon step m mixing operation)
{
    nearby==1; /* while placing the mixers, it will make sure that the mixers whose products mix in the next stage are nearby*/
}
}
}
Get_Critical_Path(m, G)
{
Min_path_length(m, G);
Calculate all possible paths from m to G with minimum path length;
}
Min_path_length(input1(x,y), input2(x,y))
{
min_path_len = _x2 − x1_ + _y2 − y1_+1; //assuming a fault free grid
}
Place_Mixers (m,G, nearby)
{
Orientation of sources is known.
Consider nearby;
```

```
Using midpoint theorem, calculate mid point of the sources and place mixer.
if ( other mixer located there)
{
Shift present mixer location by 2 electrodes towards any one of the sources)
}
}
```

17.5 Integrated Testing, Scheduling, and Resource Allocation

Testing, reconfiguration, scheduling, and resource allocation strategies have to be integrated to enable an effective biochip. In this section, these strategies are combined to form off-line and on-line testing methodologies. While off-line testing of the biochip implies that the testing and optimization of architectures mapped to the chip are performed in a sequential manner, on-line testing implies that the fault testing of the system runs concurrently with the optimized execution of various bioassays.

17.5.1 Off-Line Testing

The chip is initially tested and based on the faults diagnosed when the biochip is reconfigured. The next step is to schedule the bioassays to perform operations over the fault-free grid space. Simulations were made to calculate the latency required by the system to perform the entire off-line testing and bioassay executions.

Both clustered and dispersed faults were created using the PRNG. The testing algorithm is used to test the chip, followed by the optimizer combined with the reconfiguration algorithms (explained in Section 17.3.2) for calculating the total latency required to execute the multiplexed bioassays shown in Figure 17.11. Three unique bioassays were simulated to execute over the biochip post testing. These multiplexed bioassays are not executed in parallel. The bioassays were programmed to execute at different time frames to check the robustness of the optimizer.

If any bioassay has to be executed at any point in time, the scheduler checks whether there are a sufficient number of sources, sinks, and required grid space to accommodate the first stage of the new bioassay. If any one of these requirements is

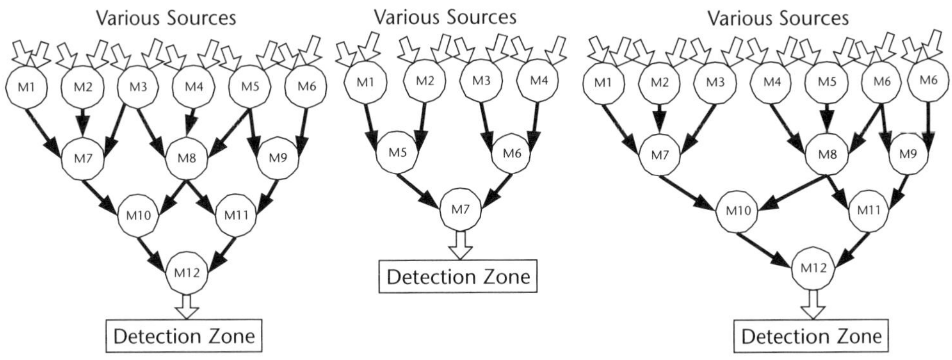

Figure 17.11 Multiplexed bioassays considered for off-line and on-line testing.

unsatisfied, it keeps a check using an ASAP (As Soon As Possible) algorithm to accommodate the pending bioassay.

During simulation, the first and second assays are dispensed right after the testing is complete. The third assay is launched after a random latency generated by the PRNG. The algorithm for the off-line testing is given below. The PRNG generates random occasions and questions the user if any bioassay is pending. If the user agrees, the next bioassay is queued to be executed. These algorithms have been implemented using direct referencing [27] and cross referencing [8] methods of transporting the droplets over the chip.

Algorithm for off-line testing:

1. ***Input*** *(total grid size of the biochip, number of sources/sinks available to dispense test droplets)*
2. ***Partition_test*** *(grid space, number of sources, time) /* mentioned in section 3.2*/ /* faults are located. Now the optimization begins*/*
3. ***Input*** *(number of sources available to dispense bioassay droplets, bioassay dependency graph)*
4. ***Simulated_annealing*** *loop*
   {
5. *Division of the bioassay dependency graph into macro steps.*
6. ***For*** *(each macro step) loop*
   {
7. ***Resource_allocation*** *(number of sources available to dispense bioassay droplets, number of input droplets of current macro step)*
8. *Calculation of location of mixers. /* done as described in [1]*/*
9. *Mixer location is checked for faulty electrodes.*
10. ***If*** *(faulty electrode/electrode is detected) then*
11. ***Reconfigure_mixer_loc*** *(mixer location, fault location/locations) /*mentioned in section 4.3*/*
12. *Calculation of the 3 shortest paths between the source and mixer location for each input droplet of the current macro step.*
13. ***PRNG*** *randomly selects any of the 3 paths as the critical path* Δ_D.
14. *Critical paths* (Δ_D) *of all droplets are checked for faulty electrodes.*
15. ***If*** *(faulty electrode/electrode is detected in any droplet's path) then*
16. ***Reconfigure*** *(fault location/locations, droplet path) /*mentioned in section 4.2*/*
17. ***Scheduling*** *(All droplets running in current macro step, time)*
18. *Total time (of that simulated _annealing iteration) = Total time (of that simulated _annealing iteration) + time /*time taken to complete all operations of current macro step*/*
    } end ***for*** *loop*
    } end ***Simulated_annealing*** *loop*
19. *Final time result =* ***Minimum*** *(Total_time) + ttime, /* final result is the time taken for fault diagnosis and optimization of architectures over the bio chip*/*

```
20. Resource_allocation (x, y)
    {
21. PRNG randomly maps x uniquely to y.
    }
22. Scheduling (All droplets running in current macro step, time)
    {
23. For (every time step of the current macro step) loop
    {
24.     time + +;
25.     Set_priority(All droplets )
26.     Compare each droplet to the other droplets and check for any clash or
    EWOD droplet violations at current time step.
27.     If (at current time step there is a clash OR EWOD droplet violation) then
28.     {
29.         Compare priority_assigned value of each droplet.
30.         The droplet with lower priority_assigned is stalled and Δ_D is incremented.
        }
    } end for loop
31. Return (time)
    }
32. Set_priority( All droplets)
    {
33. priority_assigned = number of electrodes remaining to be traversed by
    every droplet
    }
```

Tables 17.2 and 17.3 show some simulation results.

17.5.2 On-Line Testing

The bioassays and the test droplets are dispensed simultaneously from their respective sources and retrieved at their respective sinks. The bioassays are sent in to execute following the optimization algorithm [1]. Similar to off-line testing, the bioassays can be scheduled at any point of time. The PRNG is programmed to randomly question the user if any bioassay is pending to be scheduled and executed. If at any point of time a fault is detected, the current assay droplets operating in the faulty region are flushed (sent back to the reservoirs or sinks). If the current assay's previous macro step was executed in the faulty region, the droplets are simply sent to the sinks and are regarded as wasted. If not, they are directed to the reservoirs. The fault location process begins. After locating the fault, the system reads through all the assays that have previously passed through the faulty region. All these assay droplets are dispensed again and scheduling for these droplets occurs again since the previous operations of these assays was incorrect. These assays are put up as high priority by the scheduler, so that as soon as there is free grid space available these assay droplets are dispensed from their scheduled sources. The on-line testing algorithm is given below.

Table 17.2 Off-Line Testing Results of the Biochip Simulator Using Direct Referencing (in Seconds)

Grid Size	*Sources = 1*		*Sources = 2*		*Sources = 4*		*Sources = 6*		*Sources = 8*			
(50, 50)	*32 faults*	*60 faults*	*32 faults*	*60 faults*	*32 faults*	*60 faults*	*32 faults*	*60 faults*	*32 faults*		*60 faults*	
	942.5	1209.18	459.7	522.75	328	422.75	306.62	391.25	286.5		320.56	
	Sources = 1		*Sources = 2*		*Sources = 4*		*Sources = 6*		*Sources = 8*		*Sources = 10*	
(100, 100)	*32 faults*	*60 faults*	*32 faults*	*60 faults*	*32 faults*	*60 faults*	*32 faults*	*60 faults*	*32 faults*	*60 faults*	*32 faults*	*60 faults*
	2545.18	3447.5	1352.96	1696.6	1140.01	1407.13	987.17	1027.22	714.4	865.7	602.03	752.14

Table 17.3 Off-Line Testing Results of the Biochip Simulator Using Cross Referencing (in Seconds)

Grid Size	*Sources = 1*		*Sources = 2*		*Sources = 4*		*Sources = 6*		*Sources = 8*			
(50, 50)	*32 faults*	*60 faults*	*32 faults*	*60 faults*	*32 faults*	*60 faults*	*32 faults*	*60 faults*	*32 faults*		*60 faults*	
	968.02	1266.11	488.32	621.93	367.56	485.06	319.01	462.68	312.02		377.49	
	Sources = 1		*Sources = 2*		*Sources = 4*		*Sources = 6*		*Sources = 8*		*Sources = 10*	
(100, 100)	*32 faults*	*60 faults*	*32 faults*	*60 faults*	*32 faults*	*60 faults*	*32 faults*	*60 faults*	*32 faults*	*60 faults*	*32 faults*	*60 faults*
	2573.8	3504.43	1392.52	1795.78	1189.19	1469.44	1088.6	1039.61	746.2	922.63	627.55	814.45

Algorithm for on-line testing:

On-line_test *( )*

1. ***Simulated_annealing*** *loop*
{
2. ***Input*** *(Total grid size of the bio-chip, number of sources/sinks available to dispense test droplets, number of sources available to dispense bioassay droplets, bioassay dependency graph)*
3. ***Partition_test*** *(grid space, number of sources, time, fault loacted) /* mentioned in section 3.2*/*
4. */* faults are located. Now the optimization begins*/*
5. *Division of the bioassay dependency graph into macro steps*
6. ***For*** *(each macro step) loop*
{
7. ***Resource_allocation*** *(number of sources available to dispense bioassay droplets, number of in-put droplets of current macro step)*
8. *Calculation of location of mixers*
9. ***If*** *(Fault located)*
10. *Previous macro steps are checked*
11. ***If*** *(previous macro step allocated droplets path passes through fault located)*
{
12. ***Flush*** *(Present macro step)*
13. *Depending which previous macro step is affected,*
macro step = macro step-x.
/ x is the number of previous executed macro steps*/*
14. *Go to step 6.*
}
15. *Mixer location is checked for faulty electrodes*
16. ***If*** *(faulty electrode/electrode is detected) then*
17. ***Reconfigure_mixer_loc*** *(mixer location, fault location/locations)*
*/*mentioned in section 4.3*/*
18. *Calculation of the 3 shortest paths between the source and mixer location for each input droplet of the current macro step*
19. ***PRNG*** *randomly selects any of the 3 paths as the critical path* Δ_D
20. *Critical paths* (Δ_D) *of all droplets are checked for faulty electrodes.*
21. ***If*** *(faulty electrode/electrode is detected in any droplet's path) then*
22. ***Reconfigure*** *(fault location/locations, droplet path)*
23. ***Scheduling*** *(All bioassay droplets running in current macro step, All test droplets running, time)*
24. *Total time (of that simulated_annealing iteration) = Total time (of that simulated_annealing iteration) + time*
*/*time taken to complete all operations of current macro step*/*
} end ***for*** *loop*
} end ***Simulated_annealing*** *loop*

```
25. Final time result = Minimum (Total_time) + ttime, /* final result is the time
    taken for fault diagnosis and optimization of architectures over the
    biochip*/
26. Resource_allocation (x, y)
    {
27. PRNG randomly maps x uniquely to y.
    }
28. Scheduling (All bioassay droplets running in current macro step, All test
    droplets running, time)
    {
29. For (every time step of the current macro step) loop
    {
30.     time + +;
31.     Set_priority (All droplets )
32.     Compare each droplet to the other droplets and check for any clash or
    EWOD droplet violations at current time step.
33.     If (at current time step there is a clash OR EWOD droplet violation) then
        {
34.         Compare priority_assigned value of each droplet
35.     The droplet with lower priority_assigned is stalled and Δ_D is incremented
        }
    } end for loop
36. Return (time)
    }
37  Set_priority(All droplets)
    {
38. If (droplet is test droplet)
39.     Priority_assigned = 100;
40.     else
41.     priority_assigned = number of electrodes remaining to be traversed by
                            every droplet
    }
42. Flush (macro step)
    {
43.     All currently running droplets are stalled
44.     3 shortest distance paths between present location of all droplets and
        their respective sinks/reservoirs are calculated
45.     PRNG selects 1 critical path for each droplet (Δ_D).
46.     All droplets traverse to the sinks following the critical paths.
    }
```

17.5.3 Comparisons between Off-Line and On-Line Testing and Limitations

Tables 17.4 and 17.5 show some simulation results. It is observed that during on-line testing, there is a possibility that a certain untested part of the chip is allocated

Table 17.4 On-Line Testing Results of the Biochip Simulator Using Direct Referencing (in Seconds)

Grid Size	*Sources = 1*		*Sources = 2*		*Sources = 4*		*Sources = 6*		*Sources = 8*			
50 × 50	*12 faults*	*20 faults*	*12 faults*	*20 faults*	*12 faults*	*20 faults*	*12 faults*	*20 faults*	*12 faults*		*20 faults*	
	1503.56	1970.06	907.18	1044.18	589.87	484.62	368.5	453.12	348.37		412.43	
	Sources = 1		*Sources = 2*		*Sources = 4*		*Sources = 6*		*Sources = 8*		*Sources = 10*	
110 × 110	*20 faults*	*36 faults*	*20 faults*	*36 faults*	*20 faults*	*36 faults*	*20 faults*	*36 faults*	*20 faults*	*36 faults*	*20 faults*	*36 faults*
	6050.43	6856.06	2627.5	2960.31	1789.12	2075.43	1289.06	1718.93	1007.62	1338.37	910.75	1139.56

Table 17.5 On-Line Testing Results of the Biochip Simulator Using Cross Referencing (in Seconds)

Grid Size	*Sources = 1*		*Sources = 2*		*Sources = 4*		*Sources = 6*		*Sources = 8*			
50 × 50	*12 faults*	*20 faults*	*12 faults*	*20 faults*	*12 faults*	*20 faults*	*12 faults*	*20 faults*	*12 faults*		*20 faults*	
	1509.5	1976.12	916.87	1049.5	594.87	489.5	374.93	462.56	353.94		417.81	
	Sources = 1		*Sources = 2*		*Sources = 4*		*Sources = 6*		*Sources = 8*		*Sources = 10*	
110 × 110	*20 faults*	*36 faults*	*20 faults*	*36 faults*	*20 faults*	*36 faults*	*20 faults*	*36 faults*	*20 faults*	*36 faults*	*20 faults*	*36 faults*
	6056	6858.25	2633.37	2964.06	1794.93	2080.12	1295	1784.37	1012.56	1342.75	926.81	1145.68

for execution of any operation. If this part turns faulty, there is a certain possibility of flooding to occur.

Also, at any point of time, there are so many test droplets operating on the chip that the optimizations of the bioassays are not completely utilized. If there is an EWOD droplet constraint violation between a test droplet and a bioassays droplet, the test droplet gets higher priority, compelling the latter to stall for a fixed number of micro steps. To schedule the test droplets along with the bioassay droplets results in the complexity of the scheduler to increase significantly. The CPU process time (*time taken by an INTEL PENTIUM 4 2.8 GHz processor*) is reported to increase by 19% as compared to off-line testing. The difference between the execution latency between on-line testing and off-line testing is a mere 3.2%. Another disadvantage of on-line testing is the requirement of storage areas where the mixtures have to be stored. Storage areas or reservoirs are required in case a bioassay is flushed during its execution. Initial volume of the bioassay source droplets requirement is greater, compared to that required by the off-line testing method.

17.6 Future Trends

Currently most of the researchers have focused on fault tolerance and architectural optimizations for individual biochips. This is mainly due to the fact that the existing biochips are prone to defects because of lack of maturity of the relevant manufacturing technologies. Future applications will require development of new materials, technologies, and integration of biochips and other components that will lead to complex embedded systems. Thus, a shift in design paradigm will be needed to develop effective system-level fault tolerance and architectural optimization strategies.

While the current demand for biochips is primarily in the area of genome mapping and sequencing, biochips are rapidly finding inroads in several other areas. For example, the pharmaceutical industry has started to recognize the potential benefits of biochips in drug discovery, since biochips could be used for high throughput screening leading to better drugs. Moreover, new applications are emerging in the areas of environmental monitoring and disease discovery and diagnostics. Environmental monitoring will require development of innovative biochips that act as sensors to detect biochemical agents. Thus, as biochip applications and the market expand into different areas, it will become critical to develop technologies—such as materials, bioinformatics, and chemistry—that will support high-throughput screening and increased complexity for a biochip to function as a lab-on-a-chip.

It has been estimated that the annual R&D spending in pharmaceutical sciences is about $30 billion in the United States, while the in vitro market in the United States is $9 billion [35], suggesting that there is a tremendous market potential for biochips. This has attracted a diverse group of researchers from industry and research organizations. For example, the semiconductor industry has identified that semiconductor devices can have significant impact on certain types of systems that fall under the categories of high margin, low volume, and low margin, high volume. However, it has been well recognized that new materials and devices will have to be developed for biochips to meet the needs of different applications.

Similarly, in Section 17.2 it was identified that complex and highly dense biochips in the future will result in thousands of control pins per unit area. It will be impossible to control individual pins and thus innovative control schemes will be required that would impose considerable constraints on how multiple bioassays can be manipulated concurrently.

Thus, to improve product yield to remain competitive, improve reliability, lifetime, and throughput of the complex biochip-based systems, continual advances in fault tolerance and architectural optimization strategies will be required.

References

[1] K. Chakrabarty and J. Zeng, "Design automation for microfluidics-based biochips," *ACM Journal on Emerging Technologies in Computing Systems*, vol. 1, pp. 186–223, 2005.

[2] J. Chandy, A. Kim, S. Ramkumar, B. Parkes, and P. Banerjee, "An evaluation of parallel simulated annealing strategies with application to standard cell placement," *IEEE Transactions on Computer Aided Design Integrated Circuits Systems*, vol. 16, pp. 398–410, 1997.

[3] A. Cassoto, F. Romeo, and A. Sangiovanni-Vincentelli, "A parallel simulated annealing algorithm for the placement of macro-cells," *IEEE Transactions on Computer Aided Design of Integrated Circuits Systems*, vol. 6, pp. 838–847, 1987.

[4] D. Davids, S. Datta, A. Mukherjee, B. Joshi, and A. Ravindran, "Multiple fault diagnosis in Digital Microfluidic based bio chips," *ACM Journal on Emerging Technologies in Computing Systems*, vol. 2, no. 4, pp. 272–276, 2006.

[5] N. Deb and R. Blanton, "Analysis of failure sources in surface-micromachined MEMS," *Proceedings of the IEEE International Test Conference*, pp. 739–749, 2000.

[6] N. Deb and R. Blanton, "Multi-modal built-in self-test for symmetric Microsystems," *Proceedings of the 22nd IEEE VLSI Test Symposium*, pp.139–147, 2004.

[7] A. Dhayni, S. Mir, and L. Ruffer. "MEMS built-in-self-test using MLS." In *Proceedings of the IEEE European Test Symposium*, pp. 66–71, 2004.

[8] S. Fan, C. Hashi, and C. Kim, "Manipulation of multiple droplets on NxM grid by cross-reference EWOD driving scheme and pressure-contact packaging," *Proceedings IEEE Conference on MEMS*, Kyoto, Japan, pp. 694–697, 2003.

[9] M. Garey and D. Johnson, *Computers and Intractability—A Guide to the Theory of NP Completeness*, Freeman, New York, 1979.

[10] International Technology Roadmap for Semiconductor (ITRS), http://public.itrs.net/Files/2003ITRS/Home2003.htm.

[11] G. Kerkhoff, "Testing philosophy behind the micro analysis system," *Proceedings of the SPIE: Design, Test and Microfabrication of MEMS and MOEMS*, vol. 3680, pp. 78–83, 1999.

[12] G. Kerkhoff and A. Hendriks, "Fault modeling and fault simulation in mixed micro-fluidic microelectronic systems," *Journal of Electronic Testing: Theory and Applications*, vol. 17, pp. 427–437, 2001.

[13] G. Kerkhoff and M. Acar, "Testable design and testing of micro-electro-fluidic arrays," *Proceedings of the IEEE VLSI Test Symposium*, pp. 403–409, 2003.

[14] S. Kirkpatrick, C. Gelatt Jr., and M. Vecchi, "Optimization by Simulated Annealing," *Science*, 220, pp. 671–680, 1983.

[15] A. Kolpekwar and R. Blanton, "Development of a MEMS testing methodology," *Proceedings of the IEEE International Test Conference*, pp. 923–930, 1997.

[16] S. Mir, B. Charlot, and B. Courtois, "Extending fault-based testing to microelectromechanical systems," *Journal of Electronic Testing: Theory and Applications*, vol. 16, pp. 279–288, 2000.

[17] M. Pollack, "Electrowetting-based microactuation of droplets for digital microfluidics," Ph.D. thesis, Duke University, Durham, NC, 2001.

[18] M. Pollack, A. Shenderov, and R. Fair, "Electrowetting-based actuation of droplets for integrated microfluidics," *Lab on a Chip*, vol. 2, pp. 96–101, 2002.

[19] C. Sachen, *VLSI Placement and Global Routing Using Simulated Annealing*, Kluwer Academic, Boston, 1988.

[20] V. Srinivasan, V. Pamula, and R.B. Fair, "An integrated digital microfluidic lab-on-a-chip for clinical diagnostics on human physiological fluids," *Lab on a Chip*, pp. 310–315, 2004.

[21] D. Stewart, and M. Barr, "Rate Monotonic Scheduling," *Embedded Systems Programming*, pp. 79–80, 2002.

[22] F. Su, W. Hwang, A. Mukherjee, and K. Chakrabarty, "Defect-oriented testing and diagnosis of digital microfluidics-based biochips," *Proceedings of the IEEE International Test Conference*, paper 21.2, 2005.

[23] F. Su and K. Chakrabarty, "Testing of droplet-based microelectrofluidic systems," *Proceedings of the IEEE International Test Conference*, pp. 1192–1200, 2003.

[24] F. Su and K. Chakrabarty, "Test planning and test resource optimization for droplet-based microfluidic systems," *Proceedings of the IEEE European Test Symposium*, pp. 72–77, 2004.

[25] F. Su and K. Chakrabarty, "Concurrent testing of droplet-based microfluidic systems for multiplexed biomedical assays," *Proceedings of the IEEE European Test Symposium*, pp. 883–892, 2004.

[26] F. Su, K. Chakrabarty, and V. Pamula, "Yield enhancement of digital microfluidics-based biochips using space redundancy and local reconfiguration," *Proceedings DATE Conference*, 2005.

[27] F. Su and K. Chakrabarty, "Defect tolerance for gracefully degradable microfluidics-based biochips," *Proceedings of IEEE VLSI Test Symposium*, 2005.

[28] F. Su, K. Chakrabarty, and V. Pamula, "Yield enhancement of digital microfluidics-based biochips using space redundancy and local reconfiguration," *Proceedings of the Design, Automation and Test Europe Conference*, 1196–1201, 2005.

[29] F. Su and K. Chakrabarty, "Architectural-level synthesis of digital microfluidics-based biochips," *Proceedings of the IEEE International Conference on Computer Aided Design*, pp. 223–228, 2004.

[30] F. Su and K. Chakrabarty, "Defect tolerance for gracefully-degradable microfluidics-based biochips," *Proceedings of the IEEE VLSI Test Symposium*, pp. 321–326, 2005.

[31] F. Su and K. Chakrabarty, "Module placement for fault-tolerant micofluidics-based biochips," *ACM Transactions on Design Automation of Electronic Systems*, vol. 11, pp. 682–710, 2006.

[32] F. Su, K. Chakrabarty, and R. Fair, "Microfluidics-based biochips: Technology issues, implementation platforms, and design-automation challenges," *IEEE Transactions on Computer-Aided Design of Integrated Circuits and Systems*, vol. 25, no. 2, pp. 211–223, 2006.

[33] T. Thorsen, S. Maerkl, and S. Quake, "Microfluidic large-scale integration," *Science*, vol. 298, no. 5593, pp. 580–584, 2002.

[34] E. Verpoorte and N.F. De Rooij, "Microfluidics meets MEMS," *Proceedings of the IEEE*, vol. 91, no. 6, pp. 930–953, 2003.

[35] T. Xu and K. Chakrabarty, "A cross-referencing-based droplet manipulation method for high-throughput and pin-constrained digital microfluidic arrays," *Proceedings of the Design, Automation and Test in Europe (DATE) Conference*, pp. 552–557, 2007.

[36] http://www.future-fab.com/documents.asp?grID=208&d_ID=2295

CHAPTER 18

Magnetotactic Bacteria as Functional Components in CMOS Microelectronic Systems

Sylvain Martel

The integration of magnetotactic bacteria (MTB) as functional components in CMOS microelectronic systems offers several advantages and possibilities. Acting as bio-actuators, these bacteria can be controlled by a microelectronic circuit to implement novel microsystems. The orientation of magnetotactic bacteria are controlled through magnetotaxis, whereby a torque is induced on a chain of single-domain magnetic nanoparticles named magnetosomes, acting as a compass embedded in each bacterium. Such torque is achieved through a directional local magnetic field created by a small electrical current circulating through selected conductors in the microelectronic circuit. Here, the motility of the bacteria providing a thrust and swimming speed exceeding 4 pN and 200 μm/s, respectively, and combined with controlled swimming paths, is exploited. This allows micro-objects or structures deposited on a CMOS microcircuit to be moved by these bacteria toward desired locations. Hence, depending upon the types and characteristics of the entities being transported, several novel microsystems can be developed. Such controlled bacterial actuation has many advantages compared to known existing methods. It allows specificity in transport or manipulation of micro-objects among other objects having similar dielectric properties. The method requires very low electrical power since the motility of the bacteria is exploited. Furthermore, high frequency electrical signals being modulated to induce forces as in other methods with the possibly of inducing errors on sensitive measurement electronics in close proximity are avoided. There is also no requirement for relatively high voltage levels and no incompatibility with voltage supplied to CMOS microelectronics, allowing further miniaturization of the microsystems.

18.1 Introduction

Especially when miniaturization is required, which is often the case, CMOS microelectronic circuits are critical components of modern microsystems in many instances such as when samples must be transported between various sensors for analysis. As such, *bacterial transport* or *bacterial actuation* where bacteria are used to move or transport samples, may provide a powerful alternative. It is well recognized that flagellated bacteria are very effective for many operations in low Reynolds number regimes [1], as it is the case in microfluidic systems. In particular, the ability to transport micro- or nanoparticles coated with agents or other samples in an aqueous medium has significant potential for applications in micro- nanorobotics and microsystems such as lab-on-a-chip and in micro-total-analysis systems (μTAS) where CMOS microelectronics can play a strategic role. In these microsystems, micromanipulation, microactuation, or transport methods based on an electrical source rely mainly on techniques such as electro-osmosis [2] or dielectrophoresis (DEP) [3]. These methods rely on the principle of electrokinetics, where electrical power is required to induce a force using relatively high frequencies and voltage amplitudes that depend on dielectric properties. The resulting voltage amplitudes are most often incompatible with the embedded electronics that tend toward lower operating voltages, resulting in larger devices through added voltage converters with further increase in the overall size of the system while decreasing electrical power efficiency. As such, controlled transport or actuation methods independent of the dielectric properties of the micro- and nanoscale objects being manipulated are needed.

As an initial proof of concept, the magnetotactic bacteria (MTB) *Magnetospirillum gryphiswaldense* were used to push microbeads in a controlled manner [4].

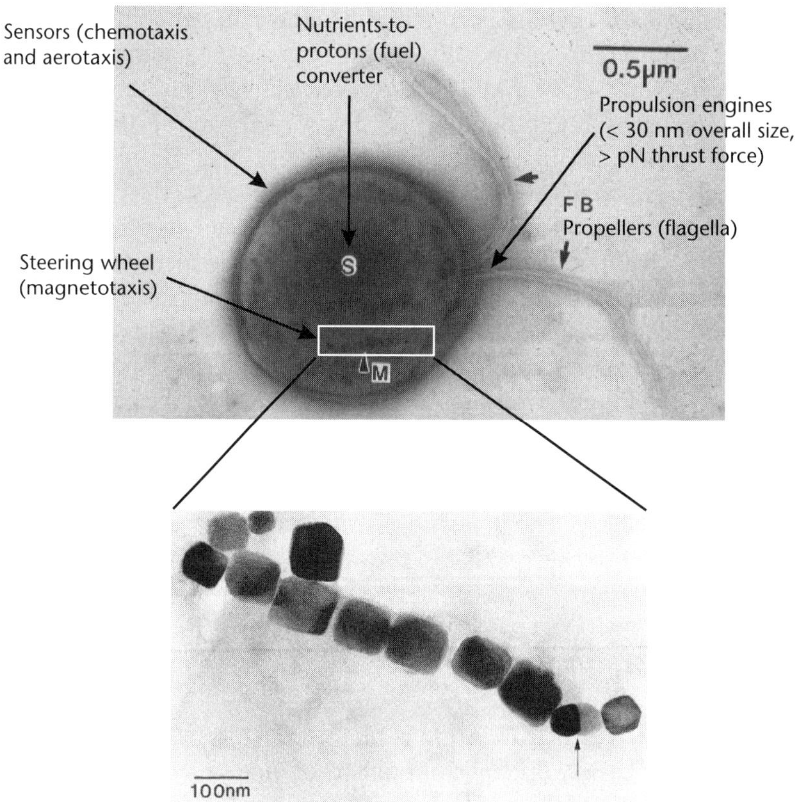

Figure 18.1 Photograph of a magnetotactic bacterium of the type MC-1 with two flagella bundles (FB) represented as a bio-actuator that can be controlled with CMOS circuitries. The chain of magnetosomes (M) is also shown. (Adapted From [12])

The experimental results suggest that MTB can be controlled to operate as micro-actuators in microsystems for various applications including but not limited to the implementation of micro-switches, micro-valves, micro-pistons, or micro-motors. Unlike most bacteria that are based on chemotaxis to detect nutrient gradients and hence influence their motility [5–7], the direction of displacement of MTB [8] with their chain of magnetosomes that are membrane-based nanoparticles of a magnetic iron, although influenced by chemotaxis and aerotaxis, can under specific conditions become mainly influenced by magnetotaxis [9–11], which represents a more suitable interface with electronics and computer-based software.

Since this chain of magnetosomes acts like a compass and enables the bacteria to orient themselves and swim along the lines of a magnetic field, the control method consists of modifying the swimming paths of the MTB with the generation of magnetic field lines using a small programmed electrical current passing through a special embedded conductor network. Compared to other traditional methods, any voltage amplitudes can be used, hence Joule heating is minimized since electrical current is only used to change the direction of the bacteria and not to induce a force on the MTB itself. As such, the power requirement can be minimized by reducing the space between the conductors and by exploiting the motility of MTB.

18.2 Selecting the Type of Magnetotactic Bacteria

All MTB studied so far are motile by means of flagella and hence can be considered for controlled means of transport in microsystems. Although several types of MTB exist and can be found all over the world, the selection process for the type of MTB to be used in microsystems is still constrained, since only a few types can be cultured in artificial or laboratory conditions. Most cultured strains belong to the genus *Magnetospirillum (M.)* and include species such as *M. magnetotactium* strain MS-1 [13], *M. gryphiswaldense* [14], *M. magneticum* strain AMB-1 [15]; the marine vibrios strains MV 1 [16] and MV-2; a marine coccus, strain MC-1 [17]; a marine spirillum, strain MMS-1 (formerly MV-4) [18]; and sulfate-reducing rod-shaped MTB known as *Defulfovibrio magneticus* strain RS-1 [19].

When interfaced to CMOS circuitries while targeting for higher throughputs, higher swimming speeds typically become one of the key factors for selecting the right MTB. In general, the magnetotactic spirilla are at the slower end (<100 μm/s) and the magnetotactic cocci are at the faster end of the range at >100 μm/s. As such, strain MC-1 seems to be a good choice (peak speeds approaching 300 μm/s have been measured experimentally by our group). If the size of the MTB is an important aspect to consider, the MV-4 bacterium is the smallest with a length of ~0.5 μm compared to ~2 μm for the MC-1, but the choice for a smaller cell is done at the cost of slower swimming speeds (in a range of ~30–80 μm/s). Both previous types have two bundles of flagella on one side of the cell and they are classified as polar MTB because they swim (in such a case normally in salt water) persistently in one direction along the magnetic field. Polar MTB, unlike axial MTB, are generally more suitable since they are usually more predictable when controlling their swimming directions for applications in microsystems. For instance, some cells have two bundles of flagella on both ends. These MTB swim in both directions along the magnetic field lines with frequent reversals of swimming directions with approximately the same number of bacteria swimming in each direction. Because of this behavior, they are classified as axial MTB. The *Magnetospirillum gryphiswaldense* bacterium is one example; it usually lives in fresh water and has a length varying between ~1 and 3 μm with a width of ~0.5 μm. This MTB has swimming speeds in the range of ~40–80 μm/s.

18.3 Bacterial Flagellated Nanomotors

Here, mechanical energy replacing electrical energy for actuation or transport in fluid is provided by the flagellated nanomotor or rotational engine of each MTB. As depicted in Figure 18 2, the shape of the bacterial flagellum consists of a 20 nanometer (nm)-thick hollow tube. It is helical in shape and has a sharp bend just outside of the outer membrane forming a "hook" that allows the helix to point directly away from the cell. A shaft runs between the hook and the basal body, passing through protein rings in the cell's membrane that act as bearings.

The bacterial flagellum is driven by a rotary engine composed of protein, located at the flagellum's anchor point on the inner cell membrane. The engine is powered by proton motive force, (i.e., by the flow of protons). The rotor transports protons across the membrane, and is turned in the process. The rotor alone can operate at 6,000 to 17,000 rpm, but with the flagellar filament attached usually only reaches 200 to 1000 rpm. Counterclockwise rotation of polar flagella thrust the cell forward

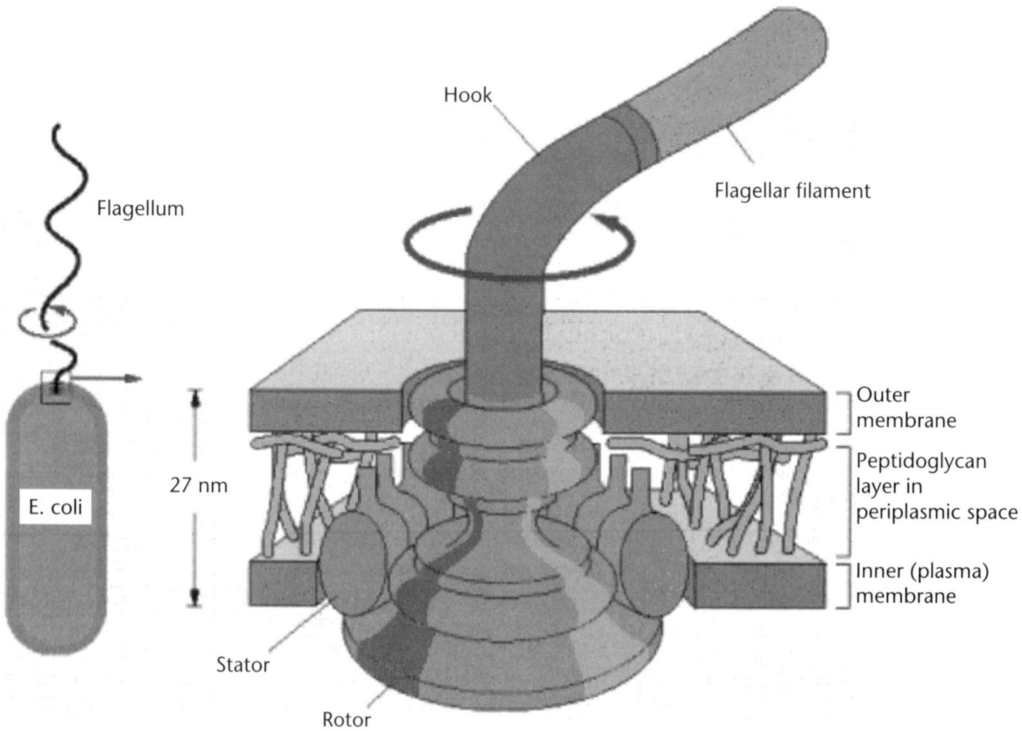

Figure 18.2 Schematic representing the bacterial flagellated nanomotor (From [http://www.ncbi.nlm.nih.gov/books/bv.fcgi?rid=mboc4.figgrp.2879]).

with the flagella trailing behind. Periodically, the direction of rotation is briefly reversed, causing what is known as a "tumble" in which the cell seems to thrash about in place. This results in the reorientation of the cell. When moving in a favorable direction, "tumbles" are unlikely; however, when the cell realizes under normal conditions that its direction of motion is unfavorable (e.g., away from a chemical attractant), a tumble may occur, with the chance that the cell will be thus reoriented in the correct direction.

18.4 Thrust Force and Terminal Velocity

For actuation or transport purpose, the thrust force provided by each MTB is the key factor to consider. The thrust force for the MC-1 MTB can be evaluated with the same equation used to compute the thrust force for a spherical object by considering the spherical shape of the cell of the MC-1 bacterium (see Figure 18.1). The thrust force can then be estimated discounting the effect of the trailing flagella from Stokes' equation as

$$F_{THRUST} = v_T 6\pi\eta r \tag{18.1}$$

with v_T and η being the terminal velocity and the viscosity of the medium, respectively. In water at room temperature, the thrust force for most flagellated bacteria is in the range of 0.3–0.5 pN. For the MC-1 MTB, because its cell size is approximately the same as other bacteria but with a much higher terminal velocity, its thrust force can be above 4 pN (peak thrust force of 4.7 pN has been recorded experimentally by our group for a small percentage of the bacterial samples), making it a very good candidate as bio-actuators in microsystems. The speed distribution of the MC-1 bacteria in an aqueous medium at room temperature and measured by our research group is depicted in Figure 18.3.

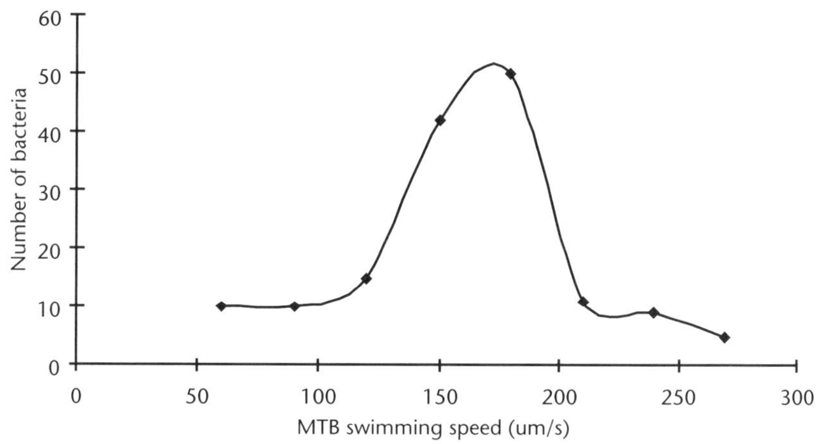

Figure 18.3 Swimming speed distribution of the unloaded and non pre-selected MC-1 bacteria in an aqueous medium at room temperature.

18.5 Controlling the Swimming Direction of MTB Through Magnetotaxis

A magnetic field will exert a torque on a ferromagnetic material (such as magnetite) or on a material with diamagnetic anisotropy. Only ferromagnets are able to produce a response to a field as weak as the geomagnetic field (0.5 Gauss) that is detectable against thermal motion. A magnetite chain in magnetotactic bacteria is rotated by a magnetic field because of the torque exerted on their magnetite particles. *Magnetospirillum gryphiswaldense* bacteria typically show the best result in term of synthesis of magnetosomes (membrane-based magnetite nanoparticles) with a longer chain than the ones typically found in other MTB. Hence, this long chain of magnetosomes imparts to the MTB a magnetic moment that generates sufficient torque so that the bacteria can align themselves to magnetic field lines. This is referred to as magnetotaxis. Compared to MC-1 and MV-4 with a number of magnetosomes varying typically between 5 and 12 or 14, the chain can have up to ~50 cubo-octahedral magnetosomes (Fe_3O_4) when grown by microaerophilic *Magnetospirillum* strains and a microaerobic fermentation procedure.

The directional magnetic field lines can be generated from a permanent magnet or in the case of interfacing with CMOS microelectronic systems, from an electrical current flowing in a conductor with directional magnetic field lines following the "right hand grip rule." We recall that the magnetic field in Tesla (T) at a radial distance r in meters from the conductor can be computed from the well-known Ampere's law as

$$B = \frac{\mu_0 I}{2\pi r} \tag{18.2}$$

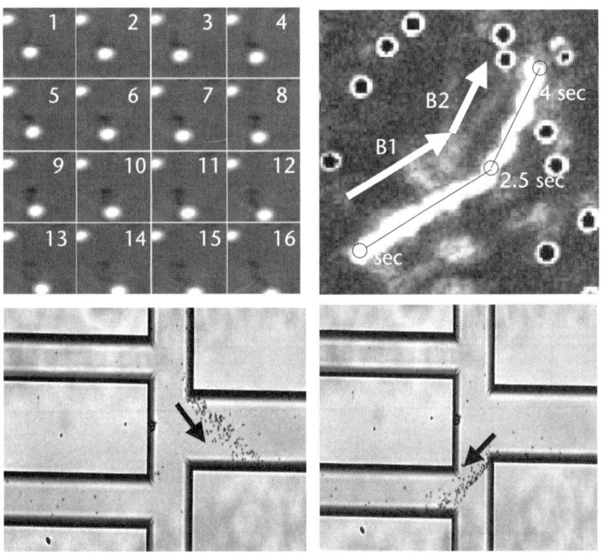

Figure 18.4 A single MTB pushing a 3 micrometer bead (top-left); the same MTB pushing the bead and directed to turn left 30 degrees after 2.5 seconds (top-right), B1 and B2 indicated direction of the magnetic field; swimming path of a swarm of MTB being controlled inside microfluidic channels (bottom).

where I is the electrical current in amperes and $\mu_0 = 4\pi \times 10^{-7}$Tm/A is the permeability of free space. We also recall that 1 T = 10,000 Gauss and that the geomagnetic field is 0.5 Gauss.

The swimming direction of MTB is influenced not only by magnetotaxis but also by aerotaxis and chemotaxis. Aerotaxis is defined as the movement of an organism, especially a bacterium, toward or away from air or oxygen, while chemotaxis is defined as directed movement of a cell or organism toward (or away from) a chemical source. Although at lower magnetic field intensities, (i.e., around the geomagnetic field of 0.5 Gauss), magnetotaxis has an influence on the swimming directions of MTB, previous experiments conducted by our group show that a higher magnetic field with a minimum value of approximately 3 Gauss (or even less) provides the best control and responses of the MTB from directional commands generated by an electrical source by making magnetotaxis the predominant factor over chemotaxis and aerotaxis.

Although electrical power is not required to provide mechanical force since the motility of the MTB is exploited, electrical power is still required when interfaced to CMOS circuitries to control the direction of motion of the MTB, (i.e., to induce a torque on the chain of magnetosomes of the MTB). From Eq. 18.2, one can see that to minimize the electrical current required for controlling the direction of motion of the MTB, the radial distance (being in this particular case the distance between the conductor and the chain of magnetosomes embedded in the MTB) must be reduced appropriately. But by doing so, the displacement speed of the MTB must be taken into account since faster responses from potential sensors and/or faster control command from the electronic system will be required.

In some cases, instead of a planar implementation, a more complex implementation on CMOS circuitries can be considered to increase the magnitude of the magnetic field while minimizing the electrical current. For instance, compared to a straight conductor, a loop would already improve the magnitude of the magnetic field produced using the same value of electrical current since the magnitude of the magnetic field at the center of a loop with a radius R is

$$B = \frac{\mu_0 I}{2R} \tag{18.3}$$

Such a loop can be implemented on a CMOS circuit as depicted in Figure 18.6. Furthermore, if the implementation complexity permits, an increase of the magnetic field can be achieved with a very small electrical current by increasing the number of loops N in a coil or micro-coil where

$$B = N\frac{\mu_0 I}{2R} \tag{18.4}$$

It is also important to understand and recall circular magnetic fields distribution and intensity when current is passed through a solid conductor. In such a case, the magnetic field strength varies from zero at the inner center of the conductor and will reach a maximum value at its surface and will decay farther away from the surface of the same conductor. Knowing for a given electrical current value that the field strength at the surface of the conductor decreases as the radius of the conductor

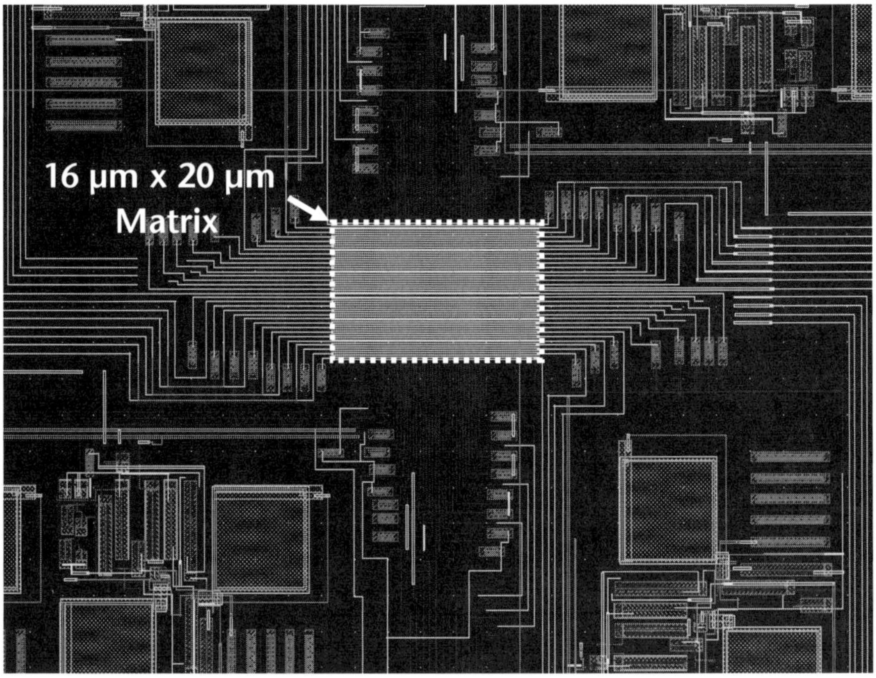

(a)

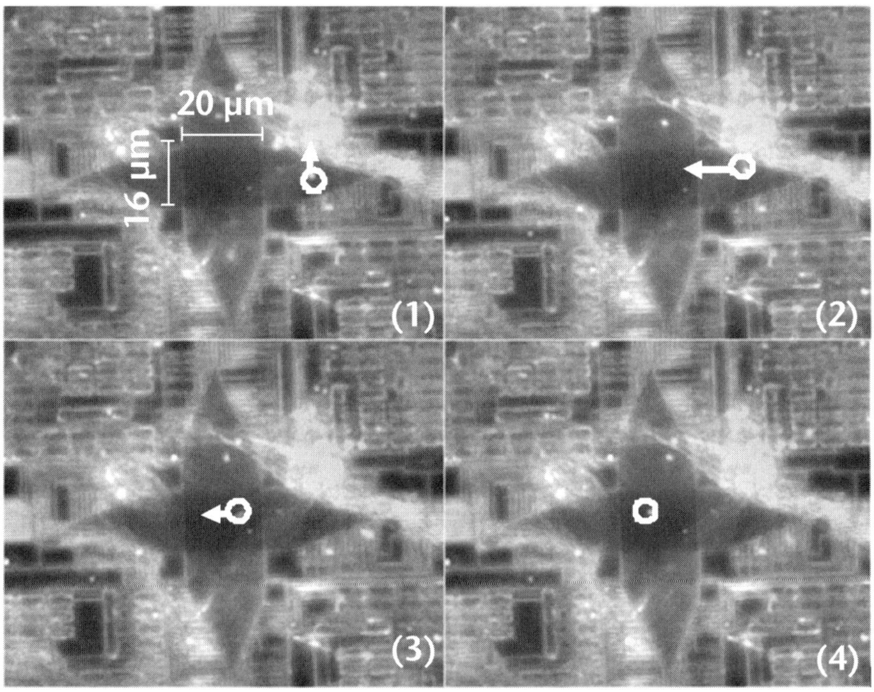

(b)

Figure 18.5 Planar implementation of a grid of conductors spaced 330 nm apart on a CMOS circuit with CAD representation (a) and the actual implementation (b). (From [20])

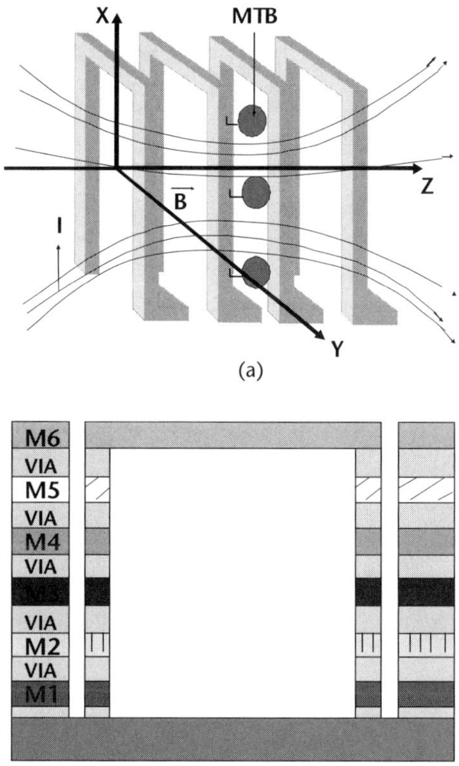

(b)

Figure 18.6 Example of the implementation of coils using the CMOS process. (a) Schematic of the coils implementation showing the orientation of the magnetic field and the MTB being trapped inside. (b) CMOS implementation of a coil showing the various stacked layers.

increases, then a reduction of the electrical power required for influencing the direction of MTB can be achieved by reducing the diameter of these conductors. On the other hand, the designer must keep in mind that reducing the diameter of the conductor will also limit the amount of current that can be carried.

In Figure 18.7, for instance, the direction of the electrical current determines in which direction the MTB will swim around the conductor. This can be exploited to create new functions. In some cases, space of only a few micrometers can be provided between the conductor and the substrate to allow 360-degree controlled rotational motion of the MTB. In other applications, the conductor can be deposited directly on the substrate providing constrained motion, 180 degrees for instance.

A technique to maintain the MTB close to the surface of the conductor to avoid the need for larger electrical currents to attract them in regions of higher field intensity is to constrain them using a thin layer of an aqueous medium around the conductor. This is depicted in Figure 18.8.

Beside rotational movements around a conductor, movement along the same conductor is also possible. Furthermore, bidirectional displacement of the MTB along the same conductor or any substrate as depicted in Figure 18.9 is also possible, providing two transport or fluidic channels for the MTB.

Furthermore, it is possible to simplify the CMOS control circuitry and requirement for directing the MTB by exploiting various geometries for the fluidic channels

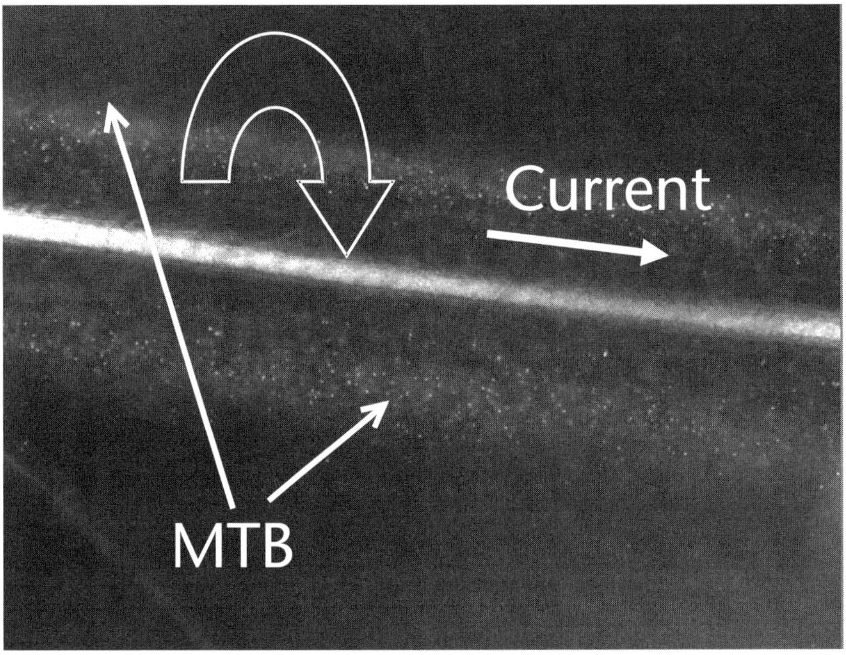

Figure 18.7 Controlled rotational motion of MTB using directional electrical current. Reversing the direction of the electrical current will reverse the rotational swimming direction of the MTB around the conductor.

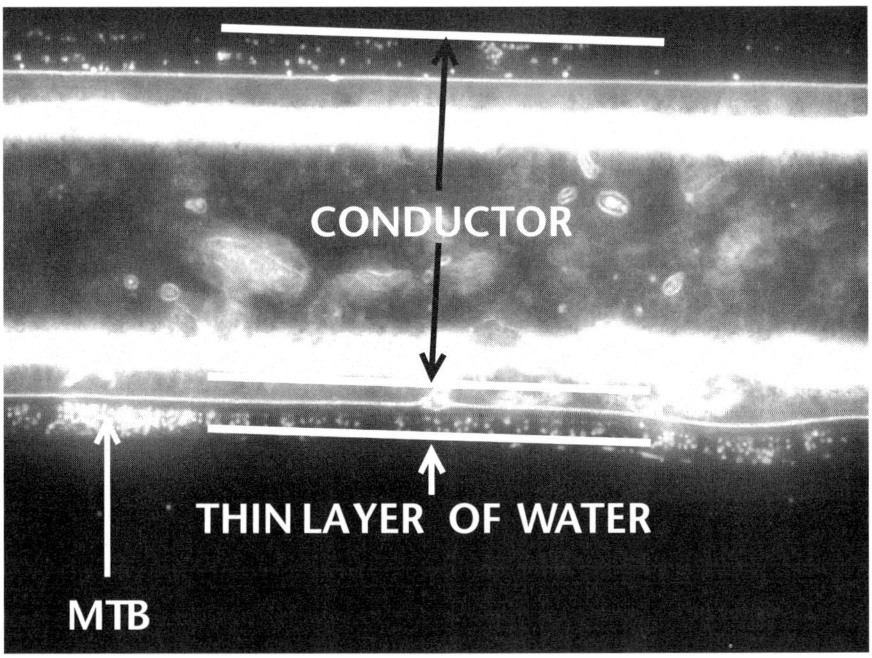

Figure 18.8 MTB being constrained near the conductor through a thin layer of water.

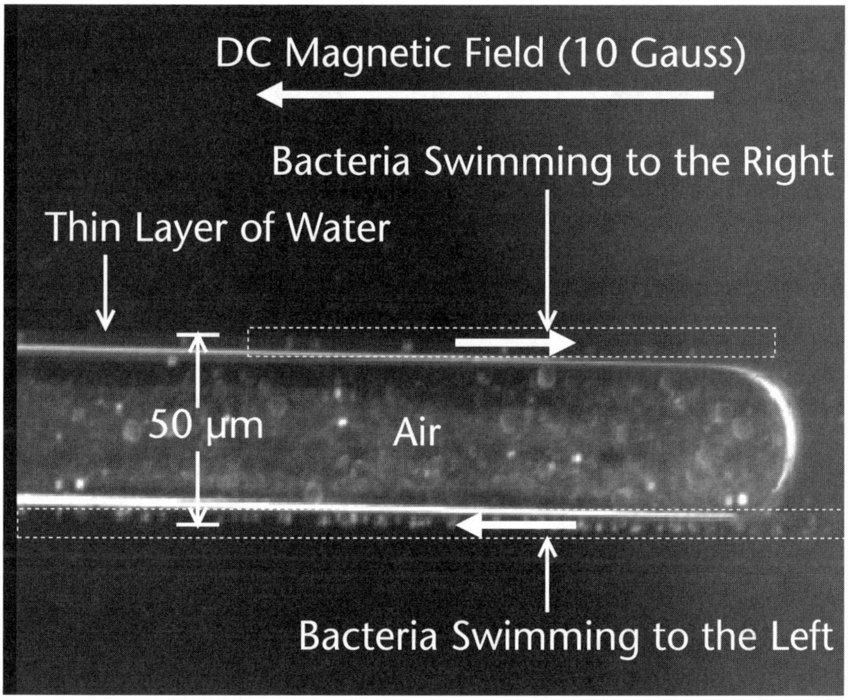

Figure 18.9 MTB swimming in both directions simultaneously.

[21]. For instance, when constrained through a thin layer of water, any angular turns of the MTB can be achieved without modifying the direction of the magnetic field or electrical current. In Figure 18.9, for instance, turns of 180 degrees in the swimming path of the MTB are achieved without changing the direction of the magnetic field.

Capillary forces can then be exploited to create more channels for the bacterial carriers as depicted in Figure 18.10. In Figure 18.10(a), four channels are created through capillary force at the corners of a square fluidic channel, thus increasing by four the density of fluidic channels where MTB can travel compared to more traditional approaches. As demonstrated in Figure 18.9 and represented schematically in

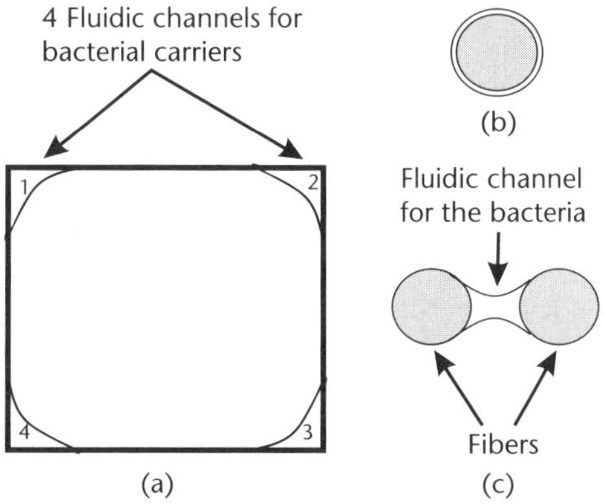

Figure 18.10 Exploitation of capillary force to increase the density of routing channels for the MTB.

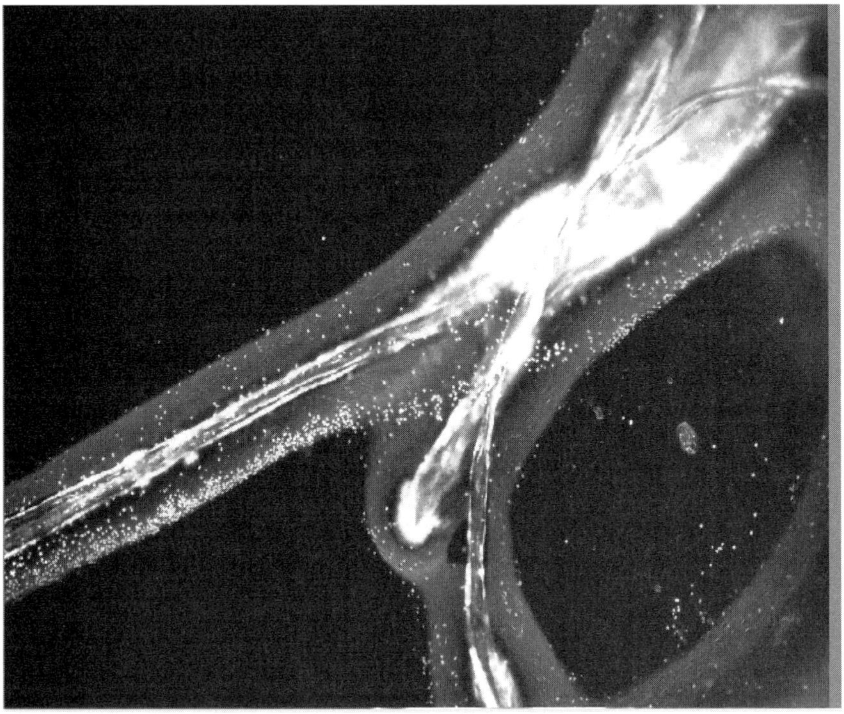

Figure 18.11 More complex pathways for MTB implemented by exploiting capillary forces. The white structures are fibers, the thin layer of water retained by capillary force can be seen as grey regions surrounding the fibers. The white dots inside the thin layer of water are MTB swimming along the fibers.

Figure 18.10(b), a thin layer of an aqueous medium can be retained on the surface of a conductor or fiber to easily create fluidic routes for the MTB. Liquid retained by capillary force between two fibers or conductors can also provide additional routes for the MTB as well as a bridge for electrical contacts. Taking advantage of the capillary forces configurations depicted in Figure 18.10(b) and Figure 18.10(c), complex routing networks that can be placed on top of CMOS circuitries can be implemented as depicted in Figure 18.11.

18.6 Controlling the Velocity of Bacterial Carriers by Modifying Viscosity and/or Temperature

From Eq. 18.1, one can see that for a given maximum potential thrust force provided by the MTB, the terminal velocity will decrease with an increase of the viscosity of the medium. Hence, it seems that one way to achieve higher actuation or bacterial transport speed is to decrease the viscosity of the medium by increasing the temperature. Most ordinary liquids have viscosities on the order of 1 to 1000 mPa·s and their values can be changed with temperature. For instance, the viscosity of water at 0, 20, 40, and 100°C is 1.79, 1.00, 0.65, and 0.28 mPa·s, respectively. On the other hand, non-pathogenic bacteria such as the MC-1 MTB are influenced by the temperature as depicted in Figure 18.12. It shows a constant reduction of the swimming speeds coupled with a significant decrease of the operational time period for bacterial actuation or transport.

Therefore, CMOS circuitries can be used to change the viscosity of the medium through Joule heating, especially for very small liquid samples. Nonetheless, this could be done at the cost of a continuous reduction in terminal velocities and lifetime of the bacterial carriers and eliminate the gain achieved when considering a reduction of the viscosity alone. On the other hand, this approach may be very attractive when velocity control using CMOS microelectronics is suitable, especially when a medium having high changes in viscosity for small temperature changes is used in order to keep MTB active for a longer time, while maintaining their maximum velocities also for a longer time. The use of glycerin as a medium is one example. The viscosity of glycerin varies as much as 1140 mPa·s between 20 and 40°C, but the large change in viscosity for a relatively small change in temperature is paid for by much lower velocities, considering that for glycerin, η = 1420 mPa·s at 20°C. Nonetheless, in all cases, attention must be paid about unwanted Joule heating generated from the CMOS circuitries despite the fact that the power requirement can be reduced when exploiting the motility of MTB.

If dynamic change in viscosity is not an issue, a liquid medium with the appropriate viscosity can be selected (or adjusted) with values ranging from 1 to 1000 mPa·s as specified earlier. One example with glycerol is depicted in Figure 18.13.

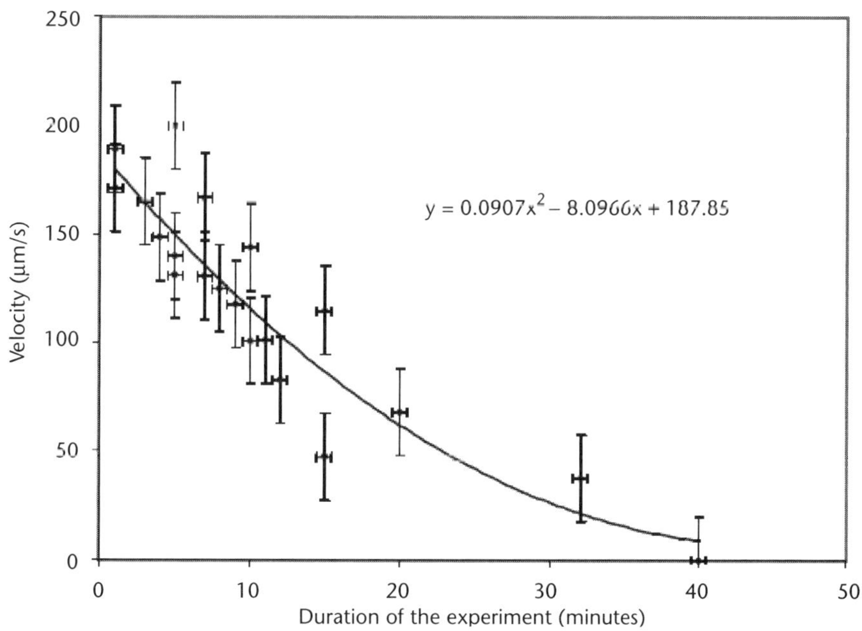

Figure 18.12 Swimming speed of unloaded MC-1 MTB in blood at 37°C. (The viscosity of blood at such temperature is 3–4 mPa·s.)

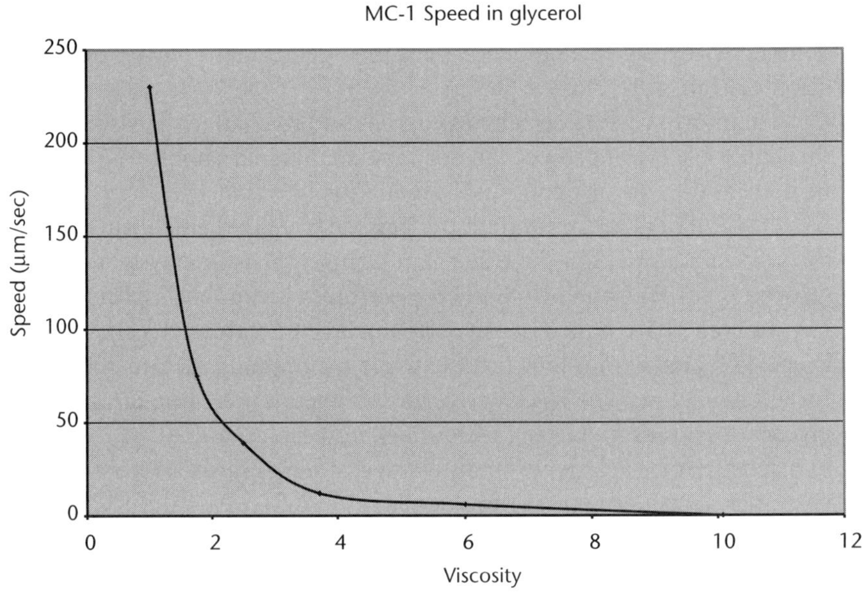

Figure 18.13 Setting the average MTB swimming speed in glycerol by modifying viscosity.

18.7 Loading the Bacterial Carriers

As each bacterium is used as a controlled carrier, the loading method is an important aspect to consider. In microsystems such as lab-on-a-chip or μTAS, beads coated with specific agents or molecules under study are often used to bring samples between sensors or analysis sites.

Bonding or attaching such beads to the cell of the MTB is typically done using polyclonal antibody produced in our particular case against MC-1. Fluorescent beads can also be used when tracking under fluoroscopy is desired. For the preparation of polyclonal antibody-coated fluorescent beads, 50 μl of Sulfate FluoSpheres® beads (2% solids) (Invitrogen) are washed three times by suspending the beads in PBS-1X, centrifuging, and removing the liquid by aspiration. Then, polyclonal anti-MC-1 antibodies are added to beads. One milliliter final volume in PBS-1X is taken and rotated overnight at 4°C. The beads are then washed three times in PBS-1X and one time with BPS-2X.

To attach the bacteria to the beads, the beads and the MC-1 bacteria are suspended in PBS solutions. The anti-MC-1 antibody-coated beads are then suspended at a working concentration of 10^9/L. MC-1 attachment is then achieved by introducing the microorganisms into the bead suspension at a concentration of approximately double that of the bead concentration. The suspension of beads and MC-1 bacteria is left for no longer than 30 minutes before experimentation or processing, by which time a sufficient number of MC-1 bacteria should be attached to the surface of the bead.

First, transport of samples can be done by attaching a single coated microbead to each MC-1 cell as depicted in the schematic in Figure 18.15(a) with a real imple-

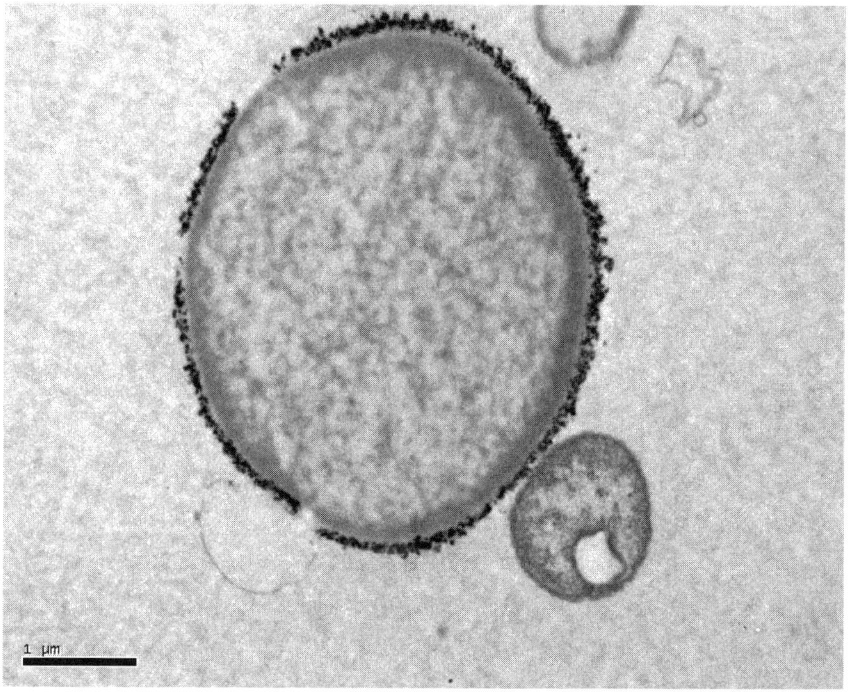

Figure 18.14 Attachment of a microbead (larger sphere in the picture) to a single MTB (smaller sphere in the photograph). The black dots around the bead are the antibodies.

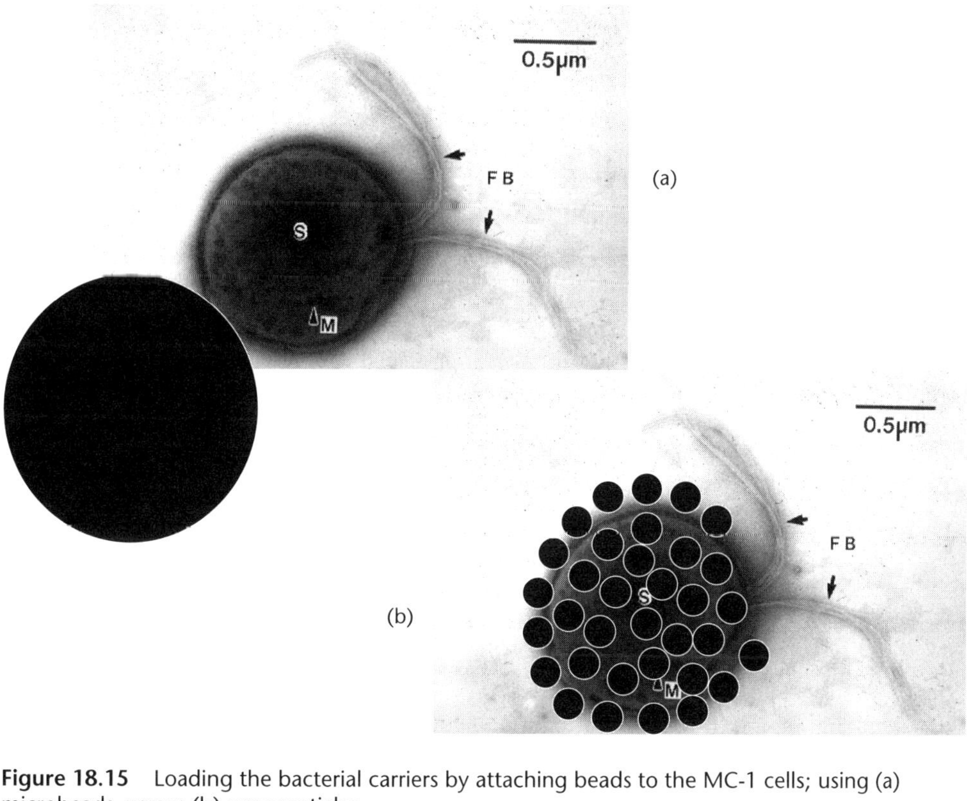

Figure 18.15 Loading the bacterial carriers by attaching beads to the MC-1 cells; using (a) microbeads, versus (b) nanoparticles.

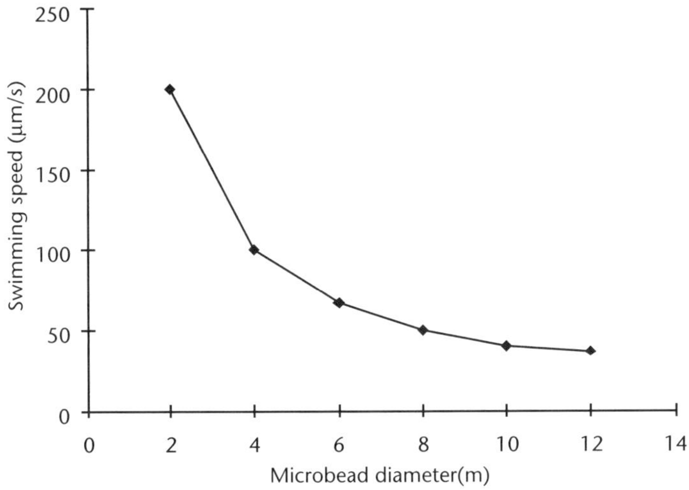

Figure 18.16 Velocity of a microbead being pushed by a single MTB for various bead diameters. The graph assumes that the swimming speed of unloaded (i.e., before being attached to the microbead) MTB is 200 μm/s. The last part with larger beads of approximately 10 micrometers is hypothetical since with such large beads, the movements of the bead being transported by a single MTB become more unpredictable.

mentation depicted in the top left portion of Figure 18.4 and in Figure 18.14 for a much larger bead. In such a case, the bacterium will push or pull the bead, depending on the conditions. If the diameter of the bead increases beyond the diameter of the MC-1 cell, (i.e., approximately 2 μm), the bacterium will experience an increase of the drag force typically leading to a more significant decrease of the swimming speed of the loaded bacterial carrier. This is illustrated in the graph of Figure 18.16.

It becomes difficult when the diameter of the bead becomes larger, to maintain adequate planned trajectories (i.e., maintaining straight swimming patterns when desired) while maintaining an adequate transport speed. To correct for such deficiencies, another approach using charged nanoparticles is shown in Figure 18.15(b). By distributing the charge or sample more evenly on the MC-1 cell, better control and speed can be achieved. The drawback is that it is difficult to maintain the same number of nanoparticles or charge among the bacterial carriers and in some cases, it may put constraints on the sensing method being used, as described in the next section.

18.8 Integrating MTB-Based Carrier Detection and Tracking in CMOS Circuits

Various sensors can be integrated in microsystems where bacterial transport is being considered. But one type of the sensor needed when open-loop control is not appropriate and closed-loop control of individual bacterial carriers is essential to synchronize navigational commands from the CMOS electronic system with the position of specific MTB, is an embedded detection and tracking system. Hence, to detect MTB, variations in impedance between the microelectrodes in microchannels often provide the most convenient method due to compatibility with CMOS electronics, low power requirement, and compactness.

In some applications, a single microbead being transported by a single MTB as depicted in Figure 18.15(a) can be coated with phages or antibodies specific to a target type of pathogenic bacteria. In this particular microsystem developed for the fast detection of pathogenic bacteria [22], agglomeration of MTB-tagged microbeads are controlled by a CMOS microelectronic circuit to sweep through a sample containing several species of bacteria. When a MTB-tagged microbead comes in contact with a target pathogenic bacterium, the latter will "stick" to it, otherwise it is repulsed, allowing specificity in the detection method. Once sweeps of the sample medium have been performed by controlling the swimming paths of the MTB-tagged microbeads, the latter are brought toward the CMOS detection circuitries embedded in the same circuit used to control the swimming paths of the MTB. This is a perfect example showing that not only MTB-tagged microbeads can be detected and hence tracked when navigating in a network of microfuidic channels, but also additional detection capability can be implemented such as the detection of target species.

In this particular example, an increase in impedance will be observed for an MTB-tagged microbead with a target bacterium attached due to the additional capacitance and resistance of the pathogenic bacteria's membrane and cytoplasm. The number of target bacteria present in a sample will then be able to be determined by detecting how many MTB-microbeads have bacteria attached after sweeping the sample. This is shown in the equivalent circuit model of the MTB carrier system in Figure 18.17. Based on the circuit model, a CMOS chip can be designed and fabricated.

Instead of directly measuring the variation in impedance, which is extremely small for a single bacterium, a circuit that could record the signal delay time due to a change in impedance can be developed. Simulation results show that micrometer-size beads or bacteria can be detected using this approach.

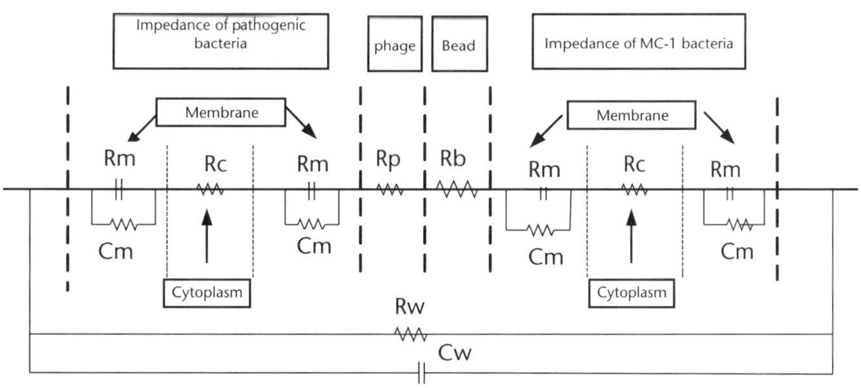

Figure 18.17 Impedance between the electrodes when a pathogenic bacterium is attached on the microbead. Parameters R_b, R_p, R_w, and R_m denote the resistance of the microbead, phage, media, and cell membrane respectively. R_c is the resistance of the cytoplasm. C_m and C_w represent the capacitance of the cell's membrane and medium between the electrodes respectively.

As such, a circuit based on resistive impedance detection can be designed. Here, two reference currents corresponding to referencing impedance are injected between a pair of electrodes and the voltage drop created gives information about the range of impedance present between the same electrodes. Impedances ranging from approximately 3 kΩ to at least 100 MΩ can be detected. Here, the detection of large impedances is limited to the operational frequencies and leakage currents.

An improved version (Figure 18.18) of the circuit in terms of sensitivity can be achieved based on the integration time of currents. Due to the presence of the double-layer capacity at low voltage, this new circuitry can use DC current to flow between a pair of electrodes. However, when one tries to inject a current between a pair of electrodes, the present capacitance charges follow a slope proportional to the value of the capacitance and with an initial voltage value proportional to the resistance between the same electrodes. Since the capacitance between electrodes is dominated by the double-layer capacitance, the overall value of the capacitance does not change according to what flows between the electrodes. Moreover, the value of resistance changes and thus the initial value of the integration curve changes. By setting a reference voltage, we can distinguish different levels of impedance between the electrodes using the time to get to that voltage.

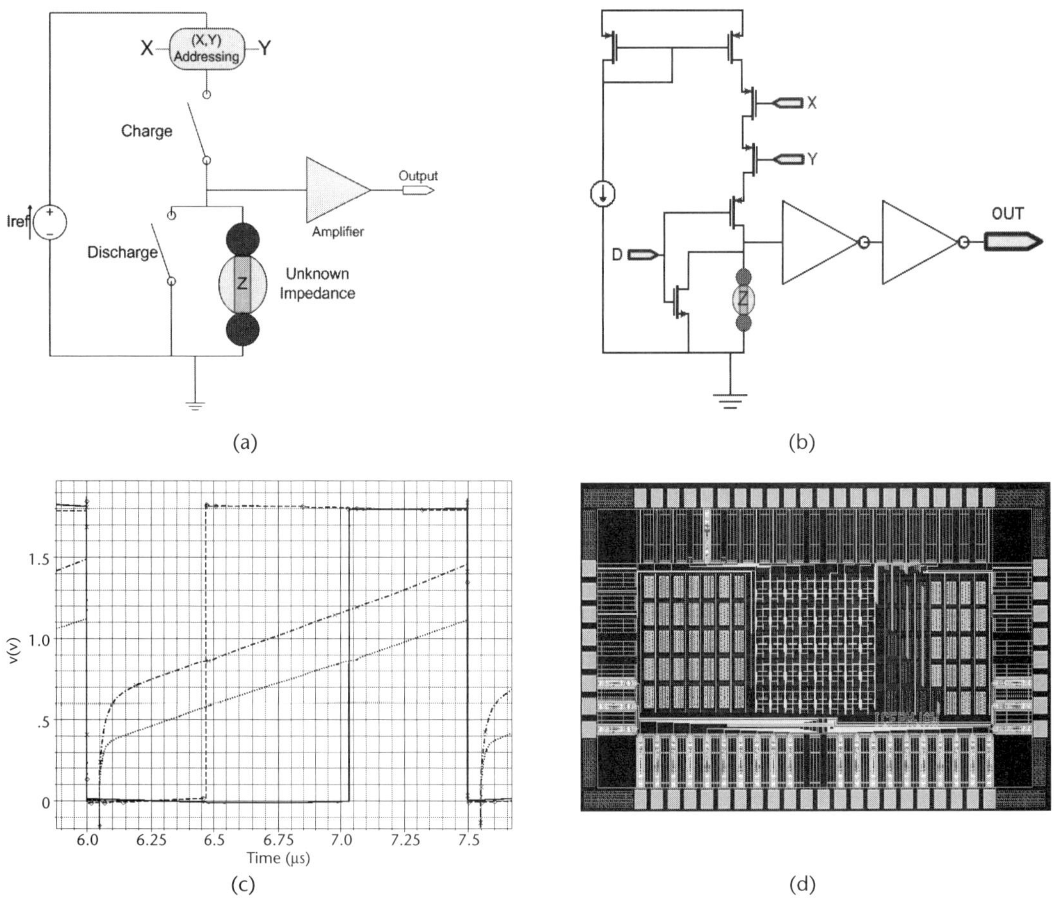

Figure 18.18 One possible version of the detection circuit; (a) Block diagram of the detection circuit; (b) Circuit schematic; (c) Results; (d) Circuit layout.

18.9 Sensing Microelectrodes

Different microfabrication techniques are available to implement microelectrodes used to detect the bacteria. Noble materials such as gold and platinum are very good candidate material for the fabrication of microelectrodes because of their good biocompatibility and anti-corrosion capability. Aluminum is also often considered due to its compatibility with conventional CMOS processes.

The sizes and geometries of microelectrodes have a direct impact on the resolution of the biosensors. Simulations based on accurate models are often used for polymer microbeads, for instance to investigate the effect of microchannel and electrode geometry, object size, and object position against sensitivity, in order to optimize the sensor prior to validation with experimental results.

It is often desirable to increase the surface area of each electrode in order to decrease the electrode's impedance. Often, bias or leakage currents from the detection circuit circulating in a too-high impedance electrode will cause the detection channel to saturate. Hence, the impedance of the electrodes is often chosen considering the characteristics of the front-end circuitries. On the other hand, although large electrodes will provide ore flexibility and ease the design of the detection circuitry, they must be small enough to be sensitive to the small objects being detected. Hence, a compromise between sensitivity, specificity, and limitations of the detection circuitries must be taken into consideration. For MTB-tagged microbeads, for instance, electrodes with overall dimensions of approximately 20 μm × 20 μm provide that kind of good compromise.

The orientation of the microelectrodes will also affect the detection sensitivity. Two fundamental orientations can be considered: planar and face to face. The results are shown in Figure 18.19. The planar electrodes are placed side by side on the bottom of the microchannel, with a center-to-center separation of 35 μm. For the face-to-face electrodes, one is placed on top of the channel and the other on the bottom of the channel (separation of 20 μm). Polymer microbeads with diameters from 2 μm to 15 μm are placed in the center of the sensing region for both electrode orientations to investigate the difference in sensitivity over a range of microbead sizes.

The volume of the sensing region also directly affects the detection threshold of the device. The sensing region volume is the volume of space in between the electrodes. In order to investigate the effect of the size of this volume, the channel depth is reduced while using face-to-face electrodes. The simulation is performed with channel depths from 20 μm down to 5 μm in 2.5 μm decrements. A polymer microbead of 4 μm in diameter is placed in the center of the sensing region and the relative impedance change calculated for each different depth. Results are shown in Figure 18.20.

The horizontal and vertical position of the microbead within the channel is investigated using face-to-face electrodes and an 8 μm polymer bead. For the vertical position, the bead is initially located 0.5 μm below the source electrode and is moved to 0.5 μm above the ground electrode in 2.75 μm increments. Results are shown in Figure 18.21. For the horizontal position, only the x-direction must be investigated, as the electric field is approximately constant in the y-direction. Here, the x-direction refers to a vector along the length of the channel and the y-direction is a vector along the width of the channel. Since the electrodes basically take up the entire width of

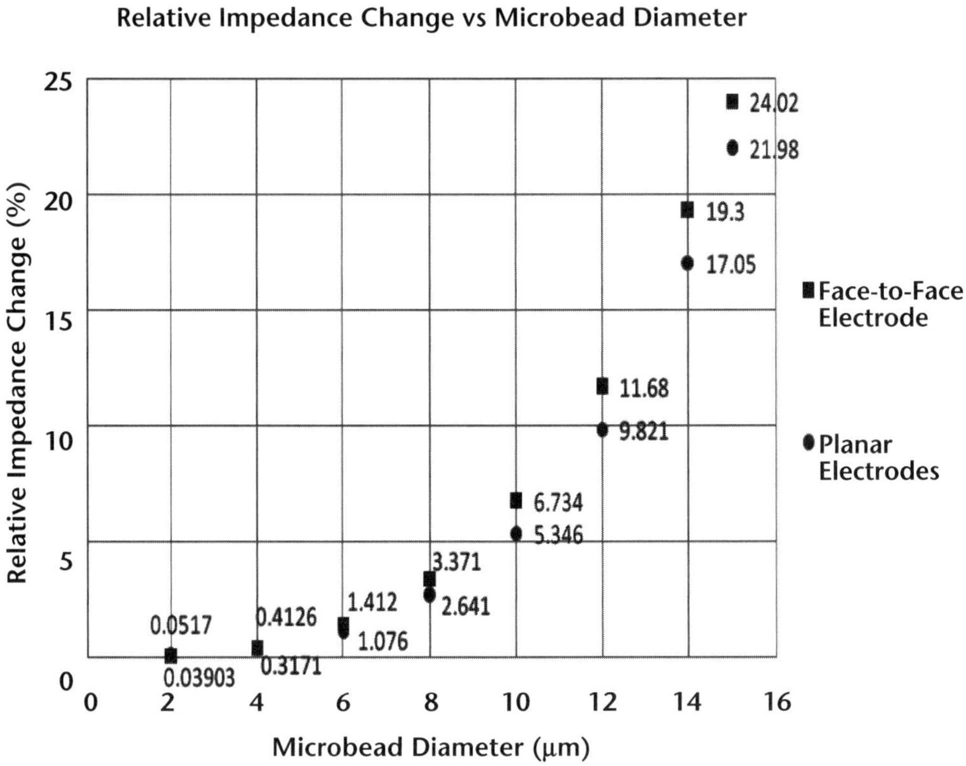

Figure 18.19 Graph of the relative impedance change at 1 MHz for microbeads of various diameters using microelectrodes in face to face and planar orientation.

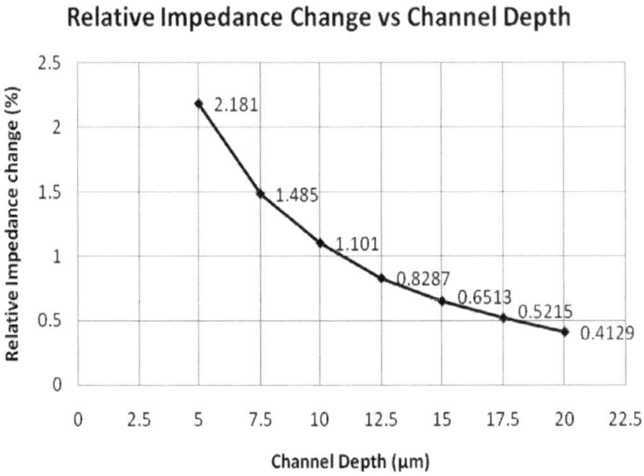

Figure 18.20 Graph of the relative impedance change at 1 MHz for a 4 μm bead with numerous different channel depths. Electrodes are in face-to-face orientation.

the channel, the y-position of the bead should not affect the impedance change because the electric field is symmetric. To investigate the effect of the x-position of the bead, only half of the electrode is considered because of the symmetry of the electric field. The bead is centered in the sensing region and moved out along the x-direction in 5 μm increments until its center is 20 μm from the center of the sensing region. Results are shown in Figure 18.22.

Validation can be done using an impedance analyzer (e.g., Agilent 4924A) to record the impedance signal across the electrodes. The impedance analyzer is programmed to produce a 0.5 V sinusoidal signal at a frequency of 1 MHz. Each measurement cycle contains 400 points. The impedance is measured by use of an auto balancing bridge method. The microchip is placed onto an optical microscope with an attached camera for observation during impedance measurements. The microchannel is filled with de-ionized water containing a low concentration of 8 μm polymer beads. The beads flow through the microchannel (or can be transported by MTB) and the impedance is recorded as the beads move between the microelectrodes.

The variation of the impedance caused by single or multiple 8 μm polymer beads is recorded. Figure 18.23(a) presents an image of the microbeads passing through a pair of electrodes. Figure 18.23(b) shows the impedance pulse recorded when such beads pass through the detection region. The observed pulse increases by approximately 2.7% when compared with the reference signal.

Other examples of microchannels that can be interfaced with CMOS MTB control and tracking/detection circuits (one example is shown in Figure 18.24) are depicted in Figure 18.25.

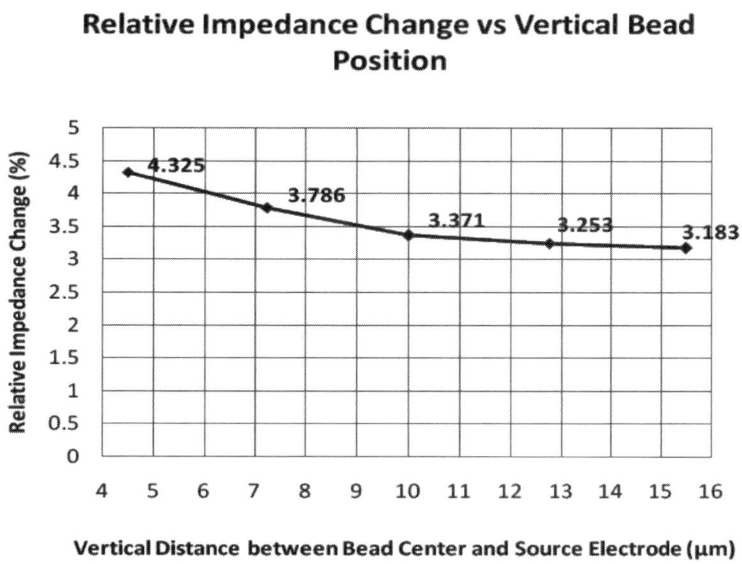

Figure 18.21 Graph of the relative impedance change for an 8 μm bead at numerous different vertical positions within the sensing region. Microelectrodes are in face-to-face orientation and results are at a frequency of 1 MHz.

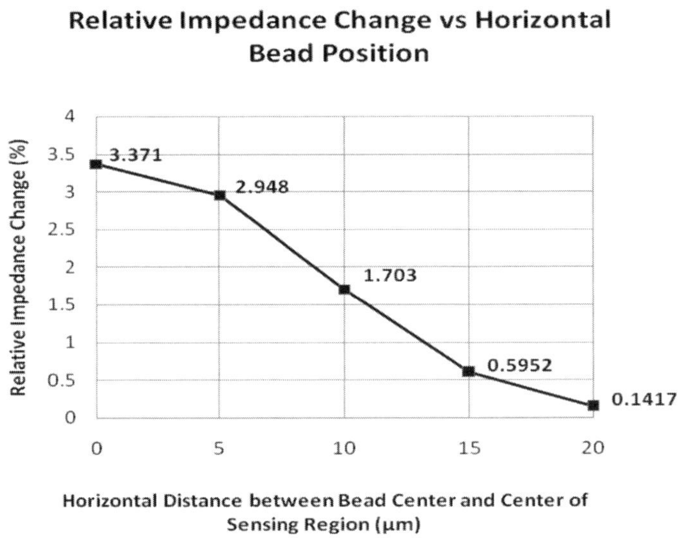

Figure 18.22 Graph of the relative impedance change for an 8 μm bead in numerous different horizontal positions within the sensing region. Electrode orientation is face-to-face and results are for a frequency of 1 MHz.

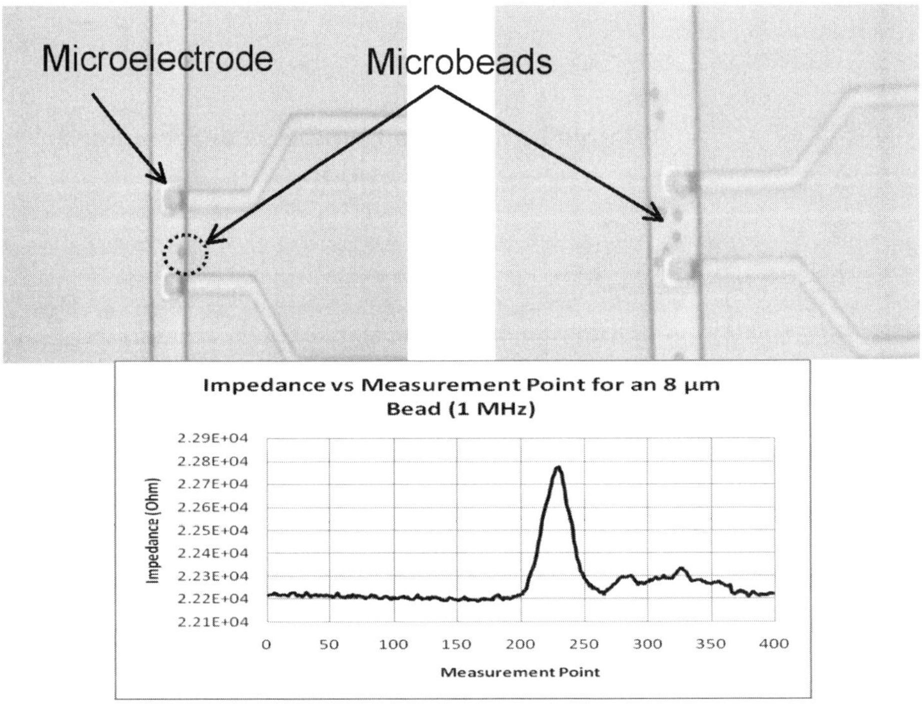

Figure 18.23 Photographs of microbeads passing between the electrodes and graph of the impedance sweep at 1 MHz as microbeads (8 μm in diam.) pass between the electrodes. Pulse height is approximately 2.7%.

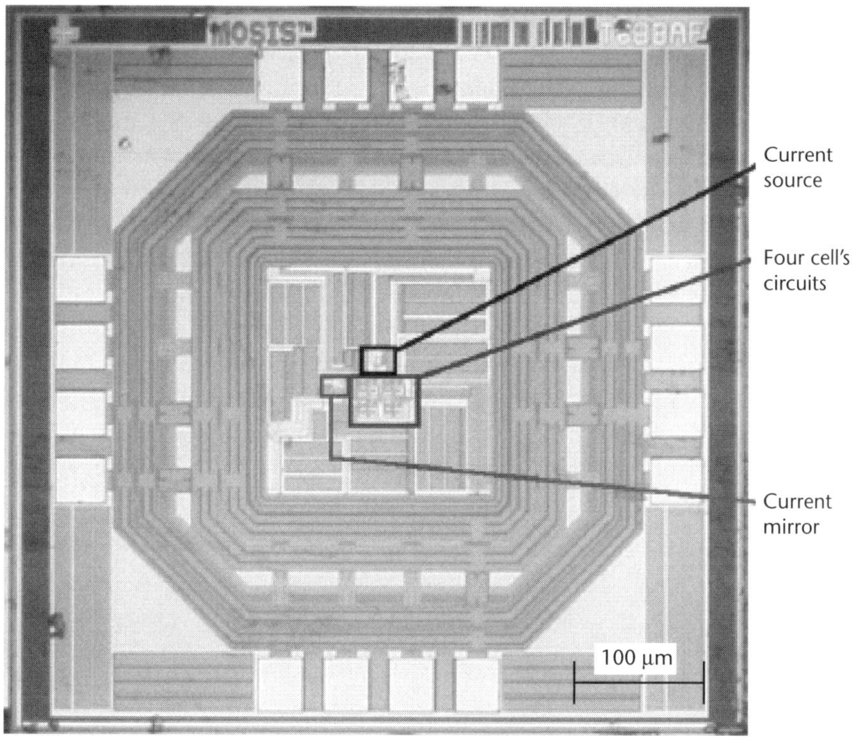

Figure 18.24 Microscope image of a fabricated CMOS chip with TSMC 0.18 μm technology.

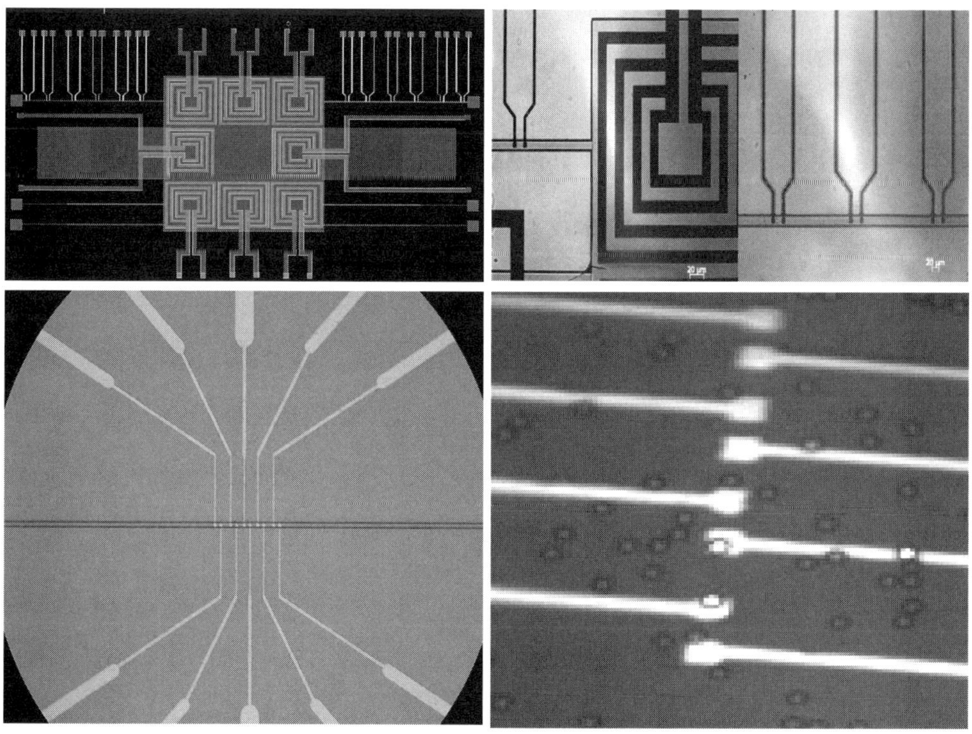

Figure 18.25 Examples of microelectrode implementations.

18.10 Conclusion and Summary

The use of Magnetotactic Bacteria (MTB) to implement MTB-tagged carriers being controlled by CMOS circuitries to transport samples for analysis in microsystems has several advantages over known traditional transport methods. Its compatibility with CMOS low-voltage operation makes it an attractive alternative for many applications. Such a bacterial transport technique can be controlled by a directional magnetic field generated by relatively small electrical currents flowing in special conductor networks. Constraining the swimming environment of the bacteria in such applications can reduce the complexity of the control circuit. Circuits linked to microelectrodes can also be used to detect and track the movement of the MTB-tagged carriers. A method to bind such beads coated with samples under study with the MTB has also been briefly described. Although not conventional, the use of biological entities and in particular MTB as functional components that can be controlled electronically offers many possibilities in the development of new CMOS-based microsystems.

References

[1] J. Happel and H. Brenner, *Low Reynolds number hydrodynamics*, Martinus Nijhoff, The Hague, the Netherlands, 1983.

[2] A. Manz et al., "Electroosmotic pumping and electrophoretic separations for miniaturized chemical analysis systems," *J. Micromech. Microeng.*, vol. 4, p. 257, 1994.

[3] H.A. Pohl, *Dielectrophoresis*, Cambridge University Press, 1978.

[4] S. Martel, C. Tremblay, S. Ngakeng, and G. Langlois, "Controlled manipulation and actuation of micro-objects with magnetotactic bacteria," *Applied Physics Letters*, 89, 233904, 2006

[5] H.C. Berg and D.A. Brown, "Chemotaxis in Escherichia coli analyzed by three-dimensional tracking," *Nature*, vol. 239, pp. 500–504, 1972.

[6] R.M. Ford, B.R. Phillips, J.A. Quinn, and D.A. Lauffenburger, "Measurement of bacterial random motility and chemotaxis coefficients. I. Stopped-flow diffusion chamber assay," *Biotech. and Bioeng.*, vol. 37(7), pp. 647–660, 1991.

[7] J.P. Armitage, "Bacterial motility and chemotaxis," *Sci. Progr.*, vol. 76, pp. 451–477, 1992.

[8] R.P. Blackmore, "Magnetotactic bacteria," *Science*, vol. 190, pp. 377–379, 1975.

[9] R.B. Frankel and R.P. Blakemore, "Navigational compass in magnetic bacteria," *J. of Magn. and Magn. Materials*, vol. 15–18 (Part 3), pp. 1562–1564, 1980.

[10] C. Denham, R. Blakemore, and R. Frankel, "Bulk magnetic properties of magnetotactic bacteria," *IEEE Trans. on Magnetics*, vol. 16(5), pp. 1006–1007, 1980.

[11] H. Debarros, D.M.S. Esquivel, and M. Farina, "Magnetotaxis," *Sci. Progr.*, vol. 74, pp. 347–359, 1990.

[12] Frankel et al. 1997.

[13] R.P. Blackmore, D. Maratea, and R.S. Wolfe, "Isolation and pure culture of a freshwater magnetic spirilum in chemically defined medium," *J. Bacteriol.*, 140:720–729, 1979.

[14] K-F. Schleifer, D. Shüler, S. Spring, M. Weizenegger, R. Amann, W. Ludwig, and M. Kohler, "The genus *Magnetospirillum* gen. nov., description of *Magnetospirillum gryphiswaldense* sp. nov. and transfer of *Aquaspirillum magnetotacticum* to *Magnetospirillum magnetotacticum* comb. nov.," *Syst. Appl. Microbiol.*, 14:379–385, 1991.

[15] T. Matsunaga, Y. Sakaguchi, and F. Tadokoro, "Magnetite formation by a magnetic bacterium capable of growing aerobically," *Appl. Microbiol. Biotechnol.*, 35:651–655, 1991.

[16] D.A. Bazylinski, R.B. Frankel, and H.W. Jannasch, "Anaerobic magnetite production by a marine, magnetotactic bacterium," *Nature*, 334:518–519, 1988.

[17] E.F. Delong, R.B. Frankel, and D.A. Bazylinski, "Multiple evolutionary origins of magnetotaxis in bacteria," *Science*, 259:803–806, 1993.

[18] F.C. Meldrum, S. Mann, B.R. Heywood, R.B. Frankel, and D.A. Bazylinski, "Electron microscope study of magnetosomes in two cultured vibrioid magnetotactic bacteria," *Proc. Roy. Soc. Lond. B*, 251:237–242, 1993.

[19] T. Sakaguchi, J.G. Burgess, and T. Matunaga, "Magnetite formation by a sulphate reducing bacterium," *Nature*, 365:4–49, 1993.

[20] W. André, B. Moufarrej, and S. Martel, "Towards bacterial microfactories," *5th International Workshop on Microfactories (IWMF)*, Besançon, France, Oct. 25–27, 2006.

[21] S. Martel and M. Mohammadi, "High throughput controlled bacterial transport using geometrical fluidic microchannels or 3D microfibers structures," *The 11th International Conference on Miniaturized Systems for Chemistry and Life Sciences (µTAS)*, Paris, France, Oct. 7–11, 2007.

[22] S. Martel, "Magnetotactic phage-based microrobotic systems for the detection of live bacteria," *1st IEEE-RAS/EMBS International Conference on Biomedical Robotics and Biomechatronics (BioRob)*, Pisa, Italy, Feb. 20–22, 2006.

List of Contributors

Mohammad M. Ahmadi
1207–30 Charles Sr. West
Toronto, ON M4Y 1R5

Luca Benini
Dipartimento di Elettronica
Informatica e Sistemistica
Facoltà di Ingegneria
Università di Bologna
Viale Risorgimento 2
40136 Bologna, Italy

Yannick Bornat
UMR 5818 CNRS, ENSEIRB
University Bordeaux 1
351 cours de la Liberation
33405 Talence, France

Sandro Carrara
Swiss Federal Institute of Technology-Lausanne (EPFL)
EPFL IC ISIM LSI1—INF 333 (Batiment INF)
Station 14
CH-1015 Lausanne, Switzerland

Gert Cauwenberghs
University of California San Diego
Pacific Hall 3100E, MC 0357
9500 Gilman Dr.
La Jolla, CA 92093-0357

Shantau Chakrabartty
2120 Engineering Building
Michigan State University
East Lansing, MI 48824
Phone: 517-432-5679
Fax: 517-353-1980

Dr. Andreas Demosthenous
Department of Electronic and Electrical Engineering
University College London
Torrington Place
London WC1E 7JE, UK

Niell G. Elvin
Michigan State University
Civil and Environmental Engineering
3573 Engineering Building
East Lansing, MI 48824

Alex Elvin
School of Civil and Environmental Engineering
University of the Witwatersrand
Private Bag 3, Wits 2050
South Africa

José Gerald
Instituto Superior Técnico (IST) and INESC-ID
Av. Rovisco Pais, 1049-001
Lisboa, Portugal

João Carlos da Palma Goes
Nova University of Lisbon, Portugal
Dept. De Engenharia Electotecnica
Faculdade de Ciencias e Tecnologica (FCT)
Universidade Nova de Lisboa
2825-114 Monte de Caparica
Portugal

Benoit Gosselin
École Polytechnique de Montréal
Montreal, Canada

Carlotta Guiducci
University of Bologna
Bologna, Italy

Maysam Ghovanloo
Georgia Institute of Technology
Van Leer Electrical Engineering Building
777 Atlantic Drive NW
Atlanta, GA 30332-0250

Reid R. Harrison
University of Utah
50 S. Central Campus Drive, Room 3280
Salt Lake City, UT 84112

Sheryl Howard
Dept. of Electrical Engineering
Northern Arizona University
P.O. Box 15600
Flagstaff, AZ 86011-5600

Krzysztof Iniewski
CMOS ET
2865 Stanley Pl.
Coquitlam, BC, V3B 7L7, Canada

Bharat Joshi
University of North Carolina at Charlotte
Charlotte, NC 28223

Graham A. Jullien
380 Old Tecumseh Road
Tecumseh
Ontario N8N 3S8, Canada

Nizar Lajnef
Michigan State University
East Lansing, Michigan

Timothée Levi
14 rue Jean Giono
33850 Leognan, France

Noëlle Lewis
351 cours de la Liberation
33405 Talence cedex
University Bordeaux
Talence, France

Xiao Liu
University College London
London, UK

Sylvain Martel
École Polytechnique de Montréal
Department of Computer and Software Engineering
P.O. Box 6079 Station Centre-ville
Montreal (Quebec) H3C 3A7, Canada

Pedram Mohseni
Case Western Reserve University
Department of EECS
Glennan Building, Room 510
10900 Euclid Avenue
Cleveland, OH 44106-7071

Mohsen Mollazadeh
Johns Hopkins University
Baltimore, MD

Arindam Mukherjee
Department of Electrical and Computer Engineering
University of North Carolina at Charlotte
9201 University City Blvd.
Charlotte, NC 28223

Kartikeya Murari
Johns Hopkins University
Baltimore, MD

Moisés Piedade
Instituto Superior Técnico (IST) and INESC-ID
Av. Rovisco Pais, 1049-001
Lisboa, Portugal

Arun Ravindran
Department of Electrical and Computer Engineering
University of North Carolina at Charlotte
9201 University City Blvd
Charlotte, NC 28223

Sylvie Renaud
University Bordeaux
Talence, France

Sylvain Saighi
University Bordeaux
Talence, France

Christian Sauer
Johns Hopkins University
Baltimore, MD

Mohamad Sawan
Department of Electrical Engineering
École Polytechnique de Montréal
POBox 6079, Station centre-ville
Montreal, QC, Canada, H3C3A7

Chris Siu
Wavelink Ltd.
1081 West 16 Avenue
Vancouver, BC
V6H 1S7, Canada

Leonel Sousa
Instituto Superior Técnico (IST) and INESC-ID
Lisbon, Portugal

Milutin Stanacevic
Department of Electrical & Computing Engineering
Stony Brook University
Stony Brook, New York 11794-2350

Claudio Stagni
University of Bologna
Bologna, Italy

Boris Stoeber
Electrical and Computer Engineering
University of British Columbia
5500—2332 Main Mail
Vancouver BC V67 1Z4
Canada

Gonçalo Tavares
Instituto Superior Técnico (IST) and INESC-ID
Lisbon, Portugal

Nitish Thakor
Traylor 701, Dept of Biomedical Engineering
Johns Hopkins University School of Medicine
720 Rutland Avenue, Baltimore, MD 21205

Jean Tomas
University Bordeaux
Talence, France

Iasonas F. Triantis
Imperial College London
London, UK

Levent Yobas
Institute of Microelectronics, (IME) Singapore
11 Science Park Road
Singapore Science Park II
Singapore 117685

About the Editor

Krzysztof (Kris) Iniewski is an Executive Director of CMOS Emerging Technologies Inc. His research interests are in VLSI circuits for biomedical applications. From 2004 to 2006, he was an Associate Professor at the Electrical Engineering and Computer Engineering Department of the University of Alberta, where he conducted research on low-power wireless circuits and systems. During his tenure in Edmonton he edited a book for CRC Press, *Wireless Technologies: Circuits, Systems and Devices*.

From 1995 to 2003, he was with PMC-Sierra and held various technical and management positions. Prior to joining PMC-Sierra, from 1990 to 1994 he was an Assistant Professor at the University of Toronto's Electrical Engineering and Computer Engineering Department. Dr. Iniewski has published over 100 research papers in international journals and conferences. He holds 18 international patents granted in the USA, Canada, France, Germany, and Japan. He received his Ph.D. degree in electronics (honors) from the Warsaw University of Technology (Warsaw, Poland) in 1988. Together with Carl McCrosky and Dan Minoli, he authored *Network Infrastructure and Architecture*, Wiley, 2008. He can be reached at kris.iniewski@gmail.com.

Index

Related Titles from Artech House

Design and Test of Digital Circuits by Quatum-Dot Cellular Automata, Fabrizio Lombardi and Jing Huang

Hybrid CMOS Single-Electron-Transistor Device and Circuit Design, Santanu Mahapatra and Adrian Mihai Ionescu

CMOS RFIC Design Principles, Robert Caverly

Adaptive Cooling of Integrated Circuits Using Digital Microfluidics, Krishnendu Chakrabarty, Philip Y. Paik, and Vamsee K. Pamula

Integrated Circuit Design for High-Speed Frequency Synthesis, John Rogers, Calvin Plett, and Fost Dai

System-in-Package RF Design and Applications, Michael P. Gaynor

Modern Microwave Circuits, Noyan Kinayman

Phase-Locked Loop Engineering Handbook for Integrated Circuits, Stanley Goldman

Advanced Production Testing of RF, SoC and SiP Devices, Joe Kelly and Michael D. Engelhardt

Microwave Differential Circuit Design Using Mixed Mode S-Parameters, William R. Eisenstadt, Bob Stengel, and Bruce M. Thompson

Introduction to DNA Self-Assembled Computer Design, Christopher Dwyer and Alvin Lebeck

Introduction to Microelectromechanical Microwave Systems, Second Editon, Héctor J. De Los Santos

Microfluidics for Biotechnology, Jean Berthier

Fundamentals and Applications of Microfluidics, Second Edition, Nam-Trung Nguyen and Steven T. Wereley

Pressure-Driven Microfluidics, Vaclav Tesar

Biomolecular Computation for Bionanotechnology, Jian-Qin Liu and Katsunori Shimohara

For further information on these and other Artech House titles, including previously considered out-of-print books now available through our In-Print-Forever® (IPF®) program, contact:

Artech House
685 Canton Street
Norwood, MA 02062
Phone: 781-769-9750
Fax: 781-769-6334
e-mail: artech@artechhouse.com

Artech House
46 Gillingham Street
London SW1V 1AH UK
Phone: +44 (0)20 7596-8750
Fax: +44 (0)20 7630-0166
e-mail: artech-uk@artechhouse.com

Find us on the World Wide Web at: www.artechhouse.com